PROVIDER MANUAL
NINTH EDITION

TNCC®

TRAUMA NURSING CORE COURSE

An ENA® Course

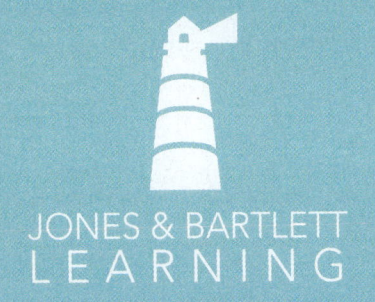

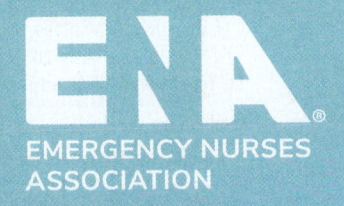

JONES & BARTLETT LEARNING

ENA
EMERGENCY NURSES ASSOCIATION

World Headquarters
Jones & Bartlett Learning
25 Mall Road
Burlington, MA 01803
978-443-5000
info@jblearning.com
www.jblearning.com

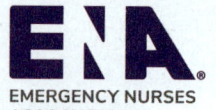

Emergency Nurses Association
930 E. Woodfield Road
Schaumburg, IL 60173
847-460-4000
education@ena.org
www.ena.org

Jones & Bartlett Learning books and products are available through most bookstores and online booksellers. To contact Jones & Bartlett Learning directly, call 800-832-0034, fax 978-443-8000, or visit our website, www.jblearning.com.

Substantial discounts on bulk quantities of Jones & Bartlett Learning publications are available to corporations, professional associations, and other qualified organizations. For details and specific discount information, contact the special sales department at Jones & Bartlett Learning via the above contact information or send an email to specialsales@jblearning.com.

Copyright © 2024 by Emergency Nurses Association (ENA)

All rights reserved. No part of the material protected by this copyright may be reproduced or utilized in any form, electronic or mechanical, including photocopying, recording, or by any information storage and retrieval system, without written permission from the copyright owner.

The content, statements, views, and opinions herein are the sole expression of the respective authors and not that of Jones & Bartlett Learning, LLC. Reference herein to any specific commercial product, process, or service by trade name, trademark, manufacturer, or otherwise does not constitute or imply its endorsement or recommendation by Jones & Bartlett Learning, LLC and such reference shall not be used for advertising or product endorsement purposes. All trademarks displayed are the trademarks of the parties noted herein. *Trauma Nursing Core Course (TNCC) Provider Manual, Ninth Edition* is an independent publication and has not been authorized, sponsored, or otherwise approved by the owners of the trademarks or service marks referenced in this product.

There may be images in this book that feature models; these models do not necessarily endorse, represent, or participate in the activities represented in the images. Any screenshots in this product are for educational and instructive purposes only. Any individuals and scenarios featured in the case studies throughout this product may be real or fictitious but are used for instructional purposes only.

The authors, editor, and publisher have made every effort to provide accurate information. However, they are not responsible for errors, omissions, or for any outcomes related to the use of the contents of this book and take no responsibility for the use of the products and procedures described. Treatments and side effects described in this book may not be applicable to all people; likewise, some people may require a dose or experience a side effect that is not described herein. Drugs and medical devices are discussed that may have limited availability controlled by the Food and Drug Administration (FDA) for use only in a research study or clinical trial. Research, clinical practice, and government regulations often change the accepted standard in this field. When consideration is being given to use of any drug in the clinical setting, the healthcare provider or reader is responsible for determining FDA status of the drug, reading the package insert, and reviewing prescribing information for the most up-to-date recommendations on dose, precautions, and contraindications, and determining the appropriate usage for the product. This is especially important in the case of drugs that are new or seldom used.

28631-1

Production Credits
Vice President, Product Management: Marisa R. Urbano
Vice President, Content Strategy and Implementation: Christine Emerton
Director, Product Management: Matthew Kane
Product Manager: Tina Chen
Director, Content Management: Donna Gridley
Content Strategist: Christina Freitas
Content Coordinator: Samantha Gillespie
Director, Project Management and Content Services: Karen Scott
Manager, Project Management: Jackie Reynen
Project Manager: Kelly Mahoney
Senior Digital Project Specialist: Angela Dooley
Content Services Manager: Colleen Lamy
Product Fulfillment Manager: Wendy Kilborn
Composition: S4Carlisle Publishing Services
Cover and Text Design: Michael O'Donnell
Senior Media Development Editor: Troy Liston
Rights & Permissions Manager: John Rusk
Rights Specialist: Maria Leon Maimone
Cover Image (Title Page, Chapter Opener): © antishock/iStockphoto.
Printing and Binding: Lakeside Book Company

Library of Congress Cataloging-in-Publication Data
Names: Emergency Nurses Association, editor.
Title: Trauma nursing core course (TNCC) provider manual / Emergency Nurses
  Association.
Other titles: TNCC. | TNCC : trauma nursing core course
Description: Ninth edition. | Burlington, MA : Jones & Bartlett Learning,
  [2024] | Preceded by: TNCC / Emergency Nurses Association ; lead editor,
  Joseph S. Blansfield. Eighth edition. [2020] | Includes bibliographical
  references and index.
Identifiers: LCCN 2023002591 | ISBN 9781284286311 (paperback)
Subjects: MESH: Wounds and Injuries--nursing | Emergencies--nursing |
  Trauma Nursing--methods
Classification: LCC RD99.24 | NLM WY 154.2 | DDC
  617/.0231--dc23/eng/20230421
LC record available at https://lccn.loc.gov/2023002591

6048

Printed in the United States of America
27 26 25 24 23   10 9 8 7 6 5 4 3 2

Contents

The Pedagogy	**xxi**
Preface	**xxiv**
Acknowledgments	**xxvi**

CHAPTER 1 — Trauma Around the World — 1

Introduction	1
Epidemiology of Global Trauma	1
Global Impact	2
Injury Risk Factors	2
Injury Prevention	4
Special Considerations	5
Snapshots of Trauma Systems Across the Globe	6
Armed Conflict and Trauma	8
Summary	9
References	9

CHAPTER 2 — Preparing for Trauma — 13

Introduction	13
Trauma Nursing	13
Trauma Nursing Education Position Statement	14
Trauma Programs	14
Trauma Team Activities	15
Trauma Nurse Roles and Responsibilities	15
Trauma Team Structure and Roles	16
Team Leader	16
Core Team Members	17
Ancillary Team Members	17
High-Performance Trauma Teams	17
Communication	17
Shared Mental Model	18
Brief	19
Huddle	19

	Debrief	19
	Effective Communication in the Trauma Bay	19
	Performance Improvement and Trauma Care	20
	Just Culture	21
	Summary	21
	References	21

CHAPTER 3 — Biomechanics and Mechanisms of Injury — 23

	Introduction	23
	Kinematics: The Physics of Energy Transfer	23
	Biomechanics: Energy Forces and Their Effect	25
	Energy Forms	25
	Kinetic Energy	25
	Types of Energy Forms	26
	Types of Injuries	27
	Blunt Trauma	27
	Penetrating Trauma	32
	Thermal Trauma	34
	Blast Trauma	34
	Emerging Trends	37
	Summary	37
	References	37

CHAPTER 4 — Initial Assessment — 39

	Introduction	39
	Preparation and Triage	40
	Preparation	40
	Triage	42
	General Impression	42
	Primary Survey	43
	A: Alertness and Airway (with Simultaneous Cervical Spine Stabilization)	43
	B: Breathing and Ventilation	45
	C: Circulation and Control of Hemorrhage	46
	D: Disability (Neurologic Status)	47
	E: Exposure and Environmental Control	48
	F: Full Set of Vital Signs and Family Presence	48
	G: Get Adjuncts and Give Comfort	49

Reevaluation ... 50
   Portable Radiograph ... 50
   Consider the Need for Patient Transfer ... 50
Secondary Survey ... 50
   H–J Steps in the Secondary Survey ... 50
   Additional Diagnostic Tests or Interventions ... 55
Post-Resuscitation Care ... 56
Definitive Care or Transport ... 56
Emerging Trends ... 56
   Computer-Aided Decision-Making in Trauma Resuscitation ... 56
   Pharmacologic Treatment to Create a Pro-Survival Phenotype ... 56
Summary ... 57
References ... 57

CHAPTER 5   Airway and Ventilation ... 63

Anatomy and Physiology of the Airway ... 63
   Upper Airway ... 63
   Lower Airway ... 64
   Physiology ... 65
Introduction ... 66
Pathophysiology as a Basis for Assessment Findings ... 66
   Airway Obstruction ... 66
   Oxygenation and Ventilation ... 66
   Inadequate Oxygenation and Ventilation ... 66
Nursing Care of the Trauma Patient with Airway and Ventilation Problems ... 68
   Preparation ... 68
   Primary Survey ... 68
Diagnostics and Interventions for Airway and Ventilation Problems ... 77
Reevaluation and Post-Resuscitation Care ... 77
Definitive Care or Transport ... 77
Summary ... 77
References ... 77
Appendix 5-1 Capnometry Devices ... 80
Appendix 5-2 Seven Ps of Rapid Sequence Intubation ... 84
Appendix 5-3 Drug-Assisted Intubation Medications ... 85
Appendix 5-4 Post-RSI Hypotension and Hypoxemia: Common Causes and Interventions ... 87

CHAPTER 6 — Shock — 89

- Introduction — 89
- The Pathophysiology of Shock — 89
- Stages of Shock — 90
  - *Compensated Shock* — 92
  - *Decompensated or Hypotensive Shock* — 92
  - *Irreversible Shock* — 92
- The Body's Compensatory Response to Shock — 93
  - *Adrenal Gland Response* — 93
  - *Pulmonary Response* — 94
  - *Cerebral Response* — 94
  - *Renal Response* — 94
  - *Systemic Inflammatory Response Syndrome* — 94
- The Trauma Triad of Death — 94
- Classification of Shock — 95
  - *Hypovolemic Shock (Volume Problem)* — 95
  - *Obstructive Shock (Mechanical Problem)* — 97
  - *Cardiogenic Shock (Pump Problem)* — 97
  - *Distributive Shock (Pipe Problem)* — 97
- Current Management Strategies — 98
  - *Tourniquets* — 98
  - *Damage Control Resuscitation* — 98
  - *Fluid Resuscitation* — 98
  - *Massive Transfusion* — 99
  - *Calcium Chloride Replacement* — 99
  - *Autotransfusion* — 99
  - *Resuscitative Endovascular Balloon Occlusion of the Aorta* — 100
  - *Damage Control Surgeries* — 100
  - *Tranexamic Acid* — 100
- Nursing Care of the Patient in Shock — 101
  - *Preparation and Triage* — 101
  - *Primary Survey and Resuscitation Adjuncts* — 101
  - *Secondary Survey* — 103
  - *Diagnostics and Interventions* — 103
- Reevaluation and Post-Resuscitation Care — 104
- Definitive Care and Transport — 104
- Emerging Trends — 104
  - *Viscoelastic Testing* — 104
  - *Whole Blood* — 105

	The Trauma Diamond of Death	105
	Freeze-Dried Plasma	105
	Bleeding Control Education and Training for the Community	105
Summary		106
References		106

CHAPTER 7   Head Trauma   109

Anatomy and Physiology of the Brain, Cranium, and Face		109
	Scalp	109
	Skull	109
	Meninges	111
	Brain	111
	Cranial Nerves	112
	Face	112
	Eyes	112
	Blood Supply for the Head	114
	Blood–Brain Barrier	114
	Cerebral Blood Flow	114
	Intracranial Pressure	115
Introduction		116
	Mechanism of Injury	117
	Risk Factors	117
Usual Concurrent Injuries		117
Types of Injury		117
Pathophysiology as a Basis for Assessment Findings		118
	Hypoxia and Hypercarbia	118
	Hypotension and Cerebral Blood Flow	118
	Intracranial Pressure	118
Nursing Care of the Patient with Head Trauma		119
	Preparation and Triage	119
	Primary Survey and Resuscitation Adjuncts	119
	Reevaluation for Transfer	123
	Secondary Survey and Diagnostics and Therapeutics for Head Trauma	123
Selected Head Injuries		126
	Coup/Contrecoup Injury	126
	Focal Brain Injuries	126
	Diffuse Injuries	129
	Penetrating Injuries	130
	Craniofacial Fractures	130

	Selected Eye Injuries	132
	Corneal Injury	132
	Orbital Fracture	132
	Retrobulbar Hematoma	132
	Globe Rupture	132
	Ocular Burns	132
	Interventions for the Patient with Head Trauma	133
	Diagnostics and Interventions for Head Trauma	136
	Radiographic Studies	136
	Laboratory Studies	136
	Reevaluation and Post-Resuscitation Care	136
	Continuous ICP Monitoring	136
	Definitive Care or Transport	137
	Emerging Trends	137
	Point of Care Ocular Ultrasonography	137
	Middle Meningeal Artery Embolization	137
	Summary	137
	References	137
CHAPTER 8	**Thoracic and Neck Trauma**	**141**
	Anatomy and Physiology of the Thoracic Cavity and Neck	141
	Respiratory System	141
	Heart and Thoracic Great Vessels	142
	Neck	143
	Introduction	144
	Epidemiology	144
	Biomechanics and Mechanisms of Injury	145
	Usual Concurrent Injuries	145
	Pathophysiology as a Basis for Assessment Findings	146
	Ineffective Ventilation	146
	Ineffective Circulation	147
	Nursing Care of the Patient with Thoracic or Neck Trauma	147
	Primary Survey	147
	Secondary Survey	150
	Selected Neck and Thoracic Injuries	150
	Tracheobronchial Injury	150
	Esophageal Injury	151
	Neck Trauma	151
	Rib and Sternal Fractures	152
	Flail Chest	152
	Simple Pneumothorax	153

Open Pneumothorax	154
Tension Pneumothorax	155
Hemothorax	156
Pulmonary Contusion	156
Blunt Cardiac Injury	157
Cardiac Tamponade	157
Aortic Disruption	158
Ruptured Diaphragm	158
Reevaluation	159
Imaging Studies	159
Other Studies	159
Chest Drainage Systems	159
Reevaluation and Post-Resuscitation Care	160
Definitive Care or Transport	160
Emerging Trends	160
Summary	160
References	160

CHAPTER 9 Abdominal and Pelvic Trauma — 163

Anatomy and Physiology of the Abdominal and Pelvic Cavity	163
Abdominal and Pelvic Cavity	163
Abdominal Solid Organs	165
Abdominal Hollow Organs	165
Pelvic Structures	166
Pelvic Organs	166
Abdomen and Pelvic Vasculature	166
Retroperitoneal Organs	166
Introduction	167
Epidemiology	168
Blunt Trauma	169
Penetrating Trauma	170
Usual Concurrent Injuries	170
Pathophysiology as a Basis for Assessment Findings	170
Hemorrhage	170
Pain	170
Nursing Care of the Patient with Abdominal and Pelvic Trauma	171
Primary Survey	171
Laboratory Monitoring	171
Secondary Survey	171
General Interventions for All Patients with Abdominal and Pelvic Trauma	172

Selected Abdominal Injuries	172
Liver Injuries	172
Spleen Injuries	173
Pancreatic Injuries	175
Small and Large Bowel Injuries	175
Rectal Injuries	176
Stomach Injuries	176
Selected Pelvic Cavity Injuries	176
Reproductive Organs	176
Male and Female Genitalia	176
Bladder and Urethral Injuries	176
Pelvic Fractures	177
Renal Injuries	179
Diagnostics and Interventions for Abdominal and Pelvic Trauma	179
Laboratory Studies	179
Imaging Studies	179
Resuscitative Endovascular Balloon Occlusion of the Aorta	181
Nonoperative Management of Penetrating Abdominal Wounds	181
Reevaluation and Post-Resuscitation Care	182
Emerging Trends	182
Abdominal Aortic Junctional Tourniquet: Go for the Green	182
Summary	182
References	182

CHAPTER 10   **Spinal and Musculoskeletal Trauma**   **187**

Anatomy and Physiology of the Spinal Cord and Vertebral Column	187
Spinal Cord	187
Motor Function	188
Vertebral Column	191
Anatomy and Physiology of Musculoskeletal System	192
Classification of Bones	194
Structure of Bone	194
Joints, Tendons, and Ligaments	194
Blood and Nerve Supply	195
Introduction	195
Epidemiology	195
Mechanisms of Injury and Biomechanics	195
Types of Injuries	196
Usual Concurrent Injuries	197

Pathophysiology as a Basis for Assessment Findings 197
   Primary Spinal Cord Injury 198
   Secondary Spinal Cord Injury 198
   Alterations in Neurovascular Exam 200
   Other Related Pathophysiologic Changes 200
Selected Vertebral Column and Spinal Cord Injuries 201
   Spinal Cord Injuries 201
   Vertebral Injuries 203
Selected Musculoskeletal Injuries 204
   Selected Fractures 204
   Amputations 207
   Crush Injury 207
   Mangled Extremity 207
   Compartment Syndrome 207
   Hyperkalemia 210
   Rhabdomyolysis 210
   Joint Dislocations 210
Nursing Care of the Patient with Spinal and Musculoskeletal Trauma 211
   Preparation and Triage 211
   Primary Survey and Resuscitation Adjuncts 211
   Interventions 215
   Diagnostics and Interventions for Musculoskeletal Trauma 218
Reevaluation and Post-Resuscitation Care 219
Definitive Care or Transport 219
Emerging Trends 219
   Stem Cell Research 219
   Hypothermia 219
Summary 219
References 220
Appendix 10-1 Clearing the Cervical Spine 224
Appendix 10-2 The NEXUS Criteria for Cervical Spine Clearance 225

CHAPTER 11   Surface and Burn Trauma   227

Anatomy and Physiology of the Integumentary System 227
   Epidermis 227
   Dermis 228
   Hypodermis/Adipose Tissue 228
   Wound Healing 228
   Capillary and Fluid Dynamics 229

Introduction	229
Surface Trauma	230
Mechanisms of Injury	230
Pathophysiology as a Basis for Assessment Findings	230
Nursing Care of the Patient with Surface Trauma	230
Primary Survey	230
Secondary Survey	230
Selected Surface Trauma Injuries	231
Abrasion	231
Avulsion	232
Contusion and Hematoma	232
Laceration	232
Puncture Wound	232
Frostbite	233
Diagnostics and Interventions for Surface and Burn Trauma	233
Radiographic Studies	233
Laboratory Studies	234
Wound Care	234
Reevaluation and Post-Resuscitation Care	235
Definitive Care or Transport	235
Burn Trauma	235
Epidemiology	235
Mechanism of Injury and Biomechanics	235
Thermal Burns	235
Chemical Burns	236
Electrical Burns	236
Radiation Burns	236
Usual Concurrent Injuries	236
Pathophysiology as a Basis for the Assessment Findings of Burn Trauma	237
Airway Patency	237
Hypoxia, Asphyxia, and Carbon Monoxide Poisoning	237
Pulmonary Injury	237
Capillary Leak Syndrome	238
Mechanical Obstruction and Circumferential Burns	238
Loss of Skin Integrity	238
Hypothermia	238
Nursing Care of the Patient with Burn Trauma	239
Primary Survey and Resuscitation Adjuncts	239
Reevaluation for Transfer	241

Reevaluation	242
Secondary Survey	242
Selected Burn Injuries	245
Electrical Burns	245
Chemical Burns	246
Reevaluation of the Patient with Burn Injury	247
Post-Resuscitation Care	247
Wound Care	247
Escharotomy	248
Emerging Trends	248
Pain Management	248
Computerized Protocol-Driven Resuscitation	248
Summary	248
References	248

CHAPTER 12 The LGBTQ+ Trauma Patient — 251

Introduction	251
A Brief History	251
Epidemiology	252
Healthcare Disparities and Access to Care	252
Mental Health	254
Risk-Taking Behaviors	254
Homelessness	254
Terms, Definitions, and Identities	255
Gender Identity and Gender Expression	255
Nursing Care of the LGBTQ+ Patient	256
Reduce Barriers	256
Family Presence	260
The Importance of Pronouns	260
Additional Care Considerations	260
Diversity, Equity, and Inclusion	261
Reevaluation and Ongoing Care	261
Summary	262
References	262

CHAPTER 13 The Pediatric Trauma Patient — 267

Introduction	267
Epidemiology	267
Mechanisms of Injury and Biomechanics	268
Childhood Growth and Development	269

Anatomic and Physiologic Differences from Adults
in Pediatric Trauma Patients — 270
Nursing Care of the Pediatric Trauma Patient — 270
- *Pediatric Readiness* — 271
- *Preparation* — 271
- *Triage* — 273
- *Primary Survey* — 274
- *Secondary Survey, Diagnostics, and Interventions* — 281
- *Selected Injuries* — 283

Reevaluation and Post-Resuscitation Care — 286
- *Patient Safety* — 286

Definitive Care or Transport — 287
Emerging Trends — 287
- *Reduction of the Use of Unnecessary Radiation* — 287
- *Motor Vehicle Design to Reduce Traumatic Injuries in Children* — 287
- *Pediatric Resuscitative Endovascular Balloon Occlusion of the Aorta* — 287

Summary — 287
References — 288
Appendix 13-1 Childhood Development — 292
Appendix 13-2 Pediatric Readiness in the Emergency Department — 295

CHAPTER 14   The Obese Trauma Patient — 297

Introduction — 297
Epidemiology — 298
Mechanisms of Injury and Biomechanics — 298
Pathophysiologic Differences in the Trauma Patient with Obesity — 299
Nursing Care of the Obese Trauma Patient — 300
- *Preparation* — 300
- *Primary Survey and Resuscitative Measures* — 300
- *Secondary Survey* — 306
- *Reevaluation Measures* — 306
- *Radiographs* — 307
- *Computed Tomography and Magnetic Resonance Imaging* — 307
- *Ultrasound/FAST Exam* — 307

Staff and Patient Safety — 307
Patient Dignity — 307
Reevaluation and Post-Resuscitation Care — 308
Definitive Care or Transport — 308
Emerging Trends — 308

	Summary	308
	References	308

CHAPTER 15 The Older Trauma Patient — 313

Introduction	313
Epidemiology	313
Mechanisms of Injury in the Older Adult	314
Falls	314
Motor Vehicle Collisions	316
Pedestrian-Related Collisions	317
Age-Related Anatomic and Physiologic Changes	320
Nonmodifiable Factors	320
Modifiable Factors	320
Nursing Care of the Geriatric Trauma Patient	321
Preparation and Triage	321
Primary Survey and Resuscitation Adjuncts	321
Resuscitation Adjuncts	323
Reevaluation	324
Secondary Survey and Reevaluation	324
Reevaluation and Post-Resuscitation Care	325
Definitive Care or Transport	325
Length of Stay and Adverse Events	325
Rib Fractures	325
Elder Maltreatment	326
Emerging Trends	327
Other Trends	327
Summary	328
References	328

CHAPTER 16 The Pregnant Trauma Patient — 331

Introduction	331
Epidemiology	332
Mechanisms of Injury and Biomechanics	332
Anatomic and Physiologic Changes During Pregnancy as a Basis for Assessment Findings	333
Cardiovascular Changes	333
Respiratory Changes	333
Hematologic Changes	334
Neurologic Changes	334
Gastrointestinal Changes	334
Renal and Genitourinary Changes	334

Reproductive Changes	334
Musculoskeletal Changes	334
Selected Injuries and Emergencies	335
Abdominal and Pelvic Injuries	335
Preterm Labor	335
Abruptio Placentae	335
Uterine Rupture	336
Maternal Cardiopulmonary Arrest	336
Nursing Care of the Pregnant Trauma Patient	337
Triage and Prioritization	337
Primary Survey	338
Secondary Survey	340
Interventions	341
Reevaluation	341
Reevaluation and Post-Resuscitation Care	343
Definitive Care or Transport	343
Summary	343
References	343

CHAPTER 17 Interpersonal Violence — 347

Introduction	347
Epidemiology	348
Risk Factors	348
Patterns of Abusive Behavior	350
Types of Interpersonal Violence	350
Child Maltreatment	350
Intimate Partner Violence	351
Physical Assault/Abuse	351
Sexual Assault	352
Interpersonal Violence During Pregnancy	352
Drug-Facilitated Sexual Assault	352
Lesbian, Gay, Bisexual, Transgender, Asexual, and Questioning Populations	353
Human Trafficking	353
Elder Abuse	354
Tools for Identification of At-Risk individuals	355
Initial Assessment for Interpersonal Violence	355
Safe Practice	355
Special Considerations for the Care of Patients with Physical Abuse	357

Considerations for the Care of Patients Who Have Experienced Sexual Violence: National Protocol for Sexual Assault Medical Forensic Examinations 359
Mandated Reporting 361
Danger and Lethality Assessment 361
Rehabilitation 361
Prevention 362
Summary 363
References 363
Appendix 17-1 Forensic Evidence Collection: Maintain Chain of Custody Preservation 367
Appendix 17-2 IPV and Human Trafficking: Resources for the Community 369
Appendix 17-3 IPV and Human Trafficking: Resources for the Healthcare Worker 370

CHAPTER 18 Psychosocial Aspects of Trauma Care 371

Introduction 371
Responses to Trauma 371
Psychosocial Nursing Care of the Trauma Patient 372
Adverse Childhood Experiences 372
Secondary Survey 372
Interventions 373
Selected Psychosocial Trauma Reactions 374
Acute Stress Reaction 374
Crisis 374
Traumatic Stress Disorders 375
Fear and Anxiety 377
Grief, Bereavement, and Mourning 377
Psychosocial Aspects of Caring for Agitated Patients and Families 380
Preventing Escalation 380
De-escalation 380
Mitigating Violence 380
Ethical Considerations in Trauma 381
Advance Directives 381
Organ and Tissue Donation 382
Psychosocial Care of the Nurse 382
Compassion Fatigue 382
Moral Injury 382
Secondary Traumatic Stress 383

Burnout	383
Vicarious Trauma	384
Social Media	384
Workplace Violence	384
Critical Incidents	384
Approach to the Care of the Trauma Team	385
Assessment Tools	385
Support and Strategies for the Trauma Team	386
Developing Resilience	386
Promoting Self-Awareness	387
Management of Stress in Healthcare Providers	387
Emerging Trends and Resources	387
Summary	387
References	387

CHAPTER 19 Disaster Management — 393

Introduction	393
Disaster Defined	393
Mitigation	394
Preparedness	394
Hospital Disaster Preparedness Plans	394
Incident Command System	395
Response	395
Patient Surge	395
Crisis Standards of Care	396
Disaster Triage	396
Evacuation	397
Shelter-in-Place	397
Children in Disasters	398
Recovery	398
Mass-Fatality Incidents	398
Family Reunification	398
Psychological Triage	399
Types of Disasters	399
Natural Disasters	399
Human-Made Disasters	401
Emerging Trends	405
Summary	405
References	405
Appendix 19-1 Triage Methods	409

Appendix 19-2 Chemical Agents	418
Appendix 19-3 Biologic Agents	420
Appendix 19-4 Acute Radiation Syndromes	422

CHAPTER 20 Transition of Care for the Trauma Patient — 425

Introduction	425
Initial Care and the Emergency Medical Treatment and Active Labor Act	426
Trauma Patients Who Require Transport	427
Decision to Transport	427
Transport Considerations	427
Modes of Transport	428
Transport Team Composition	428
Intrafacility	428
Interfacility	428
Risks of Transport	430
Nursing Considerations for Transport	430
Equipment for Transport	430
Emergency Department Boarding	431
Emerging Trends	431
Summary	431
References	431

CHAPTER 21 Post-Resuscitation Care Considerations — 433

Introduction	433
Operational Considerations	433
ED Boarding	434
Throughput	434
The Primary Assessment	434
Airway	434
Breathing and Ventilation	435
Circulation	435
Disability (Neurologic Status)	435
Exposure and Environmental Control	435
Trauma Triad of Death	435
Hypothermia	436
Acidosis	436
Coagulopathy	437
Monitoring Adjuncts	438
Mechanical Ventilators	438
Capnography	438

Contents

Post-Resuscitation Care of Selected Injuries and Illnesses	439
Rib Fractures	439
Flail Chest	439
Pulmonary Contusion	439
Pneumothorax	440
Hemothorax	440
Blunt Cardiac Injury	440
Cardiac Tamponade	440
Diaphragmatic Injury	440
Deep Vein Thrombosis	440
Venous Thromboembolism	441
Pulmonary Embolism	442
Fat Embolism	442
Acute Lung Injury/Acute Respiratory Distress Syndrome	442
Pneumonia and Aspiration	443
Abdominal Trauma	444
Shock	445
Disseminated Intravascular Coagulopathy	445
Abdominal Compartment Syndrome	445
Rhabdomyolysis	447
Systemic Inflammatory Response Syndrome	447
Sepsis	447
Increased Intracranial Pressure	448
Mental Health and Substance Use Disorders	448
Musculoskeletal Trauma	449
Missed and Delayed Injuries	449
Missed Injuries	450
Delayed Injuries	450
Emerging Trends	450
Extracorporeal Membrane Oxygenation	450
Use of Whole Blood	451
Use of Thromoelastography	451
Summary	451
References	451
APPENDIX A **Trauma Nursing Process**	**457**
Index	**467**

The Pedagogy

These features of the provider manual support your learning.

Objectives Each chapter begins with a list of the chapter learning objectives.

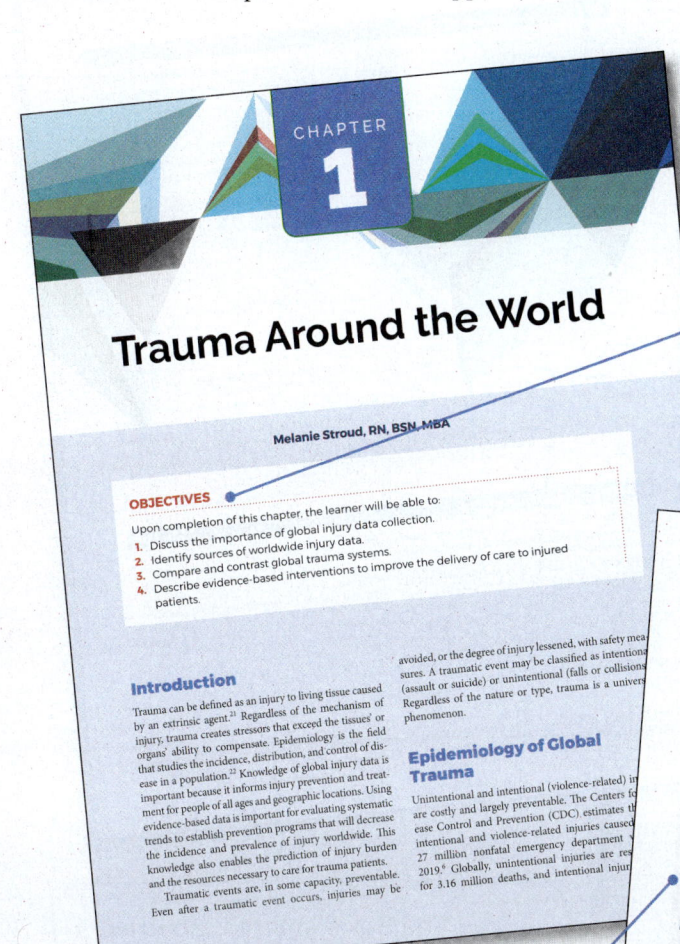

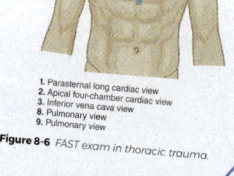

Figures Full-color illustrations, diagrams, and photographs aid your learning.

Clinical Pearls Each Clinical Pearl emphasizes an important point of clinical practice.

The Pedagogy

Notes The Note element provides brief but important bits of information that do not fit neatly into the flow of the text.

Boxes The Box element is another type of sidebar or aside for exploring additional points or concepts requiring longer, more expansive explanations.

Red Flags The Red Flag element flags anything that could become a serious threat to health.

The Pedagogy

Tables Tables summarize multidimensional information in clear, succinct fashion.

TABLE 3-3 Energy Forces

Energy Force	Description	Example
Tension	Two balancing forces causing extension (e.g., stretching by pulling at opposite ends).	Tensile strength describes the tissue's ability to resist pulling apart when stretched. Tendons, ligaments, and muscles can tear when they are overstretched (e.g. Achilles tendon).
Compression	Compression forces injure by squeezing together.	Compression injuries to organs occur when the organs are crushed from surrounding internal organs or structures; an example is a seat belt worn up across the abdomen, causing compression of the small bowel or a fracture to the lumbar spine.
Bending	Loading about an axis. Bending causes compression on the side the person is bending toward and tension to the opposite side.	A force moves from a straight form to a curved form, such as bending forward from a standing position.
Shearing	Shearing forces cause damage by tearing or bending; force is exerted on different parts in opposite directions at the same time within a structure.[28]	Shear strength describes the tissue's ability to resist a force applied parallel to the tissue. An aortic tear is an example. Shear force along a mobile portion of the aorta causes the vessel to tear away from a fixed attachment point.[9]
Torsion	Torsion forces twist ends in opposite directions.	Twisting motion depends on the body's ability to resist applied torque (e.g. a golfer's spine twisting when swinging a golf club).
Combined loading	Any combination of tension, compression, torsion, bending, and/or shear.	The combination of forces may increase the magnitude of the stress.

- **Muscle density:** Muscle density surrounding bone absorbs energy. Tensile strength is augmented by the strength of opposing muscles.
- **Organ structures:** Refer to Table 3-3.
- Solid organs tolerate pressure-wave energy better than air-filled organs do.
- Air-filled organs can resist shear forces better than solid organs.

Types of Injuries

Trauma-related injuries are classified into the following types:
- Blunt trauma
- Penetrating trauma
- Thermal trauma (see Chapter 11, "Surface and Burn Trauma," for more information)
- Blast trauma

Blunt Trauma

Blunt injuries are very common and result from a range of energy impacts. With blunt trauma applied, and energy is transferred in...

Emerging Trends The Emerging Trends section features new evidence or procedures that may eventually make their way into everyday practice.

References The information in the chapters is evidence-based and extensively documented through citations and the corresponding references.

Preface

Excellence in trauma nursing contributes to optimal patient outcomes and the prevention of complications, long-term consequences, and death for patients. The purpose of the Trauma Nursing Core Course (TNCC) is to provide registered nurses with the evidence-based core knowledge, assessments, and skills involved in the assessment and management of injured patients. The trauma nursing process (TNP) reinforces a systematic and standardized approach to trauma nursing care using an integrated approach to trauma teamwork, communication, and collaboration (see Appendix A, "Trauma Nursing Process"). TNCC empowers nurses with the knowledge and critical-thinking skills necessary to provide expert care for trauma patients.

TNCC consists of instructional materials and activities designed to teach essential trauma nursing knowledge and skills. The following sections provide an overview of the course, evaluation process, and learning materials.

Course Learners

Healthcare workers involved in the care of trauma patients may benefit from this course. It is expected that the course learner will have generic nursing knowledge, understand emergency care terminology, and be familiar with standard emergency equipment. Less experienced learners can acquire essential knowledge and skills. Postcourse application, mentoring, and support are essential to further developing trauma nursing expertise and mastering skills. Experienced learners can refresh their knowledge base with updated evidence-based content to validate and improve established practice.

Course Description

The program consists of various modes of instruction, including a comprehensive provider manual, interactive online learning modules, a study guide, skills videos, and instructor-facilitated classroom time. The framework of TNCC is based on the TNP, which is emphasized throughout the program. The required precourse online modules and study guide prepare learners to fully engage in the classroom.

It is essential that all learners read the TNCC provider manual and complete the study guide and online modules before attending the course. This provides learners with a foundational understanding of the concepts that will be applied to scenario-based classroom activities. Classroom activities and discussion highlight critical concepts from the provider manual to reinforce learning and application of the TNP. Skill stations use simulated patient care scenarios to transfer learning, helping learners incorporate the educational content into their nursing practice.

Learner Evaluation

Evaluation of learners consists of an electronic 50-question multiple-choice examination and the TNP testing station. Both evaluations include content from the precourse materials, provider manual, and classroom activities. These evaluations are designed to assess acquisition of cognitive knowledge, essential skills, and critical thinking.

Registered nurses (RNs) who score a minimum of 80% on the cognitive examination and demonstrate all critical skill steps with a minimum score of 70% in the TNP testing station are verified as TNCC providers for 4 years. TNCC verification validates successful completion of the course and is not a certification or credential. Non-RNs are welcome to attend TNCC and participate in testing but are not eligible for verification. All participants can complete an evaluation to obtain nursing professional development contact hours commensurate with their participation as a full course or challenger student. The challenger option is available at the course director's discretion. A one-day course will be available as a renewal option.

What's New and Different

The ninth edition of Trauma Nursing Core Course expands the opportunity for application of trauma knowledge and skills by increasing the TNP teaching activities from six to eight scenarios. These interactive activities are interwoven throughout the classroom time. The content in the prelearning activities has been completely reshaped and revised and now includes a communication module. The provider manual now leads off with a chapter titled "Trauma Around the World," and a new chapter, "The LGBTQ+ Trauma Patient," has been added.

The Emergency Nurses Association (ENA) recognizes that health outcomes are directly affected by systemic racism, bias, and stigmatizing language. In turn, ENA is committed to promoting diversity, equity, and inclusivity, with a focus on achieving health equity. Throughout the TNCC course, efforts have been made to change language and content to better represent and respect all patients. For example, describing skin as "pink, warm, and dry" does not encourage nurses to consider what pallor looks like in patients with darker skin tones. There are subtle but important differences in introductions starting with, "What do you like to be called?," as opposed to, "What are your chosen or preferred pronouns?" The word "chosen" or "preferred" is much less accepting of the individual, whereas "What do you like to be called?" promotes openness and the opportunity to engage in respectful communication. ENA welcomes feedback on how we can continue to improve the content we teach and the language we use in ENA educational materials.

Acknowledgments

TNCC Ninth Edition Work Team

Michael Bailey, PhD, MSN/Ed, RN, CCRN-K, NPD-BC
Market Professional Development Coordinator
HCA West Florida
Brooksville, Florida

Tibor Bajor, MSN, RN, ACNP-BC, MSN, CPEN
Staff Nurse/Quality Improvement Coordinator
University of Chicago Hospitals
Orland Hills, Illinois

Erin Beck, MS, RN, TCRN, CCRN, CEN
Clinical Nurse Educator, Trauma Services
Avera McKennan Hospital
Sioux Falls, South Dakota

Melody Campbell, DNP, RN, CEN, CCRN, CCNS, TCRN
Trauma Program Manager/Clinical Nurse Specialist/Lead APP
Kettering Health, Main Campus
Kettering, Ohio

Alexandra Carpenter, MHA, BSN, RN, TCRN, CPEN
Trauma Program Manager
Summa Health System, Akron Campus
Akron, Ohio

Roger Casey, MSN, RN, CEN, FAEN, TCRN
Staff Nurse
Kadlec Regional Medical Center
Kennewick, Washington

Sara Daykin, DNP, RN, CPEN, TCRN, CNEcl
Assistant Professor
College of Nursing, University of New Mexico
Albuquerque, New Mexico

Carolyn Dixon, DNP, MS, RN, FNP-BC, CEN, TCRN
Emergency Department Nurse Educator
Staten Island University Hospital
Staten Island, New York

Evan Edminster, MSN, RN, CNL, CFRN, TCRN, CEN, NHDP-BC
Trauma Clinical Education, Injury Prevention, Outreach Coordinator
Kaiser Permanente Vacaville Medical Center
Vacaville, California

Steven Jacobson, MSN, RN, CEN, CFRN
Flight Nurse
CALSTAR Air Medical Services
San Francisco, California

Cynthia Joseph, BSN, RN, CPEN
Simulation Education Specialist
UCHealth
Loveland, Colorado

Kristen Kaiafas, DNP, RN, CEN, CPEN
Nursing Faculty
Fayetteville Technical Community College
Fayetteville, North Carolina

Nycole Oliver, DNP, APRN, RN, FNP-C, ACNPC-AG, CEN, FAEN
Advanced Practice Registered Nurse
Baptist Health, Fort Smith
Fort Smith, Arkansas

Candice Palmisano, MSN, RN, CEN
Clinical Nurse Specialist
Los Angeles County USC Emergency Department
Los Angeles, California

Christopher Parker, MSN, RN, CEN, CPEN, CFRN, TCRN, NPD-BC, CNL, NRP
Clinical Professional Development Manager
Centra Health
Lynchburg, Virginia

Victor M. Pearson, MSN-ED, RN, CEN, CPEN, TCRN, CTRN, CCRN
United States Navy
San Diego, California

Danielle Sherar, MBA, BSN, RN, TCRN
Trauma Program Manager
JPS Health Network
Fort Worth, Texas

Judy Stevenson, DNP, MS, APRN-CNS, ACCNS-AG, RN-BC, CCRN, CEN, CSRN, CPEN, TCRN, NH, DP-BC
Tulsa, Oklahoma

Melanie A. Stroud, BSN, MBA, RN
Director of Pediatric Trauma
Stanford Medicine Children's Health
Menlo Park, California

Steven Talbot, MSN, RN, CEN, TCRN
Director of Trauma Services
HCA Houston Healthcare Clear Lake
Webster, Texas

Milagros Tabije-Ebuen, DNP, MSN, RN, CEN, PCCN, CCRN
Assistant Professor of Nursing & Nurse Supervisor
Moorpark College/CSUCI/Los Robles Hospital & Medical Center
Camarillo, California

Alisyn P. Vander Wal, DNP, RN, ACNS-BC, CEN
Clinical Nurse Specialist
Trinity Health Oakland
Pontiac, Michigan

Kai Yeung Cheung, DNURS, RN, FHKAN (Emergency)
Nurse Consultant (Emergency Care)
Hong Kong

Reviewers

Brian Aeschliman, BSN, RN, EMT-P, CEN, TCRN
Trauma Outreach and Education Coordinator
Stormont Vail Health
Topeka, Kansas

Jami Blackwell, BSN, BS, RN, CEN, TCRN, MBA
Director of Trauma and Acute Care Surgery
Cox Health
Springfield, Missouri

Amy Boren, MS, BSN, RN, CEN, CPEN, TCRN
Clinical Educator of Nursing
UCHealth
Greeley, Colorado

Cam Brandt, MS, RN, CEN, CPEN
Fenton, Michigan

Melanie Crowley, MSN, RN, CEN, TCRN
Trauma Program Manager
Providence Holy Cross Medical Center
Mission Hills, California

Paula L. Davis, MSN, APRN, CEN, CPEN, CFRN, FNP-BC, TCRN
Advanced Practice Registered Nurse
Primary Care Rural Healthcare
Newberry, Florida

Angela Dean, BSN, RN, CEN, TCRN, CPEN
Simulation Education Specialist
WakeMed Health & Hospitals
Raleigh, North Carolina

Melanie Doster, MSN, BSN, RN, CEN
Clinical Nurse IV
WakeMed Health & Hospitals
Cary, North Carolina

Sonya Drechsel, BSN, RN, CEN, TCRN
Trauma Educator
TNCC/ENPC Course Instructor/Director
Sanford Emergency Center
Moorhead, Minnesota

Jodie Flynn, PhD, MSN, RN, CNE, SANE-A, SANE-P, D-ABMDI
Curriculum and Instruction Developer
Chamberlain University
Mansfield, Ohio

Shawntay Harris, MSN, MHA, MBA, RN, CEN, TCRN, CPEN, CFRN, CTRN, NEA-BC, NE-BC
Chief Nurse Executive
Eminent Healthcare Resources, Inc.
Killeen, Texas

Janet Jenista, MSN, RN
Edvoke Education
Kingston Foreshore, ACT
Australia

Patricia Kunz Howard, PhD, RN, CEN, CPEN, TCRN, NE-BC, FAEN, FAAN
Enterprise Director of Emergency Services
UK HealthCare
Lexington, Kentucky

Steadman McPeters, DNP, CPNP-AC, CRNP, RNFA
Assistant Dean of Faculty
Chamberlain University
Chicago, Illinois

Julie Miller, BSN, RN, CEN
Nurse Manager Subspecialty Medicine
Stormont Vail Health Manhattan Campus
Manhattan, Kansas

Stefanie Miller, MSN, RN, CEN
Unit Director
UPMC Pinnacle Health
Richland, Pennsylvania

Joan Michelle Moccia, DNP, MSN, RN, ANP-BC, GS-C
Senior ER, Program Director and ANP
St. Mary Mercy Hospital
Livonia, Michigan

Ryan Oglesby, PhD, MHA, RN, CEN, CFRN, NEA-BC
Principal
Phillips Healthcare Transformation Services
Wilton Manors, Florida

Claudia Phillips, MSN-ED, RN, CEN, CPEN
Emergency Department Registered Nurse
Sandoval Regional Medical Center
Rio Rancho, New Mexico

Wendy Reynolds, MSN, BSN, RN, CEN, TCRN
U.S. Army
EL Paso, Texas

Brenda Sierzant, BSN, RN, CPEN
Staff Nurse
Memorial University Medical Center
Savannah, Georgia

Sheila Silva, DNP, RN, CEN, TCRN
Assistant Professor of Nursing
Emmanuel College
Boston, Massachusetts

Ashellee Street, BSN, RN
Simulation Center Coordinator
Sanford Health
Fargo, North Dakota

Tiffiny Strever, BSN, RN, CEN, TCRN, FAEN
Trauma Program Manager
Abrazo West Campus
Goodyear, Arizona

Rebecca VanStanton, MSN, RN, CEN, CPEN, TCRN
Pediatric Trauma Clinical Reviewer
University of Michigan C.S. Mott Children's Hospital
West Bloomfield, Michigan

Jennifer Williams-Cook, BSN, RN, CEN, CPEN, CFRN, CTRN, NRP, TCRN
Flight Nurse/Paramedic
NMMC, CareFlight
Nettleton, Mississippi

Diversity, Equity, and Inclusivity Committee

Justin J Milici, MSN, RN, CEN, CPEN, CCRN, CPN, TCRN, FAEN
Clinical Editor
Elsevier Clinical Solutions
Dallas, Texas

International Advisory Council

Nurul'Ain Ahayalimudin, PhD, RN, CEN, OHN
Assistant Professor
International Islamic University Malaysia
Pahang, Malaysia

Alison Day, PhD, MSN, BS, RN, FAEN
Assistant Professor in Emergency Nursing
Coventry University
Warwick, United Kingdom

Adam Johnston, BAN, RN, CEN, CPEN, NPD-BC
Registered Nurse Clinical Educator
Sanford Health
West Fargo, North Dakota

Walter Sergio Lugari, BSN, RN, ATCN, FKP-NP
Emergency Nurse
Städtisches Klinikum Solingen
Solingen, Germany

Vientiane Melchizedek Pajo, BSN, RN, CEN, TCRN
Rapid Response Team Registered Nurse
Ascension Sacred Heart Pensacola
Pensacola, Florida

Dawn Peta, BN, RN, ENC(C)
Clinical Instructor
Alberta Health Services
Lethbridge, Canada

ENA Staff

Katrina Ceci, MSN, RN, TCRN, CPEN, NPD-BC, CEN
Nursing Content Specialist
Emergency Nurses Association
Schaumburg, Illinois

Sharon Graunke, MSN, APRN, CNS, CEN
Exam Development Specialist
Emergency Nurses Association
Schaumburg, Illinois

Deb Jeffries, MSN, RN, CEN, CPEN, TCRN, FAEN
Nursing Content Specialist
Emergency Nurses Association
Schaumburg, Illinois

Yolanda Mackey, BA, PMP
Education Project Manager
Emergency Nurses Association
Schaumburg, Illinois

Chris Zahn, PhD
Senior Developmental Editor
Emergency Nurses Association
Schaumburg, Illinois

CHAPTER 1

Trauma Around the World

Melanie Stroud, RN, BSN, MBA

OBJECTIVES

Upon completion of this chapter, the learner will be able to:
1. Discuss the importance of global injury data collection.
2. Identify sources of worldwide injury data.
3. Compare and contrast global trauma systems.
4. Describe evidence-based interventions to improve the delivery of care to injured patients.

Introduction

Trauma can be defined as an injury to living tissue caused by an extrinsic agent.[21] Regardless of the mechanism of injury, trauma creates stressors that exceed the tissues' or organs' ability to compensate. Epidemiology is the field that studies the incidence, distribution, and control of disease in a population.[22] Knowledge of global injury data is important because it informs injury prevention and treatment for people of all ages and geographic locations. Using evidence-based data is important for evaluating systematic trends to establish prevention programs that will decrease the incidence and prevalence of injury worldwide. This knowledge also enables the prediction of injury burden and the resources necessary to care for trauma patients.

Traumatic events are, in some capacity, preventable. Even after a traumatic event occurs, injuries may be avoided, or the degree of injury lessened, with safety measures. A traumatic event may be classified as intentional (assault or suicide) or unintentional (falls or collisions). Regardless of the nature or type, trauma is a universal phenomenon.

Epidemiology of Global Trauma

Unintentional and intentional (violence-related) injuries are costly and largely preventable. The Centers for Disease Control and Prevention (CDC) estimates that unintentional and violence-related injuries caused nearly 27 million nonfatal emergency department visits in 2019.[6] Globally, unintentional injuries are responsible for 3.16 million deaths, and intentional injuries cause

1.25 million deaths each year.[34] Approximately 1 in 3 injury-related deaths are due to road traffic collisions, 1 in 6 are a result of suicide, 1 in 10 are due to homicide, and 1 in 61 result from armed conflict.[34] Injuries worldwide account for 3 of the top 5 causes of death.[34] Homicide resulted in approximately 475,000 deaths globally in 2019; nearly 80% of the victims were male, and the majority were between 20 and 29 years of age. Worldwide, men over 60 years of age had the highest rate of suicide.[34]

In the United States, 278,345 people died from injury in 2020.[6] Unintentional injury is the leading cause of death in individuals ages 1–44 years (**Figure 1-1**) and the fourth leading cause of death across all age groups in the United States.[7] In 2019, the CDC estimated that the cost of injury in the United States skyrocketed to $4.2 trillion, which resulted from healthcare costs, lost productivity, loss of quality of life, and lives lost associated with trauma.[26] **Figure 1-2** displays the number of deaths by cause over time.[8] It indicates that the number of unintentional deaths has been increasing over time. **Figure 1-3** shows the leading causes of preventable injury death worldwide.[25]

Significant disparity exists in the incidence of global injuries; some locations have experienced a 50% increase in injuries, while other areas have seen a 51% decrease.[34]

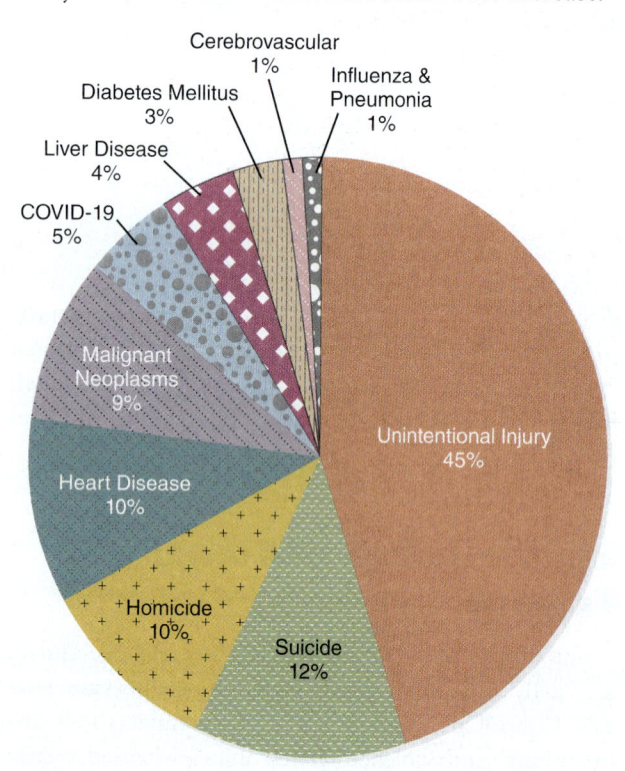

Figure 1-1 *Leading causes of death for individuals younger than age 45, United States.*

Data from Centers for Disease Control and Prevention, National Center for Injury Prevention and Control. (n.d.). *Leading causes of death visualization tool.* Web-Based Injury Statistics Query and Reporting System (WISQARS). https://wisqars.cdc.gov/data/lcd/home

Further injury facts from the World Health Organization include the following[34]:

- Intentional and unintentional injuries account for 8% of all deaths.
- Injuries and violence are the cause of almost 10% of all years lived with a disability.
- Injuries and violence place a huge burden on national economies, costing countries billions each year for healthcare and law enforcement, and in lost productivity.
- Prevention of injuries and violence will facilitate the achievement of several sustainable development goal targets created by the United Nations to decrease poverty, protect our environment, and enhance lives.

Global Impact

Caring for trauma patients is not confined solely to the treatment of physical injuries; it also includes recognition of the lifelong impact of trauma, especially in children. Some consequences include an increased risk of the following:

- Mental illness
- Alcohol and substance abuse
- Suicide
- Smoking
- Chronic illness such as diabetes, cancer, and heart disease

Sociologic variables also play a role in trauma prevalence and incidence. The risk of intentional and unintentional injury is worsened by poverty; approximately 90% of deaths due to trauma occur in low- to middle-income countries.[34] Factors influencing injuries within this demographic include working, living, and going to school in dangerous areas; limited access to hospital and emergency care; limited rehabilitation services; and limited or absent injury prevention programs.[34] Additionally, many parts of the world have poor safety frameworks, inadequate criminal justice systems, and an absence of national injury prevention policies.[34]

Injury Risk Factors

Risk factors contributing to injury worldwide include the following[34]:

- Inadequate supervision of children
- Alcohol and substance abuse
- Economic and gender inequality
- Poverty
- Unsafe work environments
- Unsafe products
- Unemployment

Global Impact 3

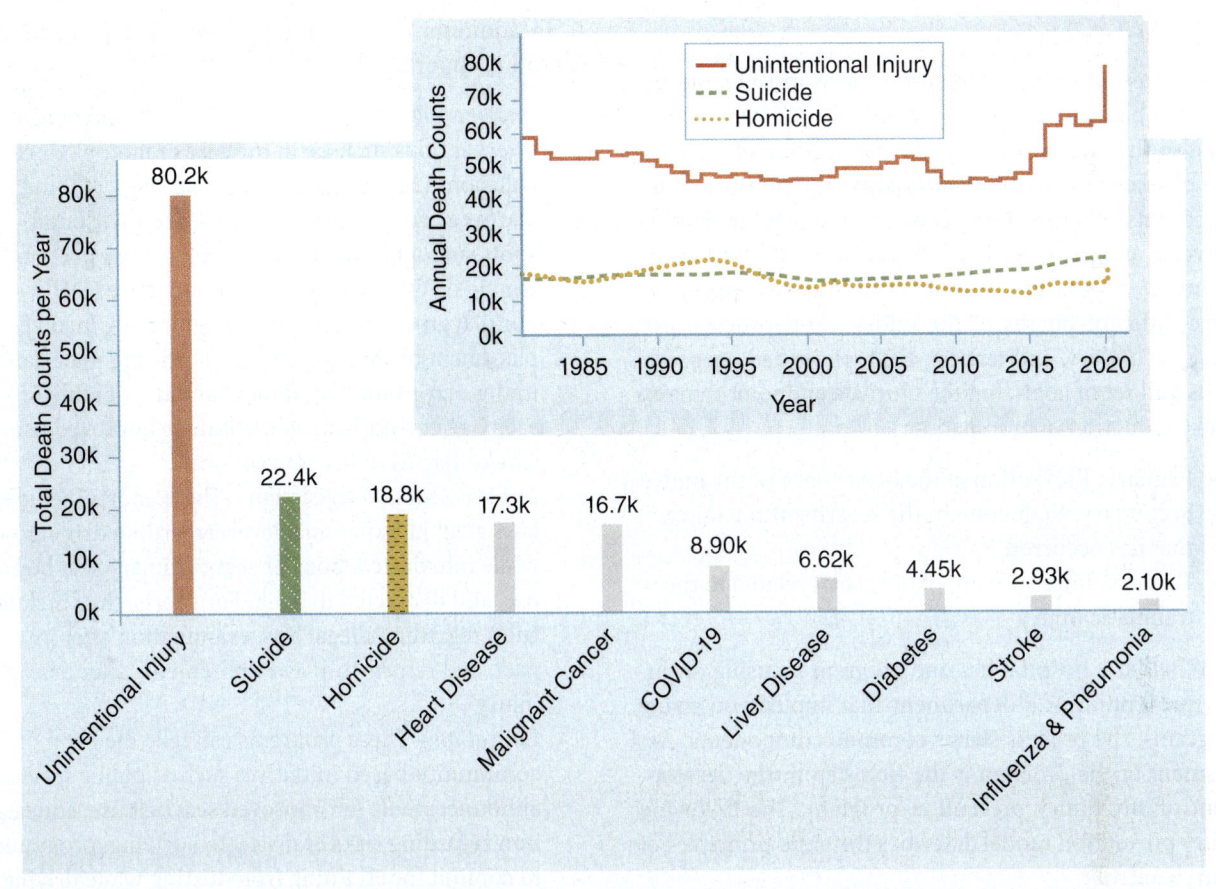

Figure 1-2 *Top 10 leading causes of death in the United States for individuals ages 1–44 years, 1981–2020, with bar chart for 2020 totals.*
Reproduced from Centers for Disease Control and Prevention, National Center for Injury Prevention and Control. (n.d.). *Injuries and violence are leading causes of death*. Web-Based Injury Statistics Query and Reporting System (WISQARS). https://www.cdc.gov/injury/wisqars/animated-leading-causes.html

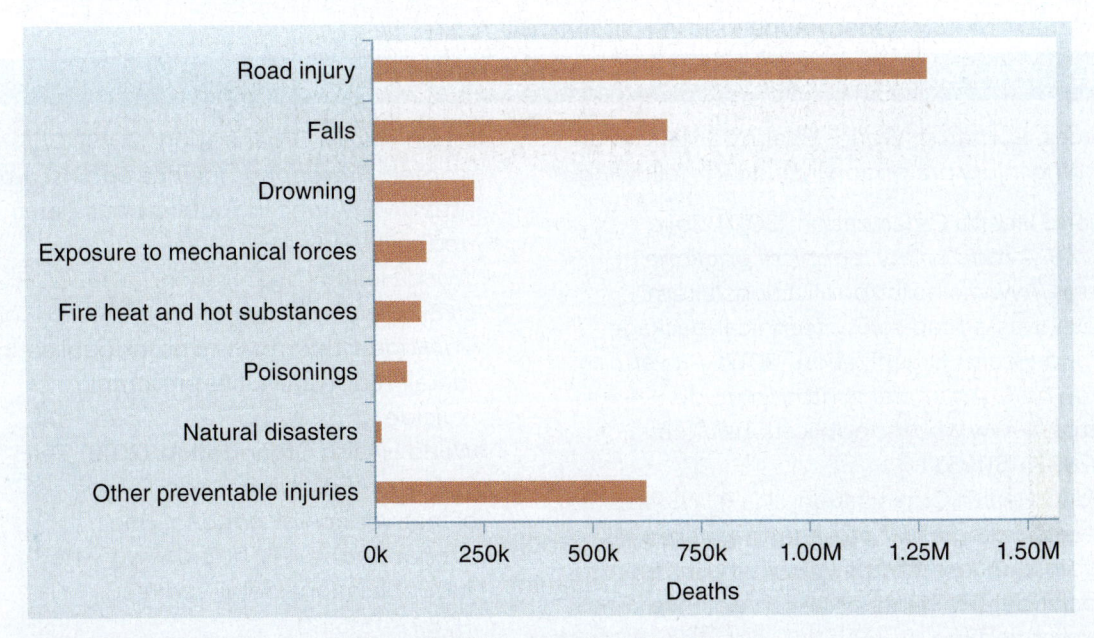

Figure 1-3 *Leading causes of deaths from preventable injuries.*
Reproduced from National Safety Council. (2021). *Injury facts*. https://injuryfacts.nsc.org/international/international-overview/#:~:text=According%20to%20the%20World%20Health,3%2C159%2C000%20died%20from%20preventable%20injuries%20

Injury Prevention

Injury prevention is an important step in reducing the financial burden of injury—not only the loss of property, but also the injured individual's loss of productivity. The aim of injury prevention is to reduce the number of injury events, whereas injury control considers the number of events and the severity of injuries when they do occur.

Injury prevention interventions can be applied to three different phases of the injury event process: primary, secondary, and tertiary. Each phase has a separate focus and set of goals, but the ultimate endpoint remains injury reduction or elimination:

- Primary: Prevention of the occurrence of the injury
- Secondary: Reduction in the severity of the injury that has occurred
- Tertiary: Improvement of outcomes related to the traumatic injury

Whether a hospital has one program focusing on injury prevention or a department that implements many programs, the process shares common components. Assessment of the problem is the first step in the development of any injury prevention program. The following injury prevention model describes the basic principles of injury control[9]:

1. Define the problem.
2. Identify risk and protective factors.
3. Develop and test prevention strategies.
4. Ensure widespread adoption

In addition, incorporation of the three Es of injury control is important:

- *Engineering*—This aspect relates to technological interventions such as, in the case of motor vehicle collisions (MVCs), side-impact air bags, automated alarms alerting drivers to vehicles in their blind spots, and ignition lock devices for those persons convicted of driving under the influence (DUI). For playgrounds and sports, engineering involves placement of shock-absorbing surfacing materials under playground equipment and use of athletic safety gear. Another intervention is improved use of smoke alarms in fire prevention.
- *Enforcement and legislation*—These efforts include laws at all jurisdictional levels regarding driving while intoxicated, booster seats, primary seat belt use, and distracted driving. For sports, they include rules regarding illegal hits, examination after impact, and return-to-play requirements after a head injury.
- *Education*—These programs can take the form of community-based initiatives such as public service announcements for improved seat belt use, education regarding risks of distracted driving, programs to commit to refraining from texting while driving, and promotions for bicycle helmet giveaways with instructions for proper use.

Injury prevention resources are available from the World Health Organization (**Box 1-1**) and other sources (**Box 1-2**).

BOX 1-1 Injury Prevention Resources: World Health Organization

Resources from the World Health Organization concerning injury prevention include the following:

- World Health Organization. (2017). *Save LIVES: A road safety technical package.* https://www.who.int/publications/i/item/save-lives-a-road-safety-technical-package
- World Health Organization. (2017). *Preventing drowning: An implementation guide.* https://www.who.int/publications/i/item/9789241511933
- World Health Organization. (2017). *INSPIRE: Seven strategies for preventing violence against children.* https://www.who.int/teams/social-determinants-of-health/violence-prevention/inspire-technical-package
- World Health Organization. (2019). *RESPECT women: Preventing violence against women.* https://www.who.int/publications-detail-redirect/WHO-RHR-18.19
- World Health Organization. (2018). *LIVE LIFE: Suicide prevention implementation package.* https://www.who.int/publications-detail-redirect/live-life-preventing-suicide
- World Health Organization. (2019). *The SAFER technical package: Five areas of intervention at national and subnational levels.* https://www.who.int/publications-detail-redirect/9789241516419

Special Considerations

Special considerations for trauma around the world include road traffic injuries, drowning, fall injuries, burn injuries, violence against children, violence against women, and violence against older people.

The Global Burden of Road Traffic Deaths

Road traffic injuries are the eighth overall cause of death for all age groups and is the leading cause of death for those 5–29 years of age.[34,38] Road traffic deaths are 3 times higher in low-income countries compared with high-income countries (**Figure 1-4**). Globally, pedestrians, motorcyclists, and bicyclists accounted for more than half of these deaths.[34,38] Recommendations for reducing road traffic deaths include the following[30]:

- Amending laws to reflect evidence-based practice to reduce speeding and increase the use of seat belts and helmets
- Requiring proper child vehicle restraints
- Improving road infrastructure
- Improving emergency service access

Driving while using a mobile phone makes the likelihood of being involved in a crash approximately 4 times greater than when not using a mobile device.[38]

BOX 1-2 Other Global Injury Prevention Resources

Other global injury prevention resources include the following:

- Primary Trauma Care Foundation. (n.d.). *What we do.* https://www.primarytraumacare.org/what-we-do/
- The University of Michigan Injury Prevention Center. (n.d.). *Area of focus: Global injury prevention.* https://injurycenter.umich.edu/global-injury/
- Harborview Injury Prevention & Research Center. (n.d.). *Global injury.* https://hiprc.org/research/global-injury/
- Global Injury Research Collaborative. (n.d.). *GIRC: Report to prevent.* https://www.globalirc.org/
- The George Institute for Global Health. (n.d.). *Injury.* https://www.georgeinstitute.org/units/injury

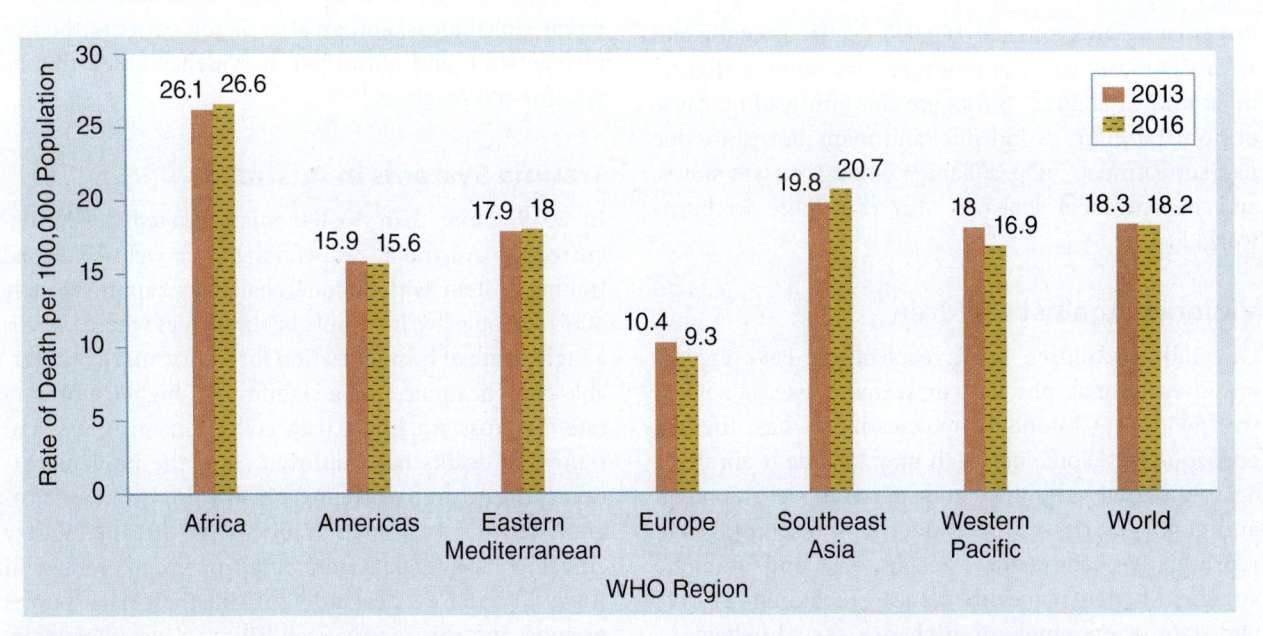

Figure 1-4 *Rates of road traffic death per 100,000 population by WHO regions: 2013, 2016.*

Reproduced from World Health Organization. (2018). *Global status report of road safety.* https://www.who.int/publications/i/item/9789241565684. License: CC BY-NC-SA 3.0 IGO.

WHO Region	2013	2016
Africa	26.1	26.6
Americas	15.9	15.6
Eastern Mediterranean	17.9	18
Europe	10.4	9.3
Southeast Asia	19.8	20.7
Western Pacific	18	16.9
World	18.3	18.2

Drowning

Every year, approximately 236,000 drowning deaths occur. It is the third leading cause of unintentional injury deaths, resulting in 7% of injury-related deaths overall.[28] These are likely underestimations because drownings from floods and water transportation may not be reported as such.[28] Most at risk are children, men, and those with greater access to water.[28] Recommendations for decreasing drownings include[28]:

- Installation of physical barriers such as fences
- Community supervision of childcare
- Teaching children to swim
- Implementing policies and legislation regarding boat safety
- Implement policies and legislation for disaster preparedness, including early flood warnings

Fall Injuries

The second leading cause of unintentional injury deaths worldwide is falls.[33] Adults over 60 years of age and children are at most risk for fall deaths. Strategies to prevent falls include education, training, research, policy, and creating safe environments. More than 37 million falls each year result in injury significant enough to require medical treatment and often result in disability.[33] It is estimated that fall prevention interventions cost 6 times less than the cost of treatment.[33]

Burn Injuries

Burns cause an estimated 180,000 deaths annually and are a significant cause of morbidity, including disfigurement and disability.[29] Burns are the fifth leading cause of nonfatal injury worldwide, and many burns are due to maltreatment.[29] Open flame cooking, unsafe stoves, and interpersonal violence also contribute to burns worldwide.[29]

Violence Against Children

One billion children 2–17 years of age have experienced emotional, physical, or sexual abuse or neglect worldwide.[31] Childhood maltreatment has lifelong consequences, some of which may include brain damage; impaired cognitive and nervous development; and abnormalities of the endocrine, musculoskeletal, reproductive, circulatory, respiratory, and immune systems.[31] Mental health issues, including anxiety and depression, smoking, high-risk sexual behaviors, and substance and alcohol misuse are common.[31] See Chapter 17, "Interpersonal Violence," for additional information.

Violence Against Women

Violence against women is a significant global public health concern. It is estimated that 30% of women have been the victim of physical or sexual intimate partner violence.[36] Violence against women has long-term consequences, affecting their physical, reproductive, and sexual health.[35] Mental health issues may include depression, anxiety, eating disorders, sleeping disorders, and suicidality.[36] See Chapter 17 for additional information.

Violence Against Older People

It is estimated that 1 in 6 people over 60 years of age and living in a community setting have been the victim of abuse.[37] It is anticipated that violence against older people will continue to worsen as the global population ages.[37] Maltreatment of older adults can include physical, sexual, psychological, and emotional abuse as well as neglect and abandonment.[37] A review and meta-analysis in 2017 suggested that nearly 16% of people aged 60 years and over had been subjected to some form of abuse (**Table 1-1**). See Chapter 17 for additional information.

Snapshots of Trauma Systems Across the Globe

Trauma systems play a vital role in decreasing morbidity and mortality associated with injury.[10,12,39] However, numerous barriers to trauma care are encountered in different global areas, and great variation exists in the implementation and utilization of evidence-based trauma systems and practices.[12,39]

Trauma Systems in Australia

In 2019, more than 13,400 injury-related deaths occurred in Australia.[1] Australia has a well-developed trauma system with unique challenges; approximately 30% of people live in remote or rural areas where there is a higher rate of hospitalization for injury, more preventable complications, and a significantly higher mortality rate.[13] Across Australia, data collection on injury and traumatic deaths has improved since the implementation of the Australian Trauma Quality Improvement Program and the Australian Trauma Registry. The registry currently receives data from 30 major trauma centers in Australia and New Zealand.[11,13] Using these data sources provides information that can help in developing intervention strategies. For example, the highest mortality and poorest outcomes are in older traumatically injured patients.[5] Western Australia uses a database called the

TABLE 1-1 World Population: Abuse of Older People

Type of Abuse	Abuse of Older People in Community Settings — Reported by Older Adults	Abuse of Older People in Institutional Settings — Reported by Older Adults and Their Proxies	Reported by Staff
Psychological abuse	11.6%	33.4%	32.5%
Physical abuse	2.6%	14.1%	9.3%
Financial abuse	6.8%	13.8%	Not enough data
Neglect	4.2%	11.6%	12.0%
Sexual abuse	0.9%	1.9%	0.7%
Overall prevalence	**15.7%**	**Not enough data**	**64.2%**

Modified from World Health Organization. (2022). *Abuse of older people.* https://www.who.int/news-room/fact-sheets/detail/abuse-of-older-people

Data Linkage System, which provides information that can be used for research, quality improvement, and the development of policies.[17]

Trauma Systems in England

England averages 40,000 cases of major trauma per year and 5,400 trauma-related deaths.[10] More than 16,000 trauma-related deaths occur annually in England and Wales combined.[3] Improvements in trauma care were noted after a transition in practice was implemented, in which injured patients were transported from the scene to the most appropriate facility, not the closest hospital.[3,10] The trauma system in England was developed by creating four trauma networks in the London region, which are led by a major trauma centers designated to treat the most seriously injured patients.[3,10] Less critically injured patients are treated at local trauma units, which are led by a major trauma center.[3] The system consists of three levels of trauma center designation: major trauma center, trauma units, and emergency departments.[10] There are 27 designated major trauma centers, five of which are pediatric specific, in England.[10] The major trauma centers have specific national standards of care that include, but are not limited to, dedicated trauma teams; multispecialty care; interventional radiology; computed tomography (CT) scan within 60 minutes of arrival; tranexamic acid, when indicated, given within 3 hours of an injury; and mass transfusion protocols.[10] Seriously injured patients have a 20–23% lower rate of mortality when treated in a region with the trauma system in place.[3,10]

Trauma Systems in Germany

More than 7 million accidents occur in Germany every year, 35,000 of which result in severe injuries.[10] Before 2009, no nationally standardized trauma system existed, and variations in survivability and standards of trauma care available varied significantly based on geographic location.[10,15] In 2009, the German Trauma Society began regionalizing the care of trauma patients with the development of the trauma network Deutsche Gesellschaft für Unfallchirugire (DGU). The system now has 51 regional trauma networks with more than 650 participating trauma centers. These centers have clearly identified standards of care and measurable data points for quality improvement processes.[10,15] The Whitebook-Medical Care of the Severely Injured, originally published in 2006 and updated in 2012, defines the criteria for trauma centers, staffing expectations, and equipment/processes.[10] Levels of trauma centers are determined based on criteria similar to those used in the United States: Level I centers are also known as supraregional trauma centers, Level II centers are also known regional trauma centers, and Level III centers are also known as local trauma centers.[15] Overall trauma-related mortality in Germany has decreased since the implementation of trauma network diagnostic-related groups.[10]

Trauma Systems in Ghana

Research is ongoing to identify areas of improvement to decrease the morbidity and mortality due to injury in Ghana.[20,23] Evidence supports the idea that some aspects of trauma care provided in high-income countries are expensive, whereas others are not.[20] It may be possible for low-cost interventions to be implemented more universally, enabling measurable improvements in care. One low-cost method, implemented at a main referral hospital with 1,500 beds in Ghana, is the preventable death review panel. This quality improvement program reviews all trauma-related deaths at that facility to determine whether the death was preventable. For those deaths determined by the panel to be preventable, specific recommendations are made to implement strategies to prevent future occurrences, accompanied by ongoing monitoring to assess the effectiveness of implemented interventions.[20] Some actions recommended by the panel include increased continuing trauma education for emergency physicians and nurses, emphasis on a systematic assessment for patients with polytrauma, protocols for the placement of an advanced airway and use of mechanical ventilation, use of cervical collars, standby surgical teams available 24 hours a day, available operating rooms, and public information on the need for early care for severely injured patients.[20] Public education for early transport to the hospital for severely injured patients is particularly important because most of those patients are transported by family members or bystanders.[20]

Trauma Systems in the Netherlands

The Netherlands has an average of 78,000 trauma patients treated in hospitals annually, with a mortality rate of 3% for in-hospital trauma-related deaths.[14,27] The Netherlands has had a standardized trauma system since 1999. This system came about following recognition of less-than-optimal outcomes as injured patients were transported from the scene to the closest hospital, not the most appropriate facility.[16,27] The implementation and continuous quality improvement of the trauma system have resulted in a 16% mortality-risk reduction.[10] The Netherlands has 11 Level I major trauma centers, 42 Level II trauma centers, and 33 Level III trauma centers.[10] In 2015, the Dutch National Health Care Institute set the expectation that at least 90% of severely injured patients will be taken to the closest major trauma center.[27] In the Netherlands, trauma surgeons, in addition to training for traditional injuries (thoracic, abdominal), also receive extensive training to care for musculoskeletal injuries and manage 75% of fracture treatment. Trauma surgeons in the Netherlands are responsible for the care throughout the patient hospital stay.[10]

Trauma Systems in Nepal

Injury is a leading cause of death and disability in Nepal.[4] The most common cause of trauma in Nepal is road traffic injuries, along with falls, occupational injuries, burns, assaults, and animal-related injuries.[4] There is a dearth of accurate information available because Nepal has not had a formal, standardized method for data collection.[24] Additionally, injuries related to road traffic collisions are believed to be significantly underreported.[19] Recently, the Nepal Injury Research Centre was established at the Kathmandu Medical College to explore factors related to injuries and identify interventions to decrease injuries in Nepal.[24] Some of the areas for improvement within the constraints of resource availability include the implementation of a web-based road accident information management system, improved prehospital communication, increased ambulance availability with appropriate equipment to provide advanced cardiac life support, enhanced training for first providers, governmental improvement of emergency medical services, and enhanced injury surveillance.[2,4,24]

Armed Conflict and Trauma

The impact of armed conflict or violence in insecure environments is far-reaching, affecting patients, healthcare facilities and systems, and medical teams responding to help those in need. According to the World Health Organization, "In order for IHL (international humanitarian law) to apply to a situation of violence, that situation must constitute an armed conflict. As different sets of rules apply to international and non-international armed conflicts, it is also important to identify the nature of the conflict."[32(p6)] There is much that must be considered and weighed when planning a response to these situations (**Table 1-2**).

The mission for medical teams responding to armed conflicts includes, but is not limited to, the following[32]:

- Save lives
- Alleviate suffering
- Protect vulnerable populations
- Mitigate the impact of war and violence in often insecure areas with limited resources
- Treat patients in a medically ethical manner at all times

The World Health Organization has published *A Guidance Document for Medical Teams Responding to Health Emergencies in Armed Conflicts and Other Insecure Environments*.[32]

TABLE 1-2 Intervention for the Wounded and Sick in an Armed Conflict

	Optimal	Austere	Dire
Location	Urban in a developed country	Poor rural area	Developing country, major destruction
Duration of trouble	Single, isolated event (e.g., act of terrorism)	Ongoing low-intensity fighting (e.g., guerrilla warfare)	Continuous heavy fighting and/or bombardment
Casualty flow	Small irregular numbers (compared with the population of the city)	Discontinuous/intermittent flow, including massive influx	Continuous but unpredictable flow, including massive influx
Infrastructure (roads, ambulance service, health facilities)	Intact and functioning	Poor or irregular (e.g., few good roads, limited number of ambulances)	Severely damaged or dysfunctional (roads damaged, debris in streets, hospitals looted, etc.)
Communications	Good	Poor to moderate irregular	None or poor
Personnel	Adequate in number and skills	Variable	Minimum available or complete lack
Materials and supplies	Adequate (in quantity and quality)	Irregular and inadequate	Irregular supply or nonexistent
Environment	Good (daytime, good weather)	Harsh	Bleak (night, cold, heat, etc.)
Evacuation	Safe and short	Predictable but long and arduous	Uncertain or unknown

Reproduced from World Health Organization. (2021). *A guidance document for medical teams responding to health emergencies in armed conflicts and other insecure environments.* https://apps.who.int/iris/rest/bitstreams/1351892/retrieve

Summary

Trauma is a preventable worldwide phenomenon with a disproportionate burden on low- and middle-income countries, where 90% of injuries occur. Effective strategies to decrease morbidity and mortality are multifactorial and include, but are not limited to, elements such as road infrastructure; vehicle safety; injury prevention policies provided by the government; financial, physical, and human resources; surveillance reports and accurate data collection; improved access to emergency care; improved health care systems; and injury prevention programs.[18,19,23,24]

References

1. Australian Institute of Health and Welfare. (2022). *Injury.* https://www.aihw.gov.au/reports-data/health-conditions-disability-deaths/injury/overview
2. Banstola, A., Smart, G., Raut, R., Ghimire, K. P., Pant, P. R., Joshi, P., Joshi, S. K., & Mytton, J. (2021). State of post-injury first response systems in Nepal—A nationwide survey. *Frontiers in Public Health, 9,* Article 607127. https://doi.org/10.3389/fpubh.2021.607127
3. Beeharry, M. W., & Moqeem, K. (2020). The London major trauma network system: A literature review. *Cureus, 12*(2), Article e12000. https://doi.org/10.7759/cureus.12000

4. Bhatta, S., Magnus, D., Mytton, J., Joshi, E., Bhatta, S., Adhikari, D., Manandhar, S., R., & Joshi, S. K. (2021). The epidemiology of injuries in adults in Nepal: Findings from a hospital-based injury surveillance study. *International Journal of Environmental Research and Public Health*, *18*(23), Article 12701. https://doi.org/10.3390/ijerph182312701

5. Cameron, P. A., Fitzgerald, M. C., Curtis, K., McKie, E., Gabbe, B., Earnest, A., Christey, G., Clarke, C., Crozier, J., Dinh, M., Ellis, D. Y., Howard, T., Joseph, A. P., McDermott, K., Matthew, J., Ogilvie, R., Pollard, C., Rao, S., Reade, M., Rushworth, N., . . . Australian Trauma Quality Improvement Program (AusTQIP) collaboration. (2020). Overview of major traumatic injury in Australia—Implications for trauma system design. *Injury*, *51*(1), 114–121. https://doi.org/10.1016/j.injury.2019.09.036

6. Centers for Disease Control and Prevention, National Center for Injury Prevention and Control. (n.d.). *Explore fatal injury data visualization tool*. WISQARS. https://wisqars.cdc.gov/data/explore-data/home

7. Centers for Disease Control and Prevention, National Center for Injury Prevention and Control. (n.d.). *Leading causes of death visualization tool*. WISQARS. https://wisqars.cdc.gov/data/lcd/home

8. Centers for Disease Control and Prevention, National Center for Injury Prevention and Control. (n.d.). *Injuries and violence are leading causes of death*. WISQARS. https://www.cdc.gov/injury/wisqars/animated-leading-causes.html

9. Centers for Disease Control and Prevention, National Center for Injury Prevention and Control. (n.d.). *Injury prevention and control: Our approach*. https://www.cdc.gov/injury/about/approach.html

10. Chesser, T., Moran, C., Willet, K., Bouillon, B., Sturm, J., Flohe, S., Ruchholtz, S., Dijkink, S., Schipper, I. B., Rubio-Suarez, J. C., Chana F., de Caso, J., & Guerado, E. (2019). Development of trauma systems in Europe—reports from England, Germany, the Netherlands, and Spain. *OTA International*, *2*(S1), Article e019. https://doi.org/10.1097/OI9.0000000000000019

11. Curtis, K., Gabbe, B., Shaban, R. Z., Nahidi, S., Pollard Am, C., Vallmuur, K., Martin, K., & Christey, G. (2020). Priorities for trauma quality improvement and registry use in Australia and New Zealand. *Injury*, *51*(1), 84–90. https://doi.org/10.1016/j.injury.2019.09.033

12. Dijkink, S., Nederpelt, C. J., Krijnen, P., Velmahos, G. C., & Schipper, I. B. (2017). Trauma systems around the world: A systematic review. *Journal of Trauma and Acute Care Surgery*, *83*(5), 917–925. https://doi.org/10.1097/ta.0000000000001633

13. Dobson, G. P., Gibbs, C., Poole, L., Butson, B., Lawton, L. D., Morris, J. L., & Letson, H. L. (2022). Trauma care in the tropics: Addressing gaps in treating injury in rural and remote Australia. *Rural and Remote Health*, *22*(1), Article 6928. https://doi.org/10.22605/RRH6928

14. Driessen, M. L., Sturms, L. M., Bloemers, F. W., ten Duis, H. J., Edwards, M. J., den Hartog, D., de Jongh, M. A., Leenhouts, P. A., Poeze, M., Schipper, I. B., Spanjersberg, W. R., Wendt, K. W., de Wit, R. J., van Zutphen, S., & Leenen, L. P. (2020). The Dutch nationwide trauma registry: The value of capturing all acute trauma admissions. *Injury*, *51*(11), 2553–2559. https://doi.org/10.1016/j.injury.2020.08.013

15. Ernstberger, A., Koller, M., Zeman, F., Kerschbaum, M., Hilber, F., Diepold, E., Loss, J., Herbst, T., Nerlich, M., & Trauma Centers of the Trauma Network of Bavaria (Traumanetzwerk Ostbayern – TNO). (2018). A trauma network with centralized and local health care structures: Evaluating the effectiveness of the first certified Trauma Network of the German Society of Trauma Surgery. *PLOS ONE*, *13*(3), Article e0194292. https://doi.org/10.1371/journal.pone.0194292

16. Hietbrink, F., Houwert, R. M., van Wessen, K. J., Simmermacher, R. K., Govaert, G. A., de Jong, M. B., Bruin, I. G., de Graaf, J., & Leenen, L., P. (2020). The evolution of trauma care in the Netherlands over 20 years. *European Journal of Trauma and Emergency Surgery*, *46*, 329–335. https://doi.org/10.1007/s00068-019-01273-4

17. Iddagoda, M. T., Burrell, M., Rao, S., & Flicker, L. (2022). Evolution of trauma care and the trauma registry in the West Australian health system. *Journal of Trauma and Injury*, *35*(2), 71–75. https://doi.org/10.20408/jti.2021.0060

18. James, S. L., Castle, C. D., Dingles, Z. V., Fox, J. T., Hamilton, E. B., Liu, Z., Roberts, N. L., Sylte, D. O., Henry, N. J., LeGrand, K. E., Abdelalim, A., Abdoli, A., Abdollahpour, I., Abdulkader, R. S., Abedi, A., Abosetugn, A. E., Abushouk, A., I., Abdebayo, O. M., Agudelo-Botero, M., Ahmad, T., . . . Vos, T. (2020). Global injury morbidity and mortality from 1990 to 2017: Results from the Global Burden of Disease Study 2017. *Injury Prevention*, *26*, i96–i114. https://doi.org/10.1136/injuryprev-2019-043494

19. Khadka, A., Parkin, J., Pilkinton, P., Joshi, S. K., & Mytton, J. (2022). Completeness of police reporting of traffic crashes in Nepal: Evaluation using a community crash recording system. *Traffic Injury Prevention*, *23*(2), 79–84. https://doi.org/10.1080/15389588.2021.2012766

20. Konadu-Yeboah, D., Kwasi, K., Donkor, P., Gudugbe, S., Sampen, O., Okleme, A., Boakye, F. N., Osei-Ampofo, M., Okrah, H., & Mock, C. (2020). Preventable trauma deaths and correction actions to prevent them: A 10-year comparative study at the Komfo Anokye Teaching Hospital, Kumasi, Ghana. *World Journal of Surgery*, *44*(11), 3643–3650. https://doi.org/10.1007/s00268-020-05683-z

21. Merriam-Webster. (n.d.). Trauma. In *Merriam-Webster.com dictionary*. Retrieved January 10, 2023, from https://www.merriam-webster.com/dictionary/trauma#medicalDictionary

22. Merriam-Webster. (n.d.). Epidemiology. In *Merriam-Webster.com dictionary*. Retrieved January 10, 2023, from https://www.merriam-webster.com/dictionary/epidemiology#medicalDictionary

23. Mesic, A., Gyedu, A., Mehta, K., Goodman, S. K., Mock, C., Quansah, R., Donkor, P., & Stewart, B. (2022). Factors contributing to and reducing delays in the provision of adequate care in Ghana: A qualitative study of trauma care providers. *World Journal of Surgery*. https://doi.org/10.1007/s00268-022-06686-8

24. National Institute for Health and Care Research. (2022). Case study: Preventing injury and improving trauma care in Nepal and worldwide. *Traffic Injury Prevention, 23*(2), 79–84. https://doi.org/10.1080/15389588.2021.2012766
25. National Safety Council. (n.d.). *Injury facts.* https://injuryfacts.nsc.org/#:~:text=In%202021%2C%2061%2C105%20weather%20events,Learn%20more...&text=The%20National%20Safety%20Council%20estimates,this%20Labor%20Day%20holiday%20period
26. Peterson, C., Miller, G. F., Barnett, S., & Florence, C. (2021). Economic cost of injury—United States, 2019. *Morbidity and Mortality Weekly Report (MMWR), 70*(48), 1655–1659. https://doi.org/10.15585/mmwr.mm7048a1
27. Sturms, L. M., Driessen, M. L., van Klaveren, D., ten Duis, H., J., Kommer, G. J., Bloemers, F. W., den Hartog, D., Edwards, M. J., Leenhouts, P. A., van Zutphen, S., Schipper, I. B., Spanjersberg, R., Wendt, K. W., de Wit, R. J., Poeze, M., Leenen, L. P., & de Jongh, M. (2021). Dutch trauma system performance: Are injured patients treated at the right place? *Injury, 52*(7), 1699–1696. https://doi.org/10.1016/j.injury.2021.05.015
28. World Health Organization. (2017). *Preventing drowning: An implementation guide.* https://www.who.int/publications/i/item/9789241511933
29. World Health Organization. (2018). *Burns.* https://www.who.int/news-room/fact-sheets/detail/burns
30. World Health Organization. (2018). *Global status report on road safety 2018.* https://www.who.int/publications/i/item/9789241565684
31. World Health Organization. (2020). *Violence against children.* https://www.who.int/news-room/fact-sheets/detail/violence-against-children
32. World Health Organization. (2021). *A guidance document for medical teams responding to health emergencies in armed conflicts and other insecure environments.* https://apps.who.int/iris/rest/bitstreams/1351892/retrieve
33. World Health Organization. (2021). *Falls.* https://www.who.int/news-room/fact-sheets/detail/falls
34. World Health Organization. (2021). *Injuries and violence.* https://www.who.int/news-room/fact-sheets/detail/injuries-and-violence
35. World Health Organization. (2021). *Violence against women.* https://www.who.int/news-room/fact-sheets/detail/violence-against-women
36. World Health Organization. (2021). *Violence against women prevalence estimates, 2018—Global fact sheet.* https://www.who.int/publications/i/item/WHO-SRH-21.6
37. World Health Organization. (2022). *Abuse of older people.* https://www.who.int/news-room/fact-sheets/detail/abuse-of-older-people
38. World Health Organization. (2022). *Road traffic injuries.* https://www.who.int/news-room/fact-sheets/detail/road-traffic-injuries
39. Zhou, J., Wang, T., Belenkiy, I., Hardcastle, T. C., Rouby, J. J., & Jiang, B. (2021). Management of severe trauma worldwide: Implementation of trauma systems in emerging countries: China, Russia, and South Africa. *Critical Care, 25,* Article 286. https://doi.org/10.1186/s13054-021-03681-8

CHAPTER 2

Preparing for Trauma

Alexandra Carpenter, MHA, BSN, RN, CPEN, TCRN

OBJECTIVES

Upon completion of this chapter, the learner will be able to:
1. Appreciate the nursing role in trauma program development and function.
2. Define the qualities of high-performance teams.
3. Describe principles of effective communication.

Introduction

Around the world, injuries account for almost 8% of all deaths, taking an estimated 4.4 million lives a year.[28] Chapter 1, "Trauma Around the World," includes examples of international strategies and initiatives to reduce trauma-related morbidity and mortality. This chapter includes guidelines from the American College of Surgeons (ACS), the Agency for Healthcare Research and Quality, and the American Heart Association to improve trauma care preparedness and teamwork. Some principles may be specific to the U.S. healthcare system. The intent is to present information that can be adapted to a variety of care settings to improve trauma patient care processes.

Trauma Nursing

Trauma nurses are one component of a team that functions within a trauma system to provide care. Within this team structure, processes and strong communication are required to provided optimal care and improve patient outcomes. Trauma nursing occurs wherever nurses care for injured patients. Nurses play a critical role throughout the continuum of care, from the prehospital environment through resuscitation, surgery, recovery, rehabilitation, and return to the community. Trauma nursing is care-specific and is not dependent on specialized care environments. It includes advocating for patient care (including at the level of the local and national legislatures), providing injury prevention education, and conducting research to further nursing practice.

The practice of the trauma nurse employs a standardized, systematic approach to care, integrating the nursing process as the foundation. Trauma nurses are skilled in the management of difficult situations; moral agency is applied to advocate for excellence in patient care, even in the face of cultural and administrative obstacles.[27]

The practice of trauma nursing involves core knowledge derived from scientific and evidence-based sources and from the nurse's personal/life experiences. It is critical that the trauma nurse gain the appropriate knowledge base and assessment skills needed to recognize the trauma patient and predict injury patterns and severity. Engaging nurses with expertise in trauma nursing in the development of trauma programs and systems promotes optimal outcomes.

Trauma Nursing Education Position Statement

The Emergency Nurses Association has stated its position on trauma nursing education, which includes the following[26(pp1-2)]:

It is the position of the Emergency Nurses Association that:

1. A standardized and organized trauma system approach improves trauma care and reduces morbidity and disability.
2. Trauma-related continuing education and certification are recommended and an important adjunct for emergency nurses who provide care to trauma patients.
3. The trauma nursing process, taught in the TNCC course, is recommended as a systematic and standardized approach for the assessment, intervention, and evaluation of the trauma patient.
4. Emergency nurses with two years of trauma nursing experience are encouraged to take the Trauma Certified Registered Nurse (TCRN) certification exam.
5. Healthcare facilities support, promote, and value the achievement of trauma nursing education and certification for emergency nurses.
6. Educating bystanders can help start emergency treatment before emergency medical services arrive. Emergency nurses are therefore encouraged to support their communities by teaching injury prevention and first aid techniques such as hemorrhage control.
7. The development and implementation of injury prevention programs and best practices are an essential component of the continuum of trauma care.
8. Emergency nurses conduct and participate in research that links clinical trauma outcomes to basic and advanced trauma nursing education.

Trauma Programs

The development of trauma centers in the United States led to the implementation of integrated systems that progress from the point of injury through recovery (**Figure 2-1**).[23] The systematic and standardized approach to trauma care has been instrumental in saving lives and improving outcomes for those affected by trauma.[6,12,15]

Trauma programs serve as the primary structure for providing care to injured patients. Their focus is to coordinate management across the continuum of trauma care, which includes the planning and implementation of clinical protocols and practice management guidelines, monitoring care of in-hospital patients, and serving as a resource for clinical practice. Trauma programs transcend normal departmental hierarchies to ensure that the injured patient receives high-quality care, from the acute resuscitation phase up through rehabilitation and/or discharge.[27]

The trauma program is responsible for providing intrafacility emergency medical services, and regional outreach, education, and professional staff development opportunities regarding trauma care. Trauma programs perform concurrent data abstraction, analysis, and reporting for injured patients through maintenance of a trauma registry. Data points collected at individual trauma centers are aggregated and analyzed at the local, state, and national levels. Trauma programs meet stringent criteria to be verified as trauma centers through the ACS or designated by regional governing bodies. Trauma centers participate in the development of trauma care

Bystander Care — to provide early first aid

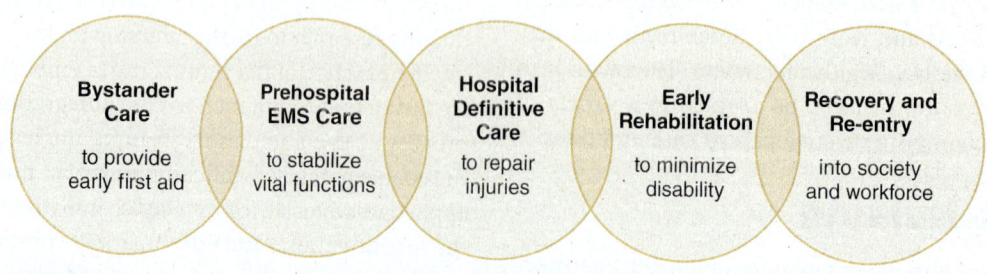

Prehospital EMS Care — to stabilize vital functions

Hospital Definitive Care — to repair injuries

Early Rehabilitation — to minimize disability

Recovery and Re-entry — into society and workforce

Figure 2-1 *Elements of the trauma system.*
Reproduced from National Academies of Sciences, Engineering, and Medicine. (2016). *A national trauma care system: Integrating military and civilian trauma systems to achieve zero preventable deaths after injury.* National Academies Press. https://doi.org/10.17226/23511

systems at the community, state, provincial, regional, or national levels and participate in injury prevention activities. The American College of Surgeons Committee on Trauma (ACS COT) recognizes three levels of trauma center designation. Each trauma center serves an important role in its community and has a critical function in the trauma system. The ACS COT expects trauma centers' commitment to quality care to be the same regardless of level. Trauma center level is a reflection of available resources. Being a trauma center is a facility-wide commitment that extends far beyond trauma resuscitation. The dedication to the ACS standards implies the entirety of care that must be available to the injured patient at the facility, along with other intentions related to education and research improvements, advancing the field, and increasing capacity.[9]

Trauma center level expectations are as follows[9(pvii)]:

- **Level I:** Level I trauma centers must be capable of providing system leadership and comprehensive trauma care for all injuries. In its central role, a Level I trauma center must have adequate depth of resources and personnel. Most Level I trauma centers are university-based teaching hospitals due to the resources required for patient care, education, and research. In addition to providing acute trauma care, these centers have an important role in local trauma system development, regional disaster planning, increasing capacity, and advancing trauma care through research.
- **Level II:** Level II trauma centers are expected to provide initial definitive trauma care for a wide range of injuries and injury severity and may take on additional responsibilities in the region related to education, system leadership, and disaster planning.
- **Level III:** Level III trauma centers typically serve communities that may not have timely access to a Level I or II trauma center and fulfill a critical role in much of the United States by serving more remote and/or rural populations. Level III trauma centers provide definitive care to patients with mild to moderate injuries, allowing patients to be cared for closer to home. These centers also have processes in place for the prompt evaluation, initial management, and transfer of patients whose needs might exceed the resources available.

Trauma Team Activities

The purpose of the trauma team activation is to provide advanced simultaneous care from relevant specialists to the seriously injured trauma patient. The primary aims of the team are to rapidly resuscitate and stabilize the patient, to prioritize, to determine the nature and extent of the injury, and to prepare the patient for transport to the site of definitive care, either within or outside the institution.

The criteria for trauma activation must be clearly defined by the hospital or trauma center. Typically, trauma centers have a tiered trauma activation protocol that is based on predetermined hospital criteria. Trauma activation criteria often include physiologic, anatomic, and mechanism of injury criteria, with consideration for special populations.[9]

While some may arrive unannounced by private vehicle, seriously injured patients largely are transported to the hospital via prehospital personnel, which allows the trauma team to be notified in advance of the patient's arrival.

The prenotification process gives the trauma team time to assemble, prepare, and anticipate needed resources before patient arrival. Regardless of the method of transport, the trauma resuscitation team should be activated as quickly as possible to provide adequate time to assemble the team and prepare. Even though nontrauma centers may not have a formal activation response, a structured and systematic approach to care of the injured patient as described throughout the TNCC course will promote optimal patient outcomes.[10]

Trauma Nurse Roles and Responsibilities

Trauma nurses are essential members of a multidisciplinary team that is structured to meet the complex needs of the trauma patient. During the trauma resuscitation, the nurse plays a critical role in ensuring team coordination, effective communication, and delivery of systematic, timely care to the injured patient. The trauma nurse coordinates the resuscitation in collaboration with the trauma surgeon and/or emergency department (ED) physician. The trauma nurse is well suited to lead the core patient-care team and support services, coordinating the care of both the patient and the team in conjunction with the team leader.[19]

Following the immediate resuscitation phase, additional trauma nursing responsibilities include ensuring that serial assessments are performed and documented, and all subtle or new findings in the patient's condition are reported. Nurses who provide direct care to trauma patients are dynamic and highly skilled professionals who demonstrate the following skills/characteristics:

- Assist in the delegation and coordination of trauma team roles and responsibilities
- Anticipate and prepare for trauma patient needs

- Document all prearrival information, primary and secondary assessment, medications, and procedures
- Provide continuous updates to the trauma team leader on changes in patient status
- Ensure that adequate protective equipment is worn by all core team members
- Prepare and administer ordered medications
- Assist with trauma interventions and procedures as needed
- Maintain order in unpredictable, and at times uncontrolled, situations
- Advocate for patients and families
- Formulate efficient and effective decisions based on limited information
- Remain focused in the face of distraction
- Exhibit strong communication and teamwork skills
- Demonstrate resiliency in a high-stress environment

During the resuscitation phase, the trauma nurse is responsible for ensuring continuity and facilitating high-quality care throughout the initial phase, until the patient's admission, discharge, or transfer.

The trauma nurse's highest priority is to ensure that the patient remains the focus of the provision of trauma care. The highly technical nature of trauma care often eclipses the simple human connection with the patient and family. Involving and communicating with the patient and family is also a key role for the trauma nurse. The trauma nurse should designate a qualified and available member of the team to fulfill this purpose if they are unable to do so.

Trauma Team Structure and Roles

Trauma resuscitation requires all team members to perform together for successful results. During the delivery of trauma care, team members respond to and provide specific expertise, with a shared goal of achieving the best possible outcomes for their patient. Teamwork is important and extends throughout all aspects of care.

Team structure dynamics exhibit the following characteristics[10]:

- Clear roles and responsibilities
- Knowing limitations
- Constructive interventions
- Knowledge sharing
- Summarizing and reevaluating
- Closed-loop communication
- Clear messaging
- Mutual respect

The size and composition of the trauma team may vary with hospital size, the severity of injury, and the corresponding level of trauma team activation. Time of day and resources available may also impact trauma team composition. Regardless of the situation, a systematic, organized approach is required by all members of the trauma team to provide optimal care for the trauma patient and family. Trauma team roles should be assigned before patient arrival. The typical composition of trauma teams includes the following members: team leader, core team members, and ancillary team members.[8,9]

Team Leader

Every high-performance team needs a leader to organize the efforts of the group. The trauma team leader is a critical component of a trauma team and the common link of communication and coordination of all personnel throughout the resuscitation. The trauma team leader should be clearly identifiable by all members of the team. All instruction and feedback to the team must go through the leader.

The role of trauma team leader involves determining the priorities, timing, and sequence of assessment and interventions throughout the resuscitative phase. The critical functions of the team leader are maintaining situational awareness, clearly communicating to the team, and encouraging mutual support. The leader should be trained in advanced trauma life support and the basics of medical management. Effective trauma team leaders[8,10]:

- Organize the team and delegate team roles and responsibilities
- Establish the preparation for the arrival of the patient to ensure that a smooth transition to the hospital environment is made
- Supervise, check, and direct the trauma assessment
- Ensure safe, timely, and thorough assessment of the trauma patient, to include obtaining the prehospital report
- Provide continuous updates on the patient status and plan of care to the team (i.e., shared mental models, brief, huddle, debrief)
- Articulate clear goals
- Coordinate patient stabilization and transfer to definitive care
- Communicate orders and instructions using closed-loop communication
- Make decisions through collective input of other team members
- Empower members to speak up and ask questions
- Model excellent team behavior
- Allocate resources

- Train and coach
- Temporarily designate another team member to take over team leadership if an advanced procedure is required
- Provide constructive feedback
- Ensure seamless transition through the phases of care

Core Team Members

This group of care providers works interdependently to manage a trauma patient from assessment to disposition.[17] Roles and responsibilities are often assigned to each member for technical skills such as airway management, procedural interventions, vascular access, transport, medication administration, and documentation. Institutional guidelines and policies specific to roles, responsibilities, and resources assist in ensuring consistent delivery of high-quality trauma care. Core team roles are best assigned before patient arrival and are reiterated during the briefing period.[8]

Core team members often include trauma surgeons and ED physicians, advanced practice providers, surgical and emergency residents, and nursing (emergency, critical care, and the operating room) and other allied health personnel (i.e., respiratory therapists, paramedic, patient care technician).

Core team member roles include the following[10]:

- Being proficient in performing their skills within their scope of practice
- Being clear about role assignments
- Being prepared to fulfill their role and responsibilities
- Having well-practiced resuscitation skills
- Being committed to success

Ancillary Team Members

These team members provide support to the core team to facilitate optimal trauma care. Ancillary team members may include individuals from anesthesia, physician consultant specialties, pharmacy, radiology, lab, blood bank, social work, case management, protective services, and pastoral care, as well as registration/clerical personnel.[8,9]

High-Performance Trauma Teams

Trauma resuscitation requires all team members to be efficient and coordinated, with the common goal of providing high-quality care. There can be little argument that the hallmark of an effective team is proficiency. The foregone conclusion is that each member of the team is proficient at the task they are assigned to perform. Effective trauma teams are collaborative, dynamic, interdependent, and adaptive, always moving toward a common goal.[18,25] High-performing teams have the following characteristics and responsibilites[1,8,10]:

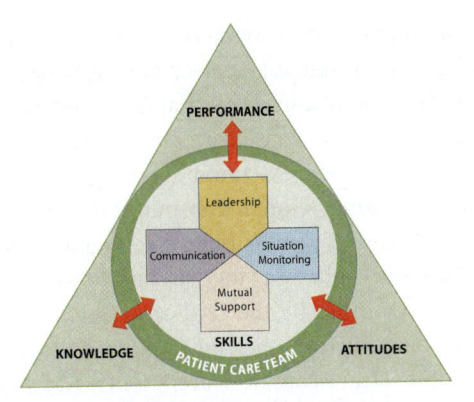

Figure 2-2 *Cornerstones of high-performance teams in trauma care.*
Reproduced from Agency of Healthcare Research and Quality. (2018). TeamSTEPPS 2.0 pocket guide: Team strategies and tools to enhance performance and patient safety. https://www.ahrq.gov/teamstepps/instructor/essentials/pocketguide.html

- Participate in ongoing updates on patient status and advocacy regarding concerns to the team (i.e., shared mental models, huddles)
- Optimize resources
- Exhibit strong team leadership
- Engage in a regular discipline of feedback
- Develop a strong sense of collective trust and confidence
- Create mechanisms to cooperate and coordinate their actions
- Optimize performance outcomes
- Are proficient in their skill set

Teamwork and interdisciplinary collaboration directly affect patient care. High-performing trauma teams have been shown to decrease mortality by reducing the time to investigation, total time in the resuscitation room, and the rate of missed injuries.[14] A growing body of supportive evidence also suggests that team training in trauma improves performance and patient outcomes.[24] Skilled communication, cooperation, and coordination are the cornerstones of high-performance teams and high-quality trauma care (**Figure 2-2**).[5]

Communication

For decades, the characteristics and behaviors associated with high-performing and low- or poor-performing teams have been observed and dissected. Experts in the fields of aerospace, the military, engineering, the social sciences, and the humanities have found that communication is potentially a team's greatest asset or gravest shortcoming.[18] Despite the general consensus that good communication is critical in healthcare, we continue to have an opportunity to improve in the execution of these principles.

Trauma teams should communicate continuously to ensure that everyone is on the same page and has a comprehensive view of the situation. Team performance is supported by the application of standardized, evidence-based communication tools and practices. The Agency for Healthcare Research and Quality's Team Strategies and Tools to Enhance Performance and Patient Safety (TeamSTEPPS) curriculum identifies three critical communication points in trauma care: briefs, huddles, and debriefs.[3] These points enable effective trauma teams to maintain a shared mental model.

Shared Mental Model

According to Floren et al., "a shared mental model is an individually held, organized, cognitive representation of task-related knowledge and/or team related knowledge that is held in common among health care providers who must interact as a team in pursuit of common objectives for patient care."[16(p506)]

The effects of teamwork on clinical settings such as trauma centers and EDs have been studied, and the quality of teamwork influences patient safety, care, and outcomes. Coordination of care and communication among teams are crucial for efficient and safe results with patient care. Trauma team members must share information and depend on each other's expertise to accomplish tasks successfully and to handle unexpected events. Team training has been a strategy to strengthen team behaviors and helps build a culture of safety. TeamSTEPPS tools are evidence-based and designed to improve patient safety through skills related to teamwork. These tools provide four core competencies (**Table 2-1**), translating teamwork into practices and checklists to enhance a shared mental model.[21]

A shared mental model is a mental picture or sketch of the relevant facts and relationships that define an event, situation, or problem. Trauma teams must all work together to achieve successful outcomes. Shared mental models or team mental models represent how the individuals within a team prioritize information given to them and how the information is then reflected back to the group. How a team processes and interprets information is validated best when the team has a shared mental model. Team members who communicate effectively with one another and understand each other's roles drive better outcomes.[22]

Shared mental models help trauma teams avoid errors or miscommunication that puts patients at risk (**Figure 2-3**).[2,11]

TABLE 2-1 TeamSTEPPS Core Competencies

Competency	Definition
Communication	The effective transmission of information and consultation among team members
Leadership	Ability to direct activities of the team, assign tasks, assess performance, motivate team members, develop team knowledge and skills, organize and plan, and establish a positive environment
Mutual respect	The ability to anticipate other team members' needs and change workload to achieve a balance
Situation monitoring	The development of common understandings of team dynamics and applying strategies to enhance team performance

Data from Lee, S. H., Khanuja, H. S., Blanding, R. J., Sedgwick, J., Pressimone, K., Ficke, J. R., & Jones, L. C. (2021). Sustaining teamwork behaviors through reinforcement of TeamSTEPPS principles. *Journal of Patient Safety, 17*(7), e582–e586. https://doi.org/10.1097/PTS.0000000000000414

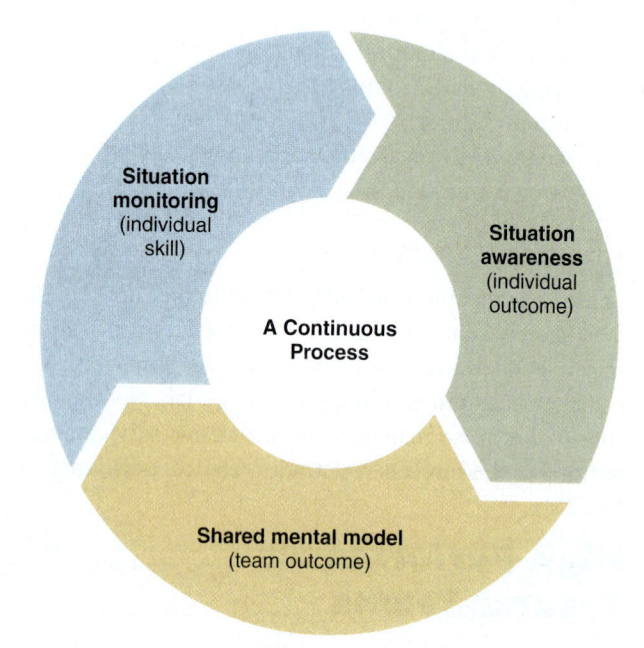

Figure 2-3 The shared mental model—a continuous process.

Reproduced from The Project Firstline program—a national training collaborative led by the Centers for Disease Control and Prevention (CDC) in partnership with the American Hospital Association and the Health Research & Educational Trust (HRET), an AHA 501(c)(3) nonprofit subsidiary.

Brief

A brief is a planned teamwork event designed to form the team, designate team roles and responsibilities, establish expectations and goals, and engage the team in short- and long-term planning.[2] Ideally, this is done at the beginning of a clinical event. Because of the unpredictable nature of trauma events, a briefing while assembling the trauma team after notification of an incoming trauma patient can help the team plan for the arrival and determine priorities of care. Briefs may also occur at designated times throughout the resuscitation to maintain situational awareness. The briefing should be performed by the trauma team leader. Elements of a briefing may include the following:

- Introductions
- Patient factors/anticipated needs
- Goals of resuscitation/set expectations
- Delegation of roles
- Concerns/potential obstacles

Huddle

Another component of team communication is a huddle. Huddles are convened as needed throughout the resuscitation to monitor and modify the plan. The purpose of a huddle is to regain situational awareness, express concerns, and make changes to the plan, with reassignment of resources as appropriate. It is important to identify and widely communicate the expectation that these team events will occur and ensure that anyone who recognizes a potential critical event or needs an update in the plan is empowered to speak up and call for a huddle.[3]

Debrief

A debrief can be a quick, informal information exchange or feedback session that occurs after the resuscitation and is designed to improve teamwork skills. A debrief checklist can be quite simple:

- What went well?
- Was communication clear?
- Were roles and responsibilities understood?
- Was situational awareness maintained?
- Were errors made or avoided?
- Were resources available?
- What might be done differently next time?
- Does anything need to be fixed right away, and who needs to know?

The debrief process should be interdisciplinary and encompass all members of the trauma team. The debriefing can be conducted in a matter of minutes and can be performed in various clinical settings. In one setting, a quick debrief may be held as the injured patient is being taken to radiology for imaging, or just after the patient is transferred to their definitive care destination. In another setting, a more formal debrief may be performed several hours or days after the resuscitation once the team members have had time to gather their thoughts. The timing varies depending on the setting and needs of the team, but the importance of the debrief occurring every time cannot be overstated. If members of the trauma team are not available for the debrief, the trauma team leader must ensure that the missing team member's feedback and concerns are gathered and included.[3]

Effective Communication in the Trauma Bay

The trauma nurse must continually develop effective communication techniques and be able to quickly recognize common pitfalls of communication during high-stress scenarios. Messages may not always be received exactly the way the sender intended, and it is important that all communicators seek feedback to check that their messages are clearly understood. Communication before, during, and after trauma resuscitation should be complete, brief, clear, concise, and timely.[1]

Barriers to effective communication during resuscitation include the following[4]:

- Perception differences among team members
  - Loss of situational awareness
- Limited information/information overload
- Inattention/distraction/noise
- Time-sensitive, high-acuity situations
- Emotionally charged/sensitive situations
- Organizational structure
  - Lack of clarity in roles/responsibilities
- Varied levels of experience

Communication Techniques During a Trauma Resuscitation

Effective communication techniques are particularly important during a resuscitation because of the potential for misunderstanding and errors, accompanied by hesitation for team members to speak up.[13] This section covers several useful techniques.

Knowledge Sharing

If resuscitative efforts are not effective, begin with the basics, and repeat the communication with the team concerning the assessment completed and patient responses to treatments already completed during the resuscitation. An example of such communication is, "We have completed the primary survey and have observed the following [repeat of information during the survey]. Has anything been missed?" High-performing team members should provide all available information about any observed changes in the patient's condition.[10]

Closed-Loop Communication

The team leader and the high-performance team members should use closed-loop communication steps[9,10,13]:

1. The leader communicates a message, order, or assignment to a specific individual team member.
2. The leader requests a clear response, using eye contact with the team member to ensure that they understand the messaging.
3. The leader confirms that the team member completed the task before assigning them another task.

An example of closed-loop communication follows:

Doctor Mike: Nurse Jane, can you call for an ICU bed for this patient?
Nurse Jane: Yes, I will call for an ICU bed.
Nurse Jane: The admissions coordinator has assigned an ICU bed.

Clear Messaging

Clear, precise messages and systematic methods of communication using a controlled voice and nonverbal behavior consistent with such a voice should be used. Unclear communication can delay treatment or cause errors.[10]

1. Deliver messages calmly and in a direct voice.
2. Do not yell, mumble, or shout.
3. Thoughts should be arranged in a sequential order and communicated accordingly.
4. Avoid the use of ambiguous statements; clearly state the question or statement and the purpose behind it.
5. Minimize distractions; identify and eliminate contributing factors as they occur (e.g., unnecessary team members, extraneous conversations).

Assertive Statement

An assertive statement is a tool used to facilitate speaking up when there is concern for patient safety. The steps involved in using an assertive statement are as follows[4]:

1. Get the individual's attention. Address them by name/formal title.
2. State, "I have a concern."
3. Provide details of the concern.
4. Offer a solution or alternate course of action if appropriate.
5. Obtain agreement and approval to implement the proposed resolution to the concern.

Another example of an assertive statement follows:

"Dr. Smith, I have a concern. I see that the patient has an oxygen saturation of 76%, and I am concerned that they will decompensate further. I would like to suggest that we pre-oxygenate for a couple minutes before the next intubation attempt. Do you agree?"

Mutual Respect

The best high-performance team members have mutual respect for each other and collegially work together in a supportive manner. These teams also create a culture that provides a safe space in which concerns and safety issues can be discussed without fear of repercussions or reprisals.[10,20]

Performance Improvement and Trauma Care

The needs of injured patients span the continuum of injury care, from prevention through rehabilitation. Injured patients are present in urban, suburban, and rural environments. In addition, they can cross geographic and political boundaries. A performance improvement process is a system of multidisciplinary reviews with a feedback loop; its purpose is to identify areas of opportunity and develop a demonstrated action plan to resolve identified issues. This requires the authority and accountability to continuously measure, evaluate, and improve care, and routinely reduce unnecessary variation in care and prevent adverse events (**Figure 2-4**). Patient outcome and quality of care provided are evaluated by a robust ongoing performance improvement program whose members meet regularly to discuss and resolve performance issues. To ensure evaluation of all aspects of

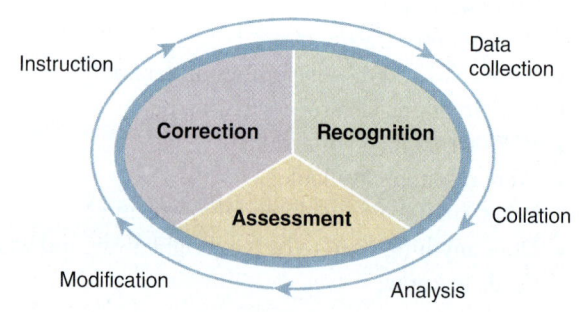

Figure 2-4 *The continuous process of performance improvement.*

Reproduced from American College of Surgeons, Committee on Trauma. (2014). Resources for optimal care of the injured patient (p. 114). https://www.facs.org/media/yu0Iaoqz/resources-for-optimal-care.pdf

trauma care, events that are addressed involve multiple disciplines. The trauma nurse may be invited to participate in performance improvement meetings, weigh in on clinical practice guidelines, protocols, and algorithm development, or initiate performance improvement projects.[7,9]

Just Culture

A foundational component of performance improvement is integration of just culture principles into evaluation of patient outcomes that are less than optimal or a situation in which errors occurred in the delivery of care. In a just culture, the focus is on systemic and cultural causes and concerns rather than individuals. It is imperative for patient safety that all members of the team feel confident that they have organizational and leadership support when reporting errors and will not be blamed or experience repercussions. It is incumbent for organizational, facility, and departmental leadership to encourage all staff to report errors and "near misses" to enable an accurate root cause analysis and successfully identify the system issues that contributed to the error. The purpose of a root cause analysis is not to change what already occurred or to assign blame, but to prevent future errors. Furthermore, an environment that embraces just culture principles may improve team collaboration and effectiveness as everyone strives for a culture of safety.

Summary

Trauma is a threat to the health and socioeconomic well-being of individuals, communities, and countries around the world. Whether a trauma event occurs in a community with a multiresource trauma center or a critical access hospital, a coordinated, collaborative, and systematic approach to the initial assessment and management of trauma is essential to ensure optimal outcomes and minimize morbidity and mortality.[9] A high-performance trauma team consistently delivers coordinated and collaborative care by clearly defining roles and responsibilities, in addition to ensuring efficiency, safety, and high-quality care delivery.

The trauma nurse is the coordinating member of the team who ensures continuity, consistency, and organization among team members. Nurses are essential members of the team and integral to trauma care and resuscitation in the ED. Nursing contributions through quality clinical care, in addition to effective communication, leadership, and teamwork, ultimately enable optimal patient outcomes.

The knowledge and skills learned in TNCC will assist nurses in systematically assessing the trauma patient, rapidly intervening and/or assisting with interventions, and communicating within the context of a trauma team. The Emergency Nurses Association supports ongoing commitments and efforts to improve injury surveillance, research, trauma system development, and patient safety, as well as garner governmental support for trauma care and injury prevention as a top priority.

References

1. Agency for Healthcare Research and Quality. (2012). *TeamSTEPPS Fundamentals Course: Module 2. Team structure*. http://www.ahrq.gov/teamstepps/instructor/fundamentals/module2/igteamstruct.html
2. Agency for Healthcare Research and Quality. (2012). *TeamSTEPPS Fundamentals Course: Module 5. Situation monitoring*. https://www.ahrq.gov/teamstepps/instructor/fundamentals/module5/igsitmonitor.html
3. Agency for Healthcare Research and Quality. (2014, March). *TeamSTEPPS Fundamentals Course: Module 4. Leading teams*. https://www.ahrq.gov/teamstepps/instructor/fundamentals/module4/igleadership.html
4. Agency for Healthcare Research and Quality. (2014, March). *TeamSTEPPS Fundamentals Course: Module 6. Mutual support*. https://www.ahrq.gov/teamstepps/instructor/fundamentals/module6/igmutualsupp.html
5. Agency for Healthcare Research and Quality. (2018). *Pocket Guide: TeamSTEPPS. Team strategies & tools to enhance performance and patient safety*. https://www.ahrq.gov/teamstepps/instructor/essentials/pocketguide.html
6. Alharbi, R. J., Shrestha, S., Lewis, V., & Miller, C. (2021). The effectiveness of trauma care systems at different stages of development on reducing mortality: A systematic review and meta-analysis. *Word Journal of Emergency Surgery, 16*, Article 38. https://doi.org/10.1186%2Fs13017-021-00381-0
7. American College of Surgeons. (2014). *Resources for optimal care of the injured patient*. https://www.facs.org/media/yu0laoqz/resources-for-optimal-care.pdf
8. American College of Surgeons. (2018). Appendix E: ATLS and trauma team resource management. In *Advanced trauma life support provider manual* (10th ed., pp. 303–314).
9. American College of Surgeons. (2022). *Resources for optimal care of the injured patient: 2022 standards*. https://www.facs.org/quality-programs/trauma/quality/verification-review-and-consultation-program/standards/
10. American Heart Association. (2020). Part 3. High performance teams. In *Advanced cardiovascular life support provider manual*.
11. American Hospital Association Center for Health Innovation. (n.d.). *Shared mental model*. https://www.aha.org/center/project-firstline/teamstepps-video-toolkit/shared-mental-model
12. Asensio, J. A., & Turnkey, D. D. (2016). Trauma systems. In J. A. Asensio & D. D. Turnkey (Eds.), *Current therapy of trauma and surgical critical care* (2nd ed., pp. 1–5). Elsevier.

13. Bhangu, A., Notario, L. N., Pinto, R. L., Pannell, D., Thomas-Boaz, W., Freedman, C., Tien, H., Nathens, A. B., & da Luz, L. (2022). Closed loop communication in the trauma bay: Identifying opportunities for team performance improvement through video review analysis. *Canadian Journal of Emergency Medicine 24*, 419–425. https://doi.org/10.1007/s43678-022-00295-z

14. Candefjord, S., Asker, L., & Caragounis, E. (2022). Mortality of trauma patients treated at trauma centers compared to non-trauma centers in Sweden: A retrospective study. *European Journal of Trauma and Emergency Surgery, 48*, 525–536. http://doi.org/10.1007/s00068-020-01446-6

15. Ciesla, D. J., Tepas, J. J., Pracht, E. E., Langland-Orban, B., Cha, J. Y., & Flint, L. M. (2013). Fifteen-year trauma system performance analysis demonstrates optimal coverage for most severely injured patients and identifies a vulnerable population. *Journal of the American College of Surgeons, 216*(4), 687–695. https://doi.org/10.1016/j.jamcollsurg.2012.12.033

16. Floren, L. C., Donesky, D., Whitaker, E., Irby, D. M., Ten Cate, O., & O'Brien, B. C. (2018). Are we on the same page? Shared mental models to support clinical teamwork among health professions learners: A scoping review. *Academic Medicine, 93*(3), 498–509. https://doi.org/10.1097/ACM.0000000000002019

17. Geyer, R. (2016). Core team members' impact on outcomes and process improvement in the initial resuscitation of trauma patients. *Journal of Trauma Nursing, 23*(2), 83–88. https://doi.org/10.1097/JTN.0000000000000191

18. Gillman, L., Brindley, P. G., Blaivas, M., Widder, S., & Karakitsos, D. (2016). Trauma team dynamics. *Journal of Critical Care, 32*, 218–221. https://doi.org/10.1016/j.jcrc.2015.12.009

19. Harvey, E., Freeman, D., Wright, A., Bath, J., Peters, V., Meadows, G., Hamill, M., Flinchum, M., Shaver, K., & Collier, B. (2019). Impact of advanced nurse teamwork training on trauma team performance. *Clinical Simulation in Nursing, 30*, 7–15. https://doi.org/10.1016/j.ecns.2019.02.005

20. Kassam, F., Cheong, A. R., Evans, D., & Singhal, A. (2019). What attributes define excellence in a trauma team? A qualitative study. *Canadian Journal of Surgery, 62*(6), 450–453. https://doi.org/10.1503%2Fcjs.013418

21. Lee, S. H., Khanuja, H. S., Blanding, R. J., Sedgwick, J., Pressimone, K., Ficke, J. R., & Jones, L. C. (2021). Sustaining teamwork behaviors through reinforcement of TeamSTEPPS principles. *Journal of Patient Safety, 17*(7), e582–e586. https://doi.org/10.1097/PTS.0000000000000414

22. Markin, N. W. (2018). Navigating to the goal: The importance of shared mental models in complex environments. *Journal of Cardiothoracic and Vascular Anesthesia 32*(6), 2618–2619. https://doi.org/10.1053/j.jvca.2018.03.019

23. National Academies of Sciences, Engineering, and Medicine. (2016). *A national trauma care system: Integrating military and civilian trauma systems to achieve zero preventable deaths after injury*. National Academies Press. https://doi.org/10.17226/23511

24. Peters, V. K., Harvey, E. M., Wright, A., Bath, J., Freeman, D., & Collier, B. (2018). Impact of a TeamSTEPPS Trauma Nurse Academy at a Level 1 trauma center. *Journal of Emergency Nursing, 44*(1), 19–25. https://doi.org/10.1016/j.jen.2017.05.007

25. Sethuraman, K. N., Chang, W. W., Zhou, A. L., Xia, B., Gingold, D. B., & McCunn, M. (2021). Collaboration and decision-making on trauma teams: A survey assessment. *Western Journal of Emergency Medicine, 22*(2), 278–283. https://doi.org/10.5811%2Fwestjem.2020.10.48698

26. Uhlenbrock, J. S. (2019). *Trauma nursing education* [Position statement]. Emergency Nurses Association. https://enau.ena.org/Users/LearningActivity/LearningActivityDetail.aspx?LearningActivityID=fw6tc2rFk4CkJCT1vumtZg%3D%3D&tab=4

27. Wolf, L. (2012). An integrated, ethically driven environmental model of clinical decision making in emergency settings. *International Journal of Nursing Knowledge, 24*(1), 49–53. https://doi.org/10.1111/j.2047-3095.2012.01229.x

28. World Health Organization. (2021, March 19). *Injuries and violence* [Fact sheet]. https://www.who.int/news-room/fact-sheets/detail/injuries-and-violence

CHAPTER 3

Biomechanics and Mechanisms of Injury

Alisyn P. Vander Wal, DNP, RN, ACNS-BC, CEN

OBJECTIVES

Upon completion of this chapter, the learner will be able to:
1. Apply concepts of biomechanics, kinematics, and mechanisms of injury to traumatic bodily injuries.
2. Describe forms of energy transfer related to trauma.
3. Compare the effects of environmental energy transfer on human tissues.
4. Predict potential injuries from specific mechanisms and patterns of injury.

Introduction

"Trauma" is the Greek word for "wound." One definition for trauma is "a physical injury or an emotional response to a distressing event." The potential for traumatic injury is present whenever energy comes into contact with the human body. The laws of physics govern the energy transferred during such events. When the intensity of the applied energy exceeds the capacity of tissue resistance, trauma occurs. Therefore, understanding the laws of physics and applying biomechanics, kinematics, and mechanism of injury (MOI) principles, along with knowledge of anatomy and physiology, can assist the trauma care nurse in anticipating the intervention and management needs of the trauma patient (**Table 3-1**).[15,16,28]

Kinematics: The Physics of Energy Transfer

Energy "at rest" is considered *potential*. However, once an object or mass starts to move, the potential energy becomes *kinetic*, meaning "in motion."[30] Kinematics, and the physics of energy transfer, can be applied to all mechanical traumas and is considered an essential element when determining traumatic injury.[28] The severity of injury depends on the amount of force that is transferred to and absorbed by the body. In relation to Isaac Newton's laws of motion, applying the basic laws of physics to the anatomic and physiologic properties of the human body can illustrate injury patterns experienced by a trauma victim.

TABLE 3-1 Terminology

Term	Definition
Biomechanics	The study of the movement of biological organisms using the methods of mechanics, engineering, and physics.
Kinematics	The branch of mechanics that considers motion without reference to the forces that act on that motion.
Mechanism of injury	The method of transfer of energy from the environment to the human body causing trauma.

Data from Merriam-Webster. (n.d.). Biomechanics. In *Merriam-Webster.com dictionary*. Retrieved January 22, 2022, from https://merriam-webster.com/dictionary/biomechanics; Merriam-Webster. (n.d.). Kinematics. In *Merriam-Webster.com dictionary*. Retrieved January 22, 2022, from https://merriam-webster.com/dictionary/kinematics; Sims, C. A., & Reilly, P. M. (2020). Kinematics. In D. V. Feliciano, K. L. Mattox, & E. E. Moore (Eds.), *Trauma* (9th ed., pp. 3–14). McGraw Hill. https://accesssurgery.mhmedical.com/content.aspx?bookid=2952&sectionid=249116077

> **CLINICAL PEARL**
>
> **Newton's Second Law of Motion**
>
> Newton's Second Law of Motion can be understood in terms of the following corollaries:
>
> - Force is increased = acceleration is increased
> - Mass is increased = acceleration is decreased
>
> An understanding of this relationship enables the trauma care provider to make an educated prediction regarding the extent of injury and the subsequent care required for a trauma patient.

Newton's laws of motion include the following[22]:

- *Newton's First Law of Motion* explains that a body at rest will remain at rest (potential energy) and a body in motion (kinetic energy) will remain in motion unless acted upon by an object.[22] When energy is transferred, alteration can occur to one or both objects.
  - *Example*: When a vehicle is parked, the force of gravity holds the car in a fixed position (potential energy). The vehicle will remain stationary until a force (e.g., collision with another vehicle) sets it in motion. The vehicle will remain in motion until acted upon by another object (e.g., tree).
- *Newton's Second Law of Motion* builds upon the first law and explains that acceleration is dependent upon two variables. An object's acceleration (a) depends directly on the net force (F) and indirectly on the mass (m) of an object. The net force equals the product of the mass multiplied by acceleration: F_{net} = mass × acceleration.[22] This law describes how momentum affects the speed of an object, depending on the acting force. As the force on an object is increased, the acceleration of the object is also increased. However, if the mass of an object is increased, the acceleration of the object is decreased.
  - *Example*: Two vehicles (a sport-utility vehicle and a compact car) have broken down on the road. The drivers are attempting to move their vehicles to the nearest exit ramp. The driver pushing the sport-utility vehicle (larger mass) will have to apply more effort compared with the driver moving the compact car (smaller mass). Therefore, the driver of the sport-utility vehicle may need greater force (more individuals to help push) to accelerate the vehicle and cause it to move.
- *Newton's Third Law of Motion* specifies that for every action (energy impact), there is an equal and opposite reaction resulting from the transfer of energy.[22] When two objects interact, they exert equal force upon each other. For every interaction, two forces are appreciated: (1) The size of the force of the first object equals the force of the second object, and (2) the direction of the force of the first object is opposite that of the second object.[28]
  - *Example*: A vehicle is driving down the road and collides with a bird, which strikes the windshield. The bird and the windshield interact with each other (equal and opposite reaction).
- Newton's laws of motion help form the *Law of Conservation of Energy*. Energy cannot be created or destroyed, only changed from one form

Question	Answer	Explanation
According to Newton's Third Law, which of these two forces is greater, size or force?	Neither. For each force, there is an *equal* and opposite reaction.	The potential demise of the bird results from the difference in the bird's *mass* and its inability to withstand greater acceleration.

to another or transferred from one object to another.[22] The total amount of energy must remain constant; that is, it is conserved over time. Therefore, if an object is isolated, the energy it has does not disappear but gets conserved, waiting to be acted upon. Trauma care providers must function as energy detectives, identifying where the stored energy put into motion has been transferred to anticipate a patient's physiological condition and needs. The amount of energy inflicted upon a body and the ability to tolerate it will determine injury and severity.[11]

- *Example:* Consider a car-versus-tree scenario (**Figure 3-1**). According to Newton's Law of Conservation of Energy, a car traveling at 60 mph (96.56 kph) (kinetic energy) collides (transferring its energy) with a tree (conserved energy), thereby creating an equal and opposite reaction that causes the vehicle to come to a sudden stop. However, the person or persons inside the vehicle will continue to travel at that same speed (60 mph [96.56 kph]), remaining in motion until acted upon by another force, transferring the energy of the person to that object (e.g., steering wheel, windshield, seat belt, air bag). Although the impact may have stopped the forward momentum of the body, the organs within the body remain in motion until they collide with another stationary force, such as the skull, abdominal wall, or chest wall.

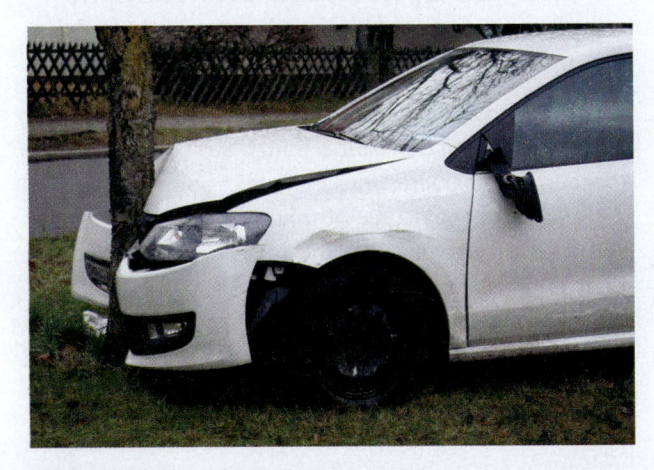

Figure 3-1 *Car versus tree.*
© Agencja Fotograficzna Caro/Alamy Stock Photo.

Biomechanics: Energy Forces and Their Effect

Understanding how energy forces affect the human body is useful for better anticipating the effects of trauma on a person.

Energy Forms

Energy can impact a person in the form of heat, motion, electricity, or some other form (**Table 3-2**). The body composition, preexisting conditions, and concomitant exposure of an individual are factors that affect the intensity of energy transfer absorption. For example, the extent of a thermal burn will vary with the temperature and duration of contact.

Kinetic Energy

The energy of a body in motion is identified as kinetic energy (KE). The amount of KE that an object has depends

TABLE 3-2	Forms of Energy
Energy Form	**Source**
Chemical	Heat energy transfer from active chemical substances such as chlorine, drain cleaner, acids, or plants
Electrical	Energy transfer from light socket, power lines, or lightning
Mechanical	Energy transfer from one object to another in the form of motion (e.g., a car hitting a tree)
Radiant	Energy transfer from blast sound waves, radioactivity such as from a nuclear facility, or rays of the sun
Thermal	Energy transfer of heat in the environment to the host

Data from U.S. Energy Information Administration. (n.d.). What is energy? https://www.eia.gov/energyexplained/what-is-energy/forms-of-energy.php

on the relationship between two variables: mass and velocity (speed). KE is equal to one-half the mass (*m*) multiplied by the square of its velocity (*v*²). While mass and velocity contribute to the energy present in a moving object, they do not have a constant ratio. When mass is doubled, so is the net energy. However, when velocity is doubled, energy is quadrupled. The KE equation is as follows[22,28]:

$$KE = \frac{1}{2}mv^2$$

While this equation may not be used to formally calculate the amount of KE involved in the trauma event when caring for a trauma patient, the comprehension of KE concepts is vital to the healthcare provider. Initial assessments in the aftermath of trauma may not identify a significant injury, but comprehension of the MOI may increase the suspicion for injuries that could have a delayed presentation.[11] This highlights the need for frequent and systematic assessments and reassessments of the trauma patient, in conjunction with understanding the transfer of energy, to identify injuries or patterns of injury.

CLINICAL PEARL

KE

Speed increases energy by the square of the velocity and can influence the extent of injury.[20] However, the absence of movement must also be considered. Speed increases the risk of injury, but the energy transfer occurs when the body stops. This causes the exertion of energy on to the tissues.

Types of Energy Forms

The degree to which tissues resist destruction under circumstances of energy transfer depends on their proximity to the impact and their structural characteristics. The basic types of energy forces are identified in **Figure 3-2** and further explained in **Table 3-3**.

In addition to the laws of physics, other factors determine the extent of traumatic injury to the body. Traumatic injury depends on the surface area to which energy is applied, tissue rigidity, and the elasticity of the structure affected by the energy force.[11] If the force applied is greater than that tolerated by the tissue, a tear or fracture will occur.[11]

External energy can be exerted by acceleration and deceleration forces. Acceleration and deceleration forces occur because of change in velocity.[1] With more sudden changes, greater force is applied, resulting in injuries.[1]

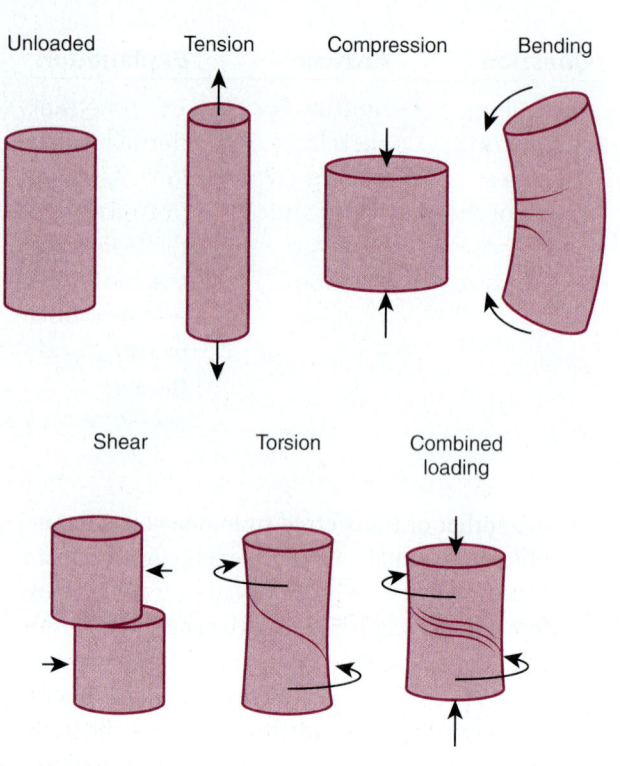

Figure 3-2 *Types of energy forces.*

- *Acceleration force:* Injury from acceleration forces occurs when applied energy causes a sudden and rapid onset of motion. For example, a pedestrian struck by a car may accelerate in the direction the car was traveling. The stationary brain is struck by the cranium that has been set in motion, causing injury.
- *Deceleration force:* Injury caused by deceleration forces occurs when energy is halted by a sudden stop. The more distance involved, the more likely a severe injury is to occur. Deceleration forces include those applied in falls and collisions where injuries are caused by a sudden stop of the body's motion.

Stress and *strain* are also exerted on the body during a traumatic event that causes injury. Stress and strain are biochemical characteristics that affect bodily tissues and directly affect the degree of injury.[27,28] When stress and strain are exerted on the body, tissues and organs change their dimensions. The degree to which tissues resist destruction depends on the amount of energy involved (high or low), as well as the structural characteristics and proximity of the organs (or tissue) to the impact. Considerations include the following:

- *Bone:* Strength and resistance to stress vary and can be augmented by adjacent muscle systems.

TABLE 3-3 Energy Forces

Energy Force	Description	Example
Tension	Two balancing forces causing extension (e.g., stretching by pulling at opposite ends).	Tensile strength describes the tissue's ability to resist pulling apart when stretched. Tendons, ligaments, and muscles can tear when they are overstretched (e.g., Achilles tendon).
Compression	Compression forces injure by squeezing together.	Compression injuries to organs occur when the organs are crushed from surrounding internal organs or structures; an example is a seat belt worn up across the abdomen, causing compression of the small bowel or a fracture to the lumbar spine.
Bending	Loading about an axis. Bending causes compression on the side the person is bending toward and tension to the opposite side.	A force moves from a straight form to a curved form, such as bending forward from a standing position.
Shearing	Shearing forces cause damage by tearing or bending; force is exerted on different parts in opposite directions at the same time within a structure.[28]	Shear strength describes the tissue's ability to resist a force applied parallel to the tissue. An aortic tear is an example: Shear force along a mobile portion of the aorta causes the vessel to tear away from a fixed attachment point.[9]
Torsion	Torsion forces twist ends in opposite directions.	Twisting motion depends on the body's ability to resist applied torque (e.g., a golfer's spine twisting when swinging a golf club).
Combined loading	Any combination of tension, compression, torsion, bending, and/or shear.	The combination of forces may increase the magnitude of the stress.

- *Muscle density*: Muscle density surrounding bone absorbs energy. Tensile strength is augmented by the strength of opposing muscles.
- *Organ structures*: Refer to Table 3-3.
- Solid organs tolerate pressure-wave energy better than air-filled organs do.
- Air-filled organs can resist shear forces better than solid organs.

Types of Injuries

Trauma-related injuries are classified into the following types:

- Blunt trauma
- Penetrating trauma
- Thermal trauma (see Chapter 11, "Surface and Burn Trauma," for more information)
- Blast trauma

Blunt Trauma

Blunt injuries are very common and result from a broad range of energy impacts. With blunt trauma, forces are applied, and energy is transferred in complex ways.[28] Understanding the distance and total surface area over which the energy transfer occurs is important for identifying an injury pattern. The more focused the impact, the greater the damage. Because blunt trauma may often appear less obvious, with minimal to no outward signs of injury as compared with other mechanisms or types of injuries, its severity may be dismissed initially, resulting in delayed treatment and increased complications. For this reason, early and frequent assessments are crucial for the trauma care provider to identify opportunities for early intervention before the trauma patient becomes unstable. The most common causes of blunt injuries involve both acceleration and deceleration forces. Common mechanisms causing blunt trauma include motor vehicle collisions (including motorcycles, bicycles, and pedestrians), falls, sports injuries, and physical assaults.[11,28]

CLINICAL PEARL

Blunt Trauma

Because blunt trauma may often appear less obvious, with minimal to no outward signs of injury as compared with other mechanisms or types of injuries, its severity may be dismissed initially, resulting in delayed treatment and increased complications.

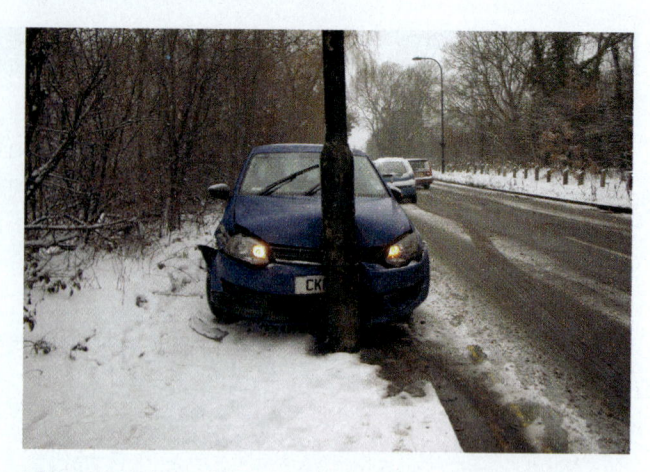

Figure 3-3 *First impact of MVC.*
© DBURKE/Alamy Stock Photo.

Motor Vehicle Impact Sequence

Motor vehicle collisions (MVCs) are the leading cause of preventable death worldwide.[19] MVCs involving collision between two or more vehicles are the most common collisions, followed by collision of a vehicle with a stationary object, collision with a pedestrian, and a non-collision, such as a rollover.[19] However, most injuries and fatalities are caused by non-collisions and collision with a stationary object.[20] MVCs commonly cause blunt trauma affecting the head, neck, chest, abdomen, and musculoskeletal system.[11]

Several impacts may occur during the progression of an MVC[11]:

- The first impact occurs when the vehicle collides with another object (e.g., a tree). The occupants experience a relative acceleration as the vehicle comes to an abrupt stop (**Figure 3-3**).
- The second impact occurs as the occupants continue to move in the original direction of travel until they collide with the interior of the vehicle or meet resistance (e.g., steering wheel, windshield, seat belt, or air bag), and the internal organs continue in motion (**Figure 3-4**).
- The third impact occurs when internal structures collide within the body cavity. The organs meet resistance from the structures that encapsulate them and/or are torn loose and may continue in motion until they meet the resistance of another structure, such as the chest wall or skull (**Figure 3-5**).

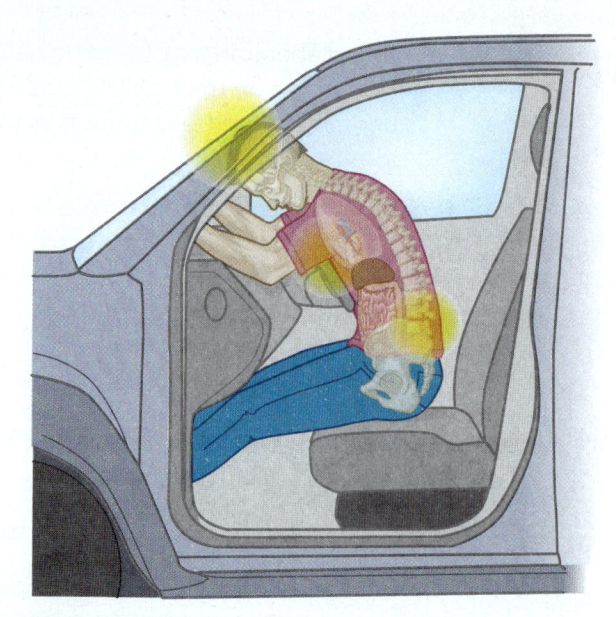

Figure 3-4 *Second impact of MVC: Example of an up and over path.*
Note: The body continues in motion until it impacts the inside of the vehicle.

MVCs involve changes in momentum, transfer of energy, and the generation of forces. Understanding these actions helps anticipate the patterns of injury. The extent of injuries is influenced by the mechanism of the crash (e.g., rollover), rate of speed, stopping distance, and deployed safety mechanisms such as seat belts, airbags, and the impact absorbency of the vehicle. See Chapter 4, "Initial Assessment," for more information related to MOI descriptions and injury patterns.

Mechanism of Injury and Potential Injury Patterns in Motor Vehicle Collisions

MOIs and potential injury patterns are associated with the type of motor vehicle involved.

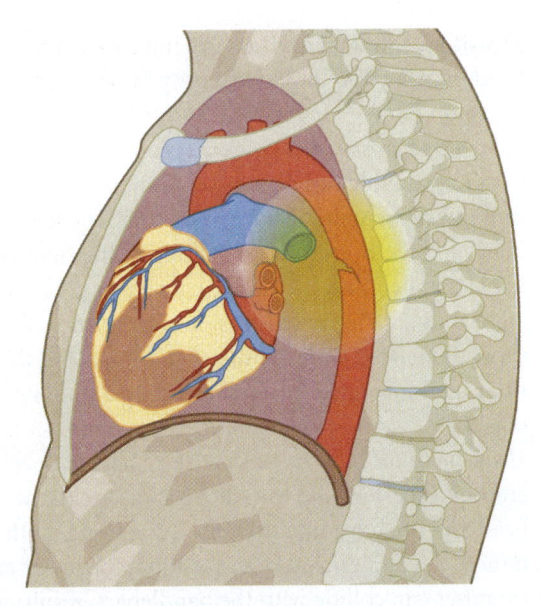

Figure 3-5 *Third impact of MVC.*

Note: Organs continue in motion and are torn away from their attachment. In this example, the aorta is torn at the ligamentum arteriosum until it impacts inside the thoracic cavity.

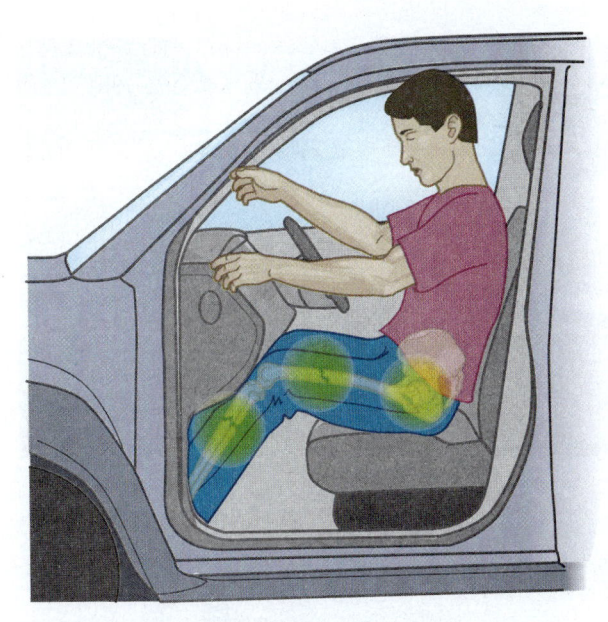

Figure 3-6 *The down and under path.*

Motor Vehicle (Auto)

Several patterns of pathway injuries are possible with collisions involving automobiles:

- In frontal collisions, the *up and over* pathway causes injuries that affect the driver and other front passengers. These injuries occur when the head and chest lead the way over the steering wheel and/or dashboard to the windshield (**Figure 3-4**). The injuries most commonly involve the head, neck, chest, and/or abdomen.[28]
- Frontal and rear-end collisions may also cause the *down and under* pathway injuries. These injuries occur when the occupants (driver or passenger) move in a downward direction under the steering wheel and/or dashboard (**Figure 3-6**). This type of collision may cause injuries from a misplaced seat belt or from contact with fixed structures under the dashboard, affecting the abdomen, spine, pelvis, and lower extremities.[5,11,28]
- *Lateral (T-bone)* impact injury patterns depend on where an individual is located in the vehicle in relation to the impact (**Figure 3-7**). This impact can cause devastating injury to the occupant of the affected compartment because of close proximity to the impact.[28] Injuries related to lateral collisions include the lateral chest, abdomen, and pelvic acetabulum.[28]
- *Rotational* impacts occur when a vehicle is struck on one corner, by either a stationary object or another vehicle going in the opposite direction, causing the rest of the vehicle to rotate around a pivot point. The impacted corner stops, but the rest of the vehicle continues to move until the energy of the vehicle is transferred. The occupant will then travel forward while the lateral side of the car extends inward and collides with the forward-moving body. The rotational impact may result in any combination of injuries that are common with frontal, rear, and lateral impacts.
- *Rollover* collisions can result in any and/or all of the injury patterns described previously. The forces that affect occupants in a rollover crash occur at random.[28]
- *Ejection* from a vehicle can be caused by many factors such as not wearing or inappropriately wearing safety restraints (i.e., seat belts). Ejection from the vehicle subjects the individual to increased morbidity and mortality because they are generally ejected at the same rate of speed that the vehicle was traveling, and strike a stationary object.[11,28]

Motorized Recreational Vehicles

Collisions involving other types of motorized recreational vehicles (MRVs)—for example, motorcycles, farm vehicles, all-terrain vehicles (ATVs), personal watercraft, snowmobiles, electric bicycles, and motorized scooters—can also cause traumatic injuries. Concerns with all MRVs include lack of regulations for use, inexperienced riders, use of alcohol and other substances, excessive speed, recklessness, and lack of restraint devices and protective gear.[3,11] Failure to use restraints increases the probability of passenger ejection. It is not the objective

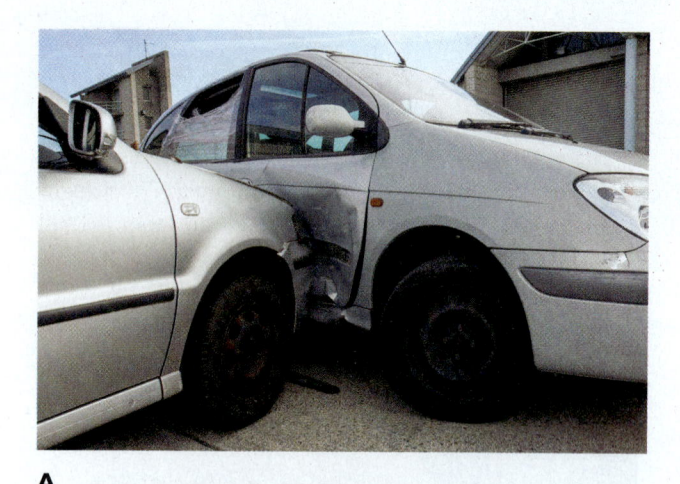

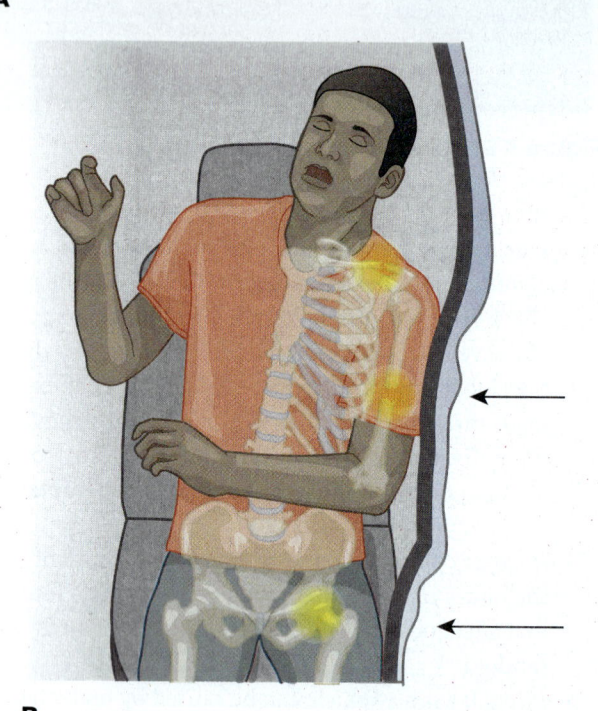

Figure 3-7 A. Lateral impact. **B.** Points of contact in a lateral impact motor vehicle collision.

Note. With a lateral T-bone accident, the greater the amount of intrusion, the greater potential for injury to the vehicle's occupants.
A. © Peter Cavanagh/Alamy Stock Photo.

of this manual to be all inclusive regarding MRV crashes. Descriptions of several crash types follow[25]:

- A *low side crash* is commonly referred to as "laying the bike down." It occurs when a motorcycle is no longer upright, with the tires leading in the direction of travel. Less speed-reducing friction is present when the motorcycle tires are no longer in upright contact with the roadway. A motorcycle sliding on its side may not slow down quickly. Therefore, impact energy experienced before and after the crash can be similar. In a low side crash, abrasions, shoulder and clavicle injuries, lateral head injuries, and lower extremity injuries are common.
- A *high side crash* occurs when a motorcycle begins to fall to the side but regains traction, placing the motorcycle in an unbalanced position. The force may vault the motorcycle, resulting in the rider being catapulted into the air. Injury patterns include all of those common to low side crashes, as well as those associated with the speed and impact of the rider landing on the ground or hitting a stationary object.
- *Head-on or topside* impacts cause an abrupt deceleration force, ejecting the rider forward with the head and torso leading the way. Depending on the motorcycle design and rider position, the lower extremities can collide with the handlebars, resulting in femur and pelvis fractures and hip dislocations. The remaining injuries depend on the subsequent collisions but are likely to involve the head, neck, chest, and extremities.
- *Lateral or angular* impacts initially result in significant lower extremity injuries, but other patterns can be present as well. The angular impact may initially crush the lower extremities but will likely cause the motorcycle to rapidly impact the ground, resulting in upper extremity, lateral head, and neck injuries. A T-bone impact to the motorcyclist may result in a lower extremity crush injury, followed by side-impact shoulder and head injuries as the rider slams into the hood and windshield of the other vehicle. The rider is then likely to tumble off the car and impact the ground.

CLINICAL PEARL

Rollover Collisions with Ejection

Ejection from the vehicle significantly increases the probability of fatal injury.[20]

Vehicle-Versus-Pedestrian Injuries

The height and speed of the vehicle, as well as the height, size, mental capacity, and distraction of the pedestrian and/or driver, may affect the severity of injuries suffered by a pedestrian who is struck by a vehicle.[28] When the vehicle collides with the adult pedestrian, crushing forces to the lower extremities may be experienced. An adult-sized individual may be catapulted onto the hood and/or windshield of the vehicle, sliding off or being propelled up and over, eventually incurring another collision with the ground (**Figure 3-8**). Adults aware of the oncoming vehicle may respond by turning to escape, resulting in the potential for lateral or posterior injuries. In contrast, children are much smaller and are much more likely to become a projectile when struck by a vehicle and have a secondary impact with the ground.[13] This causes a distinct pattern of injury to the pediatric patient known as the Waddell triad (**Figure 3-9**). The Waddell triad includes injuries that involve the head, thorax, and lower extremities.[13]

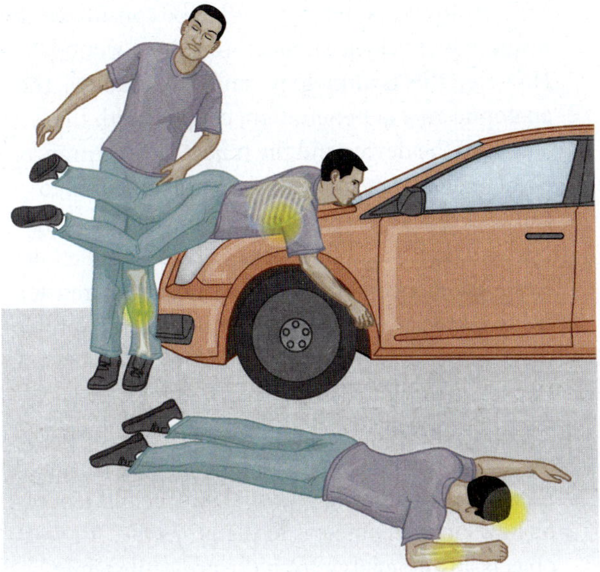

Falls

Falls involve acceleration/deceleration principles as described earlier, as well as Newton's laws of motion. As an example, consider an older adult who becomes dizzy and falls from a standing position. The energy transfer begins as the patient begins to collapse. When the patient collides with the ground, the impact causes energy transfer and injuries related to the following[28]:

- The point of impact on the patient's body determines the major point of energy transfer and underlying injuries or tissues impacted (e.g., head, hip, outstretched arm).
- The type of surface that is hit and the extent to which this surface can absorb the energy affect injuries. Carpet and grass can help to absorb energy better than a hard surface such as tile or concrete.
- The tissue's ability to resist also affects potential injuries. Bone is less flexible than soft tissue. Air-filled organs may rupture; solid organs may fracture.
- The trajectory of force influences the injuries experienced. If a person is pushed or accidentally knocked down, acceleration increases, causing additional transfer of energy that results in a greater impact on deceleration.

Consider a construction worker who falls from greater than 20 feet (6.10 m): The greater distance increases acceleration, thereby producing greater energy force, transfer of energy, and impact on deceleration. In the pediatric patient, mortality is increased if the fall is from greater than 10 feet (3.05 m).[13] Additionally, because the head is

Figure 3-8 *Pedestrian struck by a vehicle.*

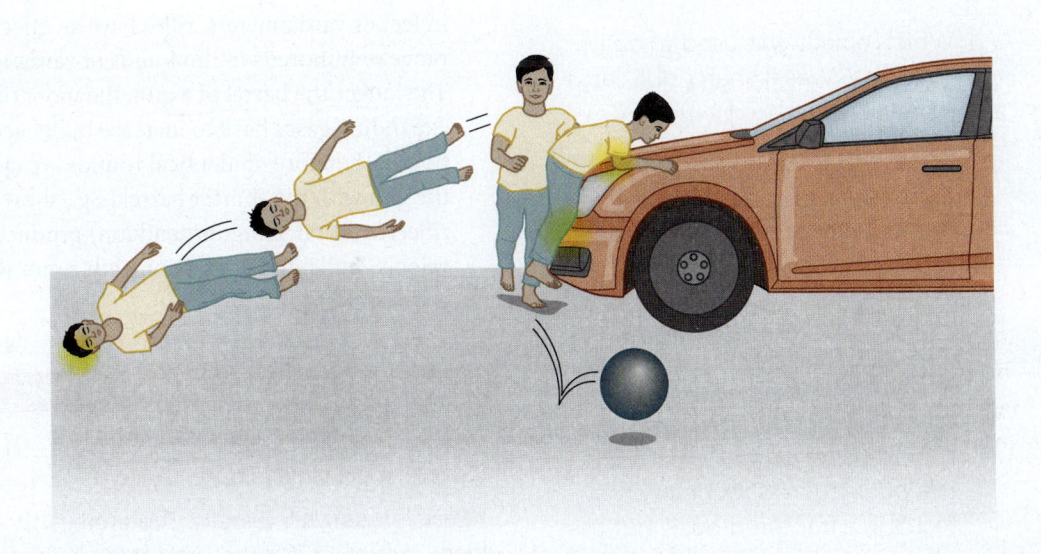

Figure 3-9 *Waddell triad.*

disproportionally larger in children than adults, there is a greater likelihood that pediatric falls will be associated with head injury.[13]

Assault

Interpersonal violence occurs in all countries and can result in blunt and/or penetrating injuries. The extent of injuries resulting from assault depends on multiple force factors, including those described in **Table 3-4**.

Penetrating Trauma

Any foreign object that enters through the skin barrier is considered penetrating. This type of injury can involve a victim's internal organs, causing hemodynamic instability (shock) and increased risk for infection.

Penetrating trauma is a notable concern in many countries, with the most common form being injuries from gunshots or stabbings. Risk factors include considerations based on age, race, gender, and geography.

The precise damage caused by penetrating mechanisms depends on several variables:

- *Point of impact:* The injury potential of a penetrating object is related to the speed and length of the penetrating object and the point of impact on the body. The density and rigidity of the body, organs, and tissues are significant in terms of determining the amount of energy transfer that occurs with a penetrating injury. Dense tissues and organs, such as the liver or kidney, absorb more energy, causing greater damage to such areas compared with less dense tissue, such as in the lung.[11,28]
- *Velocity and speed of impact:* The velocity of the object can be classified by the amount of energy generated. Medium- and high-velocity injuries may result from the use of firearms and explosives. The simplest injury patterns can often be considered the result of low-velocity impacts (e.g., stab wounds). However, this terminology can be misleading. The anatomic area of penetration, coupled with the length of the device and the trajectory of entrance of low-velocity mechanisms, has the potential to cause significant injury.[11] Although velocity is significant, the speed of the projectile (e.g., bullet) creates high energy transfer.[11,27,28] The energy transfer from a projectile is not uniform because the projectile may ricochet or deform while in transit or upon impact; the point of impact, such as tissue, bone, organs, or protective clothing, can also influence the extent of injury.[11,27,28]
- *Proximity:* Wounding potential may be influenced by how close an object is to the projectile. Air and objects absorb energy from the projectile while it is in flight, thus slowing its speed. In very close proximity (less than 3 feet [less than a meter]), the burning particulate and expanding gases that propel the projectile may also cause injury. Whereas handguns have an effective (lethal) range measured in feet or yards/meters, rifles have an effective range of hundreds to thousands of yards/meters. The longer the barrel of a gun, the more time the expanding gases have to increase bullet acceleration.[11] Therefore, if identical rounds are ejected, the gun with the shorter barrel (e.g., short-barreled rifle/sawed-off shotgun/handgun) produces a lower velocity bullet in comparison with a gun with a longer barrel.[11,14]

TABLE 3-4 Assault Force Factors and Results

Force Factor	Result
Amount	The larger the mass, the greater the force.
Distance	Force that travels from a distance is dissipated over that distance.
Object	Which object was used to deliver the force? Was it sharp, dull, large, small, . . . ?
Involved tissue	What is the ability to absorb the force? Consider the difference in the tissue affected, such as the skull versus the abdomen.
Object trajectory	Consider the difference between a boxer who is struck square in the nose versus a boxer who takes a glancing blow as he moves just enough to "roll" with the punch. The direct blow may result in a fractured nose, but the glancing blow may result in only a bruise or contusion.

> **CLINICAL PEARL**
>
> **Velocity and KE Are Positively Correlated with Destruction**
>
> KE increases with velocity. Therefore, although velocity is relative, it is the projectile's KE that causes damage by transferring energy to the tissue.

Bullet-Related Considerations

As described earlier in this chapter, in the equation $KE = mv^2/2$, KE is the kinetic energy, m is the projectile mass, and v is the bullet velocity. The velocity is squared, so an increase in velocity has a greater effect on the bullet's energy than an increase in its mass.[22] Bullets travel at their fastest when leaving the muzzle of the firearm and are then slowed by the effect of drag when they enter the air.[23]

The direction of a bullet is described as its rotational axis, while the deviation is the yaw. The yaw of a bullet is often described as the "tumbling" that happens as the bullet is oscillating linearly around the axis of its trajectory.[27]

The materials that compose the exterior and interior of the bullet, as well as any modifications made to the bullet, may influence the extent of tissue damage. Characteristics of common bullet types are briefly summarized here[11,23,28]:

- *Full metal jacket* (FMJ) bullets are made of a dense, heavy metal that covers the bullet from base to tip. They are often seen used in assault rifles and lose only a small amount of initial velocity as they travel farther from the barrel. The FMJ bullet often penetrates through a target, resulting in minimal tissue deformation on impact. When assessing the patient, the trauma team may notice lead splatter or a snowstorm pattern on radiographic imaging.
- *Soft-nose* bullets are non-jacketed. The impact energy of these bullets is designed to expand outward, but at a slower rate than with hollow-point bullets. Although soft-nose bullets can rapidly disable an individual, they are less likely to penetrate through the body to injure another person.
- *Hollow-point* bullets have a hollow cavity in the tip and jacket and are designed to produce maximal energy transfer upon contact. On impact, the bullet tip is forced backward, flattening and widening, and thereby doubling its surface area. This action is often referred to as an *expanding* round or *mushrooming*. The hollow-point bullet design is often seen in law enforcement firearms and in some cases is required in hunting to provide a more humane death for animals.
- *Frangible* bullets are designed to break apart when they impact a surface harder than the bullet. This bullet design disintegrates with rapid energy transfer, dissipating within the target and causing multiple chaotic fragment paths. Scoring a bullet makes it more likely to fragment. These designs can be controversial and were developed for close-quarters defense and law enforcement use.

Cavitation

As indicated by the KE equation, increased velocity of a projectile causes more damage than increased mass; therefore, when a projectile passes through tissue, it transfers its high-pressure KE, creating a cavity (**Figure 3-10**).[26-28] Cavitation may be temporary or permanent.

A temporary cavity is created when a high-pressure object (e.g., bullet) enters the soft tissue of the body. As the object decelerates, it transfers its energy to the surrounding tissue. The tissue then accelerates, stretching and displacing outward away from the entering object; this creates a vacuum that draws inward air and surface contaminants such as soil, clothing, and skin.[17] Although the size of the cavity may diminish, the damage that can occur via cavitation from the crushing, tearing, and shearing forces on the tissue may be significant. Damaged tissues may include subcutaneous tissue, blood vessels, organs, and bone.

In permanent cavitation, the cavity created by the path of the penetrating object remains, leaving a permanent track and potential loss of tissue.[24,27] The alterations to the body depend on the characteristics of the tissue being affected. For example, the amount of energy transferred may increase with denser tissue.[27] Air-filled organs, such as the lungs and stomach, are elastic. Therefore, this type of tissue tolerates high-velocity cavitation relatively well compared

> **CLINICAL PEARL**
>
> Cavitation can be seen when an unrestrained driver hits a steering wheel. As the chest pushes inward from the resistance of the steering wheel, a temporary cavity is created.

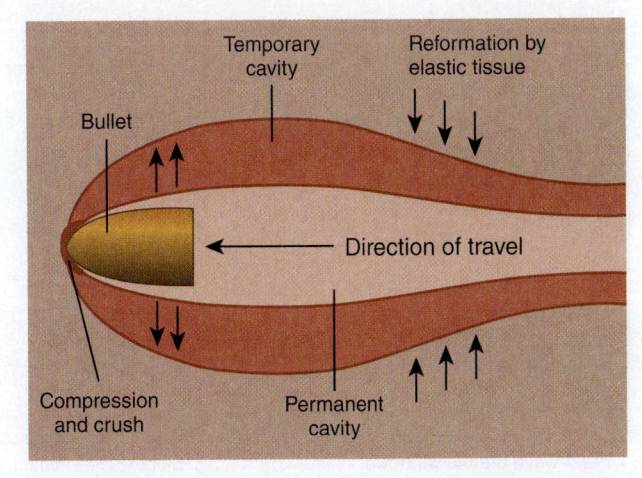

Figure 3-10 *Cavitation caused by a bullet.*
Modified from Science Direct: Imraan Sardiwalla, I., Govender, M., Matsevych, O., & Zacharia Koto, M. (2016). Indirect ballistic injury to the liver: Case report and review of literature. *International Journal of Surgery Open, 5,* 23–26. Retrieved from https://www.sciencedirect.com/science/article/pii/S240585721630050X

with denser tissues. Solid organs, such as the liver, have a greater propensity to shear or tear under the same forces (**Figure 3-11**). Permanent cavitation also depends on the type of projectile, with permanent cavitation occurring in association with larger or fragmented projectiles.[27]

Thermal Trauma

Chapter 11, "Surface and Burn Trauma," discusses the impacts and injuries associated with thermal trauma.

Blast Trauma

Although most commonly associated with the military, blast injuries can strike anywhere. They have occurred in industrial settings, mining industries, shipping industries, and chemical plants. Most recently, blasts have been associated with terrorist attacks. An explosion occurs when energy, in the form of light, heat, and sound, is released rapidly. The blast pressure expands outward in all directions at a rate greater than the speed of sound (**Figure 3-12**).[29]

The U.S. Department of Defense classifies blast injuries into five levels.[29] The effects of an explosion on the human body are numerous, as outlined in **Table 3-5**. These injuries can result from a combination of blunt or penetrating trauma and include possible exposure to chemical, thermal, physical, and radioactive agents. Blast injuries tend to affect the ears, lungs and musculoskeletal system.[31]

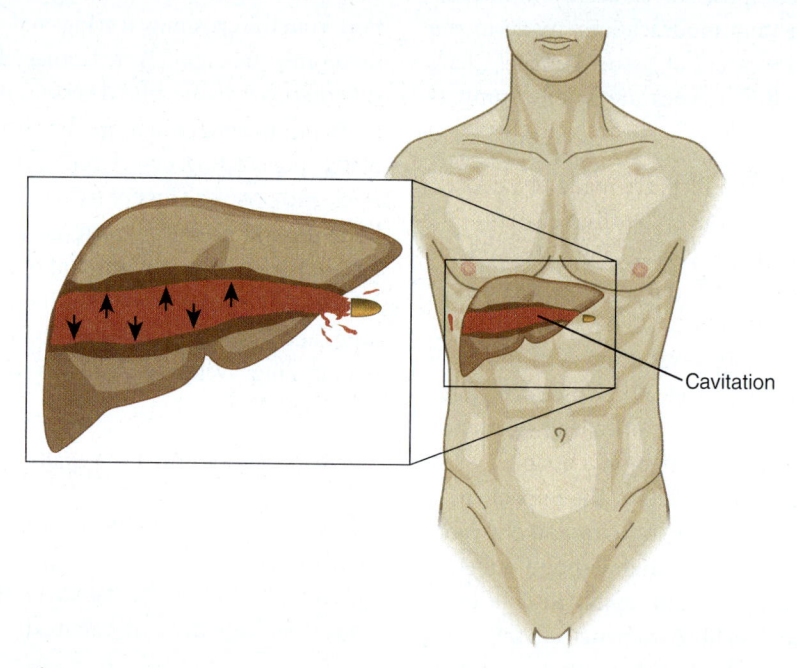

Figure 3-11 *Traumatic cavitation of the liver.*

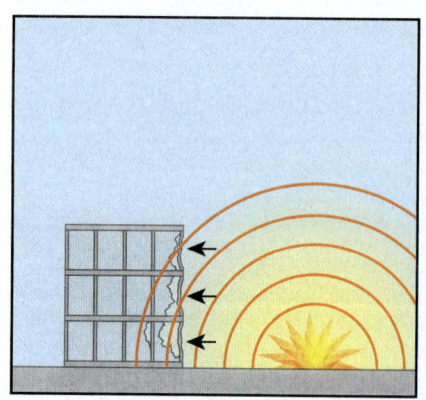

1. Blast wave breaks windows
   Exterior walls blown in
   Columns may be damaged

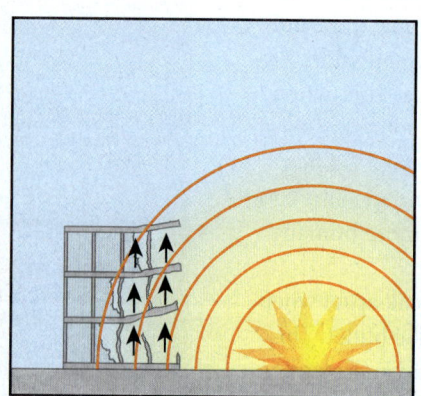

2. Blast wave forces floors upward

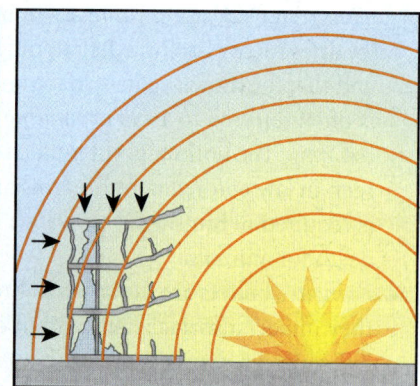

3. Blast wave surrounds structure
   Downward pressure on roof
   Inward pressure on all sides

Figure 3-12 *Blast pressure effects on a structure.*
Modified from Federal Emergency Management Agency. (2003). Explosive blast. In *Reference manual to mitigate potential terrorist attacks against buildings* (pp. 4-1-4-20). Retrieved from Unit VI - Explosive Blast (fema.gov).

TABLE 3-5 Effects of Explosions on the Human Body

Effects	Impact	Mechanism of Injury	Types of Injuries
Primary	Direct blast effects (over- and underpressurization)	› Direct tissue damage from the blast overpressure › Interaction of blast effect with body › Gas-filled structures are at high risk › Complex stress and shear waves produce injury or body dismemberment and dissemination	Blast lung (pulmonary barotrauma) Tympanic membrane rupture and middle ear damage Abdominal hemorrhage and perforation Globe (eye) rupture Mild traumatic brain injury (TBI; TBI without physical signs of head injury)
Secondary	Projectiles propelled by explosion	Wounds produced by: › Primary fragments from exploding weapon and shrapnel › Secondary fragments: projectiles from the environment (e.g., debris, vehicular metal)	Penetrating ballistic (fragmentation) or blunt injuries Eye penetration (can be occult) Closed and open brain injury
Tertiary	Results from individuals being thrown by the blast wind (propulsion of body onto a hard surface or object)	Displacement of body and structural collapse	Whole or partial body translocation from being thrown against a hard surface: › Blunt/penetrating trauma › Fractures › Traumatic amputations › Closed and open brain injury
Quaternary	All explosion-related injuries, illnesses, or diseases not due to primary, secondary, or tertiary mechanisms (heat and/or combustion fumes)	› Burns and toxic injuries from fuel › Metals › Septic syndromes from soil and environmental contamination	All other injuries associated with the blast: › External and internal burns › Crush injuries › Asthma, chronic obstructive pulmonary disease, or other breathing problems from dust, smoke, or toxic fumes › Angina › Hyperglycemia, hypertension
Quinary	Associated with exposure to hazardous materials from radioactive, biologic, or chemical components of a blast (e.g., dirty bomb)	Contamination of tissues from: › Bacteria › Radiation › Chemical agents › Contaminated tissue from bystander or assailant	Variety of health effects depending on the agent

Data from U.S. Department of Defense. (2019, June 18). What is blast injury? Blast Injury 101. https://blastinjuryresearch.amedd.army.mil/

Identifying the space in which an explosion happens can be helpful for the trauma care provider. When a blast occurs within an enclosed space, the release of energy is contained. If an individual is located within the confined space during an explosion, the resulting injuries may be increased because of the expanded pressure being transferred to the victim.[11,27,28] Suspect the possibility of internal hemorrhage and have a greater concern for fractures when there is evidence of penetrating injuries.[27,31] It is not uncommon for explosion victims to have a combination of injuries, including those involving multiple penetrating and blunt mechanisms.

Table 3-6 provides an overview of injuries commonly associated with explosions.[10]

> **CLINICAL PEARL**
>
> The explosion that occurs in an enclosed space has an increase in pressure relative to the explosion that occurs in an open environment. The increased pressure compounds the blast effects and potentially increases internal and external injury severity.

TABLE 3-6   Overview of Explosion-Related Injuries

System	Injury or Condition	System	Injury or Condition
Auditory	Cochlear damage Ossicular disruption Foreign body Tympanic membrane rupture	Circulatory	Blunt cardiac injury Myocardial infarction from air embolism Air embolism–induced injury Shock Vasovagal hypotension Peripheral vascular injury
Eye, orbit, face	Perforated globe Foreign body Fractures Air embolism	Central nervous system	Concussion Spinal cord injury Closed and open brain injury Air embolism–induced injury Stroke
Respiratory	Blast lung Hemothorax Pneumothorax Pulmonary contusion	Renal	Renal contusion Hypotension Laceration Hypovolemia Acute kidney injury due to rhabdomyolysis
Digestive	Bowel perforation Hemorrhage Mesenteric ischemia from air embolism Ruptured liver or spleen	Extremity	Traumatic amputation Lacerations Fractures Crush Acute arterial occlusion Compartment syndrome Air embolism–induced injury Burns

Data from Jorolemon, M. R., Lopez, R. A., & Krywko, D. M. (2022, May 2). Blast injuries. *StatPearls*. StatPearls Publishing. https://www.ncbi.nlm.nih.gov/books/NBK430914/

Emerging Trends

In an effort to decrease collision morbidity and mortality, several automotive safety features have been developed. As much as 94% of MVCs are associated with driver error.[20] Automotive safety initiatives such as automatic steering, parking, and antilock braking systems have been introduced, as well as driving sensors that detect objects located within blind spots, and speed limit and lane parameters.[2,20] The inclusion of side-impact air bags and decreased air bag deployment time have been implemented in an effort to reduce injuries to vehicle drivers and passengers.[17,20]

However, despite all the automotive advancements, the distracted driver remains an important factor with regard to occupant safety. Technology has improved our electronic devices, such as our smartphones and navigational systems. The U.S. Department of Transportation's National Highway Traffic Safety Administration (NHTSA) estimates that more than 4,000 deaths and approximately 276,000 injuries annually are due to distracted driving.[21] And while an estimated 96% of Americans think distracted driving is a threat, 60% report using devices while driving. Other forms of vehicular distraction include verbal conversation, eating while driving, applying makeup, and being lost in thought. The NHTSA is working toward decreasing the distraction associated with use of electronic devices while driving. Its initiatives include collaboration with the automotive industries to develop hands-free (e.g., Bluetooth) technology in vehicles, as well as laws and restrictions to reduce the use of these technologies while driving.[7,21]

The motorcycle industry has also experienced advancement in safety devices. One notable change involves improvements in motorcycle helmets. Modern helmets have replaced the older, softer materials such as leather; improved designs use several layers of foam covered in plastic or fiberglass to protect the head against impact. Despite the lack of global acceptance for requiring helmet use for all riders, helmet laws have been implemented in some jurisdictions.[6,18]

Despite improvements related to recreational equipment user safety, the recent proliferation of MRVs in the form of electric bicycles and motorized stand-up scooters has increased the incidence of blunt trauma in adults and children.[3,8] Electric bicycles and scooters tend to cause more severe injuries than their traditional counterparts.[4,12] The head, face, and upper extremities are the most likely to be affected.[3] Clearly these devices are an increasing public health concern, and injury prevention and regulations for safe use are needed.[3,4]

Summary

Trauma can be the result of a variety of forces, such as blunt, penetrating, thermal, or blast forces. Energy remains in a potential state until a force acts upon it, turning it into KE. Trauma care providers must remember the laws of energy because this will aid in anticipating a patient's physiological condition and needs.

The extent of injury can be affected by multiple factors, including the type and amount of force, the object and its distance traveled, and the point of impact and velocity. Cavitation can occur with both blunt and penetrating trauma; the resulting changes to the body depend on the characteristics of the tissue being impacted. With any significant injury, hemodynamic stability can be compromised. The materials that compose the exterior and interior of a projectile determine the extent of tissue damage on impact. Blast injuries also occur in patterns and can be the result of direct or indirect exposure to an explosion. Being in a confined space during an explosion can also increase the likelihood of severe injury.

Understanding the MOI and energy transfer can assist the prepared trauma provider in evaluating and anticipating damage. The ability to predict potential injury and provide early intervention with assessment improves patient survival rates.

As individual awareness and knowledge expand, safety improvements are also anticipated to advance. When an innovation for improved personal safety is developed, there is a human element to consider with its compliance usage: If the technology is present, will the individual utilize the safety knowledge and/or device as intended? A trauma care provider has the responsibility to provide required, up-to-date education and guidance on the importance of safety, usage of safety devices, and the consequences that may occur if these devices are not utilized.

References

1. Agarwal, H., & Kumar, A. (2019). Acceleration-deceleration injury. *Indian Journal of Surgery, 82*(1), 108–109. https://doi.org/10.1007/s12262-019-01942-z
2. Crash Test. (2018). *Crash test*. https://www.crashtest.org
3. Dhillon, N. K., Juillard, C., Barmparas, G., Lin, T., Kim, D. Y., Turay, D., Seibold, A. R., Kaminski, S., Duncan, D. Y., Diaz, G., Saad, S., Hanpeter, D., Benjamin, E. R., Tillou, A., Demetriades, D., Inaba, K., & Ley, E. J. (2020). Electric scooter injury in Southern California trauma centers. *Journal of the American College of Surgeons, 231*(1), 133–138. https://doi.org/10.1016/j.jamcollsurg.2020.02.047

4. DiMaggio, C. J., Bukur, M., Wall, S. P., Frangos, S. G., & Wen, A. Y. (2020). Injuries associated with electric-powered bikes and scooters: Analysis of U.S. consumer product data. *Injury Prevention, 26*, 524–528. https://doi.org/10.1136/injuryprev-2019-043418
5. Dowdell, J., Kim, J., Overley, S., & Hecht, A. (2018). Biomechanics and common mechanisms of injury of the cervical spine. *Handbook of Clinical Neurology, 158*, 337–344. https://doi.org/10.1016/B978-0-444-63954-7.00031-8
6. Government of Canada. (n.d.) *Motorcycle safety—The rider and the gear.* https://www2.gov.bc.ca/gov/content/transportation/driving-and-cycling/road-safety-rules-and-consequences/motorcycle-safety
7. Government of Canada. (2020). *Distracted driving from Transport Canada.* https://tc.canada.ca/en/road-transportation/stay-safe-when-driving/distracted-driving
8. Hermon, K., Capua, T., Glatstein, M., Scolnik, D., Tavor, O., & Rimon, A. (2018). Pediatric electrical bicycle injuries: The experience of a large urban tertiary care pediatric hospital. *Pediatric Emergency Care, 36*(6), e343–e345. https://europepmc.org/article/med/29324633
9. Igiebor, O. S., & Waseem, M. (2021, December 18). Aortic trauma. *StatPearls.* StatPearls Publishing. https://www.ncbi.nlm.nih.gov/books/NBK459337/
10. Jorolemon, M. R., & Lopez, R. A., & Krywko, D. M. (2022, May 2). *Blast injuries. StatPearls.* StatPearls Publishing. https://www.ncbi.nlm.nih.gov/books/NBK430914/
11. Klein, J. D., Weiglet, J., & Cipra, E. (2020). Mechanism of injury. In K. A. McQuillan & M. B. Flynn Makic (Eds.), *Trauma nursing: From resuscitation through rehabilitation* (5th ed., pp. 144–166). Elsevier.
12. Lee, K. C., Naik, K., Wu, B. W., Karlis, V., Chuang, S., & Eisig, S. B. (2020). Are motorized scooters associated with more severe craniomaxillofacial injuries? *Journal of Oral Maxillofacial Surgery, 78*, 1583–1589. https://doi.org/10.1016/j.joms.2020.04.035
13. Liu, R. W., & Hardesty, C. K. (2020). The multiply injured child. In G. A. Mencio & S. L. Frick (Eds.), *Green's skeletal trauma in children* (6th ed., pp 64–89). Elsevier.
14. Maitre, M., Chiaravalle, A., Horder, M., Chadwick, S., & Beavis, A. (2021). Evaluating the effect of barrel length on pellet distribution patterns of sawn-off shotguns. *Forensic Science International, 320*, Article 110685. https://doi.org/10.1016/j.forsciint.2021.110685
15. Merriam-Webster. (n.d.). Biomechanics. In *Merriam-Webster.com dictionary*. Retrieved January 22, 2022, from https://merriam-webster.com/dictionary/biomechanics
16. Merriam-Webster. (n.d.). Kinematics. In *Merriam-Webster.com dictionary*. Retrieved January 22, 2022, from https://merriam-webster.com/dictionary/kinematics
17. National Highway Traffic Safety Administration. (n.d.). *Air bags.* U.S. Department of Transportation. https://www.nhtsa.gov/equipment/air-bags
18. National Highway Traffic Safety Administration. (n.d.). *Motorcycle safety.* U.S. Department of Transportation. https://www.nhtsa.gov/road-safety/motorcycles
19. National Safety Council. (n.d.). *International.* https://injuryfacts.nsc.org/international/international-overview/
20. National Safety Council. (2019). *Injury facts.* https://injuryfacts.nsc.org
21. National Safety Council. (2020). *Free report: Understanding driver distraction.* https://www.nsc.org/road/safety-topics/distracted-driving/distracted-brain
22. Newton, I. (1995). *The Principia.* Prometheus Books.
23. Penn-Barwell, J. G., & Helliker, A. E. (2017). Firearms and bullets. In J. Breeze, J. G. Penn-Barwell, D. Keene, D. O'Reilly, J. Jeyanathan, & P. Mahoney (Eds.), *Ballistic trauma: A practical guide* (4th ed., pp. 7–20). Springer.
24. Penn-Barwell, J. G., & Stevenson, T. (2017). The effects of projectiles on tissues. In J. Breeze, J. G. Penn-Barwell, D. Keene, D. O'Reilly, J. Jeyanathan, & P. Mahoney (Eds.), *Ballistic trauma: A practical guide* (4th ed., pp. 35–46). Springer.
25. Petit, L., Zaki, T., Hsiang, W., Leslie, M., & Wiznia, D. (2020). A review of common motorcycle collision mechanisms of injury. *EFFORT Open Reviews, 5*(9), 544–548. https://doi.org/10.1302%2F2058-5241.5.190090
26. Sardiwalla, I., Govender, M., Matsevych, O., & Koto, M. Z. (2016). Indirect ballistic injury to the liver: Case report and review of literature. *International Journal of Surgery Open, 5*, 23–26. https://doi.org/10.1016/j.ijso.2016.09.006
27. Schmitt, K., Niederer, P. F., Cronin, D. S., Morrison, B., III, Muser, M. H., & Walz, F. (2019). *Trauma biomechanics: An introduction to injury biomechanics* (5th ed.). Springer. https://doi.org/10.1007/978-3-030-11659-0
28. Sims, C. A., & Reilly, P. M. (2020). Kinematics. In D. V. Feliciano, K. L. Mattox, & E. E. Moore (Eds.), *Trauma* (9th ed., pp. 3–14). McGraw Hill. https://accesssurgery.mhmedical.com/content.aspx?bookid=2952&sectionid=249116077
29. U.S. Department of Defense. (2019, June 18). *What is blast injury? Blast Injury 101.* https://blastinjuryresearch.amedd.army.mil/index.cfm/blast_injury_101
30. U.S. Energy Information Administration. (n.d.). *What is energy?* https://www.eia.gov/energyexplained/what-is-energy/forms-of-energy.php
31. Weinman, S. (2020). Blast incidents and their sequela. *Journal of Emergency Nursing, 46*(1), 129–133. https://doi.org/10.1016/j.jen.2019.10.013

CHAPTER 4

Initial Assessment

Kristen N. Kaiafas, DNP, MSN-Ed, CEN, CPEN

> **OBJECTIVES**
>
> Upon completion of this chapter, the learner will be able to:
> 1. Demonstrate the components of the initial assessment process.
> 2. Differentiate between the goals of the primary and secondary surveys.
> 3. Identify actual and potential threats to life and limb and the appropriate interventions using the initial assessment process.

Introduction

The approach to the care of a trauma patient requires a process to identify life-threatening injuries and treat or stabilize those injuries in a patient in an efficient and timely manner. Time is critical, so an approach that is systematic, yet easy to learn and implement, is most effective. This process is labeled *initial assessment*.

For clarity and ease of flow, the initial assessment is divided into the following process points[4]:

- Preparation and triage
- General impression
- Primary survey (ABCDE) with corresponding interventions as required (FG)
- Reevaluation (consideration of transfer/need for higher level of care)
- Secondary survey (HI) with corresponding interventions as required
- Reevaluation and post-resuscitation care (J)
- Definitive care or transfer to an appropriate trauma center

The **A–J** mnemonic delineates the components of the initial assessment (**Box 4-1**). This process helps the nurse rapidly assess for life-threatening injuries and intervene in a systematic manner, and it is the basis for the trauma nursing process (TNP). Each step will be discussed in depth throughout this chapter and throughout this manual.

> **NOTE**
>
> **Who Does the Initial Assessment?**
>
> We recognize that the initial assessment in many settings is more commonly conducted by physicians, advanced practice nurses, or a team of healthcare providers. However, it is important for all trauma nurses to be competent in performing the initial assessment so they can anticipate the next steps in care and function more efficiently as members of the trauma team. Additionally, the trauma nurse may not have access to other team members during transfer of the patient to other departments within the hospital or transport to another facility. When working in a remote location, it is important for the trauma nurse to conduct a baseline assessment to facilitate recognition of changes in patient status, if and when they occur.

BOX 4-1 Initial Assessment A–J Mnemonic

The initial assessment A–J mnemonic stands for the following:

- **A** = **A**lertness and **A**irway (with cervical spinal motion restriction as indicated)
- **B** = **B**reathing and ventilation
- **C** = **C**irculation and **C**ontrol of hemorrhage
- **D** = **D**isability (neurologic status)
- **E** = **E**xposure and **E**nvironmental control
- **F** = **F**ull set of vital signs and **F**amily presence
- **G** = **G**et adjuncts and **G**ive comfort using the mnemonic **LMNOP**
- **H** = **H**istory and **H**ead to toe
- **I** = **I**nspect posterior surfaces
- **J** = **J**ust keep reevaluating

Preparation and Triage

Initial assessment begins with preparation and triage.

Preparation

The approach to trauma care typically begins with notification that a trauma patient is or will soon be arriving in the emergency department (ED). Whether notification is from prehospital providers or the triage nurse, it is the trauma nurse's responsibility to prepare to receive that patient.

Safe Practice, Safe Care

When preparing to receive a trauma patient in the ED, keep the following tenet in mind: *Safe practice, safe care*.

Safe practice means taking into consideration the protection of the team, including the following:

- Observing universal precautions for every patient
- Donning personal protective equipment, such as gown, gloves, mask, and other equipment, as necessary, before the patient's arrival
- Maintaining situational awareness to mitigate potential violence against the patient or staff

Safe practice also includes consideration of any potential patient exposure to hazardous material that may put the trauma team, other patients, and the ED and hospital at risk. Some patients may require decontamination before entering the trauma resuscitation room. See Chapter 19, "Disaster Management," for additional information.

Safe care means ensuring that the patient gets to the *right* hospital in the *right* amount of time for the *right* care. The trauma triage criteria developed by the American College of Surgeons Committee on Trauma serve as the international standard for identifying the trauma patient who would benefit from resuscitation and care at *the right trauma facility* with appropriate resources. Educating prehospital providers on triage criteria guidelines for transport to a trauma center and access to air medical transport can mitigate delays in appropriate transport in rural areas.[28] Globally, research exploring trauma triage criteria for children has been limited.[28,31,58] There is also significant variation in activation criteria between rural and urban locations, as well as designated versus nondesignated pediatric trauma centers.[28,31,58] Often it is the trauma nurse or charge nurse who calls for trauma team activation as indicated. See Chapter 2, "Preparing for Trauma," for additional information.

The *right time* has long been referred to as the "golden hour." However, patients who present with certain serious injuries will not survive an hour for definitive treatment. Timely, effective, and efficient interventions facilitate improved outcomes for trauma patients.[4] Prehospital providers play a key role in the trauma patient's survival. Optimal outcomes result when time in the field is minimized, and care is focused on airway maintenance, control of hemorrhage, basic shock therapy, and spinal motion restriction (SMR) when necessary.[7,72] Field triage is key to the appropriate use of community resources, with the most severely injured patients being transported directly to the highest level of trauma care available in the community (**Figure 4-1**).[63,72]

RED CRITERIA
High Risk for Serious Injury

Injury Patterns

- Penetrating injuries to head, neck, torso, and proximal extremities
- Skull deformity, suspected skull fracture
- Suspected spinal injury with new motor or sensory loss
- Chest wall instability, deformity, or suspected flail chest
- Suspected pelvic fracture
- Suspected fracture of two or more proximal long bones
- Crushed, degloved, mangled, or pulseless extremity
- Amputation proximal to wrist or ankle
- Active bleeding requiring a tourniquet or wound packing with continuous pressure

Mental Status and Vital Signs

All Patients
- Unable to follow commands (motor GCS <6)
- RR <10 or >29 breaths/min
- Respiratory distress or need for respiratory support
- Room-air pulse oximetry <90%

Age 0–9 years
- SBP <70 mm Hg + (2 × age in years)

Age 10–64 years
- SBP <90 mm Hg or
- HR >SBP

Age 65 years
- SBP <110 mm Hg or
- HR >SBP

Patients meeting any one of the above RED criteria should be transported to the highest-level trauma center available within the geographic constraints of the regional trauma system

YELLOW CRITERIA
Moderate Risk for Serious Injury

Mechanism of Injury

- High-Risk Auto Crash
  – Partial or complete ejection
  – Significant intrusion (including roof)
    • >12 inches occupant site OR
    • >18 inches any site OR
    • Need for extrication for entrapped patient
  – Death in passenger compartment
  – Child (age 0–9 years) unrestrained or in unsecured child safety seat
  – Vehicle telemetry data consistent with severe injury
- Rider separated from transport vehicle with significant impact (e.g., motorcycle, ATV, horse, etc.)
- Pedestrian/bicycle rider thrown, run over, or with significant impact
- Fall from height >10 feet (all ages)

EMS Judgment

Consider risk factors, including:

- Low-level falls in young children (age ≤5 years) or older adults (age ≥65 years) with significant head impact
- Anticoagulant use
- Suspicion of child abuse
- Special, high-resource healthcare needs
- Pregnancy >20 weeks
- Burns in conjunction with trauma
- Children should be triaged preferentially to pediatric capable centers

If concerned, take to a trauma center

Patients meeting any one of the YELLOW CRITERIA WHO DO NOT MEET THE RED CRITERIA should be preferentially transported to a trauma center, as available within the geographic constraints of the regional trauma system (need not be the highest-level trauma center)

Figure 4-1 *2021 National Guideline for the Field Triage of Injured Patients.*

For the red criteria transport recommendations, patients in extremis (e.g., unstable airway, severe shock, traumatic arrest) may require transport to the closest hospital for initial stabilization, before transport to a Level I or II trauma center for definitive care. Pediatric patients meeting the red criteria should be preferentially triaged to pediatric-capable trauma centers. The EMS judgment criteria should be considered in the context of resources available in the regional trauma system, including consideration of online medical control for further direction. Examples of special, high-resource healthcare needs include patients with tracheostomy with ventilator dependence and cardiac assist devices, among others. If possible, patients with combined burns and trauma should be transported to a trauma center with burn care capability; if this is not available, a trauma center takes precedence over a burn center. Specific age used to define children is based on local system resources and practice patterns.

Reproduced from Newgard, C. D., Fischer, P. E., Gestring, M., Michaels, H. N., Jurkovich, G. J., Lerner, E. B., Fallat, M. E., Delbridge, T. R., Brown, J. B., Bulger, E. M., & the Writing Group for the 2021 National Expert Panel on Field Triage. (2022). National guideline for the field triage or injured patients: Recommendations of the National Expert Panel on Field Triage, 2021. *Journal of Trauma and Acute Care Surgery*, 93(2), e49-e60. https://doi.org/10.1097/TA.0000000000003627

The *right resources* to care for the trauma patient are outlined by the American College of Surgeons Committee on Trauma.[8] This process begins by activating the team and preparing the trauma room. The right resources include essential trauma team members with an appropriate skill mix, having the necessary equipment readily available, appropriate surgical care, skilled post-resuscitation care, and rehabilitation and support services.[4,7] Delays in patient transport to the *right* hospital with the *right* resources may result in less-than-optimal outcomes.[28,39]

Preparation in the Trauma Room

Information from the prehospital report can facilitate the initial assessment process and enable the trauma team to anticipate and prepare for interventions likely to be required to care for the patient.[4,72] The trauma nurse begins by preparing the room to ensure that resuscitation equipment is readily available and in working order. This is done on a regular basis as defined by ED policy—minimally, at the beginning of the shift and after each use of the trauma room. The prehospital report should be documented in a location that is visible for easy review by all trauma team members. Many prehospital providers use electronic templates for their patient care reports, and, as a result, they may no longer leave a hard copy behind. These "perishable data" must be captured verbally by the team to help guide the care given. Emergency medical services (EMS) may also offer digital photos of the scene that, whenever possible and in accordance with organizational policy, are incorporated into the medical record.

Triage

Triage involves the sorting of patients based on their need for treatment and the resources available to provide that treatment.[4] Triage also pertains to sorting patients in the field and is based on one or more of the following (Figure 4-1)[63]:

- Mechanism of injury (MOI)
- Mental status and vital signs with specific criteria for different age groups
- Injury patterns
- EMS judgment

The updated field triage guidelines integrate the prior field triage categories of anatomic and physiologic criteria into the new categories of injury patterns (anatomic), and mental status and vital signs (physiologic).[63] Patients meeting criteria as "high risk" should be transported to the highest level trauma center within the geographic location whenever possible.[6,63] Air medical transport should be considered, if available, to enable more rapid transport. Additionally, air transport teams often include advanced care providers, potentially allowing for a higher level of care during transport.[63]

Whether patients present via EMS or on their own, the priorities for the identification of life-threatening injuries are guided by the primary survey (ABCDE).

General Impression

The formation of the general impression begins immediately upon the patient's arrival and is completed as the patient is brought into the room. This evaluation enables a rapid determination of the patient's overall physiologic status and identification of any uncontrolled external hemorrhage. Obvious uncontrolled external hemorrhage or unresponsiveness/apnea necessitates immediate reprioritization and initiation of appropriate interventions. During the general impression and primary survey, the main goal is to immediately identify all life-threatening conditions within the first few minutes of arrival. These conditions *must* be treated upon discovery.[4] While the patient is safely transferred to a trauma stretcher, the team is given an update on the patient's condition from prehospital personnel or accompanying family or friends.

> **NOTE**
>
> **Uncontrolled Hemorrhage**
>
> Uncontrolled hemorrhage is a major cause of preventable death after injury.[4,30,48,50] If uncontrolled external hemorrhage is noted during the general impression or as the patient is being transferred to the trauma room stretcher, it may be appropriate to reprioritize C-ABC. The traditional approach to emergency care is ABC(D). Many national and international trauma centers have implemented the C-ABC approach, where C represents starting transfusion first when uncontrolled hemorrhage exists.[37] The current civilian approach to trauma resuscitation typically involves multiple trauma team members, enabling several priorities to be addressed simultaneously. The first priority remains *treating the condition posing the greatest threat to life first*.[4,36]

> **NOTE**
>
> **Assessment: Double-Starred Criteria**
>
> The double-starred criteria (**) must be completed in order before moving to the next step in the TNP. The double-starred criteria include the following:
>
> - Alertness (AVPU [alert, verbal, responds to pain, unresponsive])
> - Airway
> - Breathing and ventilation
> - Circulation and control of hemorrhage
> - Disability (neurologic status)
> - Exposure and environmental control

> **NOTE**
> **Primary Survey**
> If any component of the airway, breathing, or circulation is compromised or absent, the immediate treatment plan is to provide it for the patient—this is an important tenet of the primary survey. For example, for an airway obstructed by the tongue, insert an oropharyngeal airway; for absent or ineffective breathing, provide bag-mask ventilations; for absent circulation, provide chest compressions; and for ineffective circulation, identify and treat the cause. Support and maintenance of the primary survey components are crucial.

For teaching purposes, the steps in this chapter are presented sequentially, in linear order of priority. In reality, the trauma team will complete the components of assessment and interventions simultaneously as team members function together to accomplish these tasks. The trauma nurse integrates the appropriate examination elements of inspection, auscultation, and palpation for assessment.

Primary Survey

The steps in the primary survey follow steps A–E, beginning with assessing alertness and the airway.

A: Alertness and Airway (with Simultaneous Cervical Spine Stabilization)

The general impression includes assessing the patient's alertness and airway while also maintaining cervical SMR.

Cervical Spinal Motion Restriction

Cervical SMR is always a part of the alertness and airway assessment and is particularly important in the patient with a significant MOI or suspected spinal injury. Patients with distracting injuries (significant blood loss, open fractures) and those with altered mental status are presumed to have sustained a spinal cord injury (SCI) until proven otherwise.[6,7,56,81] The most recent recommendations[7] are for a noncontrast multidetector computed tomography (MDCT) scan to evaluate for spinal cord injury because of the low sensitivity associated with plain radiographs. See Chapter 10, "Spinal and Musculoskeletal Trauma," for additional information on cervical spine clearance and spinal injuries.

SMR can be accomplished by either of the following techniques:

- Manual stabilization: Two hands hold the patient's head and neck in alignment
- A correctly sized, semi-rigid cervical collar is securely fastened. Apply SMR to the entire spine until further clearance is obtained.[7]

The spine board is primarily a prehospital transportation device. Therefore, the patient is removed from the spine board as soon as possible; the team maintains cervical spine stabilization during spine board removal and continues SMR with the use of a semi-rigid cervical collar until cervical spine injury has been definitively ruled out.[7,36] After removing the spine board, using a slide board under the patient may be helpful to facilitate movement from the stretcher.

All SMR and transfer devices should be removed at the earliest appropriate time. Extreme care should be taken when removing a helmet from patients who have a potential cervical spine injury (CSI). Helmet removal requires a coordinated effort by two people: One person maintains manual inline stabilization of the patient's head and neck while the second person removes the helmet.[4,7,61,89]

During the entire initial assessment and identified required interventions, protection of the cervical spine is essential until a SCI is ruled out.

Assessment of Alertness

Assessment of alertness is a **double-starred criterion** in the TNP because this assessment helps in the evaluation of the patient's ability to protect their own airway.

The mnemonic **AVPU** can help the nurse quickly assess the patient's level of alertness. Its use at the beginning of the initial assessment can be an important aid to the nurse in selecting the appropriate airway intervention. The components of AVPU are as follows:

- **A:** Alert. If the patient is alert, they are more likely to be able to maintain their own airway. If the patient is alert and interactive, there is no need to proceed beyond this point. If the patient is not alert, go to the V component of the mnemonic.
- **V:** Responds to verbal stimuli. If the patient needs verbal stimulation to respond, an airway adjunct could be needed to keep the tongue from obstructing the airway. If the patient does not respond to voice, proceed to the P component.

- **P:** Responds to pain. If the patient responds only to pain, they may not be able to maintain their airway, and an airway adjunct may need to be placed while further assessment is made to determine the need for a definitive airway (intubation). If the patient does not respond to pain, proceed to the U component.
- **U:** Unresponsive. If the patient is unresponsive, announce it loudly to the team and direct someone to check whether the patient is pulseless while assessing whether the cause of the problem is the airway or something depressing respiratory function in the brain. Consider reprioritizing the assessment priority to C-ABC.[4,35]

> **NOTE**
>
> **AVPU: Assessing Alertness**
> - **A: A**lert and oriented
> - **V:** Responds to **V**erbal stimuli
> - **P:** Responds only to **P**ainful stimuli
> - **U: U**nresponsive

Assessment of Airway: Inspect, Auscultate, and Palpate

Assessment of the airway is a **double-starred criterion** in the TNP. If an airway issue is identified, appropriate interventions must be executed and reassessment of the airway completed before proceeding to the B component of the assessment.

- If the patient is alert or responds to verbal stimuli, ask the patient to open their mouth.
- If the patient is unable to open their mouth, responds only to pain, or is unresponsive, use the jaw-thrust maneuver to open the airway and assess for obstruction (actual or potential). In the patient with suspected CSI, the jaw-thrust procedure is recommended and is performed by two providers: One provides manual stabilization of the cervical spine, and the second performs the jaw-thrust procedure.[2]

Inspect for the following:

- Vocalization
- Tongue obstruction
- Loose or missing teeth
- Foreign objects
- Fluids (blood, vomit, or secretions)
- Edema
- Burns or evidence of inhalation injury

Auscultate or listen for the following:

- Adventitious airway sounds such as snoring, gurgling, or stridor, which may indicate obstruction

Palpate for the following:

- Maxillofacial bony deformity
- Subcutaneous emphysema[55]

Interventions

The information that follows represents the general approach for all trauma patients. Chapter 5, "Airway and Ventilation," provides additional information regarding specific airway devices and interventions.

If the airway is patent, efforts are aimed at supporting and maintaining a patent airway:

- If the patient is awake and has a patent airway, they may be allowed to assume a position that facilitates adequate air exchange unless contraindicated. Remember to maintain cervical spine stabilization if CSI is suspected.

If the airway is not patent, efforts must be undertaken to provide a patent airway. Use of appropriate interventions for airway obstruction and subsequent reevaluation of the airway is a **double-starred criterion** in the TNP.

- Suction the airway.
  - Use care to avoid stimulating the gag reflex.
  - If the airway is obstructed by blood, vomitus, or other secretions, use a rigid suction device to remove these obstructions.
  - If a foreign body is noted, carefully remove it with forceps or by another appropriate method.
- The patient's tongue may be the cause of the obstruction. Consider an airway adjunct, which may be required to alleviate obstruction by the tongue. See Chapter 5, "Airway and Ventilation," for additional information.
  - The jaw-thrust maneuver can be used to open the airway while maintaining SMR.
  - A nasopharyngeal airway can be used in patients who are conscious or unconscious. They are used only in patients with no evidence of midface fractures. See Chapter 5, "Airway and Ventilation," for additional information.
  - An oropharyngeal airway can only be used in patients without a gag reflex. See Chapter 5, "Airway and Ventilation," for additional information.
- Anticipate use of a definitive airway (endotracheal intubation).

B: Breathing and Ventilation

Assessment of breathing and ventilation is a **double-starred criterion** in the TNP.

Assessment

If an issue with breathing/ventilation is identified, provide the appropriate intervention, and reassess breathing/ventilation before proceeding to the C component of the primary survey. To assess breathing, expose the patient's chest and complete the assessment procedures outlined in the rest of this section.

Inspect for the following:

- Spontaneous breathing
- Symmetrical rise and fall of the chest
- Depth, pattern, and general rate of respirations
- Increased work of breathing, such as the use of accessory muscles, diaphragmatic breathing, or pursed lip breathing
- Skin color (normal, pale, flushed, dusky, cyanotic)
- Contusions, abrasions, or deformities that may be a sign of underlying injury
- Open pneumothorax (sucking chest wound)
- Jugular venous distention and the position of the trachea (tracheal deviation and jugular venous distention are late signs that may indicate a tension pneumothorax)
- Signs of inhalation injury (singed nasal hairs, carbonaceous sputum)

Auscultate for the following:

- Presence, quality, and equality of breath sounds bilaterally at the second intercostal space midclavicular line and the bases at the fifth intercostal space at the anterior axillary line

Palpate for the following:

- Integrity of or injury to the bony structures and ribs (which may affect ventilation)
- Subcutaneous emphysema, which may be a sign of a pneumothorax
- Soft-tissue injury
- Jugular venous pulsations at the suprasternal notch or in the supraclavicular area[83,85]

If the patient has a definitive airway in place, assess for proper placement of the airway device before moving to the next step of the primary survey. Assessment for proper placement of a definitive airway includes the following three steps:

1. Attachment of a CO_2 detector device; after 5 or 6 breaths, assessment for presence of exhaled CO_2
2. Observation of adequate rise and fall of the chest with assisted ventilation
3. Auscultation for absence of gurgling over the epigastrium and presence of bilateral breath sounds

Intervention

See Chapter 5, "Airway and Ventilation," for additional information. If breathing is absent, initiate the following interventions:

- After opening the airway using the jaw-thrust maneuver (while maintaining SMR), insert an airway adjunct (oropharyngeal airway or nasopharyngeal airway as indicated)
  - If the patient remains apneic, assist ventilations with a bag-mask device.
  - Prepare for a definitive airway and continue breathing support with mechanical ventilation.

If breathing is present, anticipate the need to support and maintain it:

- Administer supplemental oxygen.[2]
  - Inability to maintain adequate oxygenation causes hypoxemia, resulting in anaerobic metabolism and acidosis.
  - Trauma patients need early supplemental oxygen. However, evidence suggests that providers should closely monitor and titrate oxygen delivery for stabilized trauma patients to avoid the detrimental physiologic effects of hyperoxia, especially in patients with significant traumatic brain injury.[32,51] See Chapter 5, "Airway and Ventilation," for additional information.
- Determine whether ventilation is effective.
  - An $ETCO_2$ measurement of 35–45 mm Hg (4.7–6.0 kPa), in addition to clinical assessment, shows effective ventilation.[2,17,20,41,79] A level greater than 50 mm Hg (6.7 kPa) signifies depressed ventilation.[17]
  - Oxygen saturation (SpO_2) in a target range of 94–98% is associated with effective, adequate oxygenation.[51]

If ventilation is ineffective, initiate the following:

- Assist ventilation with a bag-mask device connected to an oxygen source at 10–15 L/minute, and administer one breath every 6 seconds (10 breaths per minute).[9]
- Determine the need for a definitive airway. It is possible that the patient may have an adequate airway but be unable to effectively ventilate. In this case, the patient will require a definitive airway to facilitate and assist ventilations.

Definitive Airway

A definitive airway is a tube securely placed in the trachea with the cuff inflated.[2]

- Cuffed tubes are now recommended for use in all patients, including children younger than 8 years.[10] See Chapter 13, "The Pediatric Trauma Patient," for more information.
- The following conditions or situations require a definitively secured airway[2]:
  - Apnea
  - Glasgow Coma Scale (GCS) score of 8 or less
  - Severe maxillofacial fractures
  - Evidence of inhalation injury (facial burns, singed nasal or facial hairs, or a hoarse voice associated with possible pulmonary burn injury and a history of exposure to smoke or products of combustion)
  - Laryngeal or tracheal injury, or neck hematoma
  - High risk of aspiration and the patient's inability to protect the airway
  - Compromised or ineffective ventilation
  - Anticipation of deterioration of neurologic status that may result in an inability to maintain or protect the airway

Difficult Airways

Injury or anatomic variations may make it difficult to successfully intubate the patient. In these cases, continue to ventilate the patient with a bag-mask device connected to oxygen at 10–15 L/minute until an alternative airway can be established. See Chapter 5, "Airway and Ventilation," for additional information.

Life-threatening pulmonary injuries require rapid identification and immediate intervention before proceeding to the next step in the primary survey.[4,83] See Chapter 8, "Thoracic and Neck Trauma," for additional information. Examples of these injuries include the following:

- Open pneumothorax
- Tension pneumothorax
- Flail chest
- Hemothorax

C: Circulation and Control of Hemorrhage

Assessment of circulation and control of hemorrhage is a **double-starred criterion** in the TNP. If an issue with circulation or hemorrhage is identified, appropriate interventions must be executed and reassessment of circulation and hemorrhage control completed before proceeding to component D.

Assessment

The major assessment parameters that produce important information regarding the patient's circulatory status within seconds of a patient's arrival are level of consciousness, skin color, and pulse.[4,72] The assessment of circulation during the primary survey includes early consideration of the possibility of hemorrhage in the abdomen and pelvis in any patient who has sustained blunt trauma, including hemodynamically stable patients.[5,27] An emergent abdominal or pelvic assessment may be performed, including a focused assessment with sonography for trauma (FAST) examination or a radiograph of the pelvis.[5,27,42]

Inspect for the following:

- Uncontrolled external bleeding
- Pale skin color (assess the tongue, lips, gums, soles of feet, and palms in patients with dark-pigmented skin)[66,72]
- Pallor in persons with darker skin tones may appear yellow-brown or ashen gray[66]
- Obvious external hemorrhage

Auscultate for the following:

- Muffled heart sounds, which may suggest pericardial tamponade[5,23]

Palpate for the following:

- Presence of carotid and/or femoral (central) pulses for rate, rhythm, and strength (bounding or weak)
  - Pulses that are strong, regular, and at a normal rate may indicate normovolemia.
  - A rapid, thready pulse may indicate hypovolemia, and an irregular pulse may warn of potential cardiac dysfunction.[5]
- Skin temperature and moisture (cool and diaphoretic or warm and dry)

If pulses are absent, be prepared to immediately provide interventions to generate pulses:

- Initiate life-supporting measures following the guidelines developed by the American Heart Association for basic life support.[9]
- If the patient is pulseless, without pausing in the primary survey, another team member may attach the patient to a cardiac monitor to assess for pulseless electrical activity. Consider and assess for the following as possible causes of pulseless electrical activity:
  - A penetrating wound to the heart
  - Pericardial tamponade
  - Rupture of great vessels
  - Intra-abdominal hemorrhage
- Assess for signs of uncontrolled internal bleeding.

Common sites for internal hemorrhage in the traumatically injured patient are the chest, abdomen, pelvis, and long bones. Significant external bleeding can occur with large wounds and amputations. Assessment of the chest, abdomen, and pelvis may be indicated at this time to determine the site of the hemorrhage.[5,42,72]

If pulses are present, but circulation is ineffective, do the following:

- Immediately assess for signs of uncontrolled internal bleeding.
- If the patient has ineffective circulation, consider common sites for hemorrhage, such as the chest, abdomen, and pelvis.[5]
    - Administer blood or blood products as ordered.
- Use a rapid infusion device per facility protocol.
- Consider the possibility of other types of shock.

Interventions

Control and treat uncontrolled external bleeding by doing the following:

- Apply direct pressure over the site.
- Elevate a bleeding extremity.
- Apply pressure over arterial sites.
- Consider a pelvic binder if an unstable pelvic fracture is suspected.[1,45] Prompt application of a pelvic binder in suspected pelvic injury has been shown to lead to shorter hospital and intensive care unit stays.[45]
- Consider the use of a tourniquet (see Chapter 6, "Shock," and Chapter 10, "Spinal and Musculoskeletal Trauma," for additional information).
- If the patient has signs of bleeding, another team member may obtain a blood pressure for baseline and trending to avoid a pause in the primary survey.

Cannulate two veins with large-caliber intravenous catheters[4,72]:

- If unable to gain venous access quickly, consider intraosseous or central venous access, depending on available resources.[5,72]
- Draw labs and obtain a blood sample for type and crossmatch.
- Initiate appropriate goal-directed therapy for the type of shock known or suspected.
- Use blood administration tubing and 0.9% sodium chloride or similar solution to facilitate blood administration, if needed.
- Consider balanced resuscitation needs. See Chapter 6, "Shock," for additional information.
- Administer blood or blood products as ordered.
- Use a rapid infusion device per facility protocol.
- Intervene in life-threatening situations:
    - Prepare and assist with emergency thoracotomy as indicated.
    - Prepare and assist with pericardial needle aspiration to relieve cardiac tamponade as indicated.
- Be prepared to expedite patient transfer to the operating suite.

Damage Control Resuscitation

Damage control resuscitation (DCR) is a process that focuses on the rapid restoration of homeostasis through the control of hemorrhage, administration of blood, and other interventions directed toward the prevention of the trauma triad of death.[21] DCR involves two strategies: hypotensive resuscitation and hemostatic resuscitation. The administration of large volumes of crystalloid solution is associated with increased bleeding and rebleeding ("popping the clot") and decreased survival rates, often as a result of hemodilution and decreased clotting factors.[5] Balanced fluid resuscitation is an approach to resuscitation that addresses all components that are lost with hemorrhage, including fluid, packed red blood cells, fresh frozen plasma, and platelets.[5,21] See Chapter 6, "Shock," for additional information on DCR, hypotensive resuscitation, hemostatic resuscitation, fluid resuscitation, and massive transfusion protocol.

D: Disability (Neurologic Status)

Assessment of disability (neurologic status) using the GCS is a **double-starred criterion** in the TNP. If an issue with the neurologic status is identified, planning for appropriate diagnostic tests and interventions should be considered at this time.

Assessment

The GCS offers a standardized method for evaluating level of consciousness. It also serves as a communication tool for members of the trauma team to convey objective information. Scores range from 3 (indicating deep unconsciousness) to 15 (indicating a patient who is alert, converses normally, and is able to obey commands).[43,67,73,74] The GCS does have limitations: It does not provide for an accurate assessment of the verbal score in intubated or aphasic patients, it is subject to interrater variability, and the complexity of use is somewhat high.[43,67,73] However, the GCS continues to be the clinical standard against which newer scales are compared and is used widely by emergency and trauma teams, medical and surgical intensive care units, and prehospital providers.[43,67,73]

Assess the GCS score upon patient arrival and repeat as necessary and according to policy. Trend analysis of GCS findings is important for detection of deteriorating or improving neurologic function. See Chapter 7, "Head Trauma," for additional information.

Assess pupils for equality, roundness, and reactivity to light (PERRL). Pupillary changes may be an indicator of increasing intracranial pressure.[4,72]

Interventions

Interventions for disability include the following:

- Anticipate the need for a computed tomography scan of the head. Consider any changes in level of consciousness to be the result of CNS injury until proven otherwise.[4,67] See Chapter 7, "Head Trauma," for additional information.
- Consider measurement of arterial blood gases (ABGs). A decreased level of consciousness may be an indicator of decreased cerebral perfusion, hypoxia, hypoventilation, or acid–base imbalance.
- Consider bedside glucose, alcohol level, and/or toxicology screening. Hypoglycemia, along with other conditions, such as the presence of alcohol, may play a role in the patient's neurologic status and need to be excluded as the primary cause.
- Unless contraindicated, consider elevation of the head of the bed greater than 30 degrees to facilitate venous return for any indication of possible increased intracranial pressure.[22] See Chapter 7, "Head Trauma," for additional information.

E: Exposure and Environmental Control

Patient exposure and environmental control is a **double-starred criterion** in the TNP. If an issue is identified, it must be addressed. Appropriate methods of temperature control must be implemented before proceeding to component F.

Assessment

Assess the patient as follows:

- Carefully and completely undress the patient to facilitate a thorough assessment. Cutting clothing using trauma shears is often the most effective way to remove garments while avoiding manipulation of the patient. Caution is advised to avoid self-injury from something on the patient or in the clothing.
- Inspect for any uncontrolled bleeding and do a quick visual scan of the visible body surfaces for any obvious injuries.

Interventions

Interventions include the following:

- If clothing may be used as evidence, preserve it according to institutional policy.[34] Cut around areas of suspected evidence, place clothing in a paper bag, and label appropriately. Maintain the chain of evidence with law enforcement as indicated.[4,34] Care of the patient always supersedes evidence collection. See Chapter 17, "Interpersonal Violence," for more information.
- If a transport device is in place, it may be removed as soon as possible.
- If there are no contraindications, the patient may be turned to quickly assess the posterior. This is deferred until after the head-to-toe assessment and imaging if needed to evaluate spinal and pelvic stability.
- Maintain body temperature as follows:
  - Cover the patient with warm blankets.
  - Keep the ambient temperature warm.
  - Administer warmed IV fluids.
  - Use forced-air warmers.
  - Use radiant warming lights.

Hypothermia, coagulopathy, and acidosis are a potentially lethal combination in the injured patient.[18,86] See Chapter 6, "Shock," for additional information.

The E assessment parameter is intentionally placed in the primary survey to ensure that aggressive measures are taken to prevent the loss of body heat and subsequent hypothermia in the trauma patient.

F: Full Set of Vital Signs and Family Presence

Vital signs and the presence of family are both essential components of the assessment of any trauma patient.

Full Set of Vital Signs

To monitor the effectiveness of the resuscitation, obtain and trend vital signs at regular intervals, including blood pressure, pulse, respirations, temperature, and SpO_2.

Family Presence

Facilitate family presence as soon as a member of the trauma team is available to act as liaison to the family. If a social worker, psychiatric nurse, or hospital chaplain is a member of the team, that person may fill this role. Honesty, sensitivity, and a trauma-informed approach are important when interacting with the patient's family and friends because this can be a stressful time. Consider factors such as the patient's age, ethnicity, cultural background, and religion when interacting with the family.

Evidence shows that patients prefer family members to be present during resuscitation.[11,26,78] In addition, strong evidence indicates that family members wish to be offered the option of being present during invasive procedures and resuscitation of a family member.[11,26,78] The Emergency Nurses Association, along with several other professional organizations, supports the option of family presence during resuscitation.

While some providers may have concerns regarding family presence during resuscitation and invasive procedures, family members should not be viewed as a problem or complication, but rather as an extension of the patient.[11,26,78] Being present at the time of a person's death is viewed in many cultures as a privilege, and trauma teams are encouraged to share this privilege with the patient's family in accordance with the patient's and family's wishes and with the facility's policies and procedures.[11,26,78]

G: Get Adjuncts and Give Comfort

Consider the mnemonic **LMNOP** to remember these resuscitation monitoring devices and supports:

- **L**: Obtain **L**aboratory studies, including ABGs or, in some cases, venous blood gases, and obtain a specimen for blood type and crossmatch.
  - Lactic acid is an excellent reflection of tissue perfusion and an endpoint measure of resuscitation effectiveness.[57,77]
  - High levels of lactic acid are associated with hypoperfusion.[57,77]
  - A lactic acid level greater than 2–4 mmol/L is associated with poor outcomes.[57,77]
  - ABGs provide values of oxygen, CO_2, and base excess, which can also be reflective of endpoint measurements of the effectiveness of cellular perfusion, adequacy of ventilation, and the success of the resuscitation.[16] Consider adding a carboxyhemoglobin to the ABGs in patients who have suffered burn trauma.
  - An abnormal base deficit may indicate poor perfusion and tissue hypoxia, which results in the generation of hydrogen ions and metabolic acidosis.
  - A base deficit equal to, or more negative than, −12 is associated with poor outcomes.[47]
  - Conduct a urine or serum pregnancy test for any female capable of pregnancy.
- **M**: **M**onitor cardiac rate and rhythm. Compare the patient's pulse to the monitor rhythm.
  - Dysrhythmias—such as premature ventricular contractions, atrial fibrillation, or ST segment changes—may indicate blunt cardiac trauma.[4,29,72]
  - Pulseless electrical activity may point to cardiac tamponade, tension pneumothorax, or profound hypovolemia.[4,29]
- **N**: **N**asogastric or orogastric tube consideration. The insertion of a gastric tube provides for evacuation of stomach contents and the relief of gastric distention. This intervention may help to optimize inflation of the lungs and prevent vomiting and/or aspiration. If midface fractures or head injury is suspected, the oral route is preferred.[2] Maintain cervical SMR and ensure that suction equipment is readily available. In the intubated patient, this is considered routine care to minimize aspiration risk.
- **O**: **O**xygenation and ventilation assessment.
  - Consider weaning oxygen based on pulse oximetry to prevent hyperoxia. Attach the patient to capnography if they are intubated or sedated.
  - Pulse oximetry detects changes in oxygenation that cannot be readily observed clinically. This noninvasive intervention measures the SpO_2 of arterial blood or percentage of bound hemoglobin. Accurate readings rely on adequate peripheral perfusion. Oximetry offers a measurement of SpO_2, but it does not provide evidence of ventilation. Additionally, oximetry readings do not differentiate between O_2 and O_1 (monoxide, which may be present in patients who have been exposed to products of combustion). Carbon monoxide tightly binds to the hemoglobin molecule and is not available for use by the cells. Patients with high levels of carboxyhemoglobin can have SpO_2 readings of 100% but still be experiencing cellular hypoxia.[65]
  - $ETCO_2$ monitoring (or capnography) provides instantaneous information about the ventilation, perfusion, and metabolism of carbon dioxide. Normal values are 35–45 mm Hg (4.7–6.0 kPa).[2,17,20,41,79]
    - Capnography should be monitored on all patients and is vital for sedated or ventilated patients.[2]
- **P**: **P**ain assessment and management. This is a **single-starred criterion** in the TNP.
  - The assessment and management of severe pain is an important part of the treatment of trauma patients; the goal is to give comfort to the patient while avoiding respiratory depression. Additionally, pain and anxiety cause the release

of epinephrine and norepinephrine, which, in turn, increases myocardial oxygen demand. It is therefore essential to treat or control both pain and anxiety as much as possible, with the aim of decreasing or controlling this increased demand.[4,44,59,71]

- Use of both pharmacologic and nonpharmacologic pain management techniques is essential in the control of pain in the trauma patient.[44,59,71,84] Injuries sustained by the trauma patient may be life-changing for both the patient and family, so it is essential that the trauma team also provide appropriate spiritual and psychosocial support.

Reevaluation

Reevaluation begins with portable radiographs.

Portable Radiograph

A portable anterior–posterior chest radiograph and pelvis radiograph can be obtained at this phase of the resuscitation, if not done previously as part of the primary survey and resuscitation. These studies are performed in the resuscitation area and may help identify or confirm suspected and potentially life-threatening injuries, such as a pneumothorax or pelvic fracture with uncontrolled internal hemorrhage. Radiographs can also be used as part of confirming placement of endotracheal tubes, chest tubes, and gastric tubes. The pelvic radiograph may be withheld if the patient's pelvis is stable on exam and if the patient is moving expeditiously to the radiology department for more definitive abdomen and pelvis imaging (CT scans).

Consider the Need for Patient Transfer

The trauma team leader gathers essential information during the primary survey and resuscitation phase that may indicate the need to transfer the patient to another facility.[4] This consideration requires a deliberate pause and moment of decision. If the patient's injuries are out of scope or beyond the capabilities of the current facility and require a higher level of care, now is the time to mobilize the transfer resources. This may be accomplished by other team members while the secondary survey is being completed. All life-threatening injuries are identified, addressed, and stabilized to the extent possible by the current facility before transferring the patient. The team leader will delegate the initial steps to begin immediate transfer and continue with ongoing evaluation and resuscitation. Follow institutional guidelines for contacting the appropriate facility that has the capability to provide care for the severely injured. See Chapter 20, "Transition of Care for the Trauma Patient," for additional information.

If the patient is not being transferred out, this is an opportune time to notify any additional services and support staff (i.e., consult services, resource nurses) who will be needed to assist in managing the patient.

Secondary Survey

After the primary survey (ABCDE) has been completed, resuscitative efforts have been initiated, vital functions have been stabilized, and additional monitoring/interventions have been considered (F and G), the secondary survey (H and I) begins.

H–J Steps in the Secondary Survey

The secondary survey begins with history taking.

H: History

The patient's condition is greatly influenced by the MOI. Certain injuries and their severity can be predicted based on the MOI.[4] See Chapter 3, "Biomechanics and Mechanisms of Injury," for more information. Additional history includes the following:

- Prehospital report: Any additional information available from prehospital providers.
- Patient history (medical records/documents): If the patient's family is present, solicit input regarding the traumatic event and the health history. If the patient is responsive, eliciting answers may assist the trauma nurse in evaluating the patient's level of consciousness and help to identify areas of pain and injury.
- The **SAMPLE** mnemonic highlights important aspects of patient history:
  - **S: S**ymptoms associated with the illness or injury
  - **A: A**llergies
  - **M: M**edications currently used, including anticoagulant therapy
  - **P: P**ast medical history (include hospitalizations and/or surgeries)
  - **L: L**ast oral intake/**L**ast output (**L**ast menstrual period if female of childbearing age)
  - **E: E**vents and **E**nvironmental factors related to the illness or injury
- When caring for patients with limited language proficiency, a qualified interpreter is necessary to ensure effective communication and equitable access to healthcare services.[15]

- When caring for a LGBTQ+ individual, ensure pertinent data collection through the health history and appropriate differential diagnostics recommended. See Chapter 12, "The LGBTQ+ Trauma Patient," for additional information.

Comorbid factors are preexisting conditions that place the patient at greater risk for complications related to the injury. These are important to note and will influence care going forward, but they do not preempt definitive care. They include the following factors[4,42,46,70,87,88]:

- Age: Risk for injury or death increases after age 55, and children require specialized pediatric care.
- Burns: Patients with burns may require early transfer to a burn facility.
- Pregnancy: Pregnant females of any gestational age warrant an early obstetric consult.
- Disabilities: Significant physical and/or mental/emotional disabilities should be noted.

H: Head-to-Toe Assessment

During this phase, a complete head-to-toe examination is performed and documented. This information is obtained primarily from inspection, auscultation, and palpation.

> **NOTE**
>
> **LACE: Soft-Tissue Injuries**
>
> Inspect for the following:
> - **L: L**acerations
> - **A: A**brasions, **A**vulsions
> - **C: C**ontusions
> - **E: E**dema, **E**cchymosis

In a noisy trauma room, percussion is difficult to perform and has been replaced in some cases by the use of FAST examinations.[4,27,42] Systematically move from the patient's head to the lower extremities and posterior surface, following the process outlined in this section to identify all injuries.

General Appearance

Note the position and posture of the patient or the presence of any spontaneous guarding. Observe for stiffness, rigidity, or flaccidity of extremities. Document specific odors, such as alcohol, gasoline, or other chemicals. Specific presentations may alert the trauma team to injuries (e.g., shortening and external rotation of a leg might suggest a hip fracture).

Head and Face

Assessment of the head and face includes the following:

- Soft-tissue injuries
  - Inspect for the following:
    - Lacerations, abrasions, avulsions, contusions, edema, or ecchymosis (LACE)
    - Puncture wounds or impaled objects
  - Palpate for the following:
    - Areas of tenderness, and crepitus
- Bony deformities
  - Inspect for the following:
    - Asymmetry of facial expression
    - Any exposed tissue or bone that may suggest disruption of the central nervous system (brain matter)
  - Palpate for the following:
    - Depressions, step-offs, angulations, areas of tenderness

Eyes

Assessment of the eyes includes the following:

- Determine gross visual acuity by holding up fingers and asking the patient to identify how many are being held up. Do this for each eye independently, and both eyes together. Remember, diplopia is a significant finding that can indicate entrapment of cranial nerves III, IV, and VI (oculomotor, trochlear, and abducens nerves, respectively).[3,54]
- Determine whether the patient uses prescription eyeglasses or contact lenses. Contact lenses should be removed before edema develops and to decrease the risk of corneal abrasions (**Figure 4-2** and **Figure 4-3**).

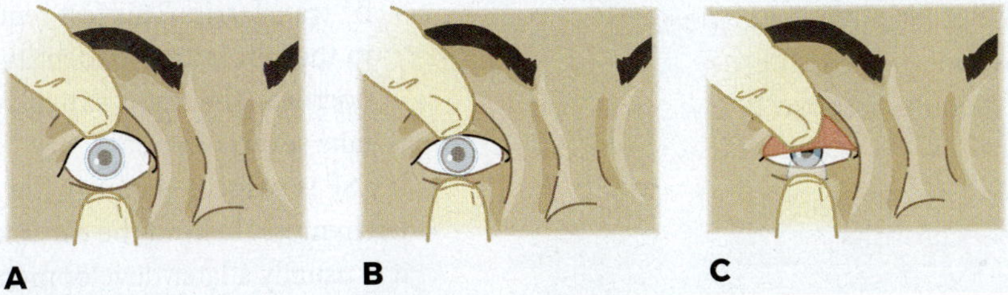

Figure 4-2 *Removal of hard contact lens.*

52   Chapter 4   Initial Assessment

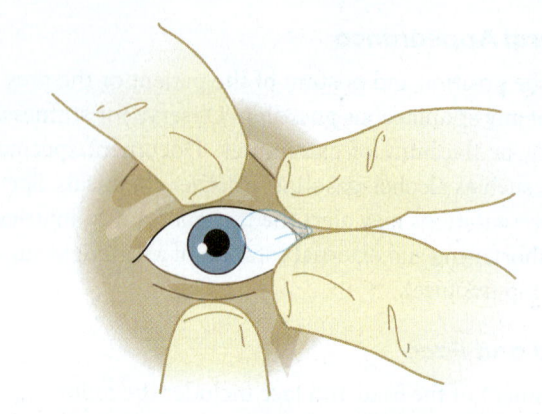

Figure 4-3 *Removal of soft contact lens.*

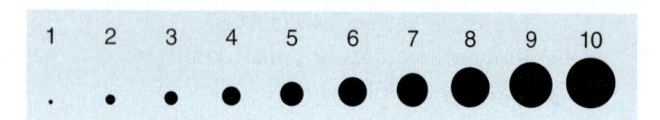

Figure 4-4 *Pupil size.*

- Inspect for the following:
  - Pupil size, equality, shape, and reactivity to light (**Figure 4-4**).
  - Muscle function: Ask the patient to follow a moving finger or penlight in the six cardinal positions (**Figure 4-5**). Assess eye movement by having the patient follow a finger as it is moved in the shape of an "H"; this is important in assessing for

> **NOTE**
>
> ### Eye Emergency Examples
>
> Specific eye emergencies, while not usually life-threatening, can be significantly life-altering. Although the initial assessment is not interrupted to immediately address these conditions, they are noted and addressed as soon as the patient is hemodynamically stable. Examples of eye emergencies include the following:
>
> - Lid lacerations (consider repair by an ophthalmologist or oculoplastic surgeon)
> - Corneal laceration
> - Corneal or intraocular foreign body
> - Orbital fracture
> - Hyphema
> - Retrobulbar hematoma
> - Globe rupture
> - Ocular burns and ultraviolet keratitis

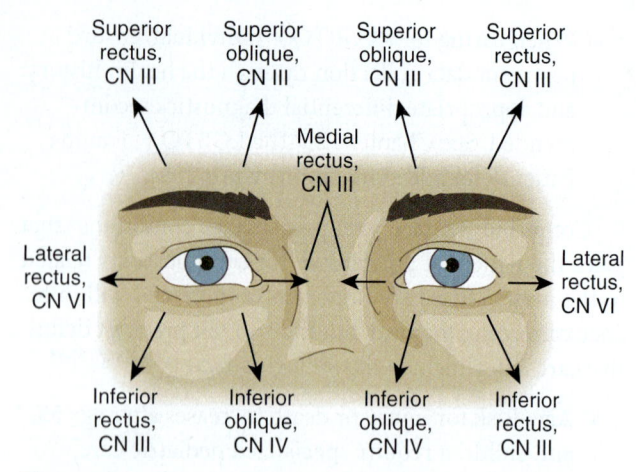

Figure 4-5 *Extraocular eye movements.*

  possible orbital fractures and entrapment of cranial nerves responsible for eye movement.
  - The presence of foreign bodies as identified by visualization or patient complaint of pain or sensation of something in the eye.

Ears

Inspect for the following:

- Look for unusual drainage, such as blood or clear fluid from the external ear. Cerebrospinal fluid (CSF) drainage from the nose or ear is due to a tear in the dura.[38] Do not pack the ear because a CSF leak may be present, and packing could increase the intracranial pressure. To test otorrhea for CSF, consider the following:
  - Two tests have historically been performed rapidly to suggest a general suspicion of CSF leak.[19,25] These two tests are neither specific nor sensitive for the detection of CSF leaks[64]:
    - Halo sign: Place the fluid on tissue or filter paper. A ring, or "halo," of clear or pink-tinged fluid will form around the area of red blood—this constitutes a positive halo sign. The test does not differentiate between CSF and other clear fluids such as saline, saliva, and water; it is considered unreliable.[19,25]
    - Test for glucose: CSF is high in glucose, and usually nasal mucus does not contain glucose.
  - β^2-transferrin: This test requires fluid to be sent to the laboratory to identify CSF otorrhea or rhinorrhea. The test is expensive, and analysis can take several days.[60,68]
- If CSF is suspected, notify the physician.
- Ecchymosis behind the ear is known as Battle sign; it is usually a later development.
- Ear avulsions or lacerations: Repairs often require the expertise of a plastic surgeon.

Nose

Inspect for the following:

- Look for unusual drainage, such as blood or clear fluid. CSF drainage from the nose or ear is due to a tear in the dura.[38] Do not pack the nose to stop clear fluid drainage because it may be CSF, and packing could increase intracranial pressure. To test rhinorrhea for CSF, refer to the information in the Ears section.
- If CSF is suspected, notify the physician, and do not insert a nasogastric tube.
- Note the position of the nasal septum.

Neck and Cervical Spine

Assume that patients with maxillofacial or head trauma have a CSI (fracture and/or ligament injury). Restrict motion of the cervical spine until adequate studies have been completed and an injury has been excluded. The absence of neurologic deficit does not exclude CSI.[24,46,56,70] See Chapter 10, "Spinal and Musculoskeletal Trauma," for more information.

Inspect for the following:

- LACE, plus signs of penetrating trauma, including presence of impaled objects or any open wounds
- The position of the trachea and the appearance of the jugular veins

Gently palpate for the following:

- Neck pain, tenderness, crepitus, subcutaneous emphysema, or step-off deformities between vertebrae
- Have a second person maintain manual SMR of the cervical spine while the collar is opened for palpation.[6] Close the collar after assessment and confirm its proper placement.
- Frequently remind the patient to remain still during palpation and examination, to verbalize areas that are painful to examination, and to avoid shaking the head or nodding.

Chest

Inspect for the following:

- Presence of spontaneous breathing; respiratory rate, respiratory depth, and degree of effort required; use of accessory or abdominal muscles; and any paradoxical chest movement
- Anterior and lateral chest walls—including the axillae—for LACE, puncture wounds, impaled objects, and scars that may indicate previous chest surgery
- Expansion and excursion of the chest during ventilation
- Facial expressions or reactions that indicate the presence of pain with inspiration and/or expiration

Auscultate for the following:

- Breath sounds, noting the presence of any adventitious sounds, such as wheezes or crackles, and equality
- Heart sounds, for the presence of murmurs, friction rubs, or muffled heart tones

Palpate for the following:

- Presence of subcutaneous emphysema
- Bony crepitus or deformities (step-offs or areas of tenderness) to the clavicles, sternum, and *all* ribs

Abdomen/Flanks

Inspect for the following:

- LACE, puncture wounds, impaled objects, and scars that may indicate previous abdominal surgery
- Evisceration
- Distention

Auscultate for the following:

- Presence or absence of bowel sounds

Palpate for the following:

- Begin light palpation in an area where the patient has not complained of pain or where there is no obvious injury.
- Note any rigidity, guarding, masses, or areas of tenderness in all four abdominal quadrants.

Pelvis/Perineum

Inspect for the following:

- LACE, puncture wounds, impaled objects, and scars that may indicate previous surgery
- Bony deformities or exposed bone
- Blood at the urethral meatus (more common in male patients because of the extraperitoneal position of the urethra), vagina, and rectum
- Priapism
- Pain and/or the urge to void but inability to do so (may indicate bladder rupture)
- Scrotal/labial hematoma

Palpate for the following:

- Instability of the pelvis: Apply gentle pressure over the iliac wings, downward and medially.[1]
- Instability of the pelvis: Place gentle pressure on the symphysis pubis. This assessment is deferred if pelvic instability has already been noted.

Valid indications for the insertion of a urinary catheter include the following[40,80]:

- Urinary obstruction or retention
- Alteration in blood pressure or volume status

- The need to determine accurate input and output, and the patient is unable to use a urinal or bedpan
- Emergency surgery or major trauma
- Urologic procedures or bladder irrigation
- Comfort care for the terminally ill

> **CLINICAL PEARL**
>
> **Monitoring Urinary Output**
>
> Urinary output reflects end-organ perfusion and is considered a sensitive indicator of the patient's volume status. Continuous or frequent monitoring is best accomplished with an indwelling urinary catheter. However, it is necessary to assess the patient's condition to determine the need for urinary catheter insertion by considering indications and contraindications. Urinary tract infection in the healthcare setting is strongly associated with the presence of an indwelling catheter, and alternative methods should be considered before a urinary catheter is placed.[40,80]

Insertion of a urinary catheter is contraindicated if urethral injury is suspected. Signs and symptoms of urethral injury include the following[4,12]:

- Blood at the urethral meatus
- Perineal ecchymosis
- Scrotal ecchymosis
- High-riding or nonpalpable prostate
- Difficulty/inability to void
- Palpable bladder distention
- Displaced pubic rami fracture
- Pelvic hematoma

Extremities

When performing the extremity assessment, it is important to evaluate neurovascular status, including circulation, motor function, and sensation.

Inspect for the following:

- Soft-tissue injuries
  - Bleeding, LACE, puncture wounds, impaled objects, deformity, and any open wounds
- Bony injuries
  - Angulation, deformity, open wounds (with or without evidence of protruding bone fragments), or edema
  - Previously applied splints for correct placement. Leave in place if correctly applied and neurovascular function is intact distal to splint.
- Skin color
- Presence of dialysis catheters or dialysis access (fistula or grafts), peripherally inserted central catheters, or other signs of complex medical history

Palpate for the following:

- Circulation
  - Skin temperature and moisture
  - Pulses
    - Always compare one side with the other and note any differences in the quality of the pulses. Assess the femoral, popliteal, dorsalis pedis, and posterior tibialis pulses in the lower extremities. Assess the brachial and radial pulses in the upper extremities.
    - Compare pulse quality in the upper extremities with pulse quality in the lower extremities. Weaker pulses in lower extremities could indicate aortic aneurysm.
- Bony injury
  - Crepitus
  - Deformity and areas of tenderness
  - Sensation
    - Determine the patient's ability to sense touch in all four extremities.
- Motor function
  - Elicit the presence or absence of spontaneous movement in the extremities.
  - Determine motor strength and range of motion in all four extremities. Compare left to right for strength and quality.

I: Inspect Posterior Surfaces

If pelvic or spinal trauma is suspected, imaging should be obtained before inspecting the patient's posterior surfaces. Logrolling can cause secondary injuries, including hemorrhage from pelvic fractures.[1,52,62,75] However, logrolling may be indicated if there is suspicion of penetrating injury causing hemodynamic instability or airway compromise.[62,75] If imaging is deferred or confirms the presence of an unstable spine, use extreme caution, with consideration of risks and benefits, for any patient movement. The healthcare team uses the safest technique possible based on the available staff and handling devices. Alternate methods to move the patient include air-assisted mattresses and the 6-plus lift-and-slide.[33,75] If there is a low index of suspicion for spinal instability, logroll the patient, and inspect and palpate the posterior surfaces.

If the patient must be turned prior to imaging, do the following while inspecting posterior surfaces:

- Support the extremities, especially those with suspected injuries.
- Logroll the patient with the assistance of members of the trauma team.

- A designated person, either the team leader or someone else (at the request of the team leader), is positioned at the patient's head. This person is responsible for maintaining cervical spine stabilization and directing the team to turn together.
- Other team members, positioned at one side of the patient, maintain the torso, hips, and lower extremities.
- Maintain the vertebral column alignment during the turning process.
- When possible, avoid rolling the patient onto the side of an injured extremity. The patient is logrolled away from the examiner so that the back, flanks, buttocks, and thighs can be visually examined.

Inspect for the following:

- LACE, puncture wounds, impaled objects, and scars along the entire posterior surface
- Presence of blood in or around the rectum

Palpate for the following:

- Deformity and areas of tenderness along the vertebral column; palpate along each spinous process and attempt to determine a vertebral body fracture, including the costovertebral angles
- Deformity and areas of tenderness over the entire posterior surface of the body, including the flanks

Assess rectal tone if indicated. This assessment is typically performed by a physician or advanced practice nurse during the secondary survey.[4,7]

- An alternative to a digital rectal exam (DRE) is to ask the alert patient to squeeze the buttocks together.
- Assess for sacral sparing.
  - The presence of perianal sensation and anal sphincter tone when seen in conjunction with focal deficits represents an incomplete SCI.[82] Note, however, that perianal sensation and anal sphincter tone may be absent until the resolution of spinal shock.
- Assess for presence of high-riding prostate.

Promote timely removal of the patient from the spine board if there are no contraindications. Consider placement of a slider board, if not already present, to facilitate patient movement on and off the stretcher.

J: Just Keep Reevaluating

Trauma patients require ongoing monitoring and evaluation. The patient may appear stable during the initial assessment, and all possible life-threatening injuries may have been identified and appropriate interventions implemented; however, this does not mean that the patient is, or will remain, stable. Once the initial assessment is completed, the nurse must continually reevaluate the patient for response to the injury as well as effectiveness of any interventions, treatments, and/or procedures performed during the initial assessment phase. Reevaluation consists of the following:

- The primary survey (ABCDE)
- The patient's vital signs (F)
- The patient's level of pain (the P in the LMNOP of G)
- The injuries you have identified in H and I

Serial assessments and analyzing trends are essential components of trauma care and the TNP. It is important to continuously reevaluate all your findings when caring for a trauma patient. The major components of the reevaluation can be recalled using the mnemonic **VIPP**:

- **V:** **V**ital signs
- **I:** **I**njuries sustained and **I**nterventions performed
- **P:** **P**rimary survey
- **P:** Level of **P**ain

These are the parameters that you will be continuously reevaluating for your patient.

Additional Diagnostic Tests or Interventions

Upon completion of the secondary survey, the trauma nurse anticipates orders for additional diagnostic tests and interventions to identify or address specific injuries. These may include the following:

- Additional laboratory studies: ABGs (if indicated and not previously done), cardiac enzymes, liver function tests, metabolic profiles, and coagulation studies
- Radiologic imaging
  - Radiographs (of any suspected skeletal injuries)
  - CT scans (of any affected body regions), including the potential for CT angiography
  - Magnetic resonance imaging
- Wound care as required
- Application of splints as indicated
- Application of traction devices as indicated
- Administration of medications:
  - Tetanus prophylaxis
  - Antibiotics
  - Anticoagulation reversal agents
  - Pain medications (part of ongoing assessment)
  - Anxiolytics
  - Neuromuscular blocking agents

- Angiography
- Contrast urography and angiography
- Bronchoscopy or esophagoscopy
- Preparation for the operating room
- Preparation for admission or transfer
- Psychosocial support

These procedures may require transportation of the patient out of the ED. Therefore, nurses should ensure that appropriately trained personnel, necessary medications, and resuscitative equipment are available during transport of the patient. Ideally, many of these procedures will not be performed until the patient is hemodynamically stabilized. Injuries identified in the primary and secondary surveys continue to be reassessed, along with pain and response to analgesics (the VIPP). Many of these interventions are metrics that are measured as part of a performance improvement program and are time sensitive, such as time of antibiotics and time to operative intervention.

Additional considerations include the following:

- Documentation: Careful and accurate documentation of the assessment, interventions, resuscitation, and patient's response is expected of the trauma nurse. Remember that any trauma patient is a potential legal case (criminal or civil), so accurate and complete documentation is vitally important.[34]
- Family support: The trauma nurse with primary responsibility for the patient can contribute to the ongoing psychosocial support of both the patient and family. Collaboration with the family support person (who is chosen by the patient and family) will ensure that needs are met and information is shared. Whenever possible, allow the family to stay with the patient, and provide adequate time for them to have their questions answered.

Post-Resuscitation Care

The post-resuscitation phase of trauma assessment includes the trauma nurse's ongoing reevaluation of the patient's response to the injury and the effectiveness of all the interventions—the J of the A–J mnemonic. Achievement of expected outcomes is evaluated, and the treatment plan is adjusted accordingly to enhance patient outcomes.

Post-resuscitation care parameters are the same as the J in the initial assessment mnemonic. The nurse will continually reevaluate the following:

- Components of the primary survey (ABCDE)
- Vital signs (F)
- Pain and response to pain medications and non-pharmacologic interventions (an item in G)
- All identified injuries and the effectiveness of the treatment or interventions (identified in H and I)

See Chapter 21, "Post-Resuscitation Care Considerations," for additional information.

Definitive Care or Transport

Definitive care includes the need for specific subspecialty care, such as neurosurgery or orthopedics, monitoring and care in an ICU, or evaluation and operative intervention by a trauma surgeon. The decision to transfer a patient to another facility depends on the patient's injuries, facility resources, and preestablished transfer agreements. This decision is a matter of medical judgment, and evidence supports the position that trauma outcomes improve if patients who are critically injured are cared for in trauma centers.[4,28,39]

Emerging Trends

As the science and evidence of trauma care continue evolving, tools to improve patient outcomes also continue to be trialed and refined. Evidence is routinely tested and replicated, and new standards of care are transitioned into practice. This section on trauma care considerations explores some of the evidence and the potential significance to trauma patient care. See each chapter for additional information on applicable emerging trends.

Computer-Aided Decision-Making in Trauma Resuscitation

Clinical decision support (CDS) tools assist providers by ensuring compliance with algorithms, reducing patient error, and increasing compliance with protocols to decrease morbidity and enhance standardization of care. CDS tools can predict critical situations and augment decision-making for clinicians in trauma resuscitation.[69] For example, CDS tools have been embedded in electronic health records to ensure adequate care for pediatric patients suffering head trauma while reducing unnecessary exposure to the ionizing radiation of CT use.[49,53]

Pharmacologic Treatment to Create a Pro-Survival Phenotype

Valproic acid has been shown to cause reversible acetylation of proteins (which creates an anti-inflammatory and pro-survival phenotype), thereby decreasing the organ damage seen as the result of hemorrhage, polytrauma, and ischemia–reperfusion injury.[13,14,76] Studies are ongoing regarding the use of valproic acid to mitigate cellular damage in trauma patients and thereby decrease morbidity and mortality.[13,14,37,76]

Summary

The use of a systematic approach to the initial assessment of the injured patient is the essence of trauma care. The initial assessment of the trauma patient is achieved through the use of a systematic, standardized approach to assessment, interventions, evaluation, and definitive care of the patient. Essential components include:

- Preparation and triage
- General impression
- Primary survey (A, B, C, D, and E)
- Full set of vital signs and family support with resuscitation and use of continuous monitoring devices (F and G)
- Reevaluation (consideration of the need to transfer patient to a higher level of care)
- Secondary survey (H and I) and performance of additional tests/diagnostics as indicated/required
- Reevaluation and post-resuscitation care (J)
- Definitive care and transfer

By using this systematic and standardized approach, nurses can be more aware of the body's pathophysiologic response to injury and proactively intervene with lifesaving, goal-directed therapies and current management strategies to promote optimal outcomes for the trauma patient.

References

1. American College of Surgeons. (2018). Abdominal and pelvic trauma. In *Advanced trauma life support: Student course manual* (10th ed., pp. 82–101).
2. American College of Surgeons. (2018). Airway and ventilatory management. In *Advanced trauma life support: Student course manual* (10th ed., pp. 22–41).
3. American College of Surgeons. (2018). Head trauma. In *Advanced trauma life support: Student course manual* (10th ed., pp. 102–126).
4. American College of Surgeons. (2018). Initial assessment and management. In *Advanced trauma life support: Student course manual* (10th ed., pp. 2–21).
5. American College of Surgeons. (2018). Shock. In *Advanced trauma life support: Student course manual* (10th ed., pp. 42–61).
6. American College of Surgeons. (2018). Spine and spinal cord trauma. In *Advanced trauma life support: Student course manual* (10th ed., pp. 128–147).
7. American College of Surgeons. (2022). *Best practices guidelines: Spine injury.* https://www.facs.org/media/k45gikqv/spine_injury_guidelines.pdf
8. American College of Surgeons. (2022). *Resources for optimal care of the injured patient: 2022 standards.* https://www.facs.org/quality-programs/trauma/quality/verification-review-and-consultation-program/standards/
9. American Heart Association. (2020). *Basic life support for healthcare providers student manual.* First American Heart Association Printing.
10. American Heart Association. (2020). *Highlights of the 2020 American Heart Association guidelines for CPR and ECC.* https://cpr.heart.org/-/media/cpr-files/cpr-guidelines-files/highlights/hghlgts_2020_ecc_guidelines_english.pdf
11. Auerbach, M., Butler, L., Myers, S. R., Donoghue, A., & Kassam-Adams, N. (2021). Implementing family presence during pediatric resuscitations in the emergency department: Family-centered care and trauma-informed care best practices. *Journal of Emergency Nursing, 47*(5), 689–692. https://doi.org/10.1016/j.jen.2021.07.003
12. Battaloglu, E., Figuero, M., Moran, C., Lecky, F., & Porter, K. (2019). Urethral injury in major trauma. *Injury, 50*(5), 1053–1057. https://doi.org/10.1016/j.injury.2019.02.016
13. Bhatti, U. F., Karnovsky, A., Dennahy, I. S., Kachman, M., Williams, A. M., Nikolian, V. C., Biesterveld, B. E., Siddiqui, A., O'Connell, R. L., Liu, B., Li, Y., & Alam, H. B. (2021). Pharmacologic modulation of brain metabolism by valproic acid can induce a neuroprotective environment. *The Journal of Trauma and Acute Care Surgery, 90*(3), 507–514. https://doi.org/10.1097/TA.0000000000003026
14. Biesterveld, B. E., Siddiqui, A. Z., O'Connell, R. L., Remmer, H., Williams, A. M., Shamshad, A., Smith, W. M., Kemp, M. T., Wakam, G. K., & Alam, H. B. (2021). Valproic acid protects against acute kidney injury in hemorrhage and trauma. *The Journal of Surgical Research, 266,* 222–229. https://doi.org/10.1016/j.jss.2021.04.014
15. Blay, N., Ioannou, S., Seremetkoska, M., Morris, J., Holters, G., Thomas, V., & Bronwyn, E. (2018). Healthcare interpreter utilisation: Analysis of health administrative data. *BMC Health Services Research, 18*(1), Article 348. https://doi.org/10.1186/s12913-018-3135-5
16. Boon, Y., Kuan, W. S., Chan, Y. H., Ibrahim, I., & Chua, M. T. (2021). Agreement between arterial and venous blood gases in trauma resuscitation in emergency department (AGREE). *European Journal of Trauma and Emergency Surgery, 47*(2), 365–372. https://doi.org/10.1007/s00068-019-01190-6
17. Bovino, L., Brainard, C., Beaumier, K., Concetti, V., Lefurge, N., Mittelstadt, E., Wilson, T., & Langhan, M. L. (2018). Use of capnography to optimize procedural sedation in the emergency department pediatric population. *Journal of Emergency Nursing, 44*(2), 110–116. https://doi.org/10.1016/j.jen.2017.10.016
18. Bozorgi, F., Khatir, I. G., Ghanbari, H., Jahanian, F., Arabi, M., Ahidashti, H. A., Hosseininejad, S. M., Ramezani, M. S., & Montazer, S. H. (2019). Investigation of frequency of the lethal triad and its 24 hours prognostic value among patients

with multiple traumas. *Open Access Macedonian Journal of Medical Sciences, 7*(6), 962–966. https://doi.org/10.3889/oamjms.2019.217

19. Broering, B. (2020). Head trauma. In V. Sweet & A. Foley (Eds.), *Sheehy's emergency nursing: Principles and practice* (pp. 401–418). Elsevier.

20. Bullock, A., Dodington, J. M., Donoghue, A. J., & Langhan, M. L. (2017). Capnography use during intubation and cardiopulmonary resuscitation in the pediatric emergency department. *Pediatric Emergency Care, 33*(7), 457–461. https://doi.org/10.1097/PEC.0000000000000813

21. Cap, A. P., Pidcoke, H. F., Spinella, P., Strandenes, G., Borgman, M. A., Schreiber, M., Holcomb, J., Chin-Nan Tien, H., Beckett, A. N., Doughty, H., Woolley, T., Rappold, J., Ward, K., Reade, M., Prat, N., Ausset, S., Kheirabadi, B., Benov, A., Griffin, E. P., . . . Stockinger, Z. (2018). Damage control resuscitation. *Military Medicine, 183*(Suppl. 2), 36–43. https://doi.org/10.1093/milmed/usy112

22. Changa, A. R., Czeisler, B. M., & Lord, A. S. (2019). Management of elevated intracranial pressure: A review. *Current Neurology and Neuroscience Reports, 19*(12), 1–10. https://doi.org/10.1007/s11910-019-1010-3

23. Chen, L. L. (2020). Under pressure. *The Nurse Practitioner, 45*(2), 5–7. https://doi.org/10.1097/01.NPR.0000651136.91775.c9

24. Chilvers, G., Porter, K., & Choudhary, S. (2018). Cervical spine clearance in adults following blunt trauma: A national survey across major trauma centres in England. *Clinical Radiology, 73*(4), 410.e1–410.e8. https://doi.org/10.1016/j.crad.2017.11.006

25. Chukwulebe, S., & Hogrefe, C. (2019). The diagnosis and management of facial bone fractures. *Emergency Medicine Clinics of North America, 37*(1), 137–151. https://doi.org/10.1016/j.emc.2018.09.012

26. Dainty, K. N., Atkins, D. L., Breckwoldt, J., Maconochie, I., Schexnayder, S. M., Skrifvars, M. B., Tijssen, J., Wyllie, J., Furuta, M., Aickin, R., Acworth, J., Atkins, D., Couto, T. B., Guerguerian, A. M., Kleinman, M., Kloeck, D., Nadkarni, V., Ng, K. C., Nuthall, G., . . . Education, Implementation and Teams Task Force. (2021). Family presence during resuscitation in paediatric and neonatal cardiac arrest: A systematic review. *Resuscitation, 162*, 20–34. https://doi.org/10.1016/j.resuscitation.2021.01.017

27. Dammers, D., El Moumni, M., Hoogland, I. I., Veeger, N., & Ter Avest, E. (2017). Should we perform a FAST exam in haemodynamically stable patients presenting after blunt abdominal injury: A retrospective cohort study. *Scandinavian Journal of Trauma, Resuscitation and Emergency Medicine, 25*(1), Article 1. https://doi.org/10.1186/s13049-016-0342-0

28. Deeb, A., Phelos, H. M., Peitzman, A. B., Billiar, T. R., Sperry, J. L., & Brown, J. B. (2020). Disparities in rural versus urban field triage: Risk and mitigating factors for undertriage. *Journal of Trauma and Acute Care Surgery, 89*(1), 246–253. https://doi.org/10.1097/TA.0000000000002690

29. Dogrul, B. N., Kiliccalan, I., Asci, E. S., & Peker, S. C. (2020). Blunt trauma related chest wall and pulmonary injuries: An overview. *Chinese Journal of Traumatology, 23*(3), 125–138. https://doi.org/10.1016/j.cjtee.2020.04.003

30. Drake, S. A., Holcomb, J. B., Yang, Y., Thetford, C., Myers, L., Brock, M., Wolf, D. A., Cron, S., Persse, D., McCarthy, J., Kao, L., Todd, S. R., Naik-Mathuria, B. J., Cox, C., Kitagawa, R., Sandberg, G., & Wade, C. E. (2020). Establishing a regional trauma preventable/potentially preventable death rate. *Annals of Surgery, 271*(2), 375–382. https://doi.org/10.1097/SLA.0000000000002999

31. Drendel, A. L., Gray, M. P., & Lerner, E. B. (2019). A systematic review of hospital trauma team activation criteria for children. *Pediatric Emergency Care, 35*(1), 8–15. https://doi.org/10.1097/PEC.0000000000001256

32. Dylla, L., Anderson, E. L., Douin, D. J., Jackson, C. L., Rice, J. D., Schauer, S. G., Neumann, R. T., Bebarta, V. S., Wright, F. L., & Ginde, A. A. (2021). A quasiexperimental study of targeted normoxia in critically ill trauma patients. *The Journal of Trauma and Acute Care Surgery, 91*(Suppl. 2), S169–S175. https://doi.org/10.1097/TA.0000000000003177

33. Emergency Nurses Association. (2016). *Avoiding the log roll maneuver: Alternative methods for safe patient handling* [Topic brief]. https://enau.ena.org/Users/LearningActivity/LearningActivityDetail.aspx?LearningActivityID=LJMRSp85WwPew%2BHMK6%2B5YQ%3D%3D&tab=4

34. Emergency Nurses Association. (2018). *Forensic evidence collection in the emergency care setting* [Position statement]. https://enau.ena.org/Users/LearningActivity/LearningActivityDetail.aspx?LearningActivityID=IbSK17mF0fIOme29ea9Gvw%3D%3D&tab=4

35. Ferrada, P., Callcut, R. A., Skarupa, D. J., Duane, T. M., Garcia, A., Inaba, K., Khor, D., Anto, V., Sperry, J., Turay, D., Nygaard, R. M., Schreiber, M. A., Enniss, T., McNutt, M., Phelan, H., Smith, K., Moore, F. O., Tabas, I., Dubose, J., & AAST Multi-Institutional Trials Committee. (2018). Circulation first—the time has come to question the sequencing of care in the ABCs of trauma: An American Association for the Surgery of Trauma multicenter trial. *World Journal of Emergency Surgery, 13*, Article 8. https://doi.org/10.1186/s13017-018-0168-3

36. Fischer, P. E., Perina, D. G., Delbridge, T. R., Fallat, M. E., Salomone, J. P., Dodd, J., Bulger, E. M., & Gestring, M. L. (2018). Spinal motion restriction in the trauma patient—A joint position statement. *Prehospital Emergency Care, 22*(6), 659–661. https://doi.org/10.1080/10903127.2018.1481476

37. Georgoff, P. E., Nikolian, V. C., Bonham, T., Pai, M. P., Tafatia, C., Halaweish, I., To, K., Watcharotone, K., Parameswaran, A., Luo, R., Sun, D., & Alam, H. B. (2018). Safety and tolerability of intravenous valproic acid in healthy subjects: A Phase I dose-escalation trial. *Clinical Pharmacokinetics, 57*(2), 209–219. https://doi.org/10.1007/s40262-017-0553-1

38. Gisness, C. M. (2020). Maxillofacial trauma. In V. Sweet & A. Foley (Eds.), *Sheehy's emergency nursing: Principles and practice* (7th ed., pp. 419–430). Elsevier.

39. Gough, B. L., Painter, M. D., Hoffman, A. L., Caplan, R. J., Peters, C. A., & Cipolle, M. D. (2020). Right patient, right place, right time: Field triage and transfer to Level I trauma

centers. *The American Surgeon, 86*(5), 400–406. https://doi.org/10.1177/0003134820918249

40. Gould, C. V., Umscheid, C. A., Agarwal, R. K., Kuntz, G., Pegues, D. A., & Healthcare Infection Control Practices Advisory Committee. (2019). *Guideline for prevention of catheter association urinary tract infections 2009*. Department of Health and Human Services, Centers for Disease Control and Prevention. https://www.cdc.gov/infectioncontrol/pdf/guidelines/cauti-guidelines-H.pdf

41. Gutiérrez, J. J., Leturiondo, M., Ruiz de Gauna, S., Ruiz, J. M., Leturiondo, L. A., González-Otero, D. M., Zive, D., Russell, J. K., & Daya, M. (2018). Enhancing ventilation detection during cardiopulmonary resuscitation by filtering chest compression artifact from the capnography waveform. *PLOS ONE, 13*(8), Article e0201565. http://doi.org/10.1371/journal.pone.0201565

42. Hooman, B-M., Fatemeh, H., Masoud, M., Babak, S., & Maryam, H. (2020). Test characteristics of focused assessment with sonography for trauma (FAST), repeated FAST, and clinical exam in prediction of intra-abdominal injury in children with blunt trauma. *Pediatric Surgery International, 36*(10), 1227–1234. https://doi.org/10.1007/s00383-020-04733-w

43. Hopkins, E., Green, S. M., Kiemeney, M., & Haukoos, J. S. (2018). A two-center validation of "patient does not follow commands" and three other simplified measures to replace the Glasgow Coma Scale for field trauma triage. *Annals of Emergency Medicine, 72*(3), 259–269. https://doi.org/10.1016/j.annemergmed.2018.03.038

44. Hsu, J. R., Mir, H., Wally, M. K., Seymour, R. B., & Orthopaedic Trauma Association Musculoskeletal Pain Task Force. (2019). Clinical practice guidelines for pain management in acute musculoskeletal injury. *Journal of Orthopaedic Trauma, 33*(5), e158–e182. https://doi.org/10.1097/BOT.0000000000001430

45. Hsu, S. D., Chen, C. J., Chou, Y. C., Wang, S. H., & Chan, D. C. (2017). Effect of early pelvic binder use in the emergency management of suspected pelvic trauma: A retrospective cohort study. *International Journal of Environmental Research and Public Health, 14*(10), Article 1217. https://doi.org/10.3390/ijerph14101217

46. Jambhekar, A., Lindborg, R., Chan, V., Fulginiti, A., Fahoum, B., & Rucinski, J. (2018). Over the hill and falling down: Can the NEXUS criteria be applied to the elderly? *International Journal of Surgery, 49*, 56–59. https://doi.org/10.1016/j.ijsu.2017.12.009

47. Javali, R. H., Ravindra, P., Patil, A., Srinivasarangan, M., Mundada, H., Adarsh, S. B., & Nisarg, S. (2017). A clinical study on the initial assessment of arterial lactate and base deficit as predictors of outcome in trauma patients. *Indian Journal of Critical Care Medicine, 21*(11), 719–725. https://doi.org/10.4103/ijccm.IJCCM_218_17

48. Kalkwarf, K. J., Drake, S. A., Yang, Y., Thetford, C., Myers, L., Brock, M., Wolf, D. A., Persse, D., Wade, C. E., & Holcomb, J. B. (2020). Bleeding to death in a big city: An analysis of all trauma deaths from hemorrhage in a metropolitan area during 1 year. *The Journal of Trauma and Acute Care Surgery, 89*(4), 716–722. https://doi.org/10.1097/TA.0000000000002833

49. Khalifa, M., & Gallego, B. (2019). Grading and assessment of clinical predictive tools for paediatric head injury: A new evidence-based approach. *BMC Emergency Medicine, 19*, Article 35. http://doi.org/10.1186/s12873-019-0249-y

50. Koh, E. Y., Oyeniyi, B. T., Fox, E. E., Scerbo, M., Tomasek, J. S., Wade, C. E., & Holcomb, J. B. (2019). Trends in potentially preventable trauma deaths between 2005–2006 and 2012–2013. *American Journal of Surgery, 218*(3), 501–506. https://doi.org/10.1016/j.amjsurg.2018.12.022

51. Leitch, P., Hudson, A. L., Griggs, J. E., Stolmeijer, R., Lyon, R. M., & Ter Avest, E., on behalf of Air Ambulance Kent Surrey Sussex. (2021). Incidence of hyperoxia in trauma patients receiving pre-hospital emergency anaesthesia: Results of a 5-year retrospective analysis. *Scandinavian Journal of Trauma, Resuscitation and Emergency Medicine, 29*(1), Article 134. https://doi.org/10.1186/s13049-021-00951-w

52. Maschmann, C., Jeppesen, E., Rubin, M. A., & Barfod, C. (2019). New clinical guidelines on the spinal stabilisation of adult trauma patients—Consensus and evidence based. *Scandinavian Journal of Trauma, Resuscitation and Emergency Medicine, 27*(1), Article 77. https://doi.org/10.1186/s13049-019-0655-x

53. Masterson Creber, R. M., Dayan, P. S., Kuppermann, N., Ballard, D. W., Tzimenatos, L., Alessandrini, E., Mistry, R. D., Hoffman, J., Vinson, D. R., & Bakken, S., for the Pediatric Emergency Care Applied Research Network and the Clinical Research on Emergency Services and Treatments Network. (2018). Applying the RE-AIM Framework for the evaluation of a clinical decision support tool for pediatric head trauma: A mixed-methods study. *Applied Clinical Informatics, 9*(3), 693–703. https://doi.org/10.1055/s-0038-1669460

54. Migliorini, R., Comberiati, A. M., Pacella, F., Longo, A. R., Messineo, D., Trovato Battagliola, E., Malvasi, M., Pacella, E., & Arrico, L. (2021). Utility of ocular motility tests in orbital floor fractures with muscle entrapment that is not detected on computed tomography. *Clinical Ophthalmology, 15*, 1677–1683. https://doi.org/10.2147/OPTH.S292097

55. Mitsusada, K., Dote, H., Tokutake, M., & Atsumi, T. (2022). Airway obstruction caused by massive subcutaneous emphysema due to blunt chest trauma. *BMJ Case Reports, 15*, Article e251068. https://doi.org/10.1136/bcr-2022-251068

56. Moeri, M., Rothenfluh, D. A., Laux, C. J., & Dominguez, D. E. (2020). Cervical spine clearance after blunt trauma: Current state of the art. *EFORT Open Reviews, 5*(4), 253–259. https://doi.org/10.1302/2058-5241.5.190047

57. Moon, J., Hwang, K., Yoon, D., & Jung, K. (2020). Inclusion of lactate level measured upon emergency room arrival in trauma outcome prediction models improves mortality prediction: A retrospective, single-center study. *Acute and Critical Care, 35*(2), 102–109. https://doi.org/10.4266/acc.2019.00780

58. Mora, M. C., Veras, L., Burke, R. V., Cassidy, L. D., Christopherson, N., Cunningham, A., Jafri, M., Marion, E., Lidsky, K., Yanchar, N., Wu, L., & Gosain, A. (2020). Pediatric

trauma triage: A Pediatric Trauma Society Research Committee systematic review. *Journal of Trauma and Acute Care Surgery, 89*(4), 623–630. https://doi.org/10.1097/TA.0000000000002713

59. Mota, M., Cunha, M., Santos, M. R., Silva, D., & Santos, E. (2019). Non-pharmacological interventions for pain management in adult victims of trauma: A scoping review protocol. *JBI Database of Systematic Reviews and Implementation Reports, 17*(12), 2483–2490. https://doi.org/10.11124/JBISRIR-2017-004036

60. Mourad, M., Inman, J. C., Chan, D. M., & Ducic, Y. (2018). Contemporary trends in the management of posttraumatic cerebrospinal fluid leaks. *Craniomaxillofacial Trauma & Reconstruction, 11*(1), 71–77. https://doi.org/10.1055/s-0036-1584890

61. Murray, J., & Rust, D. A. (2017). Cervical spine alignment in helmeted skiers and snowboarders with suspected head and neck injuries: Comparison of lateral C-spine radiographs before and after helmet removal and implications for ski patrol transport. *Wilderness & Environmental Medicine, 28*(3), 168–175. https://doi.org/10.1016/j.wem.2017.03.009

62. National Institute for Health and Care Excellence. (2017). *Fractures (complex): Assessment and management.* https://www.nice.org.uk/guidance/ng37

63. Newgard, C. D., Fischer, P. E., Gestring, M., Michaels, H. N., Jurkovich, G. J., Lerner, E. B., Fallat, M. E., Delbridge, T. R., Brown, J. B., Bulger, E. M., & the Writing Group for the 2021 National Expert Panel on Field Triage. (2022). National Guideline for the Field Triage of Injured Patients: Recommendations of the National Expert Panel on Field Triage, 2021. *Journal of Trauma and Acute Care Surgery, 93*(2), e49-e60. https://doi.org/10.1097/TA.0000000000003627

64. Newton, E., & Taira, T. (2022). Head trauma. In K. Bakes, J. Buchanan, M. Moreira, R. Byyny, & P. Pons, *Emergency medicine secrets* (7th ed., pp. 491–485). Elsevier.

65. Nisar, S., Gibson, C. D., Sokolovic, M., & Shah, N. S. (2020). Pulse oximetry is unreliable in patients on veno-venous extracorporeal membrane oxygenation caused by unrecognized carboxyhemoglobinemia. *ASAIO Journal, 66*(10), 1105–1109. https://doi.org/10.1097/MAT.0000000000001144

66. Nnedu, C. C. (2021). Nigerian Americans. In J. N. Giger & L. G. Haddad (Eds.), *Transcultural nursing* (8th ed., pp. 589–611). Elsevier.

67. Nuttall, A. G., Paton, K. M., & Kemp, A. M. (2018). To what extent are GCS and AVPU equivalent to each other when assessing the level of consciousness of children with head injury? A cross-sectional study of UK hospital admissions. *BMJ Open, 8*(11), Article e023216. https://doi.org/10.1136/bmjopen-2018-023216

68. Oh, J. W., Kim, S. H., & Whang, K. (2017). Traumatic cerebrospinal fluid leak: Diagnosis and management. *Korean Journal of Neurotrauma, 13*(2), 63–67. https://doi.org/10.13004/kjnt.2017.13.2.63

69. Osterhoff, G., Pförringer, D., Scherer, J., Juhra, C., Maerdian, S., Back, D. A., & Arbeitsgruppe Digitalisierung der Deutschen Gesellschaft für Orthopädie und Unfallchirurgie. (2020). Computerassistierte Entscheidungsfindung beim Traumapatienten [Computer-assisted decision-making for trauma patients]. *Der Unfallchirurg, 123*(3), 199–205. https://doi.org/10.1007/s00113-019-0676-y

70. Paykin, G., O'Reilly, G., Ackland, H. M., & Mitra, B. (2017). The NEXUS criteria are insufficient to exclude cervical spine fractures in older blunt trauma patients. *Injury, 48*(5), 1020–1024. https://doi.org/10.1016/j.injury.2017.02.013

71. Porter, K., Morlion, B., Rolfe, M., & Dodt, C. (2020). Attributes of analgesics for emergency pain relief: Results of the Consensus on Management of Pain Caused by Trauma Delphi initiative. *European Journal of Emergency Medicine, 27*(1), 33–39. https://doi.org/10.1097/MEJ.0000000000000597

72. Prehospital Trauma Life Support Committee of the National Association of Emergency Medical Technicians, & American College of Surgeons Committee on Trauma. (2020). Golden principles, preferences, and critical thinking. In *Prehospital trauma life support* (9th ed., pp. 21–44). Jones & Bartlett Learning.

73. Ramazani, J., & Hosseini, M. (2019). Comparison of full outline of unresponsiveness score and Glasgow Coma Scale in medical intensive care unit. *Annals of Cardiac Anaesthesia, 22*(2), 143–148. https://doi.org/10.4103/aca.ACA_25_18

74. Reith, F., Lingsma, H. F., Gabbe, B. J., Lecky, F. E., Roberts, I., & Maas, A. (2017). Differential effects of the Glasgow Coma Scale Score and its components: An analysis of 54,069 patients with traumatic brain injury. *Injury, 48*(9), 1932–1943. https://doi.org/10.1016/j.injury.2017.05.038

75. Rodrigues, I. F. (2017). To log-roll or not to log-roll—That is the question! A review of the use of the log-roll for patients with pelvic fractures. *International Journal of Orthopaedic and Trauma Nursing, 27*, 36–40. https://doi.org/10.1016/j.ijotn.2017.05.001

76. Russo, R., Kemp, M., Bhatti, U. F., Pai, M., Wakam, G., Biesterveld, B., & Alam, H. B. (2020). Life on the battlefield: Valproic acid for combat applications. *The Journal of Trauma and Acute Care Surgery, 89*(Suppl. 2), S69–S76. https://doi.org/10.1097/TA.0000000000002721

77. Safari, E., & Torabi, M. (2020). Relationship between end-tidal CO_2 ($ETCO_2$) and lactate and their role in predicting hospital mortality in critically ill trauma patients: A cohort study. *Bulletin of Emergency and Trauma, 8*(2), 83–88. https://doi.org/10.30476/BEAT.2020.46447

78. Sağlık, D. S., & Çağlar, S. (2019). The effect of parental presence on pain and anxiety levels during invasive procedures in the pediatric emergency department. *Journal of Emergency Nursing, 45*(3), 278–285. https://doi.org/10.1016/j.jen.2018.07.003

79. Sandroni, C., De Santis, P., & D'Arrigo, S. (2018). Capnography during cardiac arrest. *Resuscitation, 132*, 73–77. https://doi.org/10.1016/j.resuscitation.2018.08.018

80. Shaver, B., Eyerly-Webb, S. A., Gibney, Z., Silverman, L., Pineda, C., & Solomon, R. J. (2018). Trauma and intensive care nursing knowledge and attitude of Foley catheter insertion and maintenance. *Journal of Trauma Nursing, 25*(1), 66–72. https://doi.org/10.1097/JTN.0000000000000344

81. Stahel, P. F., & VanderHeiden, T. (2017). Spinal injuries. In E. E. Moore, D. V. Feliciano, & K. L. Mattox (Eds.), *Trauma* (8th ed., pp. 455–472). McGraw Hill.

82. Stacy, K. M. (2022). Neurologic anatomy and physiology. In L. D. Urden, K. M. Stacy, & M. E. Lough (Eds.), *Critical care nursing: Diagnosis and management* (9th ed., pp. 534–564). Elsevier.

83. Sulton, C. D., Middlebrooks, L. S., & Taylor, T. (2020). The pediatric airway and rapid sequence intubation. *Pediatric Emergency Medicine Reports, 25*(1). https://www.reliasmedia.com/articles/145479-the-pediatric-airway-and-rapid-sequence-intubation

84. Torabi, J., Kaban, J. M., Lewis, E., Laikhram, D., Simon, R., DeHaan, S., Jureller, M., Chao, E., Reddy, S. H., & Stone, M. E., Jr. (2021). Ketorolac use for pain management in trauma patients with rib fractures does not increase of acute kidney injury or incidence of bleeding. *The American Surgeon, 87*(5), 790–795. https://doi.org/10.1177/0003134820954835

85. Tulaimat, A., & Trick, W. E. (2017). DiapHRaGM: A mnemonic to describe the work of breathing in patients with respiratory failure. *PLOS ONE, 12*(7), Article e0179641. https://doi.org/10.1371/journal.pone.0179641

86. van Veelen, M. J., & Maeder, M. B. (2021). Hypothermia in trauma. *International Journal of Environmental Research and Public Health, 18*(16), Article 8719. https://doi.org/10.3390%2Fijerph18168719

87. Viviano, S. L., Hoppe, I. C., Halsey, J. N., Chen, J. S., Russo, G. J., Lee, E. S., & Granick, M. S. (2017). Pediatric facial fractures: An assessment of airway management. *The Journal of Craniofacial Surgery, 28*(8), 2004–2006. https://doi.org/10.1097/SCS.0000000000004036

88. Walrath, B. D., Harper, S., Barnard, E., Tobin, J. M., Drew, B., Cunningham, C., Kharod, C., Spradling, J., Stone, C., & Martin, M. (2018). Airway management for trauma patients. *Military Medicine, 183*(Suppl. 2), 29–31. https://doi.org/10.1093/milmed/usy124

89. Warth, R. J., Hays, M. R., Dodd, C. T., Rao, M., Kumaravel, M., Lowe, W. R., & Prasarn, M. L. (2019). On-field removal of large anti-concussive football helmets using current guidelines leads to increased passive cervical lordosis. *Orthopaedic Journal of Sports Medicine, 7*(Suppl. 5). https://doi.org/10.1177/2325967119S00405

CHAPTER 5

Airway and Ventilation

Evan Edminster, MSN, RN, CNL, CFRN, TCRN, CEN, NDHP-BC

OBJECTIVES

Upon completion of this chapter, the learner will be able to:
1. Describe pathophysiologic changes as a basis for assessment of the trauma patient with actual or potential airway and ventilation complications.
2. Demonstrate airway and ventilation assessment of the trauma patient.
3. Plan appropriate interventions and evaluate their effectiveness for actual or potential airway and ventilation complications.

Knowledge of normal anatomy and physiology serves as a foundation for understanding anatomic derangements and pathophysiologic processes that may result from trauma. Anatomy is not emphasized in the classroom, but it is the basis of physical assessment and skill evaluation, as well as the foundation of questions for testing purposes.

Anatomy and Physiology of the Airway

The pulmonary system consists of both the upper and lower airways. The upper airway includes the nose, mouth, pharynx, larynx, epiglottis, and trachea (**Figure 5-1**). These structures humidify, filter, and transport inhaled air from the atmosphere to the alveoli. The lower airway is composed of the lungs, bronchi, and alveoli. The alveoli serve as the primary location for the diffusion of oxygen into the capillary network, where it then enters the arterial system and is transported to organs, tissues, and cells.[17]

Upper Airway

The nasal passages are the primary entryway for air into the lungs.[6] Coarse hairs line the outer nasal passages and filter dust and other particles. The mucous membrane within the nasal cavity contains tiny blood vessels and provides warmth and moisture.[6] The mouth is the secondary passageway for inhaled air into the lungs (**Figure 5-2**). The presence of swelling, blood, vomitus, or foreign objects in the mouth may cause mechanical obstruction and prevent adequate ventilation. In unconscious patients, airway obstruction is commonly caused by the tongue.[46]

The nasopharynx and oropharynx meet at the base of the skull and extend to the lower border of the cricoid

Figure 5-1 *Upper airway structures.*

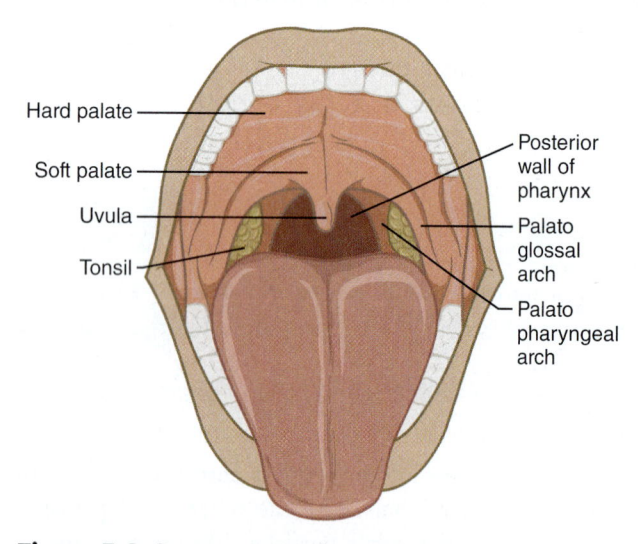

Figure 5-2 *Structures in the mouth.*

cartilage. The structures within the posterior oropharynx serve as guides to locate the trachea during the intubation process. The epiglottis is a cartilaginous structure that lies superior to the larynx. This protective structure allows air into the lungs and prevents the aspiration of liquids and solids during swallowing.

The larynx is a tubular structure composed of cartilage that connects the oropharynx to the trachea. The primary function of the larynx is to serve as a conduit for air to enter the trachea. The larynx is a heavily innervated sensory structure (**Figure 5-3**). The vagus nerve (cranial nerve X) serves as the primary parasympathetic nerve; stimulation during intubation can lead to a vagal response, including bradycardia and hypotension, especially in infants and young children (Figure 5-3).[3,24,35]

Below the larynx is the cricothyroid membrane, which extends from the upper surface of the cricoid cartilage to the inferior border of the thyroid cartilage (Adam's apple). The cricothyroid membrane is approximately 2 mm in height and 3 mm in width.[33] In adult females, the neck is relatively smaller, and the cricoid cartilage is located slightly higher than in adult males. The trachea begins just below the larynx and ends at the carina; the length and diameter of the trachea are typically shorter and smaller in females compared with males. The trachea is significantly shorter in infants and children, leading to easy obstruction of the trachea or displacement of endotracheal tubes with head movement.[3,35]

Lower Airway

The lower airway is located within the thoracic cage and includes the lungs and the bronchial tree.[6] The carina, located where the two primary bronchial branches

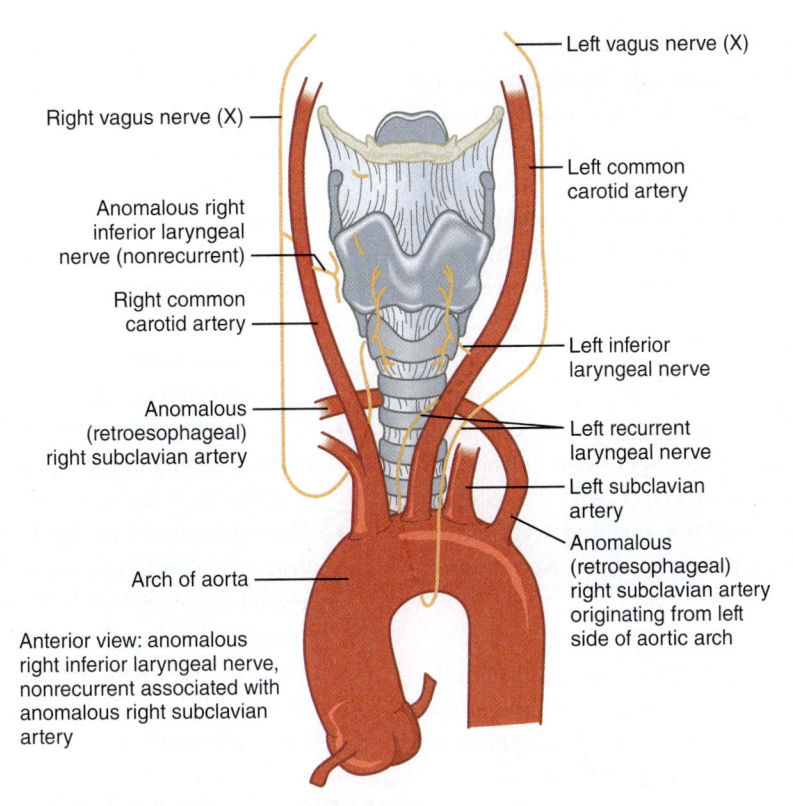

Figure 5-3 *Innervation of the larynx by the vagus nerve.*

meet, is composed chiefly of nerves. When the carina is stimulated—by deep suctioning, for instance—bronchospasm or severe coughing may result.

Each lung is divided into sections called lobes, with three lobes in the right lung and two lobes in the left lung. The smaller number of lobes on the left side is attributed to sharing space in the chest with the heart. The bronchi branch many times into smaller airways called bronchioles. Large airways are held open by semiflexible cartilage. In contrast, the smaller airways have a thin, circular layer of smooth muscle lining that can dilate or constrict to change airway diameter as needed.[6,42]

The bronchi and the bronchioles, composed primarily of epithelial tissue and smooth muscle, conduct atmospheric air to the alveoli, where gas exchange occurs. Certain anatomic features of the bronchi are clinically significant. Specifically, the right main bronchus is shorter and broader than the left and branches off from the carina at an almost straight angle.[42] These structural characteristics enable easy introduction of an endotracheal tube, resulting in an unintentional right mainstem bronchus intubation.

The mediastinum is bordered anteriorly by the sternum, posteriorly by the 12 thoracic vertebrae, and inferiorly by the diaphragm. The diaphragm serves the critical respiratory function of controlling the rate and volume of inspiration. The base of each lung rests against the diaphragm. The apex of each lung extends approximately 2 to 3 cm above where the clavicle meets the sternum.

Physiology

Three processes transfer oxygen from the air to the lungs and bloodstream[6,42]:

- *Ventilation:* The active, mechanical movement of air into and out of lungs
- *Diffusion:* The passive movement of gases from an area of higher concentration to an area of lower concentration
- *Perfusion:* The movement of blood to and from the lungs as the delivery medium of oxygen to the entire body

Ventilation

Ventilation, or breathing, begins with inhaling air through the upper airway.[42] It is the mechanical process of air movement into and throughout the lungs. Ventilation relies heavily on signals from the nervous system, in conjunction with adequately functioning lungs. Signals from the brain stem direct the pharyngeal muscles to open the pharynx during inhalation. During inspiration, the diaphragm contracts inferiorly toward the abdomen and flattens, thereby increasing the size of the thorax and extending it into the 10th or 12th intercostal space.

During expiration, the diaphragm relaxes superiorly toward the lungs and the lungs recoil, decreasing the size of the pleural cavity to the fourth intercostal space. The external intercostal muscles also assist with ventilation by enlarging the rib cage, which increases the anterior-to-posterior diameter of the thoracic cavity and expands the lungs. Conversely, the anterior-to-posterior diameter decreases as the internal intercostal muscles contract, enabling the passive exhalation of air from the lungs.

Diffusion

Diffusion is the movement of gases (such as oxygen and carbon dioxide) from an area of higher concentration to an area of lower concentration. Gases cross the relatively thin alveolar–capillary membrane, enabling oxygen to enter the alveoli and carbon dioxide to escape from them.[42]

Perfusion

Perfusion is the movement or flow of blood through the circulatory system (including the heart and lungs) that results in the oxygenation of tissues. Adequate perfusion depends on many factors, including the following:

- Airway patency
- Ventilatory effort
- Gas exchange in the alveoli
- Hemoglobin's oxygen-carrying capacity
- Cardiac output

Introduction

The priority for managing a trauma patient after controlling obvious life-threatening external hemorrhage is to ensure a patent, protected airway. Knowledge of effective airway and ventilatory management is crucial to supporting the delivery of oxygenated blood to the brain and other vital organs.[1,6,42]

Pathophysiology as a Basis for Assessment Findings

Abnormal airway pathophysiology may include airway obstruction, inadequate oxygenation, or inadequate ventilation, alone or in combination.

Airway Obstruction

The obstruction of a trauma patient's airway may be caused by one or more of the following[13]:

- Altered level of consciousness:
  - The tongue falling posteriorly into the oropharynx: This is a common cause of obstruction in patients who are not alert.
- Alcohol or other substances: Patients under the influence may have an altered level of consciousness, which may inhibit their ability to maintain a patent airway.
- Blood, secretions, or vomit: Patients with an altered level of consciousness may lack the ability to clear blood, secretions, or vomit by swallowing or coughing.
- Maxillofacial trauma: May cause edema, increased secretions, bleeding, or dislodged teeth/dentures within the oral cavity.
- Neck or laryngeal trauma: May cause vascular injuries, resulting in expanding hematomas that can compress and obstruct the airway.
- Obese patients are at significant risk for airway obstruction and hypoventilation because of increased fat deposition in the pharyngeal tissues and pharyngeal wall collapse when given medications that depress the central nervous system.[13,38] See Chapter 14, "The Obese Trauma Patient," for additional information.

Oxygenation and Ventilation

To ensure understanding of oxygenation and ventilation terminology, review **Table 5-1** before proceeding.[25,45]

Inadequate Oxygenation and Ventilation

Once a patent airway is established and confirmed, the next priority becomes ensuring adequate oxygenation and ventilation. The following factors may contribute to inadequate oxygenation and ventilation:

- Altered mental status: Due to brain injury, prolonged loss of consciousness, increased intracranial pressure, hypoxia, medications, alcohol or substance use or misuse.
- Cervical spine trauma or spinal cord injury: Can disrupt sympathetic nervous system.
- Blunt thoracic trauma: May result in chest wall instability and ineffective oxygenation and ventilation. See Chapter 8, "Thoracic and Neck Trauma," for additional information.
- Penetrating thoracic trauma: May result in a hemothorax, pneumothorax, or both. See Chapter 8, "Thoracic and Neck Trauma," for additional information.
- Underlying pulmonary comorbidities: Conditions such as chronic obstructive pulmonary disease may alter the response to injuries and interventions.[15]
- Advanced age: Older patients have decreased vital capacity, tidal volume, and functional reserve. See

TABLE 5-1 Oxygenation and Ventilation Terminology

Component	Definition	Measurement	Normal Range
Oxygenation			
SaO_2	The percentage of oxygen-saturated hemoglobin in arterial blood	ABG	> 95%
SpO_2	Noninvasive measurement of the percent of saturated hemoglobin in the capillary bed	Co-oximetry with a pulse oximeter	> 94%
PaO_2	Amount of oxygen dissolved in plasma	ABG	> 80 mm Hg (10.7 kPa)
Ventilation			
$PaCO_2$	Partial pressure of carbon dioxide (CO_2) in arterial blood	ABG	35–45 mm Hg (4.7–6.0 kPa)
$ETCO_2$	Maximum concentration of CO_2 at the end of each breath	Colorimetric CO_2 detector	Purple for $ETCO_2$ < 3 mm Hg (0.4 kPa); tan for 3–15 mm Hg (0.4–2.0); yellow for > 15 mm Hg (2.0 kPa)
		Capnometer or capnography device	35–45 mm Hg (4.7–6.0 kPa)
Delivery			
FiO_2	Fraction (as a percentage) of oxygen in the air mixture that is delivered to the patient	Manual setting adjusted by the operator	0.21 (room air) to 1% (100% oxygen)
Room air	Ambient air oxygen concentration	Manual setting adjusted by the operator	21% (0.21 FiO_2)
Condition			
Hypoxemia	Inadequate level of oxygen either to the body as a whole (general hypoxia) or to a specific region (tissue hypoxia). Can be caused by hypoventilation, ventilation–perfusion mismatch, right-to-left shunt, diffusion impairment, reduced inspired oxygen tension, genetic disorders of hemoglobin oxygen affinity, and other hemoglobin issues that affect oxygen delivery.	PaO_2	80–100 mm Hg (10.7–13.3 kPa)
Hyperoxia	Excess of supplemental oxygen in blood	PaO_2	100 mm Hg (13.3 kPa)

ABG = arterial blood gas.

Data from Krauss, B., Falk, J. L., & Ladde, J. G. (2020). Carbon dioxide monitoring (capnography). *UpToDate*. Retrieved January 6, 2022, from https://www.uptodate.com/contents/carbon-dioxide-monitoring-capnography?search=carbon%20dioxide%20monitoring%20(capnography)&source=search_result&selectedTitle=1~150&usage_type=default&display_rank=1; Theodore, A. (2022, January 19). Measures of oxygenation and mechanisms of hypoxemia. *UpToDate*. Retrieved February 10, 2022, from https://www.uptodate.com/contents/measures-of-oxygenation-and-mechanisms-of-hypoxemia?search=Arterial%20blood%20gases%20definitions&topicRef=1648&source=see_link#H9

Chapter 15, "The Older Trauma Patient," for additional information.
- Tachypnea: A sign of compensation when a person experiences diminished oxygenation and perfusion.

Nursing Care of the Trauma Patient with Airway and Ventilation Problems

Refer to Chapter 4, "Initial Assessment," for the systematic approach to the care of the trauma patient. The following assessment parameters are specific to airway and ventilation.

Preparation

Preparation includes safe practice and triage.

Safe Practice, Safe Care

A patent airway, accompanied by effective oxygenation and ventilation, is an essential component of an optimal outcome in the trauma patient. Preparation for the arrival of the trauma patient with potential airway or ventilation compromise includes the following:

- Equipment: Ensure the availability and good working order of airway equipment and supplies in various sizes to accommodate all patients.
- Communication: Determine whether the appropriately trained personnel are all present, whether anyone else needs to be alerted to the trauma resuscitation, who will function in which roles, and who will perform identified tasks.
- Education: Trauma education includes a review of airway and ventilation, as well as hands-on practice in management of the airway, early identification of changes or deterioration in patient condition, and proficiency with utilizing and troubleshooting relevant equipment.

Triage

The prehospital report can provide clues to potential risks for airway and/or ventilation compromise and should include the following:

- Mechanism of injury
- Injuries sustained:
  - Facial, neck, or thoracic trauma
  - Head trauma
  - Inhalation injury and/or thermal or chemical burns
- Signs and symptoms
  - Altered mental status
  - Complaints of dyspnea, dysphagia, or dysphonia
  - Indications of substance use
  - Nausea or vomiting

Primary Survey

The primary survey begins with assessing the patient's alertness and airway.

A: Alertness and Airway (with Simultaneous Cervical Spine Stabilization)

Failure to adequately assess the airway and recognize when an airway intervention is needed can result in a preventable death.[1,40] After recognition of and intervention for any life-threatening external hemorrhage, identifying any airway problem is the next essential step. Once a problem has been identified, lifesaving interventions are implemented.

Cervical Spinal Motion Restriction

Cervical spinal motion restriction is *always* a part of the alertness and airway assessment, and it is particularly important in the patient with a significant mechanism of injury or suspected spinal injury. Patients with distracting injuries (significant blood loss, open fractures) and those with an altered mental status are presumed to have sustained a spinal cord injury until proven otherwise.[2,4,34,43] See Chapter 10, "Spinal and Musculoskeletal Trauma," for additional information on cervical spine clearance and spinal injuries.

Minimizing unwanted movement of the spine[14] can be accomplished by using either of the following techniques:

- Manual stabilization: Two hands holding the patient's head and neck in alignment.
- Spinal motion restriction (SMR): A correctly sized, semi-rigid cervical collar securely fastened. Apply spinal motion restriction to the entire spine until further clearance is obtained.[4]

Assess for Alertness

Use the **AVPU** mnemonic to determine the patient's level of alertness (**Table 5-2**). If the patient is not alert, their ability to protect their airway may be lost.

Open the Airway

Until injury to the cervical spine is ruled out, it is essential to maintain SMR. See Chapter 4, "Initial Assessment," for additional information. While maintaining SMR, assess the airway for patency:

- Talk to the patient. Asking the patient their name, current location, and whether they are able to open

Nursing Care of the Trauma Patient with Airway and Ventilation Problems

TABLE 5-2 Using the AVPU Mnemonic

Letter	Level	Description
A	Alert	The patient is alert and responsive.
V	Verbal	The patient responds to verbal stimulation.
P	Pain	The patient responds only to painful stimulation.
U	Unresponsive	The patient is unresponsive.

- To perform the jaw-thrust maneuver, do the following:
  1. Stand at the head of the bed.
  2. Place your index fingers under the angle of the lower jaw on each side of the patient's face, palms close to or on each cheekbone for stabilization.
  3. Gently move the mandible upward (vertically). This technique makes the airway more visible and creates space for an oropharyngeal airway (OPA), if indicated.[46]
- SMR must be maintained to minimize the risk of further injury in any patient with a suspected cervical spine injury. Spinal motion restriction is best achieved when two people perform the jaw-thrust procedure: One person maintains SMR while the second person performs the jaw-thrust procedure as previously described.

Once the airway is open, continue with the airway assessment. Inspect for the following:

- Deformities
- Lacerations
- Edema
- Blistering of the lips and oral mucosa from inhalation injury
- Fluids (blood, vomit, secretions)
- Foreign objects and loose or missing teeth (including dentures)
- Tongue obstruction

Listen for the following:

- Abnormal sounds (snoring, gurgling, stridor)
- Vocal quality abnormalities (hoarse voice, straining)

Palpate for the following:

- Maxillofacial bony deformity
- Subcutaneous emphysema[32]

If the patient has a definitive airway in place, assess for correct placement of the airway device before moving to the next step of the primary survey. Assessment for proper placement of a definitive airway includes the following three steps:

1. Attachment of a CO_2 detector device; after 5 to 6 breaths, assessment for the presence of exhaled CO_2 (**Appendix 5-1**).
2. Observation of adequate rise and fall of the chest with assisted ventilation.
3. Auscultation, first for absence of gurgling over the epigastrium, and then for presence of bilateral breath sounds.

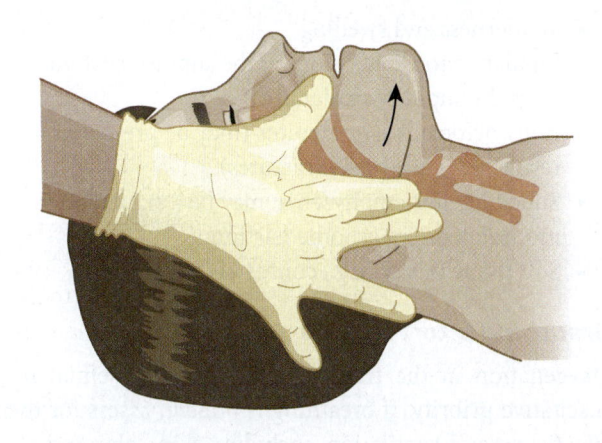

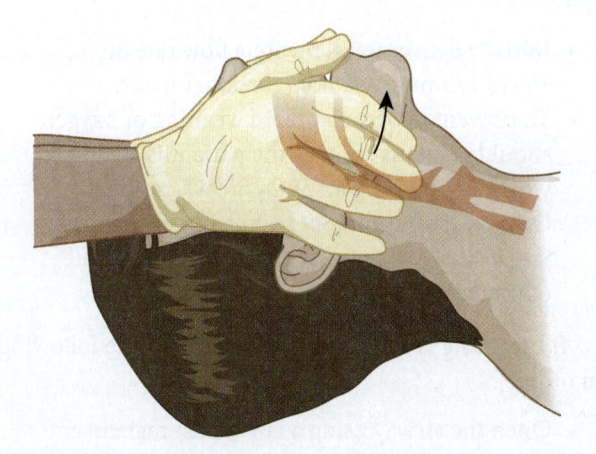

Figure 5-4 *Jaw-thrust maneuver.*

their mouth is a simple technique for determining whether the patient is alert.

- If the patient is unable to open their mouth, responds only to pain, or is unresponsive, use the jaw-thrust maneuver (**Figure 5-4**)[37] to open the airway and assess for obstruction.

Airway Interventions

If the airway is patent, proceed with the following understanding:

- An airway that is currently patent is not guaranteed to stay that way. It is essential to continuously monitor airway patency.
  - Note any potential risks for airway obstruction, such as injury to the mouth or lips; active bleeding; evidence of electrical, chemical, or thermal burns; nausea or vomiting; or decreasing level of consciousness.

If the airway is *not* patent, do the following:

- Use the jaw-thrust maneuver to safely open the airway while maintaining spinal motion restriction.
- Suction for blood, vomitus, or secretions; use care not to stimulate the gag reflex because this can cause vomiting, leading to aspiration risk.
- The tongue may be the cause, and further intervention might be warranted.
- Insert an airway adjunct (see the section "Airway Adjuncts" in this chapter):
  - Oral and nasal airways can be used to support the patient's spontaneous breathing and optimize the effectiveness of artificial ventilations when using a bag-mask device.
  - Keep in mind that basic airway adjuncts are temporary measures. If an airway adjunct is tolerated by the patient, a definitive airway (see the section "Definitive Airways" in this chapter) must be considered.
- Always reassess the effectiveness of any airway intervention.

B: Breathing and Ventilation

To assess breathing, expose the patient's chest and complete the steps outlined in this section.
Inspect for the presence of:

- Spontaneous breathing
- Symmetric, adequate rise and fall of the chest
- Depth, pattern, and rate of respiration
- Work of breathing, including the use of accessory muscles; diaphragmatic or abdominal breathing in the adult patient; and suprasternal, substernal, or intercostal retractions in the pediatric patient
- Nasal flaring, grunting, or head bobbing
- Skin color: observe for pallor, duskiness, or cyanosis
- Jugular venous distention and position of the trachea
- Signs of inhalation injury: singed nasal hairs, facial burns
- Open pneumothorax (also known as a sucking chest wound)

Auscultate for the following:

- Diminished or absent breath sounds, which can be the result of bronchoconstriction, airway obstruction, or inadequate ventilation as a response to pain, pneumothorax, or hemothorax
- When auscultating lung sounds, listen bilaterally at the second intercostal space midclavicular line and at the fifth intercostal space at the anterior axillary line.

Palpate for the following:

- Tenderness and swelling
- Jugular venous pulsations at the suprasternal notch or in the supraclavicular area
- Bony deformities or crepitus (may be present as a result of sternal or rib fractures)
- Subcutaneous emphysema: may be a sign of pneumothorax or pneumomediastinum
- Soft tissue injury (e.g., contusion, lacerations)

Breathing Interventions

Oxygenation in the trauma patient is an essential resuscitative priority. If breathing is *present,* assess for the effectiveness of ventilation, including skin color and respiratory effort.

- Initially deliver oxygen with a flow rate of 10–15 L/minute via nonrebreather mask.
- To prevent hyperoxia, rapid weaning of oxygen should occur as soon as the patient is stabilized, while maintaining an SpO_2 of 94% or greater. Oxygen saturation (SpO_2) in a target range of 94–98% is associated with effective, adequate oxygenation.[27]

If breathing is absent or inadequate, do the following in order:

- Open the airway using a jaw-thrust maneuver (while maintaining SMR) and insert an airway adjunct (OPA or NPA as indicated).
- If the patient remains apneic or without adequate ventilation, assist ventilations with a bag-mask device.
  - Attach the bag-mask device to an oxygen source and administer one breath every 6 seconds (10 breaths per minute).[5] Deliver each breath over 1 second.[5]

Using two providers is the most effective way to open the patient's airway while maintaining an adequate mask seal. If possible, use the two-person bag-mask method and do the following[46]:

- Provider 1 covers the patient's nose and mouth with the mask portion of the bag-mask device (the mask should not extend beyond the chin or cover the eyes).
  - Position the fingers so that the last three digits (pinky, ring, and middle) spread along the mandible, forming the letter "E." The last digit should be placed by the angle of the jaw with the middle finger under the chin, lifting the jaw upward.[5]
  - Place the thumb and index finger on top of the mask so they form the letter "C" around the neck of the mask, pressing the mask onto the patient's face and ensuring a good seal.[5]
- Provider 2 operates the operates the bag-mask device by slowly squeezing just enough to produce visible chest rise and fall every 6 seconds.[5]
- If only one person is available, they should be positioned at the head of the bed and use the "C-E" placement of the fingers and hand, as previously described. Using this technique, the rescuer creates an adequate seal between the mask and face with one hand while delivering the breaths with the other, as already described.
- Excessive volume delivered with the bag-mask and rapid rates have been associated with gastric distention, which can cause vomiting and aspiration, as well as barotrauma.[9]
- Life-threatening issues identified in the breathing portion of the primary assessment require rapid identification and immediate intervention before proceeding to the next step in the primary survey. These injuries can include the following (see Chapter 8, "Thoracic and Neck Trauma"):
  - Tension pneumothorax
  - Flail chest
  - Hemothorax
  - Open pneumothorax
- Consider other conditions as a source of inadequate ventilation, such as the following:
  - Preexisting pulmonary disease
  - Circumferential burns to the chest
  - Pain
  - Spinal cord injury (depending on location, can often cause diaphragmatic breathing, inadequate ventilation, and paralysis of the intercostal muscles)
  - Multiple rib fractures and possible flail segment(s)
  - Blunt thoracic trauma

Airway Adjuncts

Simple airway adjuncts, such as nasopharyngeal or oropharyngeal airways, are invaluable for establishing airway patency. They work by stenting open the upper airway to enable spontaneous patient respirations or to help facilitate artificial ventilation with a bag-mask device.

Nasopharyngeal Airway

A nasopharyngeal airway (NPA), also known as a nasal trumpet, is a hollow, soft, flexible tube that is inserted into the naris and down into the posterior pharynx. An NPA can be used in patients who are conscious, semiconscious, or unconscious and have an intact gag reflex.[5] An NPA is contraindicated in any patient with facial trauma or a basilar skull fracture because of the risk of placing it into the cranial cavity.[5] When inserting an NPA, consider the following[5,46]:

- Use the largest diameter that can easily be inserted into the naris.
  - Compare the outer circumference of the NPA with the lumen of the naris. If the NPA causes sustained blanching to the naris, it is too large.[5]
- Select the correct length by measuring from the tip of the patient's nose to the tip of the patient's earlobe.
  - An NPA that is too long may enter the esophagus, causing gastric distention and decreased effectiveness of ventilation.[46]
  - Improper sizing often causes traumatic epistaxis, increasing the risk for blood or clot aspiration.[46]
- Apply a water-soluble lubricant to the NPA before insertion, and then do the following:
  - Insert the NPA with the bevel facing the nasal septum.
  - Advance the NPA toward the posterior pharynx until the flange rests against the naris.
  - If resistance is met, rotate the NPA slightly away from the septum and attempt to advance toward the posterior pharynx.
- After insertion, reassess airway patency, ventilation, and oxygenation, and determine the need for a definitive airway. If ventilation or oxygenation is inadequate, consider the use of bag-mask ventilation to support the patient.

Oropharyngeal Airway

An oropharyngeal airway (OPA) is used in the unresponsive patient without a gag reflex as a temporary measure to open the airway and facilitate ventilation until the airway can be definitively secured (see the section "Definitive Airways"). A correctly sized OPA will hold the tongue in its normal anatomic position and follows its natural curvature.[46] If the OPA is too large, it may occlude the patient's airway, hinder the use of the face mask, or damage laryngeal structures. If it is too small, it may travel posteriorly and become an occlusive foreign body, or it can occlude the airway by pushing the tongue backward. When inserting an OPA, consider the following[5,46]:

- An OPA should only be used in an unresponsive patient who does not have a gag reflex and cannot maintain their airway. Use of an OPA in a responsive patient or a patient with gag reflex could result in vomiting and aspiration.
- Measure the correct size by placing the proximal end (flange) of the OPA at the corner of the mouth; the tip should just reach the angle of the mandible.
- Depress the tongue using a tongue blade or a rigid suction device. Advance the OPA straight over the tongue, or insert the OPA at a 90-degree angle, and then turn the OPA while avoiding trauma to the palate.
  - With either method, it is essential to take care not to push the tongue backward, causing it to occlude the airway.
- After insertion, reassess airway patency, ventilation, and oxygenation, and anticipate the need for a definitive airway. If ventilation or oxygenation is inadequate, consider the use of bag-mask ventilation to support the patient.

Extraglottic Airways

Extraglottic airway (EGA) devices can be used for initial airway management, after other failed airway attempts, or when unsuccessful intubation is anticipated. These devices are inserted blindly (without direct visualization) and are positioned above or posterior to the larynx to facilitate immediate ventilation and oxygenation. Some newer EGAs also have a port to allow gastric decompression, which may decrease the risk of aspiration.[26] Extraglottic airway devices can be divided into two categories: supraglottic and retroglottic[20,26]:

- Supraglottic airway (SGA)
  - The devices are placed above the glottis and seal the glottic opening.
  - SGAs do provide protection against aspiration.
  - The i-gel and laryngeal mask airway (LMA) (**Figure 5-5**) are examples of an SGA. Some LMAs enable intubation through the LMA, which is advantageous in emergency airway situations.

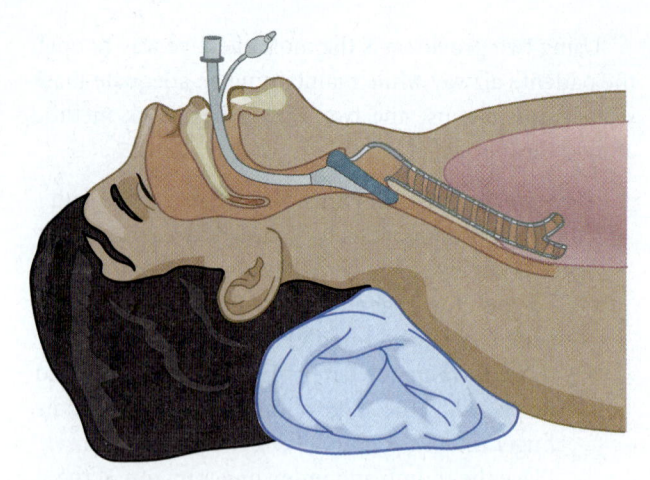

Figure 5-5 *Supraglottic airway.*
Modified from Olson, K. (2018). 3.1 ABCs of poisoning care – Resuscitation. WikiTox. https://www.wikitox.org/doku.php?id=wikitox:3.1_abcs_resuscitation

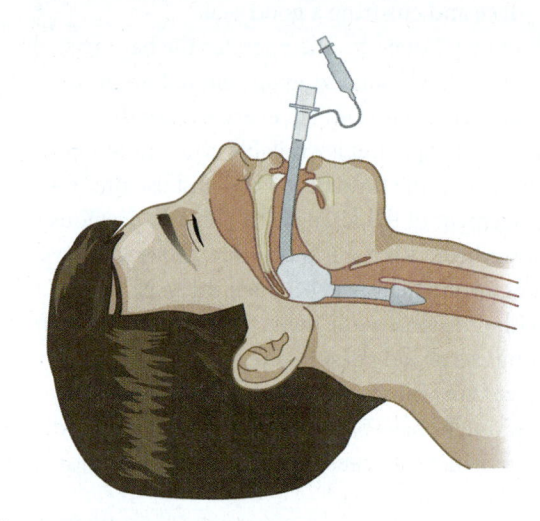

Figure 5-6 *Retroglottic airway.*

- Retroglottic airway (RGA)
  - This device sits in the upper esophagus, posterior to the glottis (**Figure 5-6**). An example of this is the King tube.
  - RGAs have two balloon cuffs: one pharyngeal and one esophageal
  - Ventilation fenestrations are located between the balloons.[26]
  - This design allows air to passively enter the lungs while preventing gastric distention.

Definitive Airways

A definitive airway is a tube that has been securely placed in the trachea with the cuff inflated below the vocal cords.[1] In an emergency or trauma situation, there are three indications for immediate definite airway management[16,31]:

- Failure of the patient to protect their airway
- Failure to maintain oxygenation or ventilation
- A specific, anticipated clinical course

Indications for securing a definitive airway in the trauma patient may include the following[1,16,31]:

- Severe oral, maxillofacial, or head trauma
- Cardiac arrest or stroke
- Hemorrhagic shock, hypoxia
- Airway disruption, compression, or respiratory distress
- Glasgow Coma Scale score ≤ 8
- Blunt or penetrating neck injury
- Expanding hematoma in or near the neck
- Smoke inhalation or caustic ingestion

Definitive airways are placed by licensed practitioners with demonstrated competency and whose practice standards include the performance of these interventions and are in accordance with organizational policies. Trauma nurses help prepare the patient and necessary equipment, assist during the procedure, and continuously reassess the patient postprocedure. Refer to **Appendix 5-2**, **Appendix 5-3**, and **Appendix 5-4** for more information regarding placing a definitive airway.

Types of Definitive Airways

An endotracheal tube (ETT) is the most commonly placed definitive airway, but other alternatives exist for patients with difficult airways.

Endotracheal Tubes

ETTs are semi-rigid, slightly curved opaque tubes designed for passage into the upper airway. Most have an inflatable cuff at the distal portion of the tube; this is designed to occlude the space between the ETT and the trachea, thereby preventing aspiration and enabling consistent delivery of tidal volumes. Other considerations include the following:

- ETTs can be inserted via the oral or nasal route.
- Oral insertion is more common.
- Nasotracheal intubation (NTI) requires a patient who is breathing.[1]
  - NTI has a higher failure rate and is not recommended in pregnant patients because of increased risk for bleeding from fragility of the nasal mucosa.
  - NTI is rarely used in the trauma setting because of the risks associated with facial and basilar skull fractures.

Endotracheal intubation (ETI) is an aerosol-generating procedure that increases transmission of certain organisms. It is imperative that full contact and airborne precautions, including the use of the appropriate mask or respirator, is used according to organization policies. When possible, ETI should be performed in an airborne infection isolation room by an experienced provider, with additional help located *outside* the room.[23]

Cricothyroidotomy

If a clinician is unable to intubate or oxygenate a patient (i.e., when less invasive techniques have failed or are deemed likely to be unsuccessful), an emergency cricothyroidotomy may be necessary.[33] A cricothyroidotomy can be performed using either a needle catheter or a surgical insertion technique. The needle insertion method involves passing an over-the-needle catheter through the cricothyroid membrane and can be performed on a patient of any age. In a surgical cricothyroidotomy, an incision is made through the patient's cricothyroid membrane, and a tracheostomy tube or ETT is inserted through the incision (**Figure 5-7**). The surgical approach is preferred in adults and children over 12 years of age because it provides more effective ventilation than an over-the-needle catheter, given the larger diameter tube.[1,33] The most common complication is bleeding.[29] Other possible complications include the following[41]:

- Laceration of the thyroid cartilage, cricoid cartilage, or tracheal rings
- Perforation of the posterior trachea
- Unintentional tracheostomy
- Tracheal trauma
- Passage of the tube into an extratracheal location (false tract)
  - The development of subcutaneous air after this procedure is highly suspicious for this issue.
- Infection

Difficult Airways

It is crucial to identify, in advance, any patient characteristics or factors that may result in a failed intubation and

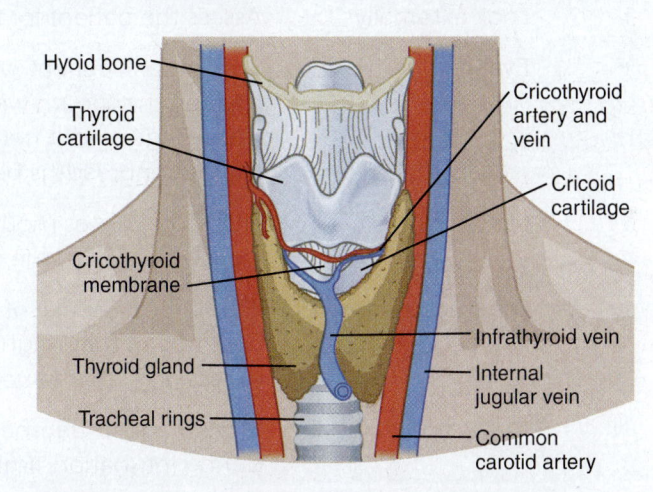

Figure 5-7 *Anterior cervical anatomy of the larynx and trachea.*

potential adverse outcome. Signs of a potentially difficult airway include the presence of any of the following:

- Cervical spine injury
- Facial trauma
- Obesity
- Signs of swelling or inflammation (stridor)
- Anatomic variations (short neck, cervical arthritis)
- Signs of inhalation injury

The **LEMON** mnemonic is one of many tools that can be used to assess for airway difficulty (**Table 5-3**).[1,8]

A video laryngoscope is a tool used to facilitate successful intubation. This approach uses a video camera at the end of the laryngoscope blade to provide visual display of the glottic opening and may decrease cervical spine motion compared with other methods of intubation.[39,44]

Drug-Assisted Intubation

Drug-assisted intubation (DAI) refers to the use of any medication(s) to facilitate intubation.[7] Rapid sequence intubation (RSI) is used in unstable patients to rapidly secure an airway by a near simultaneous administration of a sedative agent followed by a neuromuscular blocking agent.[7,11] The purpose of this approach is to minimize the time between the loss of protective airway reflexes and endotracheal intubation in order to decrease the risk of aspiration while increasing the likelihood of successful intubation.[7] The sedative (induction agent) is always given before the neuromuscular blocking agent, otherwise the patient may be fully aware and experiencing pain but be unable to respond. Chemical paralysis without sedation may cause adverse physiological responses, including tachycardia, hypertension, and increased intracranial pressure.[11]

Administration of the induction agent and the neuromuscular blocking agent will render the patient apneic. Therefore, preoxygenation is an important component in preparation for DAI because it prolongs the time to hypoxia. To prepare the patient for this apneic phase, high-flow oxygen is administered at the maximum concentration for at least 3 minutes prior to intubation attempts.[19] The high concentration of oxygen replaces other mixed gases in the lungs and creates a reserve of oxygen.[7] This reserve enables the patient to maintain the oxygen saturation during the apneic phase of intubation (also known as apneic oxygenation).[7,19] See Appendix 5-2, Appendix 5-3, and Appendix 5-4 for additional information regarding DAI and RSI.

Breathing Intervention (Intubation) Reassessment

After intubation, the cuff is inflated, and placement is confirmed using the following:

1. A CO_2 detector device is attached. After 5 to 6 breaths, assessment for the presence of exhaled CO_2 is conducted.
2. Rise and fall of the chest with assisted ventilation is observed for adequacy.

TABLE 5-3 The LEMON Mnemonic for Assessing a Difficult Airway

Letter	Step	Description
L	Look externally	Assess the patient for facial trauma, deformity, or abnormal anatomy.
E	Evaluate	3-3-2 rule. A patient who will not be a difficult intubation will be able to open the mouth wide enough to allow three fingers. There will be a three-finger width between the chin and the neck. Finally, there will be two finger breadths between the neck/mandible junction and the hyoid.
M	Mallampati score	This score relates mouth opening to the size of the tongue. It ranges from I (easy) to IV (extreme difficulty).
O	Obstruction/obesity	Assess for presence of hematoma, upper airway injury, or another obstruction that might obstruct tube passage. Obese patients have an excess of glottic tissue, which may make intubation difficult.
N	Neck mobility	Most, if not all, trauma patients require inline cervical spine stabilization during intubation, limiting the ability to visibly inspect the glottis.

Data from Brown, C. A., III, & Walls, R. M. (2018). Identification of the difficult and failed airway. In C. A. Brown III, J. C. Sakles, & N. W. Mick (Eds.), *The Walls manual of emergency airway management* (5th ed., pp. 10–16). Wolters Kluwer.

3. Auscultation for absence of gurgling over the epigastrium and presence of bilateral breath sounds is conducted as follows:
   - Listen over the epigastrium first because gurgling may indicate that the tube is in the esophagus.
   - Listen for the presence of bilateral breath sounds at the midaxillary and midclavicular lines.
     - If breath sounds are absent, there is no rise and fall of the chest, gurgling is heard at the epigastrium, and there is no evidence of exhaled CO_2, remove the ETT and oxygenate the patient before another intubation attempt.
     - If breath sounds are only heard on the right side, the ETT is likely in the right mainstem bronchus and has been inserted too far. It should be pulled back slowly until equal breath sounds are heard bilaterally.
     - If breath sounds are heard bilaterally, and there is positive evidence of exhaled CO_2 on the colorimetric or capnography monitor, then secure the ETT and note the measurement at the teeth or gums and document.
   - Prepare for mechanical ventilation.
   - Monitor the patient's skin color for improvement.
   - A chest radiograph for verification of ETT depth should be obtained after the secondary survey.

G: Get Adjuncts and Give Comfort

Pulse oximetry and capnography are used in conjunction with the primary survey and ongoing assessments to assess for adequacy of oxygenation and effectiveness of ventilation. See Chapter 4, "Initial Assessment," for additional information regarding adjuncts and comfort.

L: Laboratory Studies

Laboratory studies should be obtained based on necessity and clinical indication.[40] Those specific to airway and ventilation may include the following:

- Arterial blood gases (ABGs) provide information through analysis of acid–base balance, lactic acid, and base excess. ABGs directly measure pH, partial pressure of oxygen (PaO_2), and carbon dioxide ($PaCO_2$), supplying information about oxygenation and ventilation. ABGs also provide indirect measure of the bicarbonate concentration (HCO_3), base deficit, and arterial oxygen saturation (SaO_2).
  - A base deficit can serve as an endpoint measurement of the adequacy of cellular perfusion and can be useful in guiding resuscitation when used in conjunction with serum lactate.[40]
- Serum lactate serves as an indicator of end-organ perfusion and tissue hypoxia, and as a guide to resuscitation.[40] A lactate that normalizes within 24 hours of injury because of resuscitation and supportive care is associated with improved outcomes and mortality rates.[22]

O: Oxygenation and Ventilation

Several methods and indicators are used to measure oxygenation during ventilation. Oxygen is weaned based on clinical condition, and the indicators presented next, to avoid hyperoxia.

Pulse Oximetry

Pulse oximetry is a noninvasive method of providing oxygenation information and detecting changes in oxygenation that cannot always be detected clinically.[18] Pulse oximetry reflects the percentage of hemoglobin that is oxygen saturated (bound) relative to total hemoglobin. It does not differentiate between oxygen and carbon monoxide.[36] See Chapter 4, "Initial Assessment," for additional information.

Unreliable readings may occur that are due to the following factors[18,30]:

- Poor peripheral perfusion caused by vasoconstriction, hypotension, or hypothermia
- Inflation of blood pressure cuff above the sensor
- Carbon monoxide poisoning (carboxyhemoglobin)
- Methemoglobinemia
- Inherited abnormalities of hemoglobin, such as sickle cell disease
- Severe dehydration
- Improper placement of sensor
- Patient movement
- Skin pigmentation
- Accuracy decreases below 83% saturation.[18]

The Oxyhemoglobin Dissociation Curve

The oxyhemoglobin dissociation curve (**Figure 5-8**) indicates the correlation between tissue oxygenation (PaO_2) and hemoglobin molecule saturation (SpO_2 or SaO_2). The P_{50} value describes the oxygen pressure when the hemoglobin molecule is 50% saturated. Normal P_{50} is 26.7 mm Hg (3.56 kPa).[30] A shift in the curve indicates a change in this relationship.

- A shift to the *right* occurs in an environment of high metabolic demand. Hemoglobin's affinity for oxygen decreases, and hemoglobin holds less tightly to the oxygen molecule, releasing it more easily to the tissues.[30]

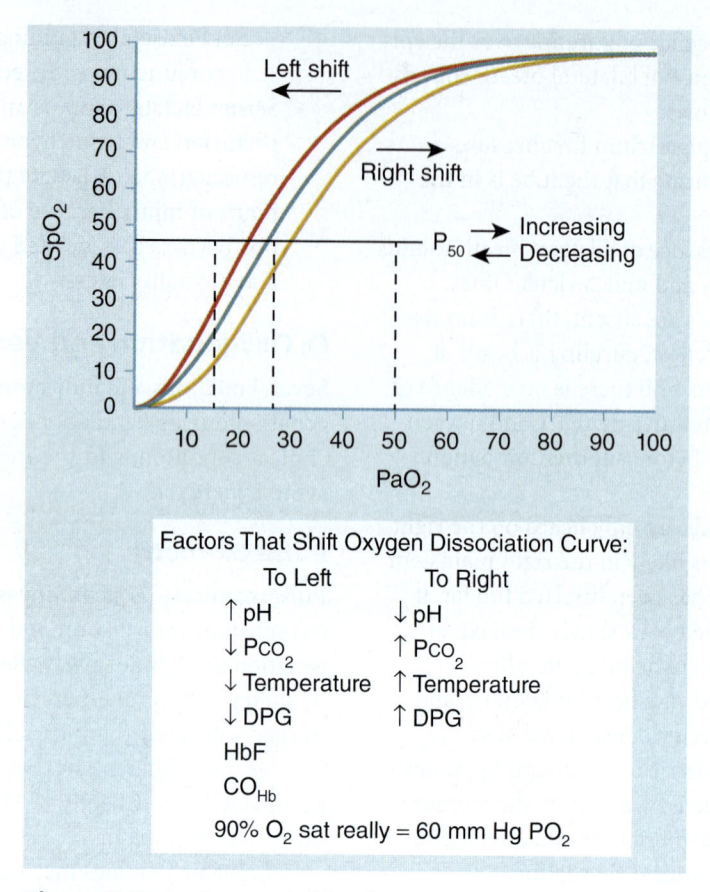

Figure 5-8 Oxyhemoglobin dissociation curve.
DPG = 2,3 diphosphoglycerate; HbF = fetal hemoglobin; CO$_{Hb}$ = carboxyhemoglobin.

- A shift to the *left* occurs in an environment of low metabolic demand. Hemoglobin's affinity for oxygen increases, and hemoglobin holds more tightly to the oxygen molecule, releasing it less easily to the tissues.[30]

It is essential that normothermia and normocarbia be maintained to improve diffusion of oxygen into the cell. See Figure 5-8 for factors that affect a shift in the oxygen dissociation curve.

Carbon Dioxide Monitoring

CO$_2$ monitoring provides instantaneous information about ventilation (pulmonary system elimination of CO$_2$), perfusion (CO$_2$ transport through the vascular system), and metabolism (CO$_2$ production from cellular metabolism). If CO$_2$ measurement is taken at the end of a breath, it is called end-tidal CO$_2$ (ETCO$_2$). CO$_2$ monitors are either qualitative or quantitative (Appendix 5-1).[25]

Qualitative devices (colorimetric detectors) use a specially treated litmus paper that changes color in the presence of CO$_2$.[25] It is used, in conjunction with physical assessment findings previously discussed, to confirm ETT placement.[25]

Quantitative monitors provide a numeric (capnometry) value and a continuous waveform (capnography), indicating both real-time measures and enabling trending over time.[25] Capnometers provide only a numeric value after each breath. There is no associated waveform. The normal range for ETCO$_2$ is 35–45 mm Hg (4.7– 6.0 kPa).[25]

ETCO$_2$ device readings may be affected by the following[25]:

- Ventilator settings and malfunctions
- Ventilator tubing disconnections and leaks
- ETT obstruction
- An improperly functioning device that was damaged or had been open to the air
- Esophageal intubation with ingestion of carbonated beverages, acidic solutions, or vinegar
- Ventilation/perfusion mismatches (e.g., acute pulmonary edema)

Diagnostics and Interventions for Airway and Ventilation Problems

A chest radiograph can determine the presence of a hemothorax, pneumothorax, or rib fractures and can help to confirm ETT placement. If the trauma patient is hemodynamically stable, a computed tomography scan may be ordered to further evaluate for intrathoracic injury. See Chapter 8, "Thoracic and Neck Trauma," for additional information.

Reevaluation and Post-Resuscitation Care

Frequent reevaluation of airway patency and adequacy of ventilation is essential and includes the following elements:

- Alertness and level of consciousness and ability to protect the airway.[28]
- Respiratory rate, pattern, work of breathing, and breath sounds.
- Vital signs, including pulse oximetry and capnography.
- ABGs.
- Response to interventions.
- Tolerance for and effectiveness of mechanical ventilation. Use the **DOPE** mnemonic to troubleshoot ventilator, capnography, or pulse oximetry alarms (**Box 5-1**).[21]
- Assess pain and sedation levels, and provide pharmacologic and nonpharmacologic interventions to facilitate effective breathing and ventilation.

> **BOX 5-1** Troubleshooting Alarms: DOPE Mnemonic
>
> The DOPE mnemonic is as follows:
>
> - **D**isplacement: ETT migration above the vocal cords or down the right mainstem
> - **O**bstruction: Patient biting on the ETT, kinking in the ETT, mucus plugs or blood clot in the ETT, aspiration, or other types of impediments
> - **P**neumothorax: Development of a new or tension pneumothorax
> - **E**quipment: Leak in ventilator tubing, ETT cuff pressure loss causing air leak, disconnection of any portion in the breathing circuit, or other electronic or mechanical malfunction

Definitive Care or Transport

Patients with airway or ventilation problems may require one of the following:

- Transfer to a higher level of care (designated trauma center)
- Admission to an inpatient unit
- Emergent transfer to the operating room/suite or interventional radiology

Summary

Maintenance of a patent airway and effective ventilation are paramount for achieving optimal patient outcomes. Assessment for and recognition of any actual or potential airway or ventilation issue are essential to the care of the trauma patient. If an airway problem is not identified during the assessment, the results can be catastrophic for the patient. Therefore, it is of the utmost importance for nurses to be able to assess and recognize life-threatening presentations and to intervene quickly and accurately. Familiarity with types of airway adjuncts and their use, as well as a thorough understanding of the anatomy and physiology associated with airway and ventilation, will assist the nurse in conducting lifesaving interventions expediently.

References

1. American College of Surgeons. (2018). Airway and ventilatory management. In *Advanced trauma life support: Student course manual* (10th ed., pp. 22–41).
2. American College of Surgeons. (2018). Initial assessment and management. In *Advanced trauma life support: Student course manual* (10th ed., pp. 2–21).
3. American College of Surgeons. (2018). Pediatric trauma. In *Advanced trauma life support: Student course manual* (10th ed., pp. 186–212).
4. American College of Surgeons. (2022). *Best practice guidelines: Spine injury*. https://www.facs.org/media/k45gikqv/spine_injury_guidelines.pdf
5. American Heart Association. (2020). Part 3: High-performance teams. In *Advanced cardiovascular life support manual* (pp. 91–164).
6. Brasher, V. L. (2020). Structure and function of the pulmonary system. In S. E. Huether, K. L. McCance, & V. L. Brasher (Eds.). *Understanding pathophysiology* (7th ed. pp. 655–669). Elsevier.
7. Brown, C. A., III, & Sakles, J. C. (2020). Rapid sequence intubation for adults outside the operating room. *UpToDate*. Retrieved January 10, 2020, from https://www.uptodate.com/contents/rapid-sequence-intubation-for-adults-outside-the-operating-room

8. Brown, C. A., III, & Walls, R. M. (2018). Identification of the difficult and failed airway. In C. A. Brown III, J. C. Sakles, & N. W. Mick (Eds.), *The Walls manual of emergency airway management* (5th ed., pp. 10–16). Wolters Kluwer.
9. Bucher, J. T., Vashisht, R., Ladd, M., & Cooper, J. S. (2022, August 10). Bag mask ventilation. *StatPearls*. StatPearls Publishing. https://www.ncbi.nlm.nih.gov/books/NBK441924/
10. Caro, D. (2020). Pretreatment medications for rapid sequence intubation in adults outside the operating room. *UpToDate*. Retrieved January 10, 2020, from https://www.uptodate.com/contents/pretreatment-medications-for-rapid-sequence-intubation-in-adults-outside-the-operating-room
11. Caro, D. (2021). Induction agents for rapid sequence intubation in adults outside the operating room. *UpToDate*. Retrieved January 10, 2020, from https://www.uptodate.com/contents/induction-agents-for-rapid-sequence-intubation-in-adults-outside-the-operating-room
12. Caro, D. (2022). Neuromuscular blocking agents (NMBAs) for rapid sequence intubation in adults outside of the operating room. *UpToDate*. Retrieved January 10, 2020, from https://www.uptodate.com/contents/neuromuscular-blocking-agents-nmbas-for-rapid-sequence-intubation-in-adults-outside-of-the-operating-room
13. Castro, D., & Freeman, L. A. (2022, September 12). Oropharyngeal airway. *StatPearls*. StatPearls Publishing. https://www.ncbi.nlm.nih.gov/books/NBK470198/
14. Fischer, P. E., Perina, D. G., Delbridge, T. R., Fallat, M. E., Salomone, J. P., & Dodd, J. (2018). Spinal motion restriction in the trauma patient—A joint position statement. *Prehospital Emergency Care, 22*(6), 659–661. https://doi.org/10.1080/10903127.2018.1481476
15. Gaasch, S., & Andersen, K. (2020). Thoracic trauma. In K. A. McQuillan & M. B. Makic (Eds.), *Trauma nursing: From resuscitation to rehabilitation* (5th ed., pp. 503–552). Elsevier.
16. Galvagno, S., & Sappenfield, J. (2022). Anesthesia for adult trauma patients. *UpToDate*. Retrieved January 10, 2020, from https://www.uptodate.com/contents/anesthesia-for-adult-trauma-patients
17. Haddad, M., & Sharma, S. (2022, July 16). Physiology, lung. *StatPearls*. StatPearls Publishing. https://www.ncbi.nlm.nih.gov/books/NBK545177/
18. Hafen, B. B., & Sharma, S. (2022, August 8). Oxygen saturation. *StatPearls*. StatPearls Publishing. https://www.ncbi.nlm.nih.gov/books/NBK525974/
19. Hagberg, C. (2022). Preoxygenation and apneic oxygenation for airway management for anesthesia. *UpToDate*. Retrieved January 10, 2020, from https://www.uptodate.com/contents/preoxygenation-and-apneic-oxygenation-for-airway-management-for-anesthesia
20. Hernandez, M. C., Aho, J. M., Zielinski, M. D., Zietlow, S. P., Kim, B. D., & Morris, D. S. (2018). Definitive airway management after pre-hospital supraglottic airway insertion: Outcomes and a management algorithm for trauma patients. *American Journal of Emergency Medicine, 36*(1), 114–119. https://doi.org/10.1016/j.ajem.2017.09.028
21. Hou, P., & Baez, A. A. (2022). Mechanical ventilation of adults in the emergency department. *UpToDate*. Retrieved January 10, 2020, from https://www.uptodate.com/contents/mechanical-ventilation-of-adults-in-the-emergency-department/print
22. Johnson, M. C., Alarhayem, A., Convertino, V. Carter, R., Chung, K., Stewart, R., Myers, J., Dent, D., Liao, L., Cestero, R., Nicholson, S., Muir, M., Schwaca, M., Wampler, D., DeRosa, M., & Eastridge, B. J. (2017). Comparison of compensatory reserve and arterial lactate as markers of shock and resuscitation. *Journal of Trauma and Acute Care Surgery, 83*(4), 603–608. https://doi.org/10.1097/ta.0000000000001595
23. Karamchandani, K., Wheelwright, J., Yang, A. L., Westphal, N. D., Khanna, A. K., & Myatra, S. N. (2021). Emergency airway management outside the operating room: Current evidence and management strategies. *Anesthesia and Analgesia, 133*(3), 648–662. https://doi.org/10.1213/ANE.0000000000005644
24. Kenny, B. J., & Bordoni, B. (2021, November 14). Neuroanatomy, cranial nerve 10 (vagus nerve). *StatPearls*. StatPearls Publishing. https://www.ncbi.nlm.nih.gov/books/NBK537171/
25. Krauss, B., Falk, J. L., & Ladde, J. G. (2020). Carbon dioxide monitoring (capnography). *UpToDate*. Retrieved January 6, 2022, from https://www.uptodate.com/contents/carbon-dioxide-monitoring-capnography
26. Laurin, E. G. (2022). Extraglottic devices for emergency airway management in adults. *UpToDate*. Retrieved January 6, 2022, from https://www.uptodate.com/contents/extraglottic-devices-for-emergency-airway-management-in-adults
27. Leitch, P., Hudson, A. L., Griggs, J. E., Stolmeijer, R., Lyon, R. M., & Ter Avest, E., on behalf of Air Ambulance Kent Surrey Sussex. (2021). Incidence of hyperoxia in trauma patients receiving pre-hospital emergency anaesthesia: Results of a 5-year retrospective analysis. *Scandinavian Journal of Trauma, Resuscitation and Emergency Medicine, 29*(1), Article 134. https://doi.org/10.1186/s13049-021-00951-w
28. Louro, J., & Varon, A. J. (2021). Airway management in trauma. *International Anesthesiology Clinics, 59*(2), 10–16. https://doi.org/10.1097/AIA.0000000000000316
29. McKenna P., Desai, N. M., & Morley, E. J. (2022, July 25). Cricothyrotomy. *StatPearls*. StatPearls Publishing. https://www.ncbi.nlm.nih.gov/books/NBK537350/.
30. Mechem, C. C. (2022, February 2). Pulse oximetry. *UpToDate*. Retrieved February 2, 2022, from https://www.uptodate.com/contents/pulse-oximetry
31. Mills, T. J., & DeBlieux, P. (2022). Emergency airway management in the adult with direct airway trauma. *UpToDate*. Retrieved February 10, 2022, from https://www.uptodate.com/contents/emergency-airway-management-in-the-adult-with-direct-airway-trauma
32. Mitsusada, K., Dote, H., Tokutake, M., & Atsumi, T. (2022). Airway obstruction caused by massive subcutaneous emphysema due to blunt chest trauma. *BMJ Case Reports, 15*(7), Article e251068. https://casereports.bmj.com/content/15/7/e251068
33. Mittal, M. K. (2021). Needle cricothyroidotomy with percutaneous transtracheal ventilation. *UpToDate*. Retrieved

February 10, 2022, from https://www.uptodate.com/contents/needle-cricothyroidotomy-with-percutaneous-transtracheal-ventilation

34. Moeri, M., Rothenfluh, D. A., Laux, C. J., & Dominguez, D. E. (2020). Cervical spine clearance after blunt trauma: Current state of the art. *EFORT Open Reviews, 5*(4), 253–259. https://doi.org/10.1302/2058-5241.5.190047

35. Nagler, J. (2023). Emergency airway management in children: Unique pediatric considerations. *UpToDate.* Retrieved February 28, 2023, from https://www.uptodate.com/contents/emergency-airway-management-in-children-unique-pediatric-considerations

36. Nisar, S., Gibson, C. D., Sokolovic, M., & Shah, N. S. (2020). Pulse oximetry is unreliable in patients on veno-venous extracorporeal membrane oxygenation caused by unrecognized carboxyhemoglobinemia. *ASAIO Journal, 66*(10), 1105–1109. https://doi.org/10.1097/MAT.0000000000001144

37. Olson, K. (2018, September 1). 3.1 ABCs of poisoning care—Resuscitation. *WikiTox.* https://www.wikitox.org/doku.php?id=wikitox:3.1_abcs_resuscitation

38. Parker, B. K., Manning, S., & Winters, M. E. (2019). The crashing obese patient. *Western Journal of Emergency Medicine, 20*(2), 323–330. https://doi.org/10.5811/westjem.2018.12.41085

39. Parotto, M., & Law, J. S. (2022). Video laryngoscopes and optical stylets for airway management for anesthesia in adults. *UpToDate.* Retrieved February 10, 2022, from https://www.uptodate.com/contents/video-laryngoscopes-and-optical-stylets-for-airway-management-for-anesthesia-in-adults

40. Raja, A., & Zane, R. D. (2022). Initial management of trauma in adults. *UpToDate.* Retrieved February 10, 2022, from https://www.uptodate.com/contents/initial-management-of-trauma-in-adults

41. Sakles, J. (2021). Emergency cricothyrotomy (cricothyroidotomy). *UpToDate.* Retrieved February 10, 2022, from https://www.uptodate.com/contents/emergency-cricothyrotomy-cricothyroidotomy

42. Stacy, K. M. (2022). Pulmonary anatomy and physiology. In L. D. Urden, K. M. Stacy, & M. E. Lough (Eds.), *Critical care nursing: Diagnosis and management* (9th ed., pp. 421–440). Elsevier.

43. Stahel, P. F., & VanderHeiden, T. (2017). Spinal injuries. In E. E. Moore, D. V. Feliciano, & K. L. Mattox (Eds.), *Trauma* (8th ed., pp. 455–472). McGraw Hill.

44. Stahl, J. L., & Miller, A. C. (2020). What's new in critical illness and injury science? A look into trauma airway management. *International Journal of Critical Illness & Injury Science, 10*(1), 1–3. https://doi.org/10.4103/IJCIIS.IJCIIS_14_20

45. Theodore, A. (2022, January 19). Measures of oxygenation and mechanisms of hypoxemia. *UpToDate.* Retrieved February 10, 2022, from https://www.uptodate.com/contents/measures-of-oxygenation-and-mechanisms-of-hypoxemia

46. Wittels, K. A. (2022). Basic airway management in adults. *UpToDate.* Retrieved February 10, 2022, from https://www.uptodate.com/contents/basic-airway-management-in-adults

APPENDIX 5-1
Capnometry Devices

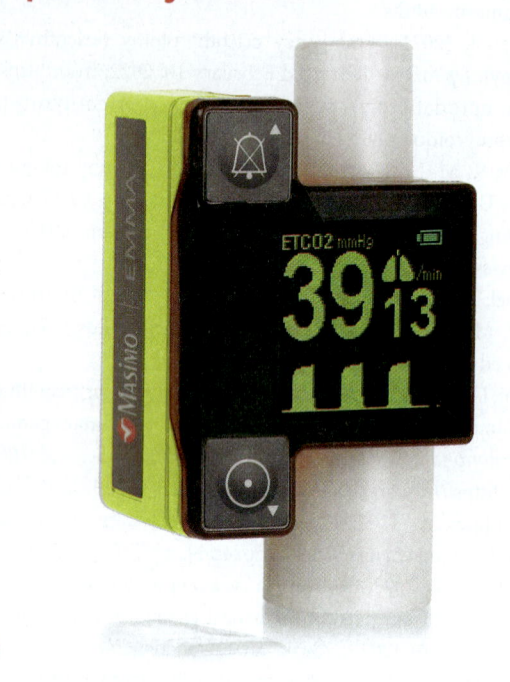

Numeric capnography devices: Measure and display ETCO$_2$ as a number on a digital or analogue monitor.

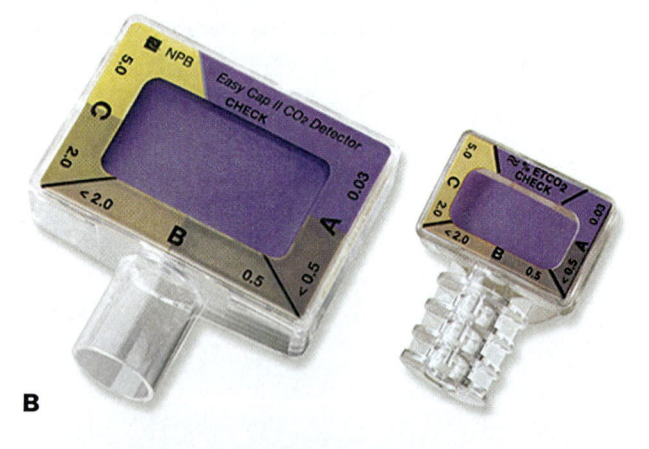

Colorimetric devices: Uses chemically treated indicators to detect exhaled carbon dioxide (ETCO$_2$).

- Evaluate the color change after 5–6 full breaths.
- Effective up to 2 hours, then discard.
- Review manufacturer instructions/color code key.

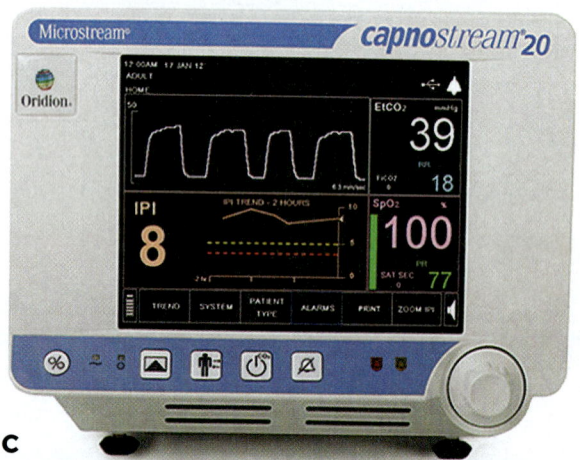

Graphical capnography devices: Provide a graphic/waveform display of the ETCO$_2$ instantaneously.

Ways to measure end-tidal carbon dioxide. **A.** *Numeric capnography device.* **B.** *Colorimetric detector.* **C.** *Capnography monitor.*

A. Courtesy of Masimo. **B, C.** © 2019 Medtronic. All rights reserved. Used with permission of Medtronic.

Appendix 5-1 Capnometry Devices

Capnography Waveforms and Their Meanings

Normal Capnography Waveform

Normal (35–45 mm Hg [4.7–6.0 kPa])

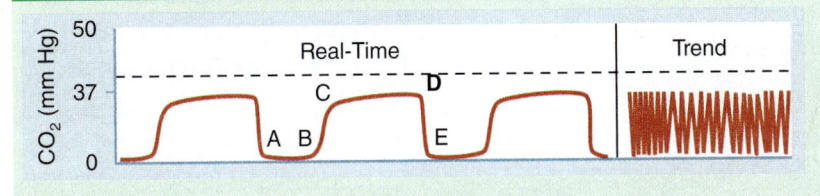

- A–B = Dead space ventilation
- B–C = Ascending expiratory phase
- C–D = Alveolar plateau
- **D = ETCO₂ value**
- D–E = Descending inspiratory phase

Breathing Variations

Hypercarbia (ETCO₂ . 45 mm Hg [6.0 kPa])

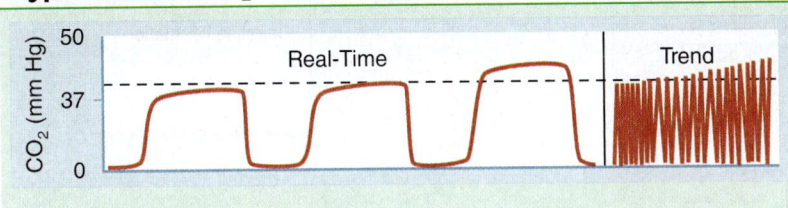

Possible causes include:
- Decrease in respiratory rate
- Decrease in tidal volume
- Increase in metabolic rate
- Rapid rise in body temperature (hyperthermia)

Hypocarbia (ETCO₂ , 35 mm Hg [4.7 kPa])

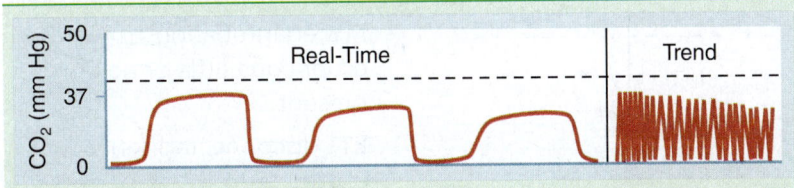

Possible causes include:
- Increase in respiratory rate
- Increase in tidal volume
- Decrease in metabolic rate
- Fall in body temperature

Muscle Relaxants Wearing Off

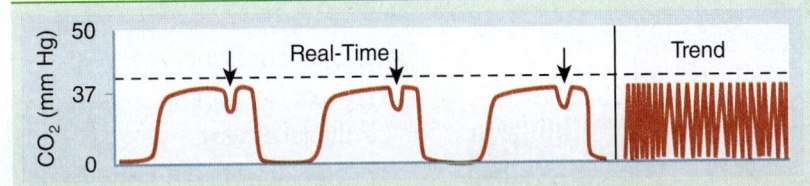

- Appear when muscle relaxants begin to subside
- Depth of cleft is inversely proportional to degree of drug activity

Apnea

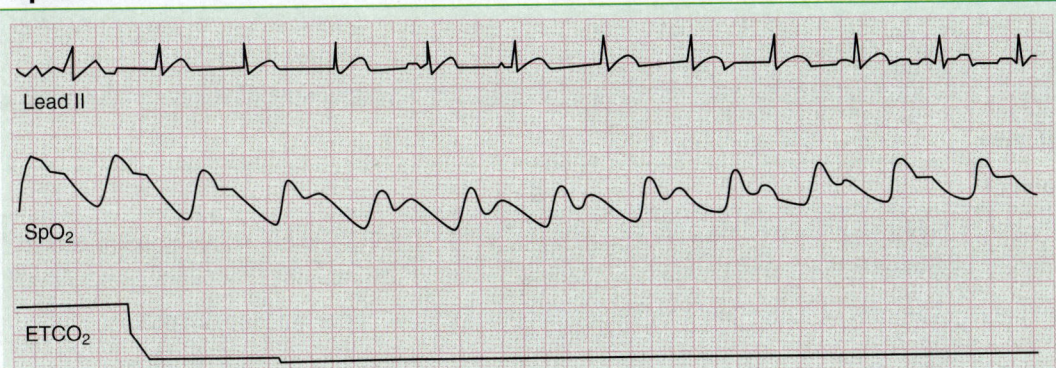

Note how in this example the SpO₂ waveform (middle waveform) continues to show an adequate oxygenation status after the patient has gone apneic but the ETCO₂ waveform (bottom waveform) abruptly drops to zero.

(continues)

Capnography Waveforms and Their Meanings (continued)

Intubation Waveforms

Right Main Stem Intubation

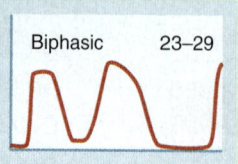

Biphasic 23–29

Biphasic waveform as a result of ETT in the right main bronchus

Esophageal Intubation

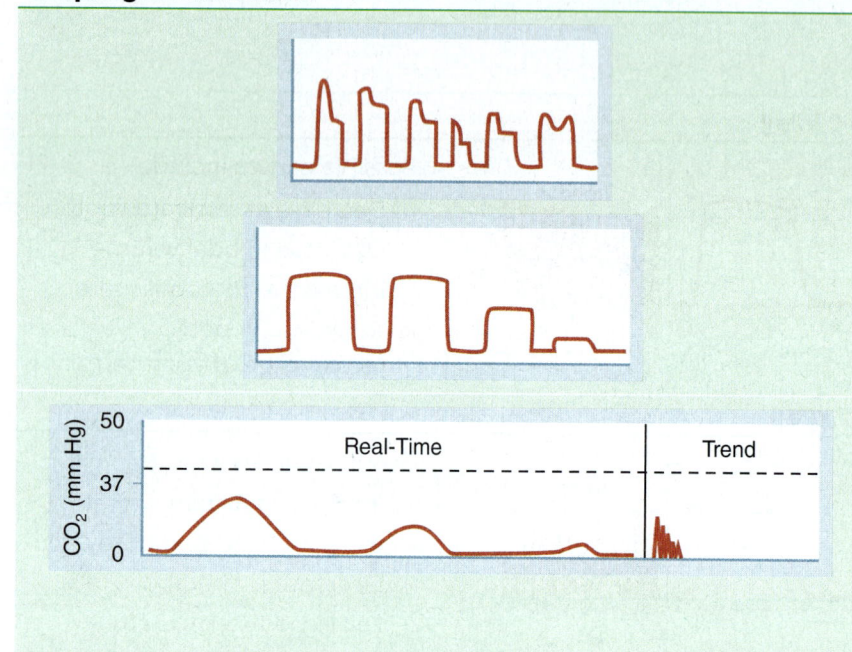

Baseline fluctuation 0–2

Possible causes include:
› Missed intubation; ETT in the esophagus, little or no CO_2 is present
› ETT disconnected, kinked, or obstructed
› Loss of circulatory function

Obstructed Airway or Breathing Circuit

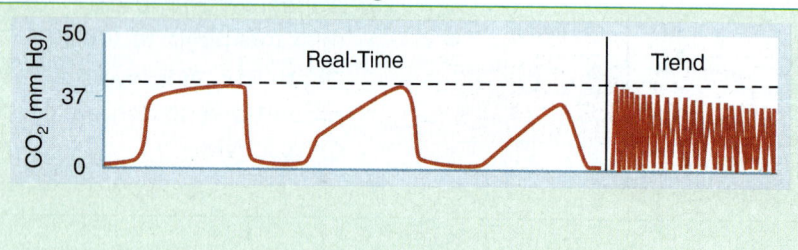

Possible causes include:
› Partially kinked or occluded artificial airway
› Presence of foreign body in the airway
› Obstruction in expiratory limb of breathing circuit
› Bronchospasm

Perfusion Waveforms

ETCO₂ Below Normal

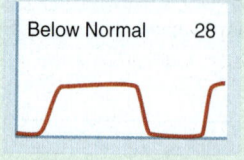

Below Normal 28

$ETCO_2$ well below normal may be due to:
› Low cardiac output
› Pulmonary embolus
› Hypothermia, etc.

Decreasing Cardiac Output

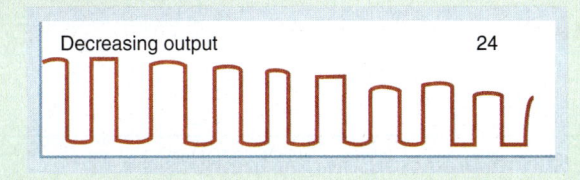

[waveform: Decreasing output, 24]	Low cardiac output and a low perfusion state will show up as a decreasing ETCO₂. A decreasing ETCO₂ waveform may also indicate a cuff leak, ETT in the hypopharynx, or a partial obstruction of the ETT.

CPR Performance: Tired Rescuer

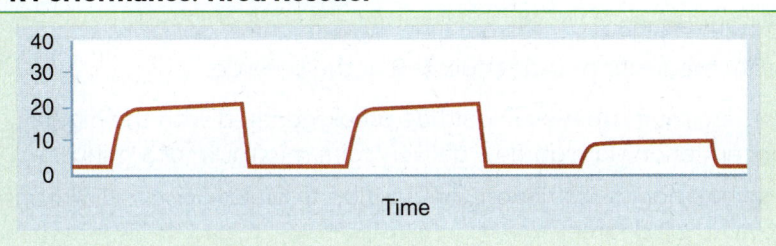

[waveform showing decreasing amplitude over Time, scale 0–40]	Adequate compressions during CPR show up on the ETCO₂ as 15–20 mm Hg (2.0–2.7 kPa), but as the rescuer fatigues, the ETCO₂ falls below 10 mm Hg (1.3 kPa). Time to rotate or change rescuers/compressors.

Return of Spontaneous Circulation

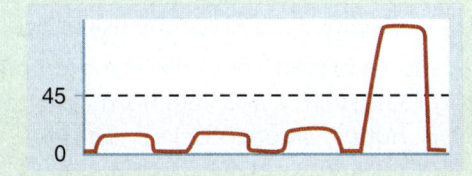

[waveform with sudden increase above 45 line]	Note the sudden increase in ETCO₂ during CPR, indicating return of spontaneous circulation.

Equipment Malfunction

Inadequate Seal Around ETT

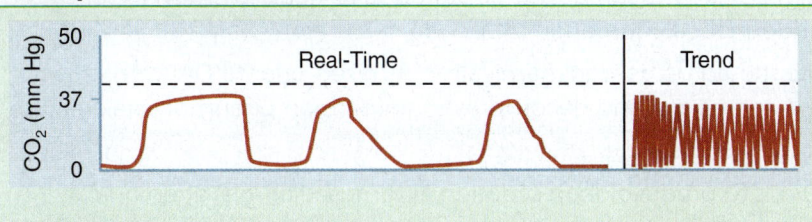

[CO₂ (mm Hg) 0–50, Real-Time and Trend waveforms, dashed line at 37]	Possible causes include: › Leaky or deflated endotracheal or tracheotomy cuff › Artificial airway too small for the patient

Rebreathing

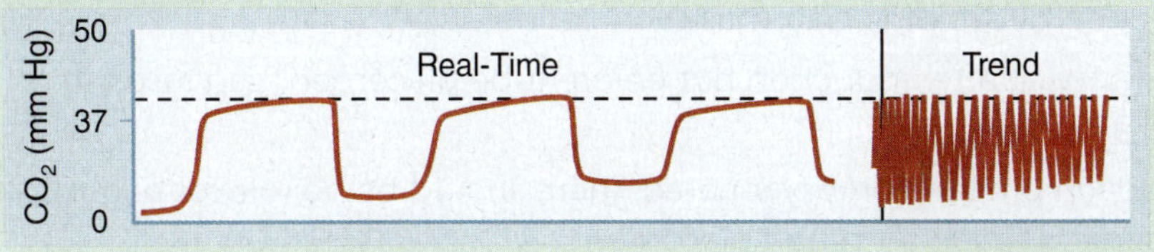

[CO₂ (mm Hg) 0–50, Real-Time and Trend waveforms, dashed line at 37]	Possible causes include: › Faulty expiratory valve › Inadequate inspiratory flow › Insufficient expiratory time › Malfunction of CO₂ absorber system

ETCO₂ = end-tidal carbon dioxide; ETT = endotracheal tube; CPR = cardiopulmonary resuscitation.

Data from Krauss, B., Falk, J. L., & Ladde, J. G. (2022). Carbon dioxide monitoring (capnography). *UpToDate*. Retrieved February 19, 2023, from https://www.uptodate.com/contents/carbon-dioxide-monitoring-capnography

APPENDIX 5-2

Seven Ps of Rapid Sequence Intubation

Phase	Description
Preparation	Ensure that all necessary personnel are assembled at the bedside.
	Ensure that all equipment is in working order and that the patient's cardiac monitor, blood pressure cuff, pulse oximetry, and end-tidal capnography are placed on the patient and functioning correctly.
	Verify patent intravenous access.
	Draw up and label DAI medications (Appendix 5-3) at the bedside.
Preoxygenation	Patients requiring emergent intubation should be preoxygenated with the highest possible oxygen concentration via high-flow delivery for a minimum of 3 minutes.
	For patients not in spinal motion restriction, the position to preoxygenate is with the head of the bed elevated 20 degrees.
	If the patient is on spinal precautions, place the bed in reverse Trendelenburg position at 30 degrees.
	Consider apneic oxygenation in all intubations to reduce the risk of hypoxemia.
	Oxygen is administered via nasal cannula placed under the standard preoxygenation device (nonrebreather mask or bag-mask) with a flow rate from 10–15 L/minute in a conscious patient and at least 15 L/minute in an unconscious patient.
	The jaw-thrust maneuver should be used to optimize oxygen flow past the upper airway and to maintain airway patency.
Preintubation optimization	During this phase, medications can be administered to mitigate the adverse effects associated with endotracheal intubation (Appendix 5-3).
	If possible, patients should be hemodynamically optimized prior to DAI with blood products, IV fluid, vasopressors, and decompression of tension pneumothorax/release of hemothorax.
Paralysis with induction	The goal during DAI is to produce deep sedation and muscular relaxation quickly (Appendix 5-3).
Positioning with protection	After the neuromuscular blocking agent is administered, the priority is to protect the airway from aspiration by avoiding bag-mask ventilation.
	Use of a bag-mask device after induction but before tube placement can result in regurgitation and aspiration.
	If the patient has been properly preoxygenated, there should be no role for bag-mask device use between induction and tube placement.
Placement with proof	Once intubation is completed, inflate the ETT cuff and secure the tube.
	Use $ETCO_2$ (colorimetric and quantitative) to confirm tube placement.
Postintubation management	Secure the ETT per institutional protocol and note the measurement at the teeth/gums.
	A postintubation chest radiograph should be obtained to determine depth of ETT insertion and for any evidence of complications.

DAI = drug-assisted intubation; IV = intravenous; ETT = endotracheal tube; $ETCO_2$ = end-tidal carbon dioxide.

Data from Brown, C. A., & Sakles, J. C. (2023). Rapid sequence intubation in adults for emergency medicine and critical care. *UpToDate*. Retrieved April 14, 2023, from https://www.uptodate.com/contents/rapid-sequence-intubation-in-adults-for-emergency-medicine-and-critical-care

APPENDIX 5-3
Drug-Assisted Intubation Medications

Onset for these medications is rapid: seconds to several minutes. Refer to current, evidence-based resources for additional information regarding these medications.[1-3]

Medication	Action	Duration	Clinical Pearls
Pretreatment			
Fentanyl	Mitigates sympathetic response (increased BP and HR) during intubation.	30–60 minutes	Can cause respiratory depression and hypotension. Administer over 60 seconds to prevent "wooden chest syndrome."
Induction			
Etomidate	Acts on the GABA receptors to block neuroexcitation and produce anesthesia.	3–12 minutes	Does not affect hemodynamic stability. Known to decrease circulating cortisol levels.
Ketamine	Acts as an agonist on GABA receptors, causing neuroinhibition and anesthesia; excites opioid receptors, causing analgesia.	10–20 minutes	Does not decrease respiratory drive. Induction agent of choice for awake intubation. Unique in that it provides analgesia.
Midazolam	Acts on GABA receptor complex to produce sedation and amnesia.	15–30 minutes	Causes 10–25% decrease in MAP in healthy individuals. Use with caution in hypovolemic and/or hypotensive patients.
Propofol	Sedative amnestic agent. Suppresses brain activity and inhibits long-term memory creation.	5–10 minutes	Causes vasodilation and decrease in MAP. Can be used for long-term sedation, procedural sedation, and anesthesia induction. Use with caution in patients with egg/soy allergies.
Paralysis			
Succinylcholine	Depolarizing agent that stimulates all cholinergic receptors (sympathetic and parasympathetic), causing depolarization and fasciculations, followed by muscular paralysis.	6–10 minutes	Absolute contraindication in patients with (or family history of) malignant hyperthermia, stroke, or burn that occurred more than 72 hours prior, rhabdomyolysis, significant hyperkalemia, myasthenia gravis, or myasthenic syndromes.
Rocuronium	Nondepolarizing agent that inhibits neuromuscular receptors, causing muscular paralysis.	45 minutes	Drug of choice when succinylcholine is contraindicated.

(continues)

Medication	Action	Duration	Clinical Pearls
Paralysis	**Paralysis**	**Paralysis**	**Paralysis**
Vecuronium	Nondepolarizing agent that inhibits neuromuscular receptors, causing muscular paralysis.	20–30 minutes	Alternative to rocuronium.

BP = blood pressure; HR = heart rate; GABA = gamma-aminobutyric acid; MAP = mean arterial pressure.

Data from Caro, D. (2020). Pretreatment medications for rapid sequence intubation in adults outside the operating room. *UpToDate*. Retrieved February 1, 2022, from https://www.uptodate.com/contents/pretreatment-medications-for-rapid-sequence-intubation-in-adults-outside-the-operating-room?source=autocomplete&index=0~2&search=pretreatment#H6; Caro, D. (2021). Induction agents for rapid sequence intubation in adults outside the operating room. *UpToDate*. Retrieved February 8, 2022, from https://www.uptodate.com/contents/induction-agents-for-rapid-sequence-intubation-in-adults-outside-the-operating-room?search=Induction%20agents%20for%20&source=search_result&selectedTitle=1~150&usage_type=default&display_rank=1; Caro, D. (2022). Neuromuscular blocking agents (NMBAs) for rapid sequence intubation in adults outside of the operating room. *UpToDate*. Retrieved February 12, 2022, from https://www.uptodate.com/contents/neuromuscular-blocking-agents-nmbas-for-rapid-sequence-intubation-in-adults-outside-of-the-operating-room?search=paralysis%20medications%20in%20rapis%20sequence%20intubation&source=search_result&selectedTitle=4~150&usage_type=default&display_rank=4

References

1. Caro, D. (2020). Pretreatment medications for rapid sequence intubation in adults outside the operating room. *UpToDate*. Retrieved February 1, 2022, from https://www.uptodate.com/contents/pretreatment-medications-for-rapid-sequence-intubation-in-adults-outside-the-operating-room
2. Caro, D. (2021). Induction agents for rapid sequence intubation in adults outside the operating room. *UpToDate*. Retrieved February 8, 2022, from https://www.uptodate.com/contents/induction-agents-for-rapid-sequence-intubation-in-adults-outside-the-operating-room
3. Caro, D. (2022). Neuromuscular blocking agents (NMBAs) for rapid sequence intubation in adults outside of the operating room. *UpToDate*. Retrieved February 12, 2022, from https://www.uptodate.com/contents/neuromuscular-blocking-agents-nmbas-for-rapid-sequence-intubation-in-adults-outside-of-the-operating-room

APPENDIX 5-4

Post-RSI Hypotension and Hypoxemia: Common Causes and Interventions

Common Causes	Clinical Findings	Interventions	Prevention/Preparation
High intrathoracic pressure › Poor bag-mask ventilation technique › Improper mechanical ventilation settings	Normal or elevated airway pressures Abnormal breath sounds (wheezing, diminished)	Slow ventilation rate (≤ 8 beats/minute) Reduce ventilation force (for BMV) Increase expiration time IVF bolus of isotonic crystalloids	Avoid overly rapid or forceful ventilation
Significant prior or ongoing hemorrhage	Blood loss Signs of shock Pallor	Blood transfusion Hemorrhage control/surgical consultation	In patients with hemorrhagic shock or at risk for hemodynamic instability, initiate blood transfusion prior to administering RSI medications
ETT malposition (dislodged; esophageal placement)	Bilateral decreased breath sounds Gastric breath sounds (esophageal intubation) Low peak inspiratory pressures	Extubate and reintubate	Waveform capnography
Mainstem intubation	Asymmetric breath sounds High resistance to bag-mask device High PIP	Withdraw ETT appropriate distance and recheck breath sounds	Insert ETT appropriate distance Keep ETT well secured
ETT cuff malfunction	Ventilator leak or low ventilation volumes Loss of pilot balloon pressure	Exchange ETT	Inflate and check cuff of primary and backup ETT prior to intubation
Mucus plugging	Increased secretions High resistance to bag-mask device High PIP	ETT suctioning	Suction frequently if heavy secretions
Pneumothorax	Asymmetric breath sounds Subcutaneous emphysema High resistance to bag-mask device High PIP	Needle thoracostomy (temporizing) Tube thoracostomy	2- to 3-inch long, 14- to 16-gauge needle or chest tube kit at the bedside for high-risk patients

BMV = bag-mask ventilation; IVF = intravenous fluid; RSI = rapid sequence intubation; ETT = endotracheal tube; PIP = peak inspiratory pressure.

Data from Brown, C. A., & Sakles, J. C. (2020). Rapid sequence intubation for adults outside the operating room. *UpToDate*. Retrieved January 6, 2022, from https://www.uptodate.com/contents/rapid-sequence-intubation-for-adults-outside-the-operating-room?search=rapid%20sequence%20intubation%20for%20adults%20outside%20the%20operating%20room&source=search_result&selectedTitle=1~150&usage_type=default&display_rank=1

CHAPTER 6

Shock

Victor M. Pearson, MSN-Ed, RN, CEN, CPEN, CTRN, CFRN, TCRN, CCRN

OBJECTIVES

Upon completion of this chapter, the learner will be able to:
1. Identify causes and characteristics of shock in the trauma patient.
2. Describe pathophysiologic changes as a basis for assessment of the trauma patient in shock.
3. Demonstrate nursing assessment priorities for the trauma patient in shock.
4. Plan appropriate interventions and assess their effectiveness shock.

Introduction

Shock is a physiologic state of inadequate tissue perfusion that results when oxygen delivery, uptake, and utilization are insufficient to meet the metabolic demands of cells and organs. This produces cellular and tissue hypoxia, causing a shift from aerobic to anaerobic metabolism. It is a dynamic process that begins when cells are hypoperfused, which sets off a series of responses to preserve homeostasis that lead to far-reaching effects on all body systems and organs.

Shock is a complex state, and its early recognition, accompanied by appropriate interventions, is the first step to managing the patient.[5] In its early stages, the presence of shock is likely to be subtle. If this condition goes unrecognized and untreated, the hypoperfused cells shift to less efficient anaerobic metabolism, leading to life-threatening acidosis, tissue ischemia, and cellular death. A basic understanding of the concepts, types, and stages of shock, as well as the physiologic response to shock, is essential to early recognition and goal-directed interventions that enable optimal care for the patient.

The Pathophysiology of Shock

Shock begins at the cellular level. For cells to perform basic metabolic functions and maintain their cellular integrity, they require the production of adenosine triphosphate (ATP) (**Figure 6-1**).[51] In the presence of oxygen, aerobic metabolism efficiently produces ATP through the breakdown of fats, carbohydrates, and proteins. This process provides a high ATP yield, which supports energy production and the maintenance of the electrical gradient known as the sodium–potassium pump.[11]

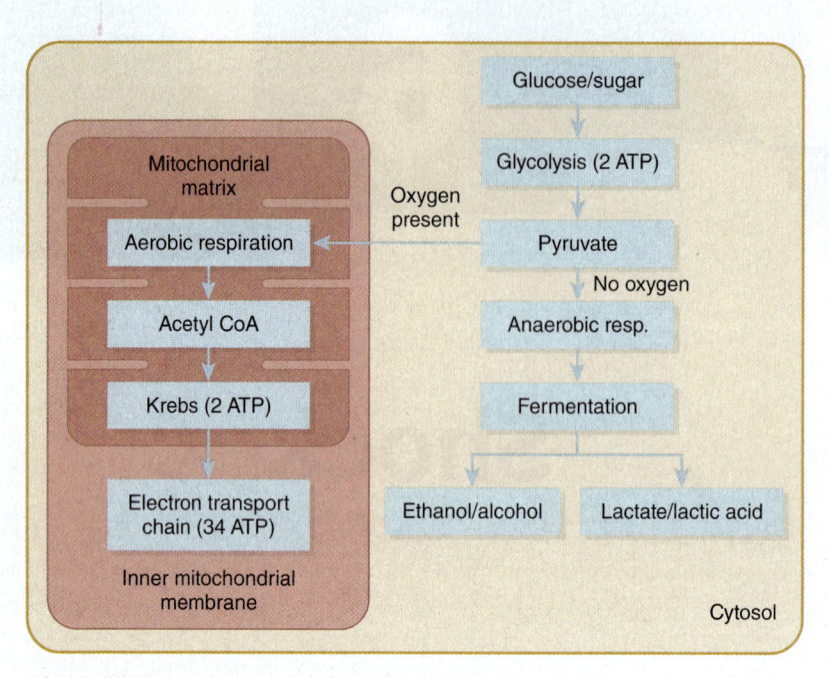

Figure 6-1 *Anaerobic and aerobic cellular metabolism.*
Modified from Wyzant. (n.d.). *Cellular respiration.* https://www.wyzant.com/resources/lessons/science/biology/cellular-respiration

Hypoperfusion deprives the cell of oxygen. As metabolism shifts from aerobic to anaerobic, lactic acid is produced, resulting in metabolic acidosis.[11,18] If shock is prolonged, and ATP cannot meet energy demand, the cell membrane loses its integrity. This results in the loss of the sodium–potassium pump, causing sodium to stay inside the cell and potassium outside the cell. The end result of this process is cellular swelling, death, and destruction (**Figure 6-2**).[11,25]

Basic cardiac function is key to maintaining cellular perfusion. Shock has many causes, classifications, and stages. Regardless of the cause, shock results from an abnormality in one or more components of cardiac output (CO), which is the volume of blood pumped by the heart per minute; CO is determined by the heart rate multiplied by the stroke volume (**Figure 6-3**).[5,39] Stroke volume is the amount of blood pumped with each cardiac contraction; it is affected by preload, afterload, and myocardial contractility.[11,18,25,39]

- Preload: The central venous pressure or volume of blood return to the heart at the end of diastole.
- Afterload: The pressure that the heart must overcome to pump blood into systemic circulation; it is a component of systemic vascular resistance (SVR).
- Contractility: The capability of the ventricles to contract, forcefully ejecting blood.

Different injuries and their sequelae can affect contractility and any component of CO.[5]

Stages of Shock

In the early stages of shock, delivery of cellular nutrients and oxygen is inadequate to meet the body's metabolic needs. To protect and maintain perfusion to essential organs, the body reacts by activating various compensatory mechanisms. In the short term, these compensatory mechanisms may improve tissue perfusion to vital organs. However, that feat is accomplished by shunting perfusion away from other organs.[14] Blood pressure alone is not an indication of cardiac output and adequate perfusion. Several other end points of resuscitation can be monitored proactively to identify early stages of shock.

If the shock state is unrecognized, untreated, or prolonged, or if the protective mechanisms fail to restore perfusion, profound effects on microcirculation and vascular permeability will ensue, and the patient will progress to irreversible shock. The cellular membrane loses its ability to maintain integrity, leading to cellular destruction and death; this is followed by a systemic inflammatory response, organ ischemia, end-organ damage, multiple organ dysfunction, and, ultimately, death. Early recognition and management are crucial, because failure to intervene will allow progression to the terminal stage of shock, in which morbidity and mortality are inevitable.[11,18,25,39]

If shock is not addressed it progresses through three stages: compensated, decompensated/hypotensive, and irreversible. These stages are illustrated in **Figure 6-4**.[14]

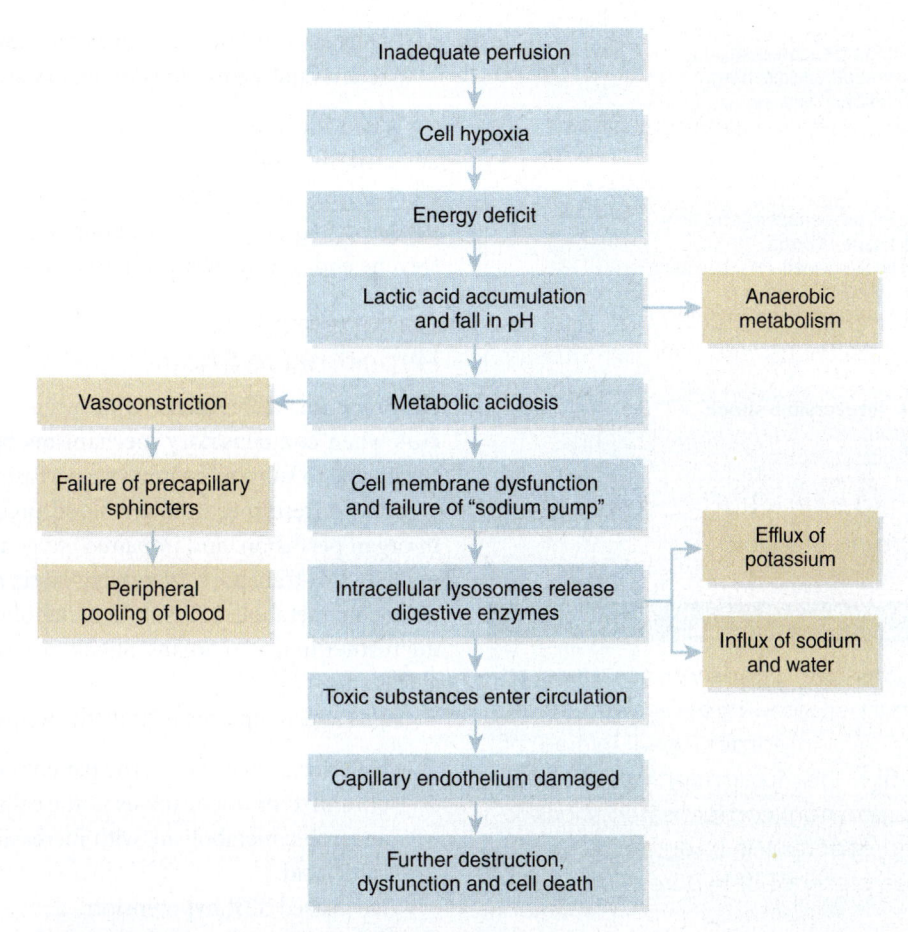

Figure 6-2 Cellular response to shock.

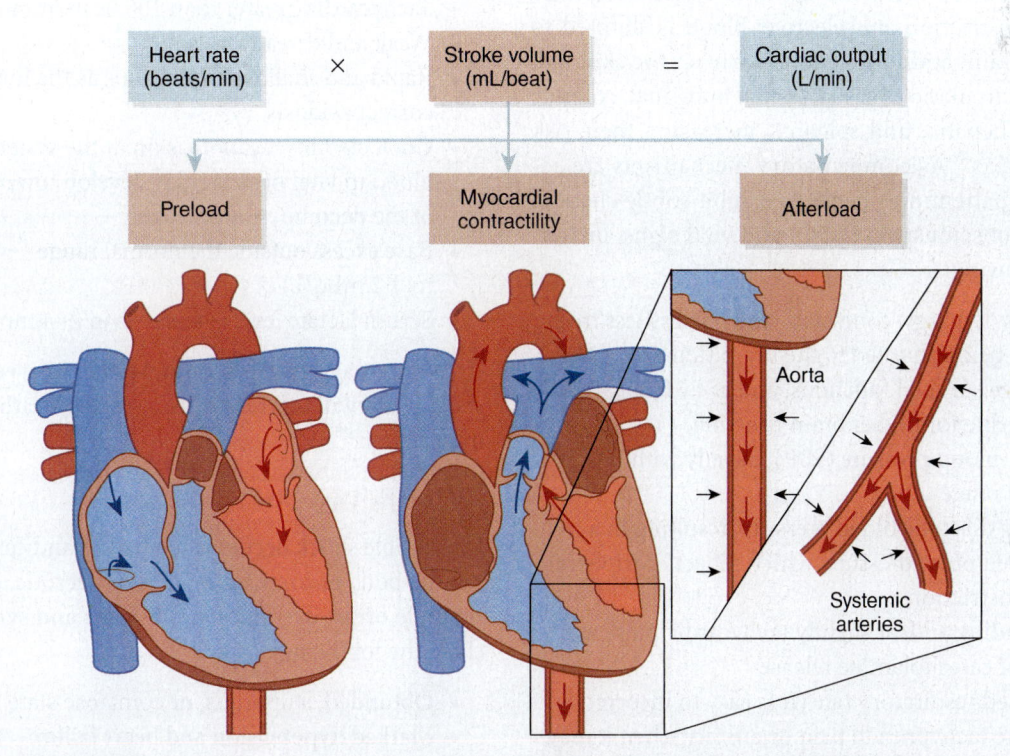

Figure 6-3 Cardiac output is the product of stroke volume and heart rate.

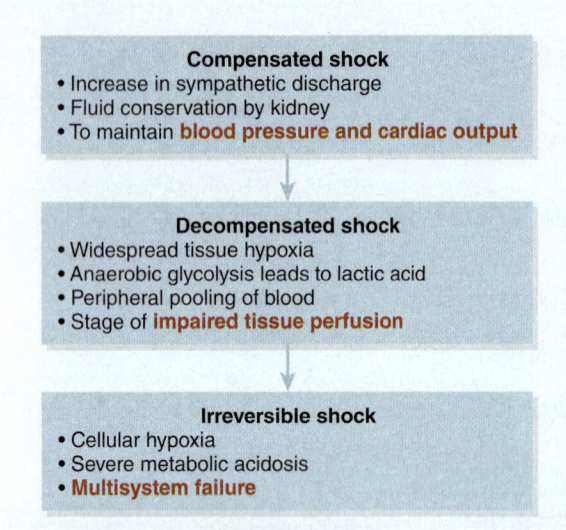

Figure 6-4 *The stages of shock.*

Compensated shock
- Increase in sympathetic discharge
- Fluid conservation by kidney
- To maintain **blood pressure and cardiac output**

Decompensated shock
- Widespread tissue hypoxia
- Anaerobic glycolysis leads to lactic acid
- Peripheral pooling of blood
- Stage of **impaired tissue perfusion**

Irreversible shock
- Cellular hypoxia
- Severe metabolic acidosis
- **Multisystem failure**

> **NOTE**
>
> The term "progressive" is sometimes used to describe decompensated/hypotensive shock, and "refractory" is sometimes used in lieu of irreversible shock.[25] The most important takeaway is that the transition from compensated shock to decompensated/hypotensive (progressive shock) is defined by the presence of hypotension.

Compensated Shock

In compensated shock, the nervous system response and vasoconstriction are selective; blood is shunted to the heart, brain, and lungs and away from the skin and splanchnic circulation (gastric, small intestinal, colonic, pancreatic, hepatic, and splenic), increasing their risk for ischemia.[14,25] As compensatory mechanisms are activated, the patient may begin to exhibit subtle changes in level of consciousness (LOC) and vital signs, including the following:

- Anxiety, lethargy, confusion, and restlessness from oxygen being shunted to the brain stem, so as to maintain survival functions, and away from areas responsible for higher brain function
- Systolic blood pressure (SBP), usually within normal range
- A rising diastolic blood pressure, resulting in a narrowed pulse pressure, which reflects peripheral vasoconstriction
- A bounding and/or slightly tachycardic pulse as a result of catecholamine release
- Increased respiratory rate (It is easy to incorrectly attribute tachypnea to pain or anxiety when it may be an early sign of shock.)
- Decreased urinary output as the kidney works to retain fluid within the circulatory system

When low blood flow and poor tissue perfusion are detected, the body responds quickly with compensatory mechanisms to maintain homeostasis. During the compensated stage, the window of opportunity to rapidly intervene and restore perfusion is narrow.

Decompensated or Hypotensive Shock

Decompensated/hypotensive or progressive shock occurs when compensatory mechanisms begin to fail and are unable to support or improve perfusion[28]: Blood flow is reduced, resulting in lower blood pressure, reduction in organ perfusion, and impaired oxygen and carbon dioxide (CO_2) transport. Increasing lactic acid levels from anaerobic metabolism result in metabolic acidosis, causing further injury to organs. Shock may still be reversible at this stage.[25,28]

Signs and symptoms include the following[14,18,25]:

- Deterioration of LOC. The patient becomes obtunded or unconscious as the cells switch to anaerobic metabolism, with increasing levels of lactic acid.
- Decreased SBP, hypotension
- Narrowing pulse pressure that continues until peripheral vascular vasoconstriction fails to provide cardiovascular support
- Tachycardia greater than 100 beats/minute
- Weak and thready pulses
- Rapid and shallow respirations as the lungs try to correct acidosis
- Cool, clammy, cyanotic skin as the system shunts blood to vital organs (may develop toward the end of the decompensated stage)
- Base excess outside the normal range (-2 mEq/L to $+2$ mEq/L)
- Serum lactate levels greater than 2–4 mmol/L

Without aggressive and immediate interventions, the shock state will worsen, causing tissue death and organ dysfunction.[48]

Irreversible Shock

Irreversible shock occurs when tissues and cells throughout the body become ischemic and necrotic, resulting in multiple organ dysfunction.[14,25] Signs and symptoms include the following[11,18,25]:

- Obtunded, stuporous, or comatose state
- Marked hypotension and heart failure
- Bradycardia with possible dysrhythmias

- Decreased and shallow respiratory rate
- Pale, cool, and clammy skin
- Kidney, liver, and other organ failure due to continued hypoperfusion and ischemia
- Severe acidosis, elevated lactic acid levels, and worsening base excess on arterial blood gases (ABGs)
- Coagulopathies with petechiae, purpura, or bleeding

Hypoperfusion leads to systemic inflammatory response syndrome, causing the release of cell mediators or cytokines and resulting in wholesale vasodilation, increased capillary permeability, and coagulopathy. In the lungs, these changes lead to acute respiratory distress syndrome. Increased permeability of the pulmonary capillaries results in noncardiogenic pulmonary edema, alveolar collapse, and ventilation–perfusion mismatch.[48] Other vital organ systems begin to fail, leading to multiple organ dysfunction syndrome.[25] The lungs, heart, and kidneys are often the first organs to be affected. Liver failure may occur later because of that organ's compensatory capacity.[14]

Despite aggressive resuscitation at this level, it becomes increasingly difficult to restore tissue perfusion, correct the coagulopathies, and minimize organ damage. Interventions in this stage of shock have minimal ability to reverse morbidity and mortality.

The Body's Compensatory Response to Shock

The human compensatory response includes a vascular component. As blood flow decreases and the arterial pressure falls below 80 mm Hg, oxygen delivery becomes impaired, resulting in decreased oxygen levels and increased CO_2 levels.[24] As a result of the lower blood pressure, a cascading response is set into motion to preserve tissue perfusion. The vascular response is activated along two different pathways:

- *Baroreceptor activation:* Baroreceptors, found in the carotid sinus and along the aortic arch, are sensitive to the degree of stretch within the arterial wall. When the baroreceptors sense a decrease in stretch, they stimulate the sympathetic nervous system to release epinephrine and norepinephrine; this causes stimulation of cardiac activity and constriction of blood vessels, which triggers a rise in heart rate, myocardial contractility, and diastolic blood pressure.[11,14,39]
- *Chemoreceptor activation*: Peripheral chemoreceptors consist of carotid and aortic bodies, whereas central chemoreceptors are located in the medulla of the brain stem. Peripheral chemoreceptors detect changes in blood oxygen levels, whereas central chemoreceptors respond to changes in CO_2 and pH. When CO_2 rises or the oxygen level or pH falls, these receptors are activated, and information is relayed to the central nervous system and to the cardiorespiratory centers in the medulla; this results in increased respiratory rate and depth, and blood pressure.[11,14]

Adrenal Gland Response

Activation of the sympathetic nervous system triggers the "fight or flight" response, which causes the adrenal glands to release the two vasoconstrictor catecholamines: epinephrine and norepinephrine[11,14]:

- High levels of epinephrine (adrenaline), produce smooth muscle relaxation in the airways and cause arteriole smooth muscle contractility (potentiating inotropic effect). Epinephrine also increases heart rate (positive chronotropic effect), peripheral vasoconstriction, and glycogenolysis (breakdown of glycogen stores in the liver into glucose for cellular use).
- Peripheral vasoconstriction manifests as a narrowed pulse pressure, causing blood to be shunted into the central circulation in order to maintain perfusion to the vital organs.
- Norepinephrine (noradrenaline), increases heart rate, vascular tone through alpha-adrenergic receptor activation, and blood flow to skeletal muscle. It also triggers the release of glucose from energy stores.[14]

> **NOTE**
>
> As diastolic pressure rises, systemic and peripheral vascular resistance (afterload) increase. A narrowing pulse pressure may be one of the first concrete measures signaling that the patient's circulatory status is compromised and the body is trying to compensate.

Changes in vital signs may present subtly, so the nurse must be observant and alert to their presence. Recognizing this early shock response can be essential to preventing further tissue injury and progression of the shock state.

In addition to the release of catecholamines, the adrenal glands stimulate the release of cortisol and aldosterone to raise blood glucose and promote renal retention of water and sodium.

Pulmonary Response

During shock, the pulmonary system responds to both hypoperfusion and acidosis. The respiratory rate increases to improve oxygen delivery to the tissues and to decrease the CO_2 level to maintain acid–base balance. Metabolic acidosis stemming from anaerobic metabolism results in the compensatory response of tachypnea and is one of the earliest responses to inadequately perfused tissue. If shock is left untreated, the pulmonary response may become ineffective, weaken, and fail, necessitating assisted ventilations. This is also the reason that tachypnea is noted in shock patients as an early response. Appropriate measurement of vital signs is crucial, including respiratory rate.[14,48]

Cerebral Response

As shock progresses, the primary goal of the body is to maintain perfusion to the vital organs—the midbrain, heart, lungs, and kidneys—by shunting blood away from liver, bowel, skin, and muscle. Sympathetic stimulation has little effect on the cerebral and coronary vessels because they are capable of autoregulation.[2] Cerebral autoregulation maintains a constant cerebral vascular blood flow as long as the mean arterial pressure is maintained in the range of 50–150 mm Hg.[2] When autoregulation in the brain fails, perfusion becomes dependent solely on systemic blood pressure.[2] See Chapter 7, "Head Trauma," for additional information.

Renal Response

Hypoperfusion of the kidneys triggers a complex compensatory mechanism in the adrenal glands to improve tissue perfusion. This mechanism includes the following steps[14,28]:

- Renal ischemia causes the kidneys to secrete renin.
- Renin accelerates the production of angiotensin I.
- Angiotensin I is converted into angiotensin II in the lungs by angiotensin-converting enzyme, which is produced by the vascular endothelium.
- Angiotensin II effects include the following:
  - Potent vasoconstriction, which increases vascular resistance and arterial pressure
  - Release of aldosterone, which increases reabsorption of sodium and water in the distal tubules to increase intravascular volume
  - Stimulation of arginine vasopressin, also known as vasopressin, argipressin, or antidiuretic hormone, which further increases retention of water

Decreased urinary output may be noted, which can be an indication of poor renal perfusion and progression of the shock state. If shock is left untreated, it will progress to oliguria and renal failure.

Systemic Inflammatory Response Syndrome

The initial posttraumatic inflammatory response is both protective and essential for survival. Tissue hypoxia activates a systemic inflammatory response, and neutrophils are sent to the injury sites, engaging signaling pathways that mobilize inflammatory cells. Tissue hypoxia also stimulates the secretion of multiple inflammatory mediators or biomarkers.[18,28]

An exaggerated immune inflammatory response can result from massive tissue injury and hemorrhage or a prolonged and untreated shock state. It can induce a generalized, acute inflammatory response that affects multiple organ systems and sets in motion a cycle of inflammation–tissue damage–inflammation that is driven by cytokines, chemokines, and products of damaged, dysfunctional, or stressed tissue.[18,20,21]

Apoptosis (programmed cell death) of neutrophils may be inhibited, leading to an accumulation of neutrophils that stimulates the release of inflammatory mediators.[18,20] In other cells, apoptosis may be magnified, increasing cell death and worsening organ function. The neutrophils change and move from the capillaries into the interstitial space and trigger further release of free oxygen radicals and tissue-destructive enzymes, leading to additional tissue injury.[21] This process may start when hypoperfusion begins or during resuscitation. If hypoxia is not corrected early, the inflammatory response becomes destructive, leading to organ failure and death.[21,47]

The Trauma Triad of Death

Resuscitation-associated coagulopathy is associated with what has been called the *trauma triad of death* (**Figure 6-5**), which, once begun, establishes a vicious cycle with catastrophic results.[42,44,49] The trauma triad of death consists of the following elements[35,42,44,49]:

- *Hypothermia*: Impairs thrombin production and platelet function. Activated protein C inhibits factors V and VIII, reducing thrombin formation, and decreases inhibition of tissue plasminogen activator, accelerating fibrinolysis and bleeding.
- *Acidosis*: Impairs thrombin production and other coagulation factors as a result of reduced pH, elevated lactate production, and increasing base deficit. Laboratory values of pH less than 7.4, elevated serum lactate, and base deficits reaching −10 mmol/L reduce the activity of various

coagulation factors by as much as 40%. Metabolic acidosis also contributes to prolonged clotting times and reduced clot strength.[37]
- *Coagulopathy*: With whole-blood loss, clotting factors are depleted, and coagulopathy is already present in 25–35% of trauma patients when they arrive at the emergency department.[37] Replacement with packed red blood cells (RBCs) and hemodilution with saline without transfusing platelets and plasma further dilute the blood's ability to clot.[5]

Hypoperfusion leads to increased levels of thrombomodulin, which inhibits thrombin and activates activated protein C. Activated protein C impairs clot formation and increases existing clot dissolution.

Acute endogenous coagulopathy begins immediately following a traumatic injury—before, and independent of, iatrogenic causes such as hypothermia and metabolic acidosis—making this a primary cause of coagulopathy after injury.[35,44] This is known as trauma-induced coagulopathy.

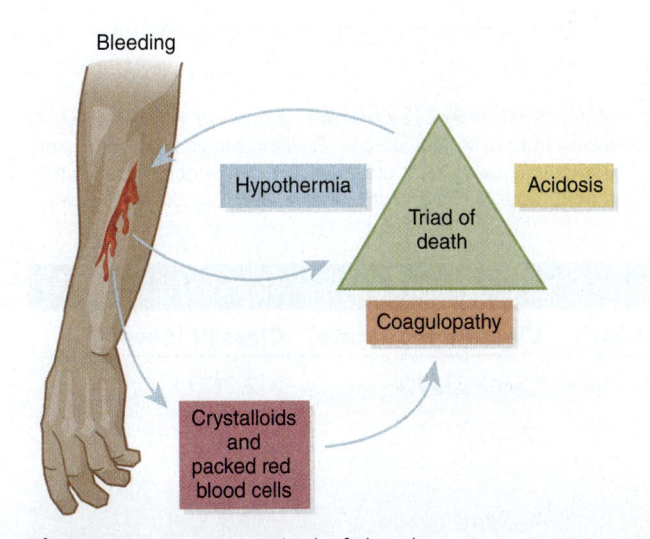

Figure 6-5 *Trauma triad of death.*

Classification of Shock

Whether the cause of shock is a volume problem (hypovolemia), a pump problem (cardiogenic), a problem with the vessels (distributive), or a mechanical problem (obstructive), the underlying issue is the same: inadequate tissue perfusion and cellular oxygenation. The etiology of the different types of shock can be traced back to an issue with one (or more) of these four components (**Figure 6-6**).[14,18,25,33] **Table 6-1** provides a summary of shock etiology; each type is discussed in the following subsections.

Hypovolemic Shock (Volume Problem)

Hypovolemia is caused by a decrease in the amount of circulating volume. In trauma, this typically results from hemorrhage but could result from a condition that leads to a precipitous loss of volume, such as vomiting, diarrhea, or burn trauma. Hemorrhage is the most common cause of shock in the trauma patient and the leading cause of preventable death in the prehospital environment.[31] Hemorrhage control is a first-line intervention, followed by restoration of circulating volume.[5]

In hypovolemic shock, decreased circulating volume results in decreased venous return and decreased preload. With less filling of the ventricles, heart muscle fibers stretch less at the end of the diastole. There is less force of contraction; this effect leads to decreased cardiac output and less oxygenated blood being transported to the tissues, resulting in hypoperfusion.[25]

The American College of Surgeons has developed a classification system for hemorrhagic shock that correlates its presentation with the volume of blood loss (**Table 6-2**).[5] This classification system is a useful tool for estimating percentage of acute blood loss. Patient

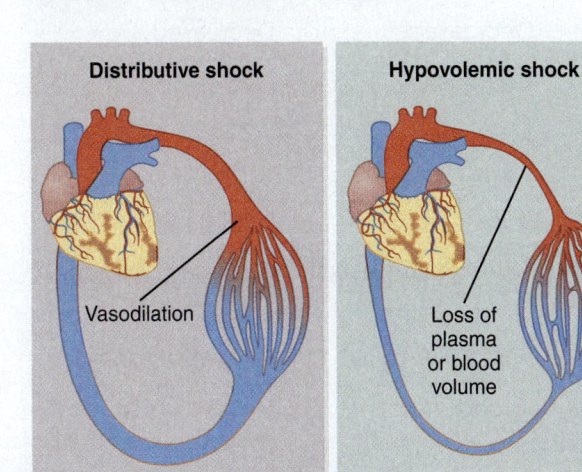

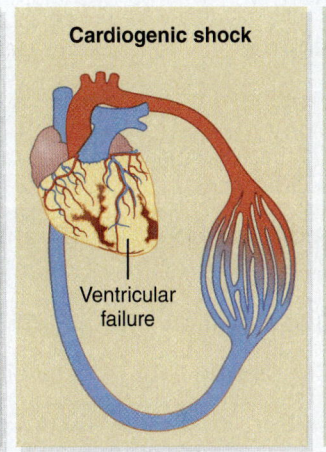

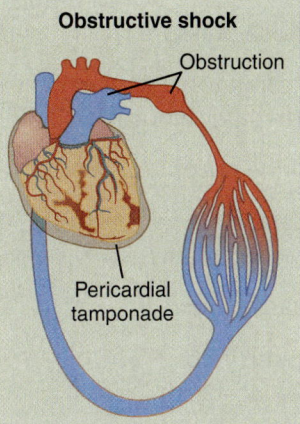

Figure 6-6 *Types of shock.*

TABLE 6-1 Classification of Shock Etiology and Underlying Defects

Classification	Etiology	Underlying Pathology
Hypovolemic	Hemorrhage	Whole-blood loss
	Burns	Plasma loss, fluid shifts
Cardiogenic	Myocardial infarction	Loss of cardiac contractility
	Dysrhythmias	Reduced cardiac output
	Blunt cardiac trauma	Loss of cardiac contractility and dysrhythmias
Obstructive	Cardiac tamponade	Compression of the heart with obstruction to atrial filling
	Tension pneumothorax	Mediastinal shift with obstruction to atrial filling
	Tension hemothorax	Combination of compression of the heart and mediastinal shift
Distributive	Neurogenic shock	Loss of vasomotor tone due to decreases in sympathetic control
	Anaphylactic shock	Vasodilation of vessels due to immune reaction to allergens (release of histamine)
	Septic shock	Mediated by systemic inflammatory response syndrome with hypotension and perfusion abnormalities

Data from Carbino, G. (2020). Shock emergencies. In V. Sweet & A. Foley (Eds.), *Sheehy's emergency nursing: Principles and practice* (7th ed., pp. 205–215). Elsevier; Dedeo, M. (2020). Traumatic shock. In K. A. McQuillan & M. B. Flynn Makic (Eds.), *Trauma nursing: From resuscitation through rehabilitation* (5th ed., pp. 167–180). Elsevier; Graham, J. K. (2022). Shock, sepsis, and multiple organ dysfunction syndrome. In L. D. Urden, K. M. Stacy, & M. E. Lough (Eds.), *Critical care nursing: Diagnosis and management* (9th ed., pp. 831–864). Elsevier.

TABLE 6-2 Estimated Blood Loss in a 70-kg Man Based on Initial Presentation

Parameter	Class I	Class II (Mild)	Class III (Moderate)	Class IV (Severe)
Blood loss (mL)	Up to 750	750–1,500	1,500–2,000	> 2,000
Blood loss (% blood volume)	Up to 15%	15–30%	31–40%	> 40%
Pulse rate (beats/minute)	< 100	100–120	120–140	> 140
Systolic blood pressure	Normal	Normal	Decreased	Decreased
Pulse pressure	Normal	Decreased	Decreased	Decreased
Respiratory rate (breaths/minute)	14–20	20–30	30–40	> 35
Urine output (mL/h)	> 30	20–30	5–15	Negligible
Central nervous system/mental status	Slightly anxious	Mildly anxious	Anxious, confused	Confused, lethargic
Base deficit	0 to −2 mEq/L	−2 to −6 mEq/L	−6 to −10 mEq/L	−10 mEq/L or more
Initial fluid replacement	Crystalloid	Crystalloid or blood	Blood	Massive transfusion protocol

Data from American College of Surgeons. (2018). Shock. In *Advanced trauma life support: Student course manual* (10th ed., pp. 42–61).

presentations may vary and may not match these classifications precisely.

Goal-directed therapy for hypovolemic shock is aimed at controlling hemorrhage and replacing the type of volume the patient has lost in an effort to restore physiologic homeostasis.[5] Not all hemorrhage involves obvious external bleeding. When solid organs (liver, spleen) and large bone structures (pelvis, femur) are injured, significant blood loss may occur internally, so it becomes imperative to consider the mechanism of injury, maintain a high index of suspicion for occult bleeding, and continually reassess for subtle signs of shock.

Obstructive Shock (Mechanical Problem)

Obstructive shock results from hypoperfusion of the tissue that is due to an obstruction in either the great vessels or the heart, resulting in decreased cardiac output.[18,48] Goal-directed therapy is aimed at relieving the obstruction and improving perfusion. Examples of obstructive shock include the following[14,18]:

- With tension pneumothorax, the increase in intrathoracic pressure leads to displacement of the vena cava, obstruction to atrial filling, decreased preload, and decreased cardiac output. See Chapter 8, "Thoracic and Neck Trauma," for additional information.
- With cardiac tamponade, an accumulation of blood within the inflexible pericardial sac impedes diastolic expansion and filling, which in turn leads to decreases in preload, stroke volume, and cardiac output. See Chapter 8 for additional information.
- A venous air embolism can occur on the right side of the heart during systole in the pulmonary artery. If it is severe enough, this embolism in the right ventricular outflow tract may precipitate an obstruction, causing a decrease in cardiac output.

Cardiogenic Shock (Pump Problem)

Cardiogenic shock results from pump failure with inadequate CO in the presence of adequate intravascular volume.[18,48] A lack of cardiac output and end-organ perfusion occurs secondary to a decrease in myocardial contractility and/or valvular insufficiency (aortic and/or mitral). The most common cause of trauma-related cardiogenic shock is blunt cardiac injury. Any injury or ischemia to myocardial tissue or the conduction system could cause a dysrhythmia and affect cardiac output.[18,34,48]

Etiologies include blunt cardiac injury, myocardial infarction, dysrhythmias, cardiomyopathy, and toxicologic pathologies. While trauma rarely causes cardiogenic shock, one of the more common etiologies may have been the precursor to a traumatic injury.

When presented with decreased cardiac output without volume loss in the context of trauma, assess the patient for signs of a myocardial infarction, dysrhythmia, or heart failure; these are more common reasons for cardiogenic shock. Goal-directed therapy includes inotropic support, antidysrhythmic medications, and correction or treatment of the underlying cause.[18,28]

Excessive volume administration or an increase in afterload can result in pulmonary edema and increased myocardial ischemia. Successful emergent stabilization includes administering controlled fluid boluses to improve preload and inotropic support to improve contractility. If signs of fluid overload are present, afterload reduction may be indicated.[9,25]

Distributive Shock (Pipe Problem)

Distributive shock occurs as a result of maldistribution of an adequate circulating blood volume with the loss of vascular tone or increased permeability. Diffuse vasodilation lowers the systemic vascular resistance, creating a relative hypovolemia, reduction of the mean systemic volume and venous return to the heart, or drop in preload, resulting in distributive shock. Causative factors include the following[14,28,48]:

- *Anaphylactic shock* typically results from a release of inflammatory mediators such as histamine, which contracts bronchial smooth muscle and increases vascular permeability and vasodilation. Treatment includes immediate removal of the allergen (if known), airway management, and early administration of epinephrine, followed by intravenous (IV) fluid administration. Epinephrine's therapeutic effects will cause vasoconstriction, increase peripheral vascular resistance and bronchodilation, and decrease release of inflammatory mediators.
- *Septic shock* is caused by the systemic release of bacterial endotoxins, resulting in increased vascular permeability and vasodilation. Treatment for septic shock includes the early administration of antibiotics and IV fluid administration; norepinephrine to vasoconstrict the peripheral vasculature, increase blood volume return to the heart, and improve cardiac output also may be needed.[28]
- *Neurogenic shock* occurs with spinal cord injury that results in the loss of sympathetic nervous system control of vascular tone, leading to venous and arterial vasodilation. Under normal homeostatic conditions, the sympathetic and parasympathetic systems oppose each other, enabling vasoconstriction and

dilation to accommodate changing vascular volumes. With the loss of sympathetic nervous system input resulting from the spinal cord injury, unopposed (parasympathetic) vagal activity may result in decreased cardiac output through bradycardia. See Chapter 10, "Spinal and Musculoskeletal Trauma," for additional information.

Close monitoring of volume status and administration of medications, such as norepinephrine, dopamine, epinephrine, phenylephrine, and vasopressin, are interventions that can be used to produce vasoconstriction and increase peripheral vascular resistance. In some cases, atropine or transcutaneous pacing may be added to counteract parasympathetic bradycardia.[25]

Current Management Strategies

Current management strategies include tourniquets, damage control resuscitation, fluid resuscitation, massive transfusion, calcium chloride replacement, autotransfusion, resuscitative endovascular balloon occlusion of the aorta (REBOA), damage control surgeries, and tranexamic acid.

Tourniquets

Extensive military experience and research have reinforced the effectiveness of tourniquet use for limb injuries with uncontrolled hemorrhage. Increased use of tourniquets in civilian trauma systems has grown as prehospital providers, first responders, and hospital providers have identified the tourniquet as a beneficial tool in controlling isolated limb exsanguination.[3] Direct pressure and pneumatic splinting devices are hemorrhage-control methods used in addition to tourniquets. Early application of the tourniquet on an actively bleeding limb will minimize the likelihood of mortality from hemorrhagic shock.[26] The rate of complications is low, and those that do occur, such as nerve palsy, distal ischemia, or amputation, are typically related to prolonged use.[3,10] However, a life saved outweighs the risk of a limb injury.[3]

Damage Control Resuscitation

Damage control resuscitation is a process that focuses on the rapid restoration of homeostasis through the control of hemorrhage, administration of blood, and other interventions directed toward the prevention of the trauma triad of death.[13] Early recognition of the patient at risk for shock facilitates the use of goal-directed therapies. Damage control resuscitation involves two strategies: hypotensive and hemostatic resuscitation.

Hypotensive Resuscitation

The administration of large volumes of crystalloid solution is associated with increased bleeding and decreased survival rates, often as a result of hemodilution and decreased clotting factors.[5] Increasing blood pressure by infusing large amounts of crystalloid solutions or blood is not a substitute for controlling hemorrhage.[5] Hypotensive resuscitation, also known as permissive hypotension, involves a more limited fluid resuscitation, enabling a lower than normal blood pressure.[13,17,36] Permissive hypotension may limit complications that lead to increased bleeding and rebleeding, informally known as "popping the clot."[17,36] Additional benefits may also include decreased hemodilution and its negative effect on coagulation, as well as decreasing the risk of hypothermia.[13,17,36] This approach is not indicated in patients with head trauma because an adequate mean arterial pressure is necessary to maintain the cerebral perfusion pressure.[17]

Hemostatic Resuscitation

The key to early goal-directed therapy is to optimize tissue and cellular oxygenation and perfusion by preventing further losses through hemodilution coagulopathy.[5,13,42] When hemorrhage occurs, clotting factors and platelets are lost along with RBCs. Excessive use of isotonic crystalloids alone or replacing blood loss with only packed RBCs can produce a hemodilution coagulopathy in which the effective concentrations of both platelets and clotting factors are significantly reduced.[5,13,41,42] It can also lead to worsening acidosis (due to anaerobic metabolism), dilution of coagulation factors, increased inflammatory response (due to large volumes of crystalloid), acute respiratory distress syndrome, abdominal compartment syndrome, and increased mortality.

- Hemorrhage control is optimized by giving component therapy, using the transfusion of both packed RBCs and fresh frozen plasma in a 1:1 ratio.[5,13,41,42] Platelets are added at a 1:1:1 ratio in the presence of actual or anticipated thrombocytopenia.[5,42]
- Balanced fluid resuscitation is an approach to resuscitation that addresses all components that are lost with hemorrhage, including fluid, packed RBCs, fresh frozen plasma, and platelets, while surgically controlling the source of bleeding.[5,13,41,42] It is crucial that hemorrhage control and balanced fluid resuscitation be initiated early.[5]

Fluid Resuscitation

Current recommendations suggest administration of a lesser volume of crystalloid solutions[36] and use of boluses to follow the principle of permissive hypotension, when indicated.[5] Large-caliber catheters for intravenous or intraosseous (IO) access are acceptable forms of vascular access. Initial fluid management for the adult trauma patient in hemorrhagic shock consists of 500-mL boluses of warmed isotonic crystalloid solution given as rapidly as possible until blood products are available or an SBP of 90 mm Hg is achieved; a maximum of 1 liter of crystalloid solution is administered. Fluids given by prehospital providers must also be considered.[5] Fluid warmer/rapid infuser devices should be used to administer warmed fluid and blood products rapidly. These devices typically require the insertion of a large-caliber IV catheter (16 or 14 gauge) or IO needle to facilitate rapid administration.

In pediatric patients, fluid management is weight based, with 20 mL/kg of warmed isotonic crystalloid solution given to pediatric patients older than 28 days. This bolus may be repeated 1 to 2 times if necessary, based on the hemodynamic response to the first bolus.[4] Neonates receive 10 mL/kg of warmed isotonic crystalloid solution. Rapid infusers are not recommended in pediatric patients weighing less than 40 kg because of the use of smaller IV catheters (24 or 22 gauge) and specific weight-based fluid boluses.[29] See Chapter 13, "The Pediatric Trauma Patient," for additional information.

Massive Transfusion

The U.S. military first demonstrated that providing a balanced resuscitation (limited use of crystalloid solution) and following a massive transfusion protocol (MTP) with a defined blood-to-plasma ratio result in hemostasis and decreased mortality in hemorrhaging patients. Similar results have been found in civilian settings, and the U.S. Department of Defense is continuing research to determine the optimal ratio of blood-to-blood products. Recognizing that a predefined MTP leads to early blood, plasma, and platelet transfusions with improved outcomes, the American College of Surgeons delineated use of MTP as a critical criterion for trauma centers in its publication *Resources for Optimal Care of the Injured Patient*.[7] Success of MTP is dependent on early recognition and implementation, using a defined ratio of one part RBCs, to one part thawed plasma, to one part platelets (1:1:1 ratio) and providing a detailed process for implementation.[13,41] Limitations associated with MTP include the timing and immediacy of implementing the protocol and the availability of thawed plasma and platelets.

Calcium Chloride Replacement

Hypocalcemia is a concern with massive transfusion because citrate is added as a preservative to banked blood to prevent coagulation. Citrate chelates (binds with) calcium, rendering it inactive. Because calcium is a vital part of the clotting cascade, hypocalcemia, as a result of massive transfusion, can worsen hypovolemic shock by permitting continued bleeding.[42] Signs of hypocalcemia include cardiac dysrhythmias, muscle tremors, and seizures.[28] If calcium administration is indicated, this therapy should be guided by the patient's serum ionized calcium levels. Excessive supplemental calcium can be harmful as well.

If the trauma patient requires more than one unit of blood every 5 minutes, anticipate citrate toxicity and hypocalcemia, and prepare to replace losses with calcium gluconate or calcium chloride. If calcium chloride is used, monitor closely for infiltration because this infusion can cause tissue necrosis. Patients who are taking calcium-channel blockers (such as diltiazem) may be predisposed to cardiac dysrhythmias. Monitoring of calcium levels may be indicated earlier for these patients.[50]

Autotransfusion

Autotransfusion, or administration of the patient's own blood from collection through a chest tube, may be an option when transfusion is needed, often for massive hemothorax.[5] Other possible indications include the inability to obtain cross-matched blood when immediate administration of blood is needed, or cases in which the patient's convictions prohibit receiving donated blood.[15,19] Follow the manufacturer's guidelines for use. Blood that has been in the chest drainage collection system for longer than 6 hours should not be used.[19]

Benefits include the following[15,19,23]:

- The patient is transfused with their own whole blood, eliminating the risk of transfusion reaction.
- Blood is warmer than room temperature, so waiting for blood products to warm is not required.
- RBCs in autotransfused blood may have better oxygen-carrying capacity, because older, banked blood may have RBCs that have begun to degrade.
- Autotransfusion has a lower cost than transfusion of banked blood.
- There is a low risk of communicable disease.
- Autotransfused blood has a lower potassium level than banked blood.

Disadvantages include the following[15,19,23]:

- There is a risk of contamination; strict adherence to sterile setup before chest tube insertion is essential.[15]
- Use is limited to patients with an isolated hemothorax without diaphragmatic perforation.
- RBCs may become hemolyzed during hemorrhage.
- Coagulation factors, including platelets and cryoprecipitate, may be destroyed, which can increase the D-dimer in the collected blood.

- Patients may develop an enhanced inflammatory response, contributing to multiple-organ failure.
- Autotransfusion is contraindicated in known malignancy; inadequate renal or hepatic function; and contamination of the wound by injury to bowel, esophagus, or stomach.[23]

Autotransfusion as an intervention for traumatic injury is typically used in the hospital setting. However, research for use in the battlefield is recommended.[30]

Resuscitative Endovascular Balloon Occlusion of the Aorta

REBOA is a technique used in trauma patients to stop life-threatening hemorrhage within the chest, abdomen, and pelvis (**Figure 6-7**). In this procedure, a balloon is inserted in the aorta, occluding blood flow below the balloon, stopping the bleeding. REBOA can temporarily restore blood pressure to within normal physiological values by increasing cardiac afterload, thereby increasing cerebral and myocardial perfusion until the patient can be taken to the operating room for definitive hemorrhage control.[8,38] See Chapter 8, "Thoracic and Neck Trauma," information.

Damage Control Surgeries

Damage control surgery is a shift from rapid definitive surgery and complete repair to surgery that is intended to stop the bleeding, restore normothermia, and treat coagulopathy and acidosis; the focus is to prevent or resolve the components of the trauma triad of death (Figure 6-5). Damage control surgery is recommended to last no longer than 90 minutes, given the high morbidity and mortality associated with surgery.[27] Definitive injury repair may be accomplished later by deferring treatment of non-life-threatening injuries until the patient has been stabilized.[42]

Tranexamic Acid

Tranexamic acid (TXA) is a synthetic version of the amino acid lysine. This antifibrinolytic agent inhibits activation of plasminogen, a substance responsible for dissolving clots. TXA has been safely used to reduce intraoperative bleeding in elective medical and dental surgery and for the control of heavy menstrual bleeding. Although commonly used, the U.S. Food and Drug Administration at this time has not given approval for use of TXA in trauma. However, this may occur in the future. Until that time, the use of TXA in trauma is considered off-label.[16]

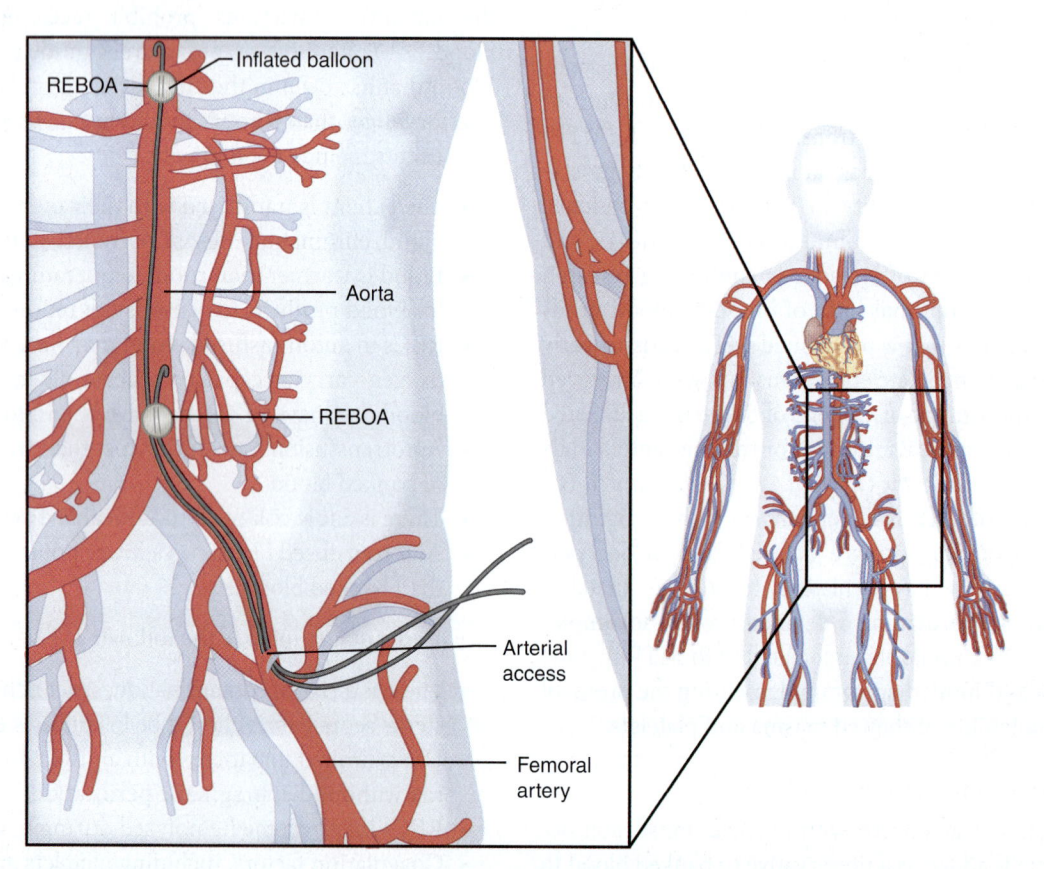

Figure 6-7 *Resuscitative endovascular balloon occlusion of the aorta.*

Nursing Care of the Patient in Shock

Nursing care of the patient in shock begins with preparation and triage.

Preparation and Triage

The American College of Surgeons Committee on Trauma considers an SBP of less than 90 mm Hg at any time to be a criterion for trauma team activation at the highest level.[7] One study found that a single SBP reading of less than 105 mm Hg was associated with severe injuries that often required operative or endovascular treatment and admission to the ICU.[45] In light of this risk, an isolated hypotensive blood pressure measurement during trauma resuscitation is considered significant.

Safe Practice, Safe Care

In the patient at risk for or experiencing shock, it is essential that assessment and intervention occur simultaneously and systematically. The primary survey is performed. Life-threatening problems are treated and reassessed before moving to the next step and before moving to the secondary survey. Integrated ongoing assessments, history, physical examination, imaging and laboratory studies, and serial assessments are crucial to optimizing patient outcomes because they involve anticipating potential blood loss from suspected or actual injuries and having a proactive management plan that anticipates the patient's potential course.

Primary Survey and Resuscitation Adjuncts

Refer to Chapter 4, "Initial Assessment," for the systematic approach to the nursing care of the trauma patient. The following assessment parameters are specific to patients with signs of shock.

A: Alertness and Airway

Considerations for assessing alertness and airway of patients with signs of shock include the following:

- Unresponsiveness in the trauma patient may be due to hypovolemia, not head trauma.
- A patient may experience decompensated shock with a blood volume loss of more than 30% before becoming unresponsive.[5]
- Use of alcohol and other substances may mask shock-induced changes in LOC in early shock and contribute to the inability to protect the airway.

B: Breathing and Ventilation

Inspect for the following:

- Increased respiratory rate and work of breathing may indicate compensation for early hypovolemic shock and respiratory correction of metabolic acidosis.
- Administer supplemental oxygen via nonrebreather mask to achieve optimal oxygenation, if not already completed as indicated in the assessment of the airway and breathing. Administer oxygen to maintain oxygen saturation (SpO_2) between 94% and 98%.

C: Circulation and Control of Hemorrhage

Inspect for the following:

- Active external bleeding
- Skin color, temperature, and moisture
- Bruised, swollen, and deformed extremities, particularly long-bone fractures
- A distended abdomen, which may indicate occult blood loss
- An unstable pelvis

Auscultate for the following:

- Diminished breath sounds (possible pneumothorax or hemothorax)
- Muffled heart tones (possible pericardial tamponade)

Palpate for the following:

- Central and peripheral pulses
  - Increased or bounding central pulses, which may indicate increased cardiac output; this can be the result of the release of catecholamines from the sympathetic nervous system to increase cardiac output.
  - A narrowing of the pulse pressure.
  - Characteristics of peripheral pulses changing in the presence of hypovolemia due to vasoconstriction; strong central pulses combined with weak peripheral pulses may indicate shock.
- Tenderness and rigidity in the abdomen and instability in the pelvis, which may be signs of occult hemorrhage

Interventions

Interventions include the following:

- Control external hemorrhage with direct pressure. Tourniquets are indicated if bleeding from an extremity is not controlled with direct pressure.[3]

- A pelvic binder or sheet is recommended for stabilization for confirmed unstable pelvic fracture. See Chapter 9, "Abdominal and Pelvic Trauma," for more information.
- Insert two large-caliber peripheral IV catheters.
  - If IV access cannot be rapidly obtained, default to IO access. Peripheral vascular access enables a more rapid infusion because the catheter length is shorter than a central line.[5]
  - Use a rapid infuser that warms the blood with blood tubing adequate to transfuse blood components.
    - Infuse blood products maintaining the 1:1:1 ratio.
    - Once hemostasis is achieved, it is estimated that one unit of packed RBCs will increase hemoglobin by 1 g/dL and hematocrit by 3%.[28]
    - Use Rh-negative blood whenever possible. If O-negative blood is limited, O-positive blood can be administered to men and postmenopausal women. If O-positive blood is administered to premenopausal women, they may become sensitized to the Rh factor, which may impact future pregnancies.
    - Consider activation of the MTP (unmatched type O blood, thawed fresh frozen plasma, and platelets). If blood is not available, infuse a 500-mL bolus of warmed isotonic crystalloid solution and reassess the patient's fluid status after each bolus.[43]
    - Vasopressors are contraindicated in early shock because they can worsen tissue perfusion.[5]

D: Disability (Neurologic Status)

Assess for loss of consciousness. A decrease may be indicative of hypoxemia and uncontrolled internal bleeding.

E: Exposure and Environmental Control

Address exposure and environmental control concerns by doing the following:

- Remove clothing to inspect for additional injuries and bleeding.
- Prevent hypothermia by warming resuscitation fluids to maintain the patient's temperature at 37°C (98.6°F).
- Other warming measures include warm blankets, warmed IV fluids, convective temperature management systems, and intravascular temperature management systems.

F: Full Set of Vital Signs and Facilitate Family Presence

Obtain a full set of vital signs and facilitate family presence.

Blood Pressure Measurements

SBP does not directly reflect cardiac output; however, trending vital signs may offer useful information regarding improved blood flow to the organs and tissue oxygenation to guide continued care. Additional measurements include the following:

- Frequent and serial blood pressure measurements to determine narrowing pulse pressure changes and monitor for signs of vascular compensatory mechanisms
- Blood pressure differences between the right and left arm, which may be a sign of thoracic aorta injury

Obtain the patient's temperature; hypothermia causes decreased tissue oxygenation, acidosis, and increased coagulopathy, resulting in increased morbidity and mortality.

Heart Rate

Heart rate may indicate the following:

- Tachycardia is one of the first signs of compensated shock in adults and especially in pediatric patients.
- Bradycardia and hypotension in combination with a spinal cord injury can reflect neurogenic shock.
- Bradycardia may indicate irreversible shock.

Respirations

Respiration may indicate the following:

- Tachypnea is an early indicator of compensated shock.
- Bradypnea may indicate irreversible shock.

G: Get Adjuncts and Give Comfort

Resuscitation adjuncts include laboratory studies, monitoring, and oxygenation.

L: Laboratory Studies

Laboratory studies used to guide resuscitative efforts in shock include the following:

- Type and cross-match
- Platelet count and clotting studies, including prothrombin time-international normalized ratio (PT-INR), partial thromboplastin time (PTT), fibrinogen, and D-dimer
- Rotational thromboelastometry (ROTEM) or thromboelastography (TEG)
- Serum lactate, anion gap, base deficit, and ABGs to assess the degree of acidosis and oxygen debt
- Toxicology screen to help assess mental status and differentiate shock from head injury

- Calcium level when rapidly infusing large volumes of blood products
- Additional blood specimens, including hemoglobin and hematocrit, electrolytes, serum osmolarity, blood urea nitrogen, creatinine, amylase, and liver enzymes. These tests may be directly correlated to the shock pathophysiology and injuries. However, unlike serum lactate, platelets, and clotting factors, they are less useful in the initial treatment and more useful in ongoing reevaluation.

M: Monitor

Place the patient on the monitor if they are hemodynamically unstable, have a suspected or known blunt cardiac injury, or have a trauma-related cardiac mechanism of injury.

O: Oxygenation

Oxygenation resuscitation adjuncts include pulse oximetry and end-tidal carbon dioxide ($ETCO_2$) monitoring.

- *Pulse oximetry*: The goal is to maintain an SpO_2 reading of 94% to 98%. Because many variables may potentially skew pulse oximeter readings, including hemodilution, carbon monoxide exposure, hypothermia, and peripheral vasoconstriction, it is essential that patient management decisions not be made on pulse oximetry values alone.
- *$ETCO_2$ monitoring*: $ETCO_2$ monitoring can be used to rapidly assess endotracheal tube placement, symptomatic pneumothoraces, or other pulmonary pathologies. It may also be used to indirectly assess cardiac output as a function of pulmonary perfusion. Continuous waveform capnography will provide a breath-to-breath analysis of both ventilation and perfusion and serve as a valuable adjunct during resuscitation and ongoing monitoring. Capnography also indirectly measures cardiac output and can be used to monitor effectiveness of cardiopulmonary resuscitation and the return of spontaneous circulation.

Additional Adjuncts

Bedside imaging may be completed emergently during B and C to evaluate for sources of shock.

Focused Assessment with Sonography for Trauma

During the primary survey, a focused assessment with sonography for trauma (FAST) examination may be used to rapidly and noninvasively assess for bleeding resulting from damage to the heart, liver, bladder, pelvis, kidneys, and spleen. The FAST examination is also increasingly used to detect pneumothorax, especially tension pneumothorax, and cardiac tamponade.[6]

Portable Radiograph

If the trauma patient is suspected of having, or being at risk for, internal hemorrhage, chest and pelvic imaging can be performed in the resuscitation room to expedite early goal-directed management. This is true for patients who may have a sequestering hemorrhage in the highly vascular pelvis.

Secondary Survey

The secondary survey begins with additional history and includes the head-to-toe assessment. See Chapter 4, "Initial Assessment," for additional information.

H: History

Additional history to be collected when the patient is at risk for shock includes the following:

- What was the estimated blood loss at the scene?
- What were the mechanism and time of injury?
- Was there any episode of SBP less than 90 mm Hg during prehospital care?
- Does the patient have changes to LOC or other symptoms that might indicate the onset of shock?
- Does the patient have complaints of chest or abdominal pain?

Additional history also includes past medical history:

- Does the patient have a history of hypertension? Does the patient take any antihypertensive medication?
- Does the patient have a history of anticoagulant therapy?
- Does the patient have a history of anemia or other blood dyscrasia (hemophilia)?

Positive responses may provide clues regarding acute blood loss, and careful inspection with close monitoring can lead to early detection of shock.

Diagnostics and Interventions

Reevaluation adjuncts include diagnostic studies and other types of studies.

Diagnostic Studies

Diagnostic studies include diagnostic peritoneal aspiration and lavage, and computed tomography (CT).

Diagnostic Peritoneal Aspiration and Lavage

Diagnostic peritoneal lavage is not used frequently but continues to be an option when FAST examination or

CT is not available or when the patient is too unstable to move for a CT scan. One of the benefits of this procedure over a FAST exam is its high sensitivity to bleeding within the abdominal cavity; it may also reveal free enteric contents.[5] Diagnostic peritoneal aspiration may be an alternative to quickly identify intraperitoneal bleeding and lessen the delay if operative intervention is indicated.

Computed Tomography

After stabilization and completion of the primary survey, CT is used to explore possible findings not seen on initial chest and abdominal radiography. An important caveat is that CT images are not required for transfer and should not delay transfer of the patient to a higher level of care if needed. Hemodynamically unstable trauma patients are high risk for deterioration during transport to radiology and imaging.

Other Studies

After achieving hemodynamic stability, echocardiography and a 12-lead electrocardiogram will provide additional cardiac assessment data.

Consider insertion of a urinary catheter to monitor urine output:

- Urine output is an important indicator of fluid volume status and organ perfusion, and it needs to be monitored hourly.
- Adequate urinary output is 0.5 mL/kg per hour (for the 70-kg adult patient).[5]
- Output of less than 0.5 mL/kg per hour for 2 consecutive hours indicates oliguria.

Reevaluation and Post-Resuscitation Care

Reevaluation specific to shock includes the following measures:

- Continued assessments of the primary survey are performed to monitor for rebleeding and previously unnoticed injuries and to ensure that sources of hemorrhage are controlled. Ongoing monitoring of hemoglobin, hematocrit, platelets, and clotting times may help to identify coagulopathy due to continued blood loss or hemodilution effects of massive volume resuscitation.[43]
- SpO_2 via pulse oximetry, $ETCO_2$ monitoring, and serial ABGs provide ongoing indicators of improved oxygenation, ventilation, and perfusion, including the following:
    - Normal serum pH
    - Decreasing serum lactate
    - Improved base excess
    - Signs of adequate perfusion to periphery
    - Adequate SpO_2
- Monitoring of urine output hourly is needed to assess effective resuscitation, and renal perfusion and function. Oliguria and an elevated blood urea nitrogen-to-creatinine ratio are signs of possible hypoperfusion.
- Continued frequent monitoring of vital signs for the following:
    - Normothermia
    - Normotension
    - Stable heart and respiratory rates

Definitive Care and Transport

Prepare the patient for surgical interventions to explore for occult blood loss and control of hemorrhage or other emergency surgical needs. Early consideration for transfer to an appropriate facility should be given. When the patient's care needs exceed the available resources at the initial facility, transport to a facility that can provide the necessary specialized or higher level of care is recommended. In an organized trauma system, severely injured trauma patients are transferred to the closest facility with appropriate resources, preferably a verified trauma center. See Chapter 20, "Transition of Care for the Trauma Patient," for additional information.

Emerging Trends

As the science and evidence of trauma care continue to evolve, tools to improve patient outcomes continue to be trialed and refined. Evidence is tested and replicated, and new standards of care are transitioned into practice. This section on care considerations for patients with shock explores some of the evidence and the potential significance to trauma patient care.

Viscoelastic Testing

Thromboelastometry (TEM) is a modification of the more traditional TEG, a blood test to evaluate the efficiency of blood clotting in an actively bleeding patient.[35,41] Unlike the standard coagulation assays, such as PT-INR and PTT, which measure only clotting factor function, TEM can also evaluate platelet function, clot strength, and fibrinolysis. Rotational TEM (ROTEM) is similar to TEM but uses rotational technology.[46] Both tests are used to guide transfusion strategies (including MTP) in the actively bleeding patient and to reduce the need for unnecessary transfusions.[35,46] Limitations include the following[35,46]:

- The tests have varying sensitivity for diagnosing hyperfibrinolysis; a body temperature of 37°C (98.6°F) is required for accuracy.
- The definitions of fibrinolysis as determined by TEM/ROTEM vary.
- Additional time is required to perform and read the test.

Whole Blood

Transfusion of whole blood, commonly used by the military and in austere environments, may be more beneficial than the use of individual blood components in treating hemorrhagic shock. Use of whole-blood transfusion for patients in hemorrhagic shock has been shown to increase survival and decrease overall blood usage.[12] Whole blood can be given quickly, however, it has limited storage time. It immediately delivers coagulation factors not found in packed RBCs alone. Precautions of giving whole blood include the risk of Rh alloimmunization during future pregnancies when given to female patients with O-positive blood. Whole blood also contains plasma with anti-A and anti-B antibodies that can cause hemolytic reactions.[32]

The Trauma Diamond of Death

The role of hypocalcemia in exacerbating each of the three components of the trauma triad of death (acidosis, coagulopathy, and hypothermia) is receiving heightened attention.[50] Calcium extensively interacts in multiple physiologic processes including, but not limited to, the electrical activity of myocardial cells, heart rate, vascular regulation, and coagulation. Hypocalcemia is detrimental to the trauma patient, leading some to transition from the trauma triad of death to the trauma diamond of death, adding hypocalcemia to acidosis, coagulopathy, and hypothermia (**Figure 6-8**).[50]

Freeze-Dried Plasma

The use of freeze-dried plasma has been adopted by the military in France and has been trialed by U.S. Army Special Forces and other sectors of the United States military.[40] The advantage of this product is that it can remain effective in its freeze-dried state for up to two years, until it is reconstituted with sterile water and administered to a patient.[22,40] Freeze-dried plasma may be most advantageous in the battlefield environment, during prehospital care when transport time is long, or in mass casualty situations.[22] Further research into this product continues.

Bleeding Control Education and Training for the Community

Just as the general public and lay community learn and perform cardiopulmonary resuscitation, education on bleeding control techniques using hands, dressings, and tourniquets is being offered in a new program available to the community that can also save a life. The American College of Surgeons Committee on Trauma and the Hartford Consensus have developed education and training for the general public on bleeding control. The "Stop the Bleed" course continues to be offered nationwide with the goal of helping to prevent death from uncontrolled bleeding.[1] See Chapter 10, "Spinal and Musculoskeletal Trauma," for more information on the "Stop the Bleed" campaign.

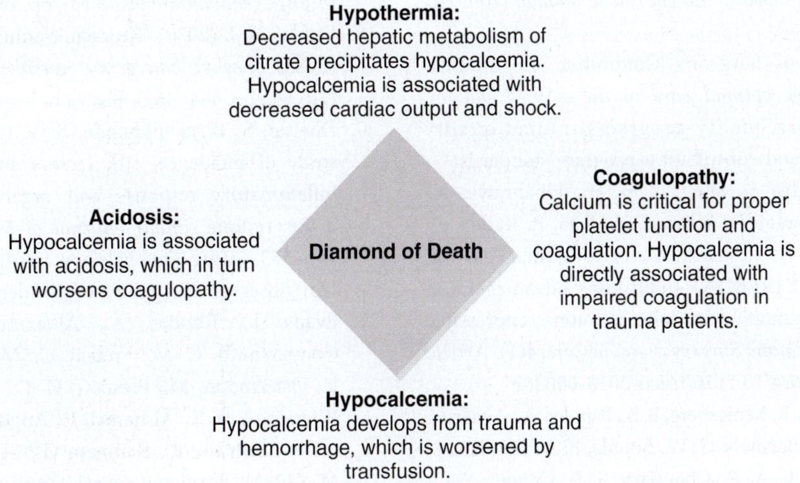

Hypothermia:
Decreased hepatic metabolism of citrate precipitates hypocalcemia. Hypocalcemia is associated with decreased cardiac output and shock.

Acidosis:
Hypocalcemia is associated with acidosis, which in turn worsens coagulopathy.

Diamond of Death

Coagulopathy:
Calcium is critical for proper platelet function and coagulation. Hypocalcemia is directly associated with impaired coagulation in trauma patients.

Hypocalcemia:
Hypocalcemia develops from trauma and hemorrhage, which is worsened by transfusion.

Figure 6-8 *Calcium and the trauma diamond of death.*

Reproduced from Wray, J., Bridwell, R., Schauer, S., Shackelford, S., Bebarta, V., Wright, F., Bynum, J., & Long, B. (2021). The diamond of death: Hypocalcemia in trauma and resuscitation. *American Journal of Emergency Medicine, 41*, 104–109. https://doi.org/10.1016/j.ajem.2020.12.065

Summary

Shock is a syndrome of impaired tissue perfusion and oxygenation. Mismatch between the supply and demand of oxygen and nutrients leads to ischemia at the cellular level, a transition from aerobic to anaerobic metabolism and resultant acidosis, and, ultimately, organ death. Shock can be classified into four main categories: hypovolemic, obstructive, distributive, and cardiogenic. Hypovolemic shock and depletion of circulating volume due to hemorrhage is the most common and primary shock state observed in trauma and a leading cause of preventable death in the prehospital environment. Early recognition and management of shock is essential to ultimately optimizing patient outcomes in traumatic shock.

References

1. American College of Surgeons. (2015). Strategies to enhance survival in active shooter and intentional mass casualty events: A compendium. *Bulletin, 100*(Suppl. 1), 16–17. https://www.stopthebleed.org/media/xt0hjwmw/hartford-consensus-compendium.pdf
2. American College of Surgeons. (2018). Head trauma. In *Advanced trauma life support: Student course manual* (10th ed., pp. 102–126).
3. American College of Surgeons. (2018). Musculoskeletal trauma. In *Advanced trauma life support: Student course manual* (10th ed., pp. 148–167).
4. American College of Surgeons. (2018). Pediatric trauma. In *Advanced trauma life support: Student course manual* (10th ed., pp. 186–212).
5. American College of Surgeons. (2018). Shock. In *Advanced trauma life support: Student course manual* (10th ed., pp. 42–61).
6. American College of Surgeons. (2018). Thoracic trauma. In *Advanced trauma life support: Student course manual* (10th ed., pp. 62–81).
7. American College of Surgeons Committee on Trauma. (2022). *Resources for optimal care of the injured patient.* https://www.facs.org/quality-programs/trauma/quality/verification-review-and-consultation-program/standards/
8. Bekdache, O., Paradis, T., Shen, Y. B. H., Elbahrawy, A., Grushka, J., Deckelbaum, D., Khwaja, K., Fata, P., Radek, T., & Beckett, A. (2019). Resuscitative endovascular balloon occlusion of the aorta (REBOA): Indications: advantages and challenges of implementation in traumatic non-compressible torso hemorrhage. *Trauma Surgery & Acute Care, 4*(1), Article e000262. https://doi.org/10.1136/tsaco-2018-000262
9. Berg, D. D., Barnett, C. F., Kenigsberg, B. B., Papolos, A., Alviar, C. L., Baird-Zars, V. M., Barsness, G. W., Bohula, E. A., Brennan, J., Burke, J. A., Carnicelli, A. P., Chaudhry, S. P., Cremer, P. C., Daniels, L. B., DeFilippis, A. P., Gerber, D. A., Granger, C. B., Hollenberg, S., Horowitz, J. M., . . . Morrow, D. A. (2019). Clinical practice patterns in temporary mechanical circulatory support for shock in the Critical Care Cardiology Trials Network (CCCTN) registry. *Circulation: Heart Failure, 12*(11), Article e006635. https://doi.org/10.1161/CIRCHEARTFAILURE.119.006635
10. Boulger, C., & Yang, B. (2018, March 1). Hemorrhage control: Advances in trauma care. *Trauma Reports.* https://www.reliasmedia.com/articles/142215-hemorrhage-control-advances-in-trauma-care
11. Brasher, V. L. (2020). Alterations of cardiovascular function. In S. E. Huether, K. L. McCance, & V. L. Brashers (Eds.), *Understanding pathophysiology* (7th ed. pp. 591–638). Elsevier.
12. Brill, J. B., Tang, B., Hatton, G., Mueck, K. M., McCoy, C. C., Kao, L. S., & Cotton, B. A. (2022). Impact of incorporating whole blood into hemorrhagic shock resuscitation: Analysis of 1,377 consecutive trauma patients receiving emergency-release uncrossmatched blood products. *Journal of the American College of Surgeons, 234*(4), 408–418. https://doi.org/10.1097/xcs.0000000000000086
13. Cap, A. P., Pidcoke, H. F., Spinella, P., Strandenes, G., Borgman, M. A., Schreiber, M., Holcomb, J., Chin-Nan Tien, H., Beckett, A. N., Doughty, H., Woolley, T., Rappold, J., Ward, K., Reade, M., Prat, N., Ausset, S., Kheirabadi, B., Benov, A., Griffin, E. P., . . . Stockinger, Z. (2018). *Military Medicine, 183*(Suppl. 2), 36–43. https://doi.org/10.1093/milmed/usy112
14. Carbino, G. (2020). Shock emergencies. In V. Sweet & A. Foley (Eds.), *Sheehy's emergency nursing: Principles and practice* (7th ed., pp. 205–215). Elsevier.
15. Catmull, S. P., & Ashurst, J. V. (2022, June 8). Autotransfusion. *StatPearls.* StatPearls Publishing. https://www.ncbi.nlm.nih.gov/books/NBK541014/
16. Chauncey, J. M., & Wieters, J. S. (2022). Tranexamic acid. *StatPearls.* StatPearls Publishing. https://www.ncbi.nlm.nih.gov/books/NBK532909/
17. Das, J. M., Anosike, K., & Waseem, M. (2022, August 7). Permissive hypotension. *StatPearls.* StatPearls Publishing. https://www.ncbi.nlm.nih.gov/books/NBK558915/
18. Dedeo, M. (2020). Traumatic shock. In K. A. McQuillan & M. B. Flynn Makic (Eds.), *Trauma nursing: From resuscitation through rehabilitation* (5th ed., pp. 167–180). Elsevier.
19. Denke, N. J. (2020). Thoracic trauma. In V. Sweet & A. Foley (Eds.), *Sheehy's emergency nursing: Principles and practice* (7th ed., pp. 444–464). Elsevier.
20. Dharap, S. B., & Ekhande, S. V. (2017). An observational study of incidence, risk factors and outcome of systemic inflammatory response and organ dysfunction following major trauma. *Indian Journal of Medical Research, 146*(3), 346–353. https://journals.lww.com/ijmr/Fulltext/2017/46030/An_observational_study_of_incidence,_risk_factors.9.aspx
21. Evans, L., Rhodes, A., Alhazzani, W., Antonelli, M., Coopersmith, C. M., French, C., Machado, F. R., Mcintyre, L., Ostermann, M., Prescott, H. C., Schorr, C., Simpson, S., Wiersinga, W. J., Alshamsi, F., Angus, D. C., Arabi, Y., Azevedo, L., Beale, R., Beilman, G., Belley-Cote, E., . . . Levy, M. (2021). Surviving sepsis campaign: International guidelines for management of sepsis and septic shock 2021. *Intensive Care Medicine, 47*, 1181–1247. https://doi.org/10.1007/s00134-021-06506-y

22. Feuerstein, S. J., Skovmand, K., Moller, A. M., & Wildgaard, K. (2020). Freeze-dried PLASMA in major hemorrhage: A systematic review. *Vox Sanguinis, 115*(4), 263–274. https://doi.org/10.1111/vox.12898
23. Gaasch, S., & Andersen, K. (2020). Thoracic trauma. In K. A. McQuillan & M. B. Flynn Makic (Eds.), *Trauma nursing: From resuscitation through rehabilitation* (5th ed., pp. 503–552). Elsevier.
24. Gitz Holler, J., Jensen, H. K., Henriksen, D. P., Rasmussen, L. M., Mikkelsen, S., Pedersen, C., & Lassen, A. T. (2019). Etiology of shock in the emergency department: A 12-year population-based cohort study. *Shock, 51*(1), 60–67. https://doi.org/10.1097/SHK.0000000000000816
25. Graham, J. K. (2022). Shock, sepsis, and multiple organ dysfunction syndrome. In L. D. Urden, K. M. Stacy, & M. E. Lough (Eds.), *Critical care nursing: Diagnosis and management* (9th ed., pp. 831–864). Elsevier.
26. Gulati, A., Jain, D., Agrawal, N. R., Rahate, P., Choudhuri, R., Das, S., Dhibar, D. P., Prabhu, M., Haveri, S., Agarwal, R., & Lavhale, M. S. (2021). Resuscitative effect of centhaquine (Lyfaquin®) in hypovolemic shock patients: A randomized, multicentric, controlled trial. *Advances in Therapy, 38*(6), 3223–3265. https://doi.org/10.1007/s12325-021-01760-4
27. Gupta, A., Kumar, S., Sagar, S., Sharma, P., Mishra, B., Singhal, M., & Misra, M. C. (2017). Damage control surgery: 6 years of experience at a Level I trauma center. *Turkish Journal of Trauma and Emergency Surgery, 23*(4), 322–327. https://doi.org/10.5505/tjtes.2016.03693
28. Holleran, R. S. (2018). Shock emergencies. In V. Sweet (Ed.), *Emergency nursing core curriculum* (7th ed., pp. 473–482). Elsevier.
29. Houston, K. A., George, E. C., & Maitland, K. (2018). Implications for paediatric shock management in resource-limited settings: A perspective from the FEAST trial. *Critical Care, 22*(1), Article 119. https://doi.org/10.1186/s13054-018-1966-4
30. Hulsebos, H., & Bernard, J. (2016). Consider autotransfusion in the field. *Military Medicine, 181*(8), e945–e947. https://doi.org/10.7205/MILMED-D-15-00046
31. Jacobs, L. M. (2015). *The Hartford Consensus III: Implementation of bleeding control*. https://bulletin.facs.org/2015/07/the-hartford-consensus-iii-implementation-of-bleeding-control/
32. Jones, A. R., Miller, J. L., Jansen, J. O., & Wang, H. E. (2021). Whole blood for resuscitation of traumatic hemorrhagic shock in adults. *Advanced Emergency Nursing Journal, 43*(4), 344–354. https://doi.org/10.1097/TME.0000000000000376
33. Katrancha, E. D., & Gonzalez, L. S. (2014). Trauma-induced coagulopathy. *Critical Care Nurse, 34*(4), 54–63. https://doi.org/10.4037/ccn2014133
34. Kislitsina, O. N., Rich, J. D., Wilcox, J. E., Pham, D. T., Churyla, A., Vorovich, E. B., Ghafourian, K., & Yancy, C. W. (2019). Shock—Classification and pathophysiological principles of therapeutics. *Current Cardiology Reviews, 15*(2), 102–113. https://doi.org/10.2174/1573403X15666181212125024
35. Kornblith, L. Z., Moore, H. B., & Cohen, M. J. (2019). Trauma-induced coagulopathy: The past, present, and future. *Journal of Thrombosis and Haemostasis, 17*(6), 852–862. https://doi.org/10.1111/jth.14450
36. Kudo, D., Yoshida, Y., & Kushimoto, S. (2017). Permissive hypotension/hypotensive resuscitation and restricted/controlled resuscitation in patients with severe trauma. *Journal of Intensive Care, 5*, Article 11. https://doi.org/10.1186/s40560-016-0202-z
37. Kushimoto, S., Kudo, D., & Kawazoe, Y. (2017). Acute traumatic coagulopathy and trauma-induced coagulopathy: An overview. *Journal of Intensive Care, 5*, Article 6. https://doi.org/10.1186/s40560-016-0196-6
38. Lee, L. O., Potnuru, P., Stephens, C. T., & Pivalizza, E. G. (2021). Current approaches to resuscitative endovascular balloon occlusion of the aorta use in trauma and obstetrics. *Advances in Anesthesia, 39*, 17–33. https://doi.org/10.1016/j.aan.2021.07.002
39. Lough, M. E. (2022). Cardiovascular anatomy and physiology. In L. D. Urden, K. M. Stacy, & M. E. Lough (Eds.), *Critical care nursing: Diagnosis and management* (9th ed., pp. 167–189). Elsevier.
40. Mok, G., Hoang, R., Khan, M. W., Pannell, D., Peng, H., Tien, H., Nathens, A., Callum, J., Karkouti, K., Beckett, A., & da Luz, L. T. (2021). Freeze-dried plasma for major trauma—Systematic review and meta-analysis. *Journal of Trauma and Acute Care Surgery, 90*(3), 589–602. https://doi.org/10.1097/TA.0000000000003012
41. Mondor, E. E. (2022). Trauma. In L. D. Urden, K. M. Stacy, & M. E. Lough (Eds.), *Critical care nursing: Diagnosis and management* (9th ed., pp. 791–830). Elsevier.
42. Ntourakis, D., & Liasis, L. (2020). Damage control resuscitation in patients with major trauma: Prospects and challenges. *Journal of Emergency and Critical Medicine, 4*, Article 34. https://doi.org/10.21037/jeccm-20-24
43. Salamea, M. J. C., Himmler, A. N., Valencia, A. L. I., Ordonez, C. A., Parra, M. W., Caicedo, Y., Guzman, R. M., Orlas, C., Granados, M., Macia, C., Garcia, A., Serna, J. J., Badiel, M., & Puyana, J. C. (2020). Whole blood for blood loss: Hemostatic resuscitation in damage control. *Colombia Médica, 51*(4), Article e4044511. http://doi.org/10.25100/cm.v51i4.4511
44. Savioli, G., Ceresa, I. F., Caneva, L., Gerosa, S., & Ricevuti, G. (2021). Trauma-induced coagulopathy: Overview of an emerging medical problem from pathophysiology to outcomes. *Medicines, 8*(16), 1–22. https://doi.org/10.3390/medicines8040016
45. Seamon, M. J., Feather, C., Smith, B. P., Kulp, H., Gaughan, J. P., & Godberg, A. J. (2010). Just one drop: The significance of a single hypotensive blood pressure reading during trauma resuscitations. *Journal of Trauma, 68*(6), 1289–1294.
46. Shaydakov, M. E., Sigmon, D. F., & Blebea, J. (2022, April 14). Thromboelastography. *StatPearls*. StatPearls Publishing. https://www.ncbi.nlm.nih.gov/books/NBK537061/
47. Sims, C. A., Guan, Y., Mukherjee, S., Singh, K., Botolin, P., Davila, A., Jr., & Baur, J. A. (2018). Nicotinamide mononucleotide preserves mitochondrial function and increases survival in hemorrhagic shock. *JCI Insight, 3*(17), Article e120182. https://doi.org/10.1172/jci.insight.120182

48. Standl, T., Annecke, T., Cascorbi, I., Heller, A. R., Sabashnikov, A., & Teske, W. (2018). The nomenclature, definition and distinction of types of shock. *Deutsches Arzteblatt International, 115*, 757–768. https://doi.org/10.3238/arztebl.2018.0757
49. van Veelen, M. J., & Maeder, M. B. (2021). Hypothermia in trauma. *International Journal of Environmental Research and Public Health, 18*(16), Article 78719. https://doi.org/10.3390/ijerph18168719
50. Wray, J., Bridwell, R., Schauer, S., Shackelford, S., Bebarta, V., Wright, F., Bynum, J., & Long, B. (2021). The diamond of death: Hypocalcemia in trauma and resuscitation. *American Journal of Emergency Medicine, 41*, 104–109. https://doi.org/10.1016/j.ajem.2020.12.065
51. Wyzant. (n.d.). *Cellular respiration.* https://www.wyzant.com/resources/lessons/science/biology/cellular-respiration

CHAPTER 7

Head Trauma

Melody R. Campbell, DNP, APRN-CNS, CEN, CCNS, CCRN, TCRN

OBJECTIVES

Upon completion of this chapter, the learner will be able to:
1. Describe mechanisms of injury associated with head trauma.
2. Describe pathophysiologic changes as a basis for assessment of the patient with head trauma.
3. Demonstrate the nursing assessment of the patient with head trauma.
4. Plan appropriate interventions for the patient with head trauma.
5. Evaluate effectiveness of nursing interventions for the patient with head trauma.

Knowledge of normal anatomy and physiology serves as the foundation for understanding anatomic derangements and pathophysiologic processes that may result from trauma. Before reading this chapter, it is strongly suggested that the learner review the following content. Anatomy is not emphasized in the classroom but is the basis of physical assessment and skill evaluation, as well as the foundation of questions for testing purposes.

Anatomy and Physiology of the Brain, Cranium, and Face

This section provides a review of the anatomy and physiology of the brain, cranium, and face.

Scalp

The scalp consists of five layers of tissue. These layers can be remembered by using the mnemonic **SCALP**: **s**kin, **c**onnective tissue, **a**poneurosis (galea aponeurotica), **l**oose areolar tissue, and **p**ericranium.[1] The scalp provides a protective covering and absorbs some energy transferred during an injury event. Because the scalp is highly vascular, lacerations or tears of it can result in profuse bleeding.[4]

Skull

The skull, which is formed by the cranial (frontal, ethmoid, sphenoid, occipital, parietal, and temporal) and facial bones, provides protection to the contents within the cranial vault (**Figure 7-1**).[55,57,73] The cranial bones are relatively thick (up to 6 mm), with the exception of the

110 Chapter 7 Head Trauma

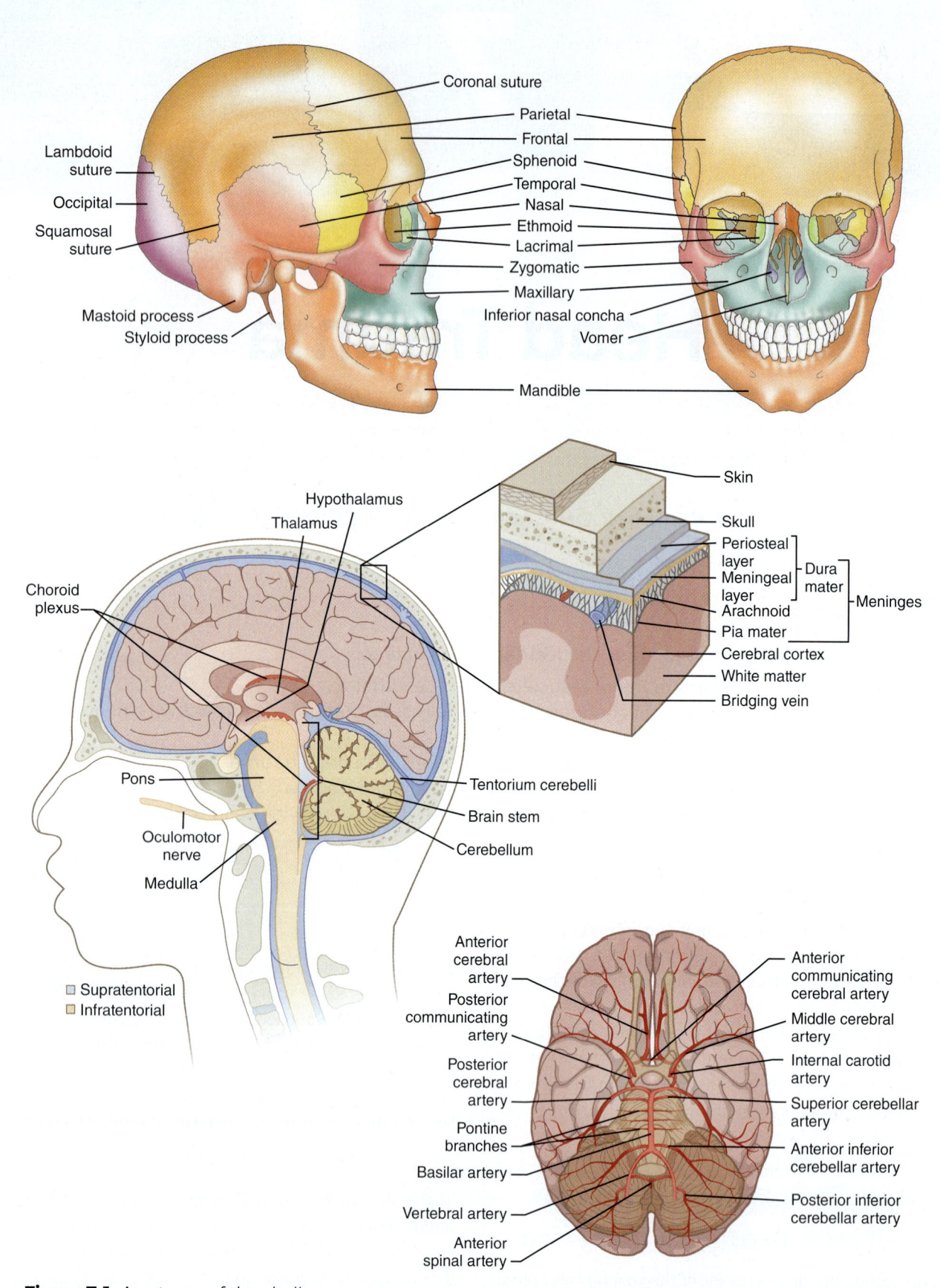

Figure 7-1 *Anatomy of the skull.*

temporal bone. Because of the thickness of the cranium, the skull may not fracture when struck by a strong excessive force. However, its lack of flexibility prevents absorption of energy, such that the force is transmitted to the parenchyma and vascular structures of the brain, often causing injury without skull fracture. Excessive force may result in fracture of the skull with resultant penetrating injury to the brain tissue.[45,54] The base of the skull forms three depressions: the anterior, middle, and posterior fossae. The internal surface of the skull base is rough and irregular. Acceleration and deceleration cause the brain to move across these rough inner surfaces, resulting in contusions, lacerations, and shearing injuries.[4]

Meninges

The meninges consist of three layers of protective coverings—the **p**ia mater, **a**rachnoid membrane, and **d**ura mater—that **PAD** the brain and spinal cord.[73] The pia mater, the innermost layer, firmly attaches to the brain and spinal cord. The arachnoid membrane is thin and transparent. The dura mater, the outermost layer, is a tough, fibrous membrane that adheres to the internal surface of the skull.[10,73]

The choroid plexus in the ventricles of the brain produces cerebrospinal fluid (CSF), which circulates around the brain beneath the arachnoid membrane (subarachnoid space) and through the central canal of the spinal cord. The CSF cushions and protects the brain and spinal cord. Arteries, including the middle meningeal arteries, are located above the dura mater. A fracture in the area of the parietal and temporal bone may cause damage to the middle meningeal artery, resulting in epidural hematoma. Small bridging veins lie beneath the dura mater. Injury to these small veins leads to the development of a subdural hematoma. The subarachnoid space is between the arachnoid membrane and the pia mater and is where large arteries enter the skull. Injury or bleeding in this area is referred to as subarachnoid hemorrhage.[73]

Tentorium

The tentorium cerebelli, which is part of the dura mater, extends from the occipital bone to the center of the cranium. The tentorium divides the cranial vault into two compartments—supratentorial and infratentorial. The supratentorial compartment contains the cerebral hemispheres in the anterior and middle fossae. The infratentorial compartment contains the lower parts of the brain stem (pons and medulla) and the cerebellum in the posterior fossa.[10,73] The upper part of the brain stem (midbrain) passes through a gap in the tentorium and the oculomotor nerve (cranial nerve [CN] III) lies against the edge of the tentorium.[4] Injury or edema near the tentorium gap may cause compression and shifting of the brain stem structures and the oculomotor nerve against the tentorium.[4]

Brain

The two cerebral hemispheres of the brain are divided into the frontal, parietal, temporal, and occipital lobes (**Figure 7-2**). The frontal lobes are responsible for judgment, reasoning, social restraint, and voluntary motor functions; the parietal lobes for sensory functions and spatial orientation; the temporal lobes for speech,

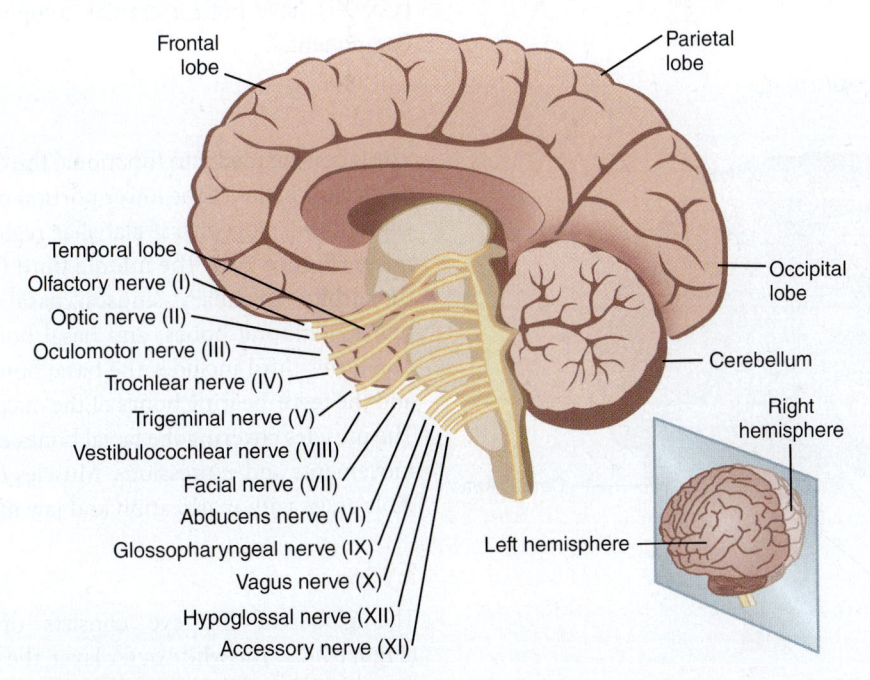

Figure 7-2 *Lobes of the brain.*

auditory, and memory functions; and the occipital lobe for vision.[55,73]

The diencephalon (**Figure 7-3**) connects the two cerebral hemispheres with the midbrain; it includes the thalamus, hypothalamus, optic chiasma, and pineal gland.[10,69] These subcortical structures play major roles in hormonal regulation and metabolic functions, including the following:

- Sensation of pain and temperature regulation
- Motor control
- Release of hormones from the pituitary gland and adrenal cortex
- Activation of the sympathetic and parasympathetic autonomic nervous systems[10,69]

The three divisions of the brain stem are the midbrain, pons, and medulla (**Figure 7-4**). The reticular activating system is composed of clusters of specialized neural tissue that originate in the midbrain and pons. The reticular activating system is primarily responsible for wakefulness or consciousness, while the medulla and the pons are responsible for vital functions such as cardiovascular function and respiration. Injury to the brain stem is associated with changes in consciousness and impairment in vital functions—specifically, blood pressure (BP), heart rate, and respiration.[10]

The cerebellum is located in the posterior fossa. The cerebellum lies behind the brain stem and beneath the cerebral hemispheres.[69] It has extensive neural connections with the spinal cord, midbrain, and cerebral hemispheres.[55] Primary functions of the cerebellum include voluntary and involuntary muscle coordination, movement, balance, and posture.[10]

Cranial Nerves

There are 12 pairs of cranial nerves (CNs) (**Figure 7-5**). The olfactory nerve (CN I) consists of a group of nerves located within a fiber tract that connect the nasal mucosa to the olfactory bulb. The optic nerve (CN II) originates in the retina and is considered a fiber tract once it leaves the optic chiasm. Millions of optic fibers then branch out to the occipital and temporal lobes. The brain stem is the point of origin for CNs III through X and XII, all of which exit via the skull foramina, leaving the cranial vault through the base of the lower brain.[73]

This shared exit pathway increases the risk for compression injury to the nerve tissue, with subsequent swelling and tissue damage.[55] The accessory nerves (CN XI) have both a cranial component and a spinal component.[73]

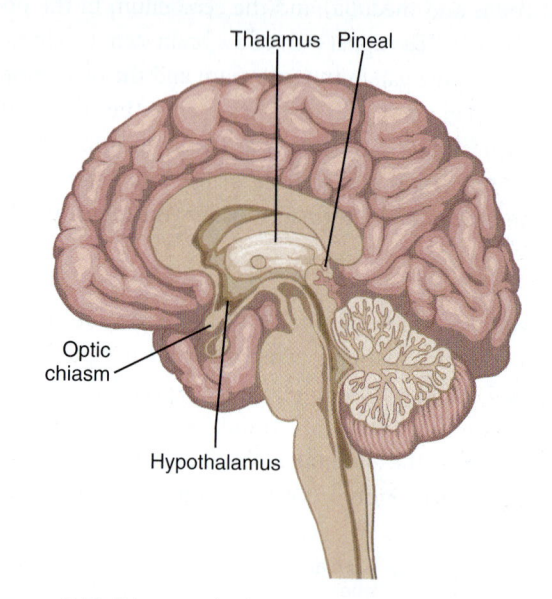

Figure 7-3 *Diencephalon.*

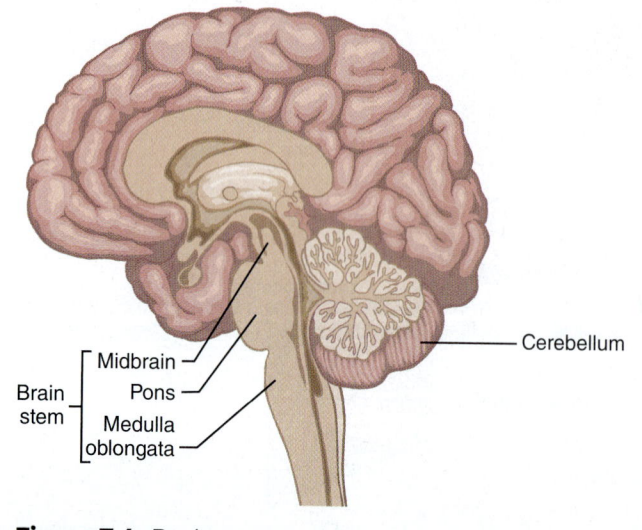

Figure 7-4 *Brain stem.*

Face

The face is divided into functional thirds. The upper third of the face includes the lower portion of the frontal bone, supraorbital ridge, nasal glabellar region, and frontal sinuses (**Figure 7-6**). The middle third (midface) includes the orbits, maxillary sinuses, nasal bone, zygomatic bones, temporal bones, and basal bone of the maxilla. The lower third includes the basal bone of the mandible and the teeth-bearing bones of the maxilla and mandible. The muscles covering the facial bones contribute to facial movements and expressions. Muscles covering the mandible assist with mastication and jaw movement.[58]

Eyes

The globe of the eye consists of multiple layers (**Figure 7-7**). The white outer layer, the sclera, can be easily seen without specialized equipment. The conjunctiva,

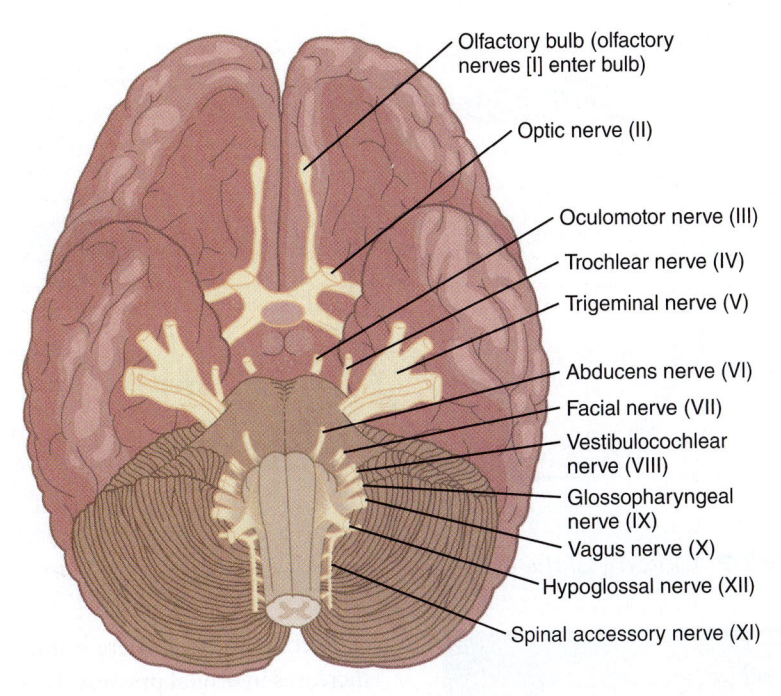

Figure 7-5 *Cranial nerves.*

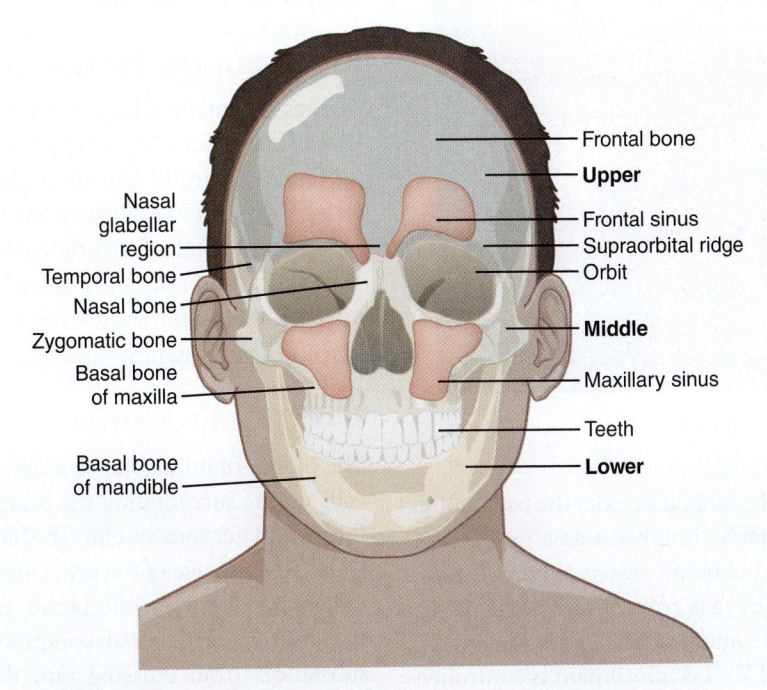

Figure 7-6 *Anatomy of the face.*

which is a mucous membrane, covers the sclera and inner surface of the eyelid.[58] Tears are secreted from the lacrimal glands in the upper eyelids and lubricate and protect the eye. These tears drain through the punctum located at the inner canthus of the eye.[28]

The cornea is an avascular layer of tissue that covers the iris and pupil. The iris is the colored portion of the eye and is positioned between the cornea and the lens; it contains the muscles responsible for constriction and dilation of the pupil. The lens separates the inside of the globe into a front segment with an anterior and posterior section filled with aqueous humor, a watery substance that supports the cornea and lens. The posterior segment contains vitreous humor.[8]

The retina is located at the back of the globe. The macula and fovea are located within the retina. The macula is the dark spot on the fundus of the eye that provides for clear and distinct vision, whereas the fovea is where

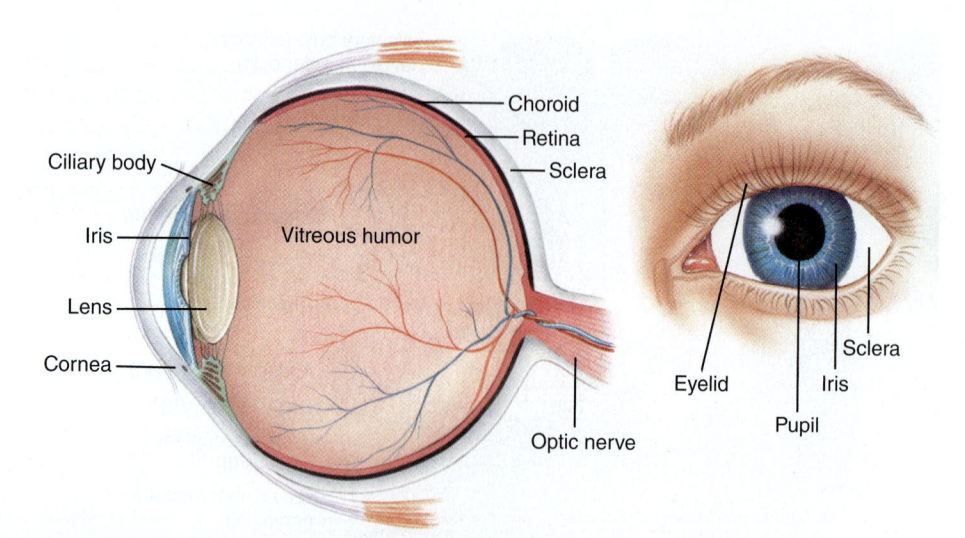

Figure 7-7 Anatomy of the eye.

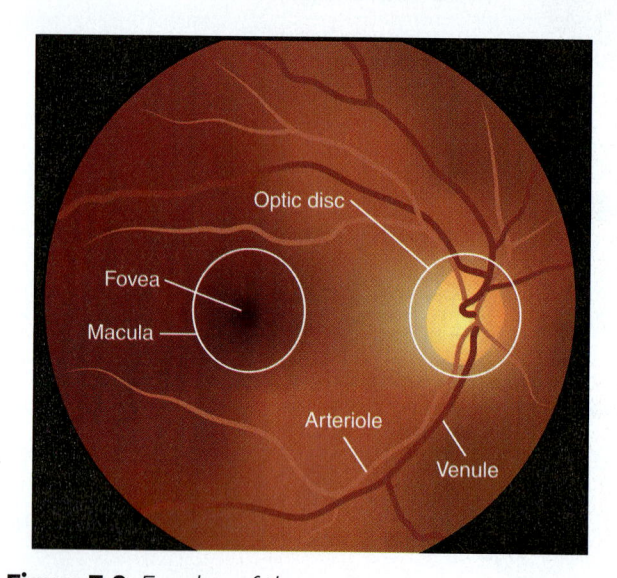

Figure 7-8 Fundus of the eye.

vision is the sharpest. The optic disc exits the back of the eye to form the optic nerve; it appears as a pale round area with a large number of blood vessels (**Figure 7-8**).

The movement of the eye is controlled by four rectus muscles and two oblique muscles. The eye is innervated by CNs II, III, IV, V, and VI. Eye movement is controlled by CNs III, IV, and VI. CN VII innervates the eyelids to close, and CN III innervates them to open. Ptosis (eyelid drooping) occurs as a result of oculomotor nerve (CN III) palsy.[10]

The blood supply to the eye comes from the ophthalmic artery, which branches off to form the central retinal artery. The majority of venous drainage occurs through the superior and inferior ophthalmic veins.[58]

The eyes are housed within a bony structure; however, this area of bone is thin and relatively easy to fracture. Additionally, because the eyes are surrounded by this rigid compartment, there is little space to accommodate increases in orbital pressure. Increases in orbital pressure due to hemorrhage and swelling may result in orbital compartment syndrome.[33]

Blood Supply for the Head

The brain contains a large vascular supply. Arterial blood travels to the brain via two pairs of arteries: the right and left internal carotid and the right and left vertebral arteries.[69] Venous blood drains via the jugular veins.[69] The blood supply to the face originates from the internal and external carotid arteries (**Figure 7-9**). Injury resulting in uncontrolled hemorrhage from any of these blood vessels may be life-threatening.

Blood–Brain Barrier

The blood–brain barrier is a network of capillaries and cells tightly surrounding the brain that act as a filter for the central nervous system. The blood–brain barrier controls the exchange of oxygen, carbon dioxide (CO_2), and metabolites between the blood and brain. This barrier makes brain capillaries less permeable, preventing some substances from crossing into the brain tissue. Other substances cross the blood–brain barrier more slowly, resulting in a lower concentration than elsewhere in the body. Traumatic brain injury (TBI) and ischemia can result in changes in permeability and blood flow, ultimately contributing to edema and increased intracranial pressure (ICP).[10,73]

Cerebral Blood Flow

The brain uses approximately 20% of the body's total oxygen supply and is heavily dependent on glucose metabolism for energy. The brain does not have the ability

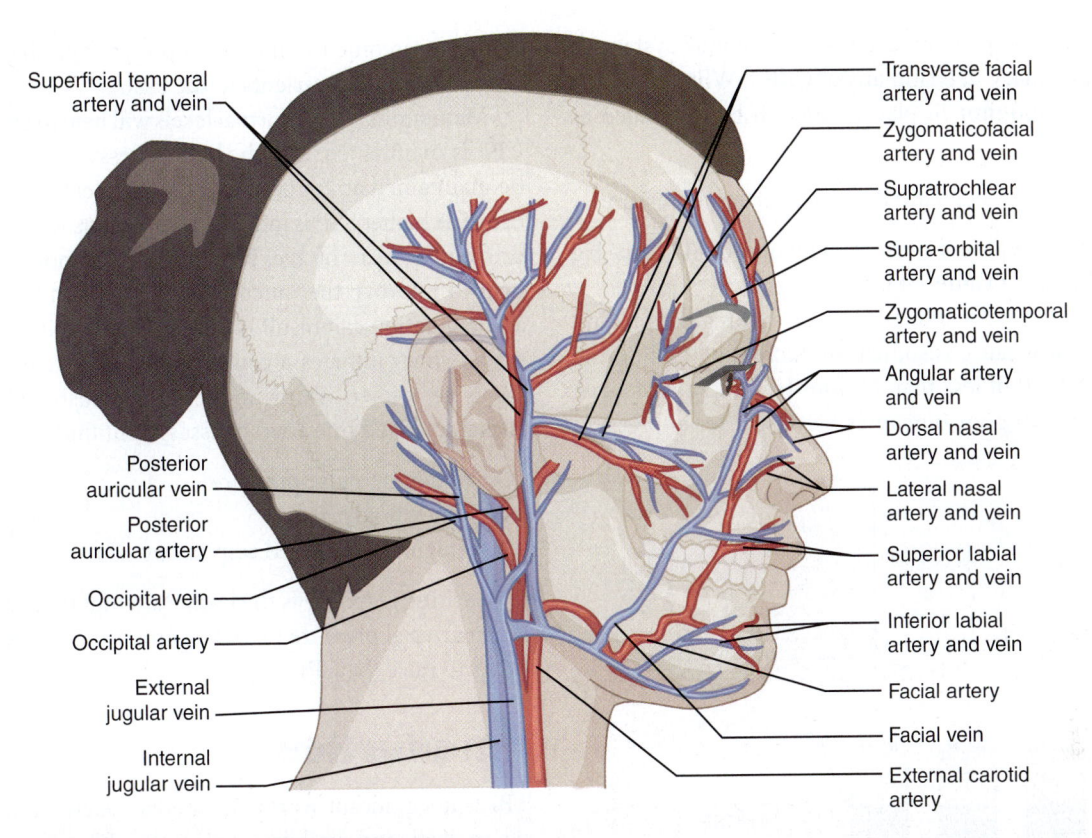

Figure 7-9 Blood supply for the head.

to store essential nutrients; therefore, it requires a continuous supply of both oxygen and glucose through the cerebral blood flow (CBF). The brain can self-regulate to maintain CBF through a process that is both complex and multifaceted. Cerebral vessels change their diameter in response to physiologic changes in the body. Hypotension, hypercarbia, and acidosis will result in cerebral vasodilation, whereas cerebral vasoconstriction results from hypertension, hypocarbia, and alkalosis.[10,54,69]

CO_2 is a primary regulator of blood flow to the brain and a strong vasodilator. At higher-than-normal levels (e.g., when a trauma patient has slow and shallow respirations), the increased partial pressure of carbon dioxide ($PaCO_2$) causes cerebral vasodilation, which increases cerebral blood volume and perfusion. Conversely, if the level of $PaCO_2$ decreases (e.g., as a result of aggressive bag-mask ventilation/hyperventilation), cerebral vasoconstriction occurs; this reduces blood volume and perfusion, subsequently decreasing ICP. The result may be inadequate oxygen and glucose delivery. Initially, the brain responds to the hypoxemia by increasing oxygen extraction from blood. When hypoxia becomes acute (partial pressure of oxygen [PaO_2] less than 50 mm Hg [6.67 kPa]), cerebral vasodilation occurs, and blood flow increases.[54,69]

Intracranial Pressure

The cranial vault contains three main components[69]:

- The brain, which occupies about 80%
- Blood (arterial and venous), which occupies about 10%
- Cerebral spinal fluid, which occupies about 10%

These volumes are relatively fixed, and together they create a normal ICP of 0–15 mm Hg (0–2 kPa).[4,68] According to the Monro–Kellie doctrine, as the volume of one component of the cranial vault triad expands, the volume of one or both of the other components must decrease to maintain a constant ICP (**Figure 7-10**). The potential for intracranial compensation is limited because the cranial vault is inflexible.[10,60] Thus, even small increases in total volume may cause significant increases in ICP, resulting in a decrease in CBF and a decrease in cerebral perfusion pressure (CPP). The recommended threshold for treatment of increased ICP is a sustained ICP of 22 mm Hg (2.93 kPa).[11,68]

Cerebral Perfusion Pressure

Adequate perfusion of oxygen and supply of nutrients (such as glucose) to the brain tissue is dependent on the CPP and CBF. CPP is defined as the pressure gradient across the brain tissue, or the difference between the pressures of the cerebral arterial and venous systems.[10] CPP is a primary determinant of CBF.[10] When a patient has an ICP monitor in place, CPP can be calculated as follows:

CPP = MAP − ICP (MAP = mean arterial pressure)

Normal CPP is in the range of 60–80 mm Hg (8–10.67 kPa)[46] (**Table 7-1**).[11,45]

In patients with intact cerebral autoregulation, hypotension will cause vasodilation, increasing CBF to the brain.[70] A CPP of less than 60 mm Hg (8 kPa) has been associated with poor outcomes because arterial pressure cannot overcome the increased pressure gradient to deliver oxygen and nutrients to the brain.[11,69]

Maintaining BP at normal levels will help to ensure that CBF is maintained. Systolic blood pressure (SBP) should be maintained at ≥ 100 mm Hg for patients 50–69 years of age. A higher SBP is indicated for patients who are 15–49 or over 70 years of age. Maintaining normotension will help to improve the outcome of the patient.[11,70] Loss of autoregulation can result in cerebral and brain stem ischemia, which initiates a central nervous system ischemic response, known as Cushing response. Cushing response is characterized by a triad of assessment findings[42]:

- Widening pulse pressure
- Reflex bradycardia
- Irregular, decreased respiratory effort

Cushing response is the body's attempt to increase the mean arterial pressure (MAP) against an elevated ICP in order to raise the CPP.

Introduction

TBI is a significant worldwide public health issue resulting in death and disability. Across the globe, an estimated 69 million people suffer a TBI each year.[22] According to recent U.S. data, 1.5 million individuals sustain a TBI annually,[26] resulting in more than 64,000 TBI-related deaths in 2020.[14] The elderly (older than 75 years) account for approximately one-third of hospitalizations and approximately

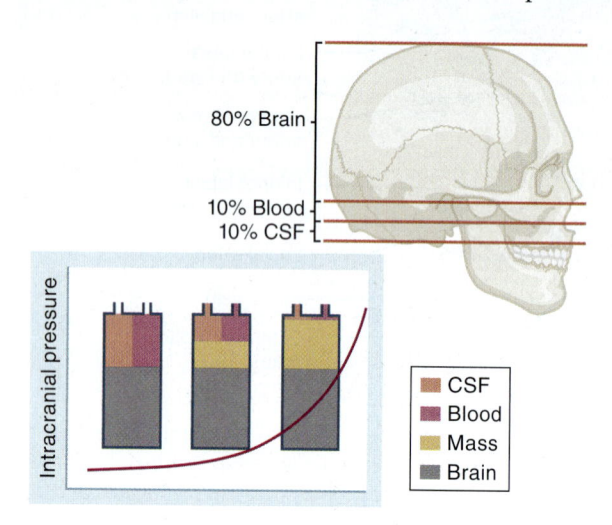

Figure 7-10 *Monro-Kellie doctrine.*
CSF = cerebrospinal fluid.

TABLE 7-1 Definitions of Terms

Term	Range	Definition
CPP	≥ 60 mm Hg (8 kPa)	The pressure gradient across the brain tissue; a measure of the adequacy of cerebral blood flow determined by the difference between MAP and ICP.
Hypercarbia	$PaCO_2$ > 45 mm Hg (6 kPa)	An increase in carbon dioxide in the bloodstream indicated by an elevated $PaCO_2$ as determined by blood gas analysis.[15]
ICP	0–15 mm Hg (0–2 kPa)	The pressure within the intracranial vault.[69]
MAP	Normal ≥ 60 mm Hg	The average arterial pressure throughout a single cardiac cycle, roughly calculated as the systolic blood pressure + (2 × the diastolic blood pressure) divided by 3.[21]

CPP = cerebral perfusion pressure; MAP = mean arterial pressure; ICP = intracranial pressure; $PaCO_2$ = partial pressure of carbon dioxide.

Data from American College of Surgeons. (2018). Head trauma. In *Advanced trauma life support: Student course manual* (10th ed., pp. 103–126); Carney, N., Totten, A. M., O'Reilly, C., Ullman, J. S., Hawryluk, G. W. J., Bell, M. J., Bratton, S. L., Chesnut, R., Harris, O. A., Kissoon, N., Rubiano, A. M, Shutter, L., Tasker, R. C., Vavilala, M. S., Wilberger, J., Wright, D. W., & Ghajar, J. (2016). *Guidelines for the management of severe traumatic brain injury* (4th ed.). https://braintrauma.org/uploads/03/12/Guidelines_for_Management_of_Severe_TBI_4th_Edition.pdf; Mondor, E. (2022). Trauma. In L. Urden, K. Stacy, & L. Mary (Eds.), *Critical care nursing* (9th ed., pp. 791–830). Elsevier; Chapman, K., & Dragan, K. E. (2022, July 4). Hypercarbia. *StatPearls*. StatPearls Publishing. https://www.ncbi.nlm.nih.gov/books/NBK559154/; Scarboro, M., Massetti, J., & Aresco, C. (2020). Traumatic brain injury. In K. McQuillan & M. Makic (Eds.), *Trauma nursing: From resuscitation through rehabilitation* (5th ed., pp. 332–409). Elsevier; DeMers, D., & Wachs, D. (2022, April 14). Physiology, mean arterial pressure. *StatPearls*. StatPearls Publishing. https://www.ncbi.nlm.nih.gov/books/NBK538226/

> **CLINICAL PEARL**
>
> **Maintain Adequate Cerebral Perfusion Pressure in the Head Trauma Patient**
>
> A CPP of less than 60 mm Hg (8 kPa) has been associated with poor outcomes because such a low arterial pressure results in inadequate delivery of oxygen and nutrients to the brain. It is advisable to maintain the CPP at greater than 60 mm Hg (8 kPa). Monitoring and supporting the BP and MAP are important methods for ensuring that CPP will be adequate.[4,11,32,70]

one-fourth of the deaths related to TBIs.[14] Men were almost two times more likely to require hospitalization and three times more likely to die from a TBI.[14] Falls lead to more than half of the hospitalizations related to TBI.[13]

Penetrating head injuries occur when a missile or object enters the skull and injures brain tissue. It is the most lethal mechanism of TBI; firearm injuries are the most common type of penetrating TBI, and more than 50% of those injuries are related to suicide.[20] The most common causes of facial fractures are assaults and motor vehicle collisions (MVCs).[17] Each year, approximately 2.4 million ocular injuries occur worldwide, and many of those result in permanent visual impairment.[8]

Mechanism of Injury

Injuries are classified as blunt, penetrating, or burns.[45]

- Blunt injuries result from the following causes:
    - Falls (the most frequent cause of TBI)
    - MVCs
    - Sports-related injuries
    - Recreation- and recreational vehicle–related injuries
- Penetrating injuries may occur from the following causes (see Chapter 3, "Biomechanics and Mechanisms of Injury," for more information):
    - Firearms
    - Exploding objects
    - Projectiles

Ocular burns may result from thermal, chemical, and radiation injury.[50] Primary injury to brain tissue may result from several factors, including the following:

- A direct blow or compression of the skull can cause a change of shape in the skull, also known as deformation, resulting in injury to brain tissue and blood vessels.[10,69]
- Acceleration/deceleration forces creating a pressure wave, resulting in energy transfer to several sites within the brain[69]
- Severe rotation or spinning that causes shearing or tensile force, resulting in tearing of cellular structures and bleeding[69]
- A blast from an explosive device, creating a pressure wave and contused tissue
- Penetrating injury from a sharp object or firearm, causing severe, irreparable damage to brain cells, blood vessels, and protective tissues around the brain[69]
- Lacerations as the brain moves across the irregular, rough base of the skull[54]
- Fractures of the skull and facial bones

Risk Factors

Certain risk factors contribute to sustaining a brain injury or having increased bleeding following the injury. These include the following:

- Gender: Compared with females, males are 1.5 times more likely to experience TBI and have a death rate 2.8 times higher.[62,69]
- Age: Children 0–4 years of age, young adults 15–19 years of age, and adults older than 75 years of age are at high risk[69]
- Anticoagulant/antiplatelet therapy
- Use of substances that may cause dizziness, imbalance, or delayed response times, such as the following[69]:
    - Alcohol
    - Medications
    - Illicit substances
    - Previous head injury

Usual Concurrent Injuries

Individuals with brain or craniofacial injuries are at risk for concurrent injuries to the cervical spinal cord and vertebral column.[5] Facial injuries may be associated with severe bleeding as a result of vascular disruption and/or airway compromise. Bony injuries may entrap nerves, causing injury to the underlying structures and presenting with ocular trauma.

Types of Injury

Brain injury is classified as a primary or secondary injury. Primary injuries result from a direct transfer of energy and include the following[4,45]:

- Skull and craniofacial fractures
- Intracranial lesions:
    - Diffuse injuries (concussion or diffuse axonal injury [DAI])
    - Focal injuries (epidural, subdural, intracerebral hematomas, or contusions)

Secondary injury is caused by complex pathophysiologic changes that include the following[4,45,69]:

- Hypotension
- Hypoxemia
- Hypercarbia
- Cerebral edema
- Increased ICP
- Decreased CPP
- Cerebral ischemia

Secondary injury increases the extent of the injury and may cause additional damage. The goal of caring for the patient who has experienced TBI is to prevent or limit secondary injury and the catastrophic cascade of events that result from those conditions, including death.[4,43]

Pathophysiology as a Basis for Assessment Findings

Pathophysiologic concepts that affect the patient with brain, cranial, or maxillofacial injuries include problems related to the following:

- Hypoxia
- Hypercarbia
- Hypotension and CBF
- Increase or decrease in ICP

Hypoxia and Hypercarbia

Signs and symptoms of hypoxia may initially be obscured by the brain's ability to compensate by extracting more oxygen from the blood. Early changes in mental status may be subtle, so it is crucial to be aware of the potential for deterioration. A single episode of hypoxemia (PaO_2 < 60 mm Hg [8 kPa]) can be detrimental to the patient's outcome.[4,82]

Carbon dioxide causes vasodilation, which can have a powerful but reversible effect on CBF. Hypercapnia causes significant dilation of cerebral arterial vasculature and increased blood flow to the brain.[31] Conversely, hypocapnia causes vasoconstriction and decreased blood flow.[54] This factor is important as it relates to assisted bag-mask ventilation and ventilator settings for the intubated patient. Hyperventilation decreases $PaCO_2$, causing cerebral vasoconstriction. This may result in hypoperfusion and cerebral ischemia. Hypercarbia ($PaCO_2$ > 45 mm Hg [6 kPa]) should be avoided because it promotes vasodilation and increases ICP.[31]

A brief period of hyperventilation may be indicated if the patient demonstrates acute signs of neurological worsening or impending herniation (unilateral or bilateral pupillary dilation, asymmetric pupillary reactivity, or abnormal posturing).[4,82] This is a temporizing measure, however, and should be maintained only until definitive interventions are implemented.[16,18,82]

> ### CLINICAL PEARL
> #### Avoid Hypoxemia in the Patient with Head Trauma
> A single episode of hypoxemia (PaO_2 < 60 mm Hg [8 kPa]) can be detrimental to the patient's outcome. Maintain pulse oximetry at 95% or greater, and obtain an arterial blood gas (ABG) measurement as soon as possible for patients with severe TBI.[61,82]

Hypotension and Cerebral Blood Flow

The brain is dependent on continuous blood flow to ensure a normal CPP. This blood flow is dependent on adequate BP. If the trauma patient is bleeding and becomes hypotensive, changes in the MAP cannot produce a perfusing CPP, and the brain tissue becomes hypoxic. The hypoperfused brain becomes ischemic and suffers irreversible damage, leading to progressively worsening neurological symptoms, with the patient eventually becoming unresponsive.[4,10] A single episode of hypotension (SBP < 90 mm Hg) can be harmful to patient outcomes.[4,82] In the context of severe head injuries, hypotension has been linked to more than double the mortality rate experienced by normotensive patients.[4]

If autoregulation fails, cerebral edema may result, which can be disastrous for the patient with TBI. Maintaining the MAP within normal limits is of the utmost importance.[4,70]

> ### CLINICAL PEARL
> #### Avoid Hypotension in the Patient with Head Trauma
> A single episode of hypotension can be harmful to patient outcomes. Maintain SBP at or greater than 100 mm Hg for patients 50–69 years old. Patients in the age range of 15–49 years, and older than 70 years should have SBP maintained at > 110 mm Hg.[4,11,70]

Intracranial Pressure

As ICP rises, CPP decreases, resulting in cerebral ischemia and secondary injury. Small elevations in BP and MAP represent attempts by the body to protect against

TABLE 7-2 Assessment Findings of Increased Intracranial Pressure

Early

Headache

Nausea and vomiting

Amnesia

Behavior changes (impaired judgment, restlessness, and drowsiness)

Altered level of consciousness (hypoarousability and hyperarousability)

Late

Dilated, nonreactive pupils

Unresponsiveness to verbal or painful stimuli

Abnormal motor posturing (flexion, extension, and flaccidity)

Cushing response

- Widening pulse pressure
  - Pulse pressure is the difference between the systolic and diastolic pressures; normal is 40–60 mm Hg
- Reflex bradycardia
- Decreased respiratory effort

Data from Broering, B. (2020). Head trauma. In V. Sweet & A. Foley (Eds.), *Sheehy's emergency nursing: Principles and practices* (pp. 401–418). Elsevier; March, K. (2018). Head injury and dysfunction. In V. Good & P. Kirkwood (Eds.), *Advanced critical care nursing* (2nd ed., pp. 218–252). Elsevier.

---

brain ischemia in a patient with elevated ICP. Intricate physiologic alterations result in a decreased PaO_2 and increased $PaCO_2$, both of which act to dilate cerebral blood vessels, increasing CBF. ICP sustained at greater than 22 mm Hg (2.93 kPa) and unresponsive to treatment is associated with poor outcomes.[4,11] Increased ICP produces signs and symptoms that are both predictable and sequential (**Table 7-2**).[4] Ultimately, increased ICP combined with an expanding hematoma, inflammation, or edema can result in brain stem herniation.[69]

> **CLINICAL PEARL**
>
> **Manage Intracranial Pressure in the Patient with Head Trauma**
>
> An ICP sustained at greater than 22 mm Hg (2.93 kPa) that is unresponsive to treatment is associated with poor outcomes.[4,32]

Nursing Care of the Patient with Head Trauma

Refer to Chapter 4, "Initial Assessment," for information on the systematic approach to the nursing care of the trauma patient. The following assessment parameters are specific to patients with head trauma.

Preparation and Triage

Anticoagulant use and bleeding disorders were previously identified as a triage parameter in the injured patient because of the potential for increased risk of bleeding.[67,79] The updated guidelines have modified this criterion to state, "In a prospective study of older adults transported by EMS, the incidence of brain hemorrhage was similar between patients taking versus not taking anticoagulants. Based on these data, the panel felt that the use of anticoagulants (including antiplatelet agents) was best considered in the context of EMS judgment."[48] However, it remains essential, as part of the prehospital report, to ask if the patient takes anticoagulation or antiplatelet medications. These medications may have the capability to cause increased hemorrhage in the trauma patient, and it is essential to identify the possible need for treating this condition in the primary survey as part of controlling hemorrhage.

Primary Survey and Resuscitation Adjuncts

The primary survey elements and resuscitation adjuncts specific to the patient with head trauma are outlined in the following sections.[4]

A: Alertness and Airway

Alertness and airway concerns include the following[3]:

- Assess the patient using the **AVPU** (**a**lert, **v**erbal, **p**ain, **u**nresponsive) mnemonic: A patient response other than "alert" may be associated with a brain injury.[42]
- Be prepared to assist with early endotracheal intubation for patients who are unable to protect their airway, especially those with facial injuries and bleeding.
  - Obtain and document a brief neurologic exam before administering sedating/paralyzing medications for intubation.[4]
- Rigid cervical collars may contribute to an increase in ICP because these devices can interfere with venous outflow and cause increased pain and discomfort to the patient.
  - The fit of the rigid collar may need to be adjusted.[69]

B: Breathing and Ventilation

Breathing and ventilation concerns include the following:

- If the patient is alert, administer oxygen at 10–15 L/minute via nonrebreather mask with a tight-fitting seal and reservoir bag.
- Obtain an ABG measurement as soon as possible.[61]
  - Titrate the oxygen for normoxia and maintain SpO_2 at 95% or greater[4] (see Chapter 5, "Airway and Ventilation," for additional information).

> **CLINICAL PEARL**
>
> **Maintain Adequate Oxygenation and Ventilation in the Patient with Head Trauma**
>
> Maintain $SpO_2 \geq 95\%$.
> Maintain end-tidal carbon dioxide ($ETCO_2$) between 35 mm Hg and 45 mm Hg (4.7–6 kPa).[4,82]

Table 7-3 presents the goals for treatment in the care of the patient with TBI.[4]

C: Circulation and Control of Hemorrhage

Concerns related to circulation and control of hemorrhage include the following:

- If applying direct pressure to bleeding sites, avoid placing pressure in the area over a depressed skull fracture.
- Avoid hypotension in patients with head trauma; hypotension has been associated with an increased mortality rate in adults.[4]
  - The goal of fluid support is to restore euvolemia. Blood products and isotonic intravenous fluid should be used to achieve SBP ≥ 100 mm Hg in patients 50–69 years of age and ≥ 110 mm Hg in patients 15–49 and older than 70 years of age.[4]
- Hypotension in the trauma patient is usually caused by bleeding. The source of bleeding should be identified and treated immediately.[69]
- Vasopressors may be indicated to maintain CPP once bleeding is controlled and the patient is adequately resuscitated.[32,42]

D: Disability (Neurologic Status)

Disability or neurologic status concerns include the following:

- Assess pupillary size and response to light.[10,69,82]
  - A unilaterally fixed and dilated pupil may indicate compression of the oculomotor nerve (CN III) from increased ICP and indicate impending herniation syndrome.
  - Bilaterally fixed and pinpoint pupils may indicate an injury at the pons or the effects of opioids.
  - A moderately dilated pupil with sluggish response may be an early sign of herniation syndrome.
  - Bilateral pupillary constriction may be caused by sedatives such as opiates.
  - Bilateral pupillary dilation may be caused by stimulants such as epinephrine or cocaine.
- Assess the Glasgow Coma Scale (GCS) score or **FOUR** (**f**ull **o**utline of **un**responsiveness) score (**Table 7-4** and **Figure 7-11**).[75,80]
  - Obtain an ABG measurement to determine and ensure adequate oxygenation and ventilation.[61]
  - Obtain a blood glucose measurement because hypoglycemia may present as lethargy or unresponsiveness.[5]
  - Intubation is recommended if the level of consciousness decreases acutely.[3]

TABLE 7-3 Goals of Treatment for Brain Injury

Pulse oximetry ≥ 95%	ICP 5–15 mm Hg (.67–2.13 kPa)	Serum sodium 135–145
PaO_2 ≥ 100 mm Hg (13.33 kPa)	$PbtO_2$ ≥ 15 mm Hg (2.13 kPa)	INR ≤ 1.4
$PaCO_2$ 35–45 mm Hg (4.66–6 kPa)	CPP ≥ 60 mm Hg[a] (8 kPa)	Platelets ≥ 75 x 10^3/mm^3
SBP ≥ 100 mm Hg[b]	Temperature 36.0–38.0°C (96.8–100.4°F)	Hemoglobin ≥ 7 g/dL
pH 7.35–7.45	Glucose 80–180 mg/dL	

ICP = intracranial pressure; PaO_2 = partial pressure of oxygen; $PbtO_2$ = brain tissue oxygen tension; INR = international normalized ratio; CPP = cerebral perfusion pressure; $PaCO_2$ = partial pressure of carbon dioxide; SBP = systolic blood pressure.
[a] Depending on the status of cerebral autoregulation.
[b] See Clinical Pearl "Avoid Hypotension in the Patient with Head Trauma" and the section "C: Circulation and Control of Hemorrhage" in this chapter for age-specific blood pressure goals.

Reproduced from American College of Surgeons. (2018). Head trauma. *Advanced trauma life support: Student course manual* (10th ed., pp. 103–126).

TABLE 7-4 Comparison of the Glasgow Coma Scale and the FOUR Score

Glasgow Coma Scale		FOUR Score	
Eye Opening		**Eye Response**	
4	Spontaneous	4	Eyelids open or opened, tracking, or blinking to command
3	To sound	3	Eyelids open but not tracking
2	To pressure	2	Eyelids closed but open to loud voice
1	None	1	Eyelids closed but open to pain
Best Verbal Response		0	Eyelids remain closed with pain
5	Oriented	**Motor Response**	
4	Confused	4	Thumbs-up, fist, or peace sign
3	Inappropriate words	3	Localizing to pain
2	Incomprehensible words	2	Flexion response to pain
1	None	1	Extension response to pain
Best Motor Response		0	No response to pain or generalized myoclonus status
6	Obeys commands	**Brain Stem Reflexes**	
5	Localizes	4	Pupil and corneal reflexes present
4	Withdraws from pressure	3	One pupil wide and fixed
3	Abnormal flexion with stimulus	2	Pupil or corneal reflexes absent
2	Abnormal extension with stimulus	1	Pupil and corneal reflexes absent
1	None	0	Absent pupil, corneal, and cough reflex
		Respiration	
		4	Not intubated, regular breathing pattern
		3	Not intubated, Cheyne-Stokes breathing pattern
		2	Not intubated, irregular breathing
		1	Breathes above ventilator rate
		0	Breathes at ventilator rate, or apnea

Glasgow Coma Scale

The GCS score ranges from 3 to 15 and provides a measure of the patient's level of consciousness. It is also a predictor of morbidity and mortality after brain injury when used in conjunction with other assessment factors.[4,34,36,76,81] The patient's total score derives from the patient's response to three aspects that are independently measured[4]:

- *Best* eye opening
- *Best* verbal response
- *Best* motor response

The initial GCS score provides a baseline score, and repeated assessments determine whether the patient's neurologic status is improving or deteriorating. The motor component of the GCS score is the most sensitive subscore for identifying patients with severe brain injury.[5,63] Refer to Chapter 4, "Initial Assessment," for a complete description of the GCS. The severity of brain injury is classified by the GCS as shown in **Table 7-5**; this classification guides management of the patient with head trauma.[4]

One or more of the patient's limbs may be immobilized from the effects of sedation, pharmacologic paralysis,

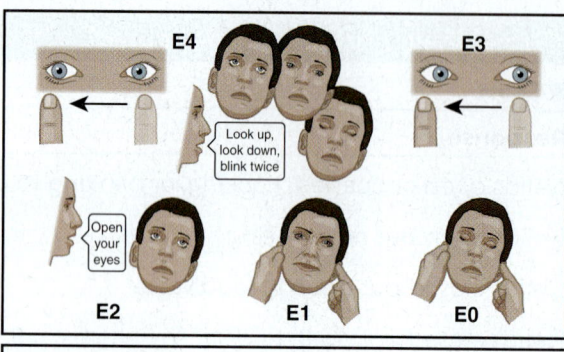

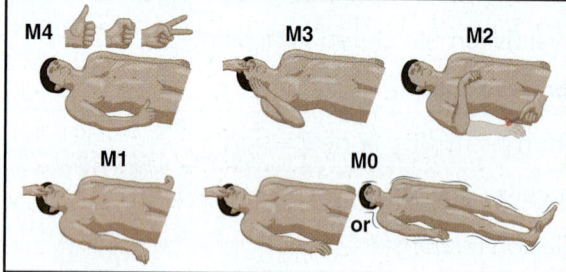

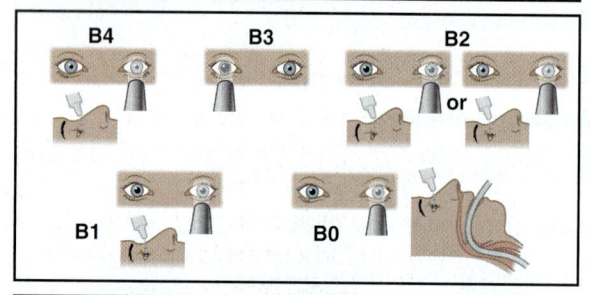

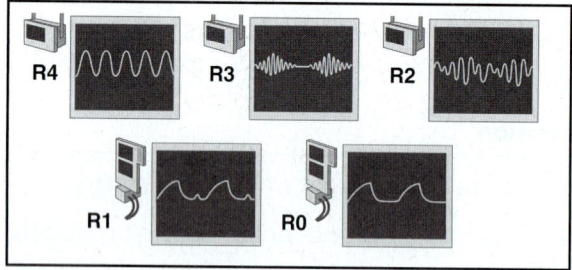

Figure 7-11 The FOUR score.
Reproduced from Mayo Foundation for Medical Education and Research. All rights reserved. For complete rationale and instructions for using the FOUR Score scale, contact the Mayo Clinic at www.mayo.edu.

Eye response
4 = Eyelids open or opened, tracking or blinking to command
3 = Eyelids open but not to tracking
2 = Eyelids closed but opens to loud voice
1 = Eyelids closed but opens to pain
0 = Eyelids remain closed with pain stimuli

Motor response
4 = Thumbs up, fist, or peace sign
3 = Localizing to pain
2 = Flexion response to pain
1 = Extension response
0 = No response to pain or generalized Myoclonus status

Brain stem reflexes
4 = Pupil and corneal reflexes present
3 = One pupil wide and fixed
2 = Pupil or corneal reflexes absent
1 = Pupil and corneal reflexes absent
0 = Absent pupil, corneal, or cough reflex

Respiration
4 = Regular breathing pattern
3 = Cheyne-Stokes breathing pattern
2 = Irregular breathing
1 = Triggers ventilator or breathes above ventilator rate
0 = Apnea or breathes at ventilator rate

TABLE 7-5 Classification of Severity of Traumatic Brain Injury by Glasgow Coma Scale Score

TBI Classification	GCS Score
Mild	13–15
Moderate	9–12
Severe	3–8

TBI = traumatic brain injury.
Data from American College of Surgeons. (2018). Head trauma. In *Advanced trauma life support: Student course manual* (10th ed., pp. 103–126).

fractures, brain or spinal cord injury, or other circumstances. Avoid misinterpreting a grasp reflex or postural adjustment as a response to a command. Remember that the *best* response is to be measured. This is particularly important when one limb's response is better than the others, or the patient moves the eyelids purposefully yet has paralysis from the neck down. If one component cannot be tested, no numeric score should be assigned; the component should be documented as nontestable, with the reason noted.[4]

FOUR Score

The FOUR score (Figure 7-11) ranges from 0 to 16, with each category score ranging from best (4) to worst (0).

The FOUR score provides greater neurologic detail compared with the GCS score but is more complex to perform.[51,53,80] The patient's total score results from a summative score of four components of response:

- Eye response (E)
- Motor response (M)
- Brain stem reflexes (B)
- Respiration (R)

All components of the FOUR score can be rated in patients with or without an endotracheal tube, so this score may have advantages in the critical care setting. Early research on the FOUR score's predictive reliability and validity is promising.[2,7,51,53,80] The scores R2–R4 are reserved for nonintubated patients.[2]

In patients who are mechanically ventilated, assessment is done preferably when $PaCO_2$ is within normal limits and no adjustments are being made to the ventilator. Assess the pressure waveform on spontaneous respiration or when the patient triggers the ventilator. A score of R1 is given to a patient who breathes at greater than the ventilator rate. A score of R0 is given to a patient who breathes only at the ventilator rate or is apneic. A standard apnea test may be needed for patients with a score of R0.[80]

E: Exposure and Environmental Control

Hypothermia in combination with shock can have a deleterious effect on oxygenation of brain tissue (see Chapter 6, "Shock," for more information). The sequela of hypothermia is well documented (trauma triad of death). However, mild hypothermia (95–97°F [35–36°C]) may be appropriate as an intervention for patients with increased ICP when other interventions have failed.[32]

F: Full Set of Vital Signs and Facilitate Family Presence

Monitoring and supporting BP and oxygenation are key components for improving outcomes of the patient with a TBI. It can be distressing for family members to see patients with altered levels of consciousness and exhibiting repetitive questioning or other symptoms. Providing psychosocial support is challenging but essential because it may be months before the patient's functional status will be known. The nurse can provide simple, realistic explanations while acknowledging the unknown to support the patient and family.[4,42,69]

G: Get Monitoring Devices and Give Comfort (LMNOP)

Be alert for bradycardia, alterations in respirations, changes in MAP, hypo- or hypertension, hypoxia, and hypercapnia with continuous monitoring. Any changes may indicate the body's attempt to compensate for increased ICP or herniation. Nasogastric tubes are contraindicated in facial trauma because some facial fractures may provide a route for the tube to pass directly into the brain. Pain management is not to be withheld, but shorter acting pain and sedation medications may be used to allow more frequent assessments of mental status.[4,69]

Reevaluation for Transfer

Determine whether the patient is a candidate for immediate surgery or meets the criteria for transport to a trauma center with neurosurgical capabilities. Any head-injured patient with evidence of neurologic deficits meets the criteria for transport if the services and expertise are not available.[4,82]

The patient's BP is a determinant for further interventions:

- Hypotension: Rarely will intracranial hemorrhage in an adult patient produce a volume of blood loss large enough to produce hypotension.
  - If hypotension is present, the priority is to determine and manage the cause of bleeding.[4]
- Normotension: With a neurologic deficit (unequal pupils or asymmetric motor examination), the priority is to obtain a computed tomography (CT) scan of the head. Secondary assessment of the patient should be completed before movement of the patient from the emergency department to radiology.
- Hypertension: Hypertension associated with increased ICP may occur as a result of Cushing reflex.[82] Treatment of pain is an element of managing intracranial hypertension.[82]

Secondary Survey and Diagnostics and Therapeutics for Head Trauma

The secondary survey and diagnostics and therapeutics for head trauma begin with the patient history and head-to-toe assessment.

H: History

History-taking questions specific to patients with suspected head trauma include the following[10,54,82]:

- If the patient is conscious, what are the patient's complaints?
  - Headache, nausea and vomiting, and amnesia may be early signs of increased ICP.
- If the patient's level of consciousness is altered, does the history suggest head trauma?
  - Impact to the head or face
  - Postinjury lucid interval (consider epidural hematoma)

- Was there any vomiting or other signs and symptoms of a brain or cranial injury?
- Was there any loss of consciousness? For how long?
- Does the patient have amnesia from the injury event?
- Does the patient take anticoagulant or antiplatelet medications? When was the last dose taken?
- What is the patient's baseline? Does the patient have dementia or preexisting neurological impairment?

Specific to Ocular Trauma

History-taking questions specific to ocular trauma include the following[50,77]:

- Was the patient wearing protective eyewear or corrective eyewear? Has it been removed?
- If a penetrating injury occurred, what material caused the injury (metallic or organic)?
  - Organic material carries a high incidence of infection.
  - Metallic foreign objects can cause permanent staining.
- Did the trauma cause a change in vision? What are those changes (e.g., blurring, double vision, or loss of vision)?
- Was there a chemical exposure? What type of chemical (acid or alkali)? Was any type of treatment or decontamination performed before patient arrival?
- Note: History taking with chemical exposure should be done concurrently with the initiation of treatment; treatment should not be delayed.[24]

H: Head-to-Toe Assessment

Inspect for the following:

- Inspect the craniofacial area for ecchymosis or contusion.
- Basilar skull fractures can produce bleeding that may not become evident until several hours after the injury.[10] These collections of blood under the tissue may become apparent in one of three areas (**Figure 7-12**):
  - Periorbital ecchymoses, also known as raccoon eyes, indicate an anterior fossa fracture.[69]
  - Mastoid process ecchymoses, also known as Battle sign, indicate a middle fossa fracture.[69]
  - Hemotympanum, blood behind the tympanic membrane, may indicate fracture of the temporal bone.[10]
- Inspect the craniofacial area for symmetry, flattening of the face, or malocclusion.[27]

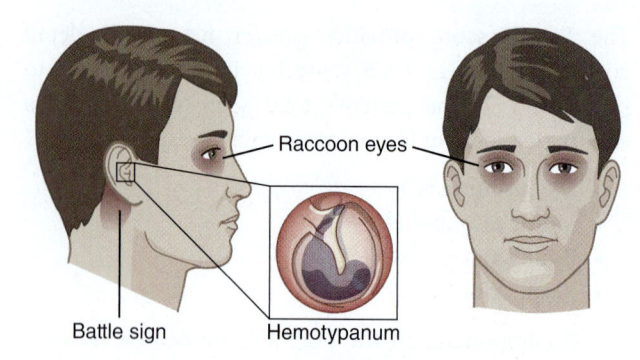

Figure 7-12 *Signs of a basilar skull fracture.*

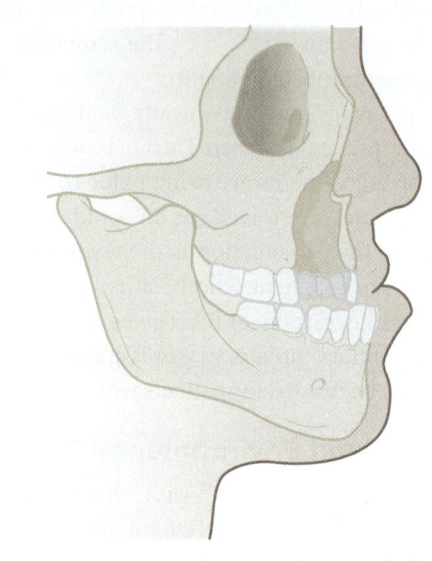

Figure 7-13 *Flattening of face due to facial fracture.*

- Asymmetrical facial appearance can indicate soft-tissue injury or facial fracture.
- Flattening of the face or a dishlike appearance is consistent with Le Fort fractures (**Figure 7-13**).
- Malocclusion may be a sign of mandibular fracture.
- Evert the upper eyelid and inspect for any potential foreign body, if needed.
- Palpate for tenderness, bony crepitus, or step-offs, which may indicate a fracture.[17]

Additional Assessments

Inspect the nose and ears for drainage. CSF drainage from the nose or ear is due to a tear in the dura.[27] To test otorrhea/rhinorrhea for CSF, consider the following:

- Two tests historically have been performed rapidly to suggest a general suspicion of CSF leak.[10,17] These two tests are neither specific nor sensitive for the detection of CSF leaks.[49]
  - Halo sign: Place the fluid on tissue or filter paper. A ring or "halo" of clear or pink-tinged fluid will form around the area of red blood—this

constitutes a "positive halo sign." The test does not differentiate between CSF and other clear fluids such as saline, saliva, and water. It is considered unreliable.[10,17]

Test for glucose: CSF is high in glucose, and nasal mucus usually does not contain glucose.[10,49] Palpate the cranial area gently for the following:

- Point tenderness
- Depressions or deformities
- Hematomas

Assess all four extremities bilaterally for the following[69]:

- Motor function
- Muscle strength
- Sensory function
- Abnormal motor posturing (abnormal flexion and abnormal extension) or flaccidity (sign of head injury)

Visual Acuity

Visual acuity is a fundamental part of the ocular assessment. Key elements to assess while performing the examination include the following:

- Ask about the patient's usual vision. Does the patient usually wear glasses or contacts?[50]
- What can the patient see? Ask the patient to describe their vision (blurry, decreased, or normal).
- Use a standard-distance Snellen chart to assess visual acuity, positioning the chart 20 feet away from the patient (**Figure 7-14**).[50,77]
- If the patient is unable to stand, use a handheld near-vision card held 14 inches away from the patient's face.[38]
- If the patient cannot read the chart, ask the patient what they can see: fingers, objects, light, or shadows.[38]
  - Assess extraocular eye movements to test the function of CNs III, IV, and VI (**Figure 7-15**). Assess smoothness of movement, symmetry, and speed. If nystagmus is present, determine whether it is the patient's baseline or began after the traumatic incident.
- In the presence of facial fractures, the inability to perform extraocular eye movements may indicate extraocular muscle entrapment.[50]

Pupil Examination

Assess pupils for shape, size, reactivity, and symmetry. As much as 10% of the general population has unequal pupils (anisocoria), which is a benign physiologic condition. Causes of abnormal anisocoria include trauma, uncal herniation, oculomotor nerve (CN III) palsy, medications, and some nebulizers (ipratropium). Pupils are normally round; an oval pupil may indicate a tumor,

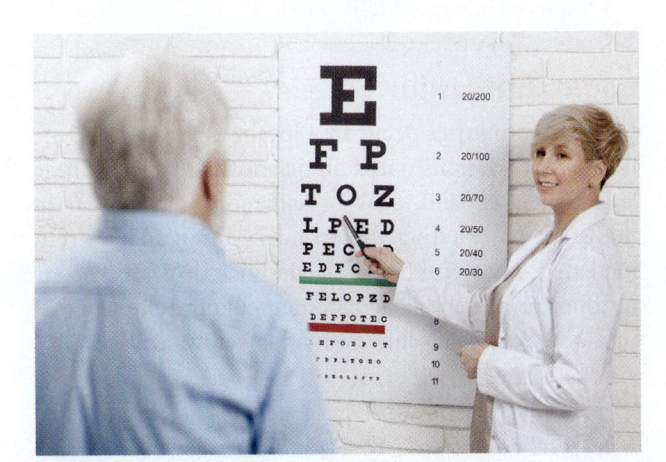

Figure 7-14 Visual acuity exam.
© Serhii Bobyk/Shutterstock.

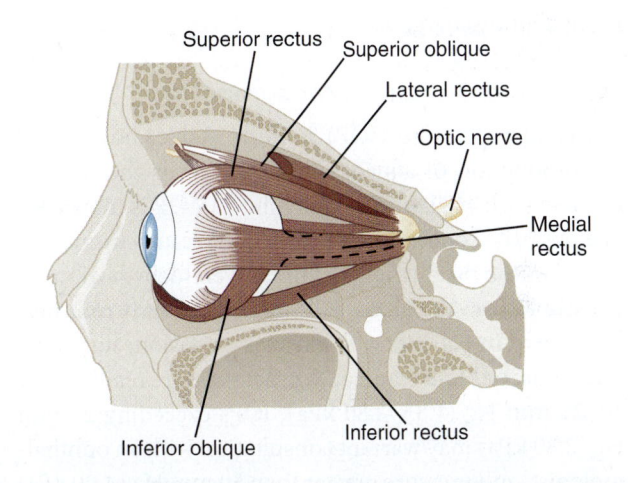

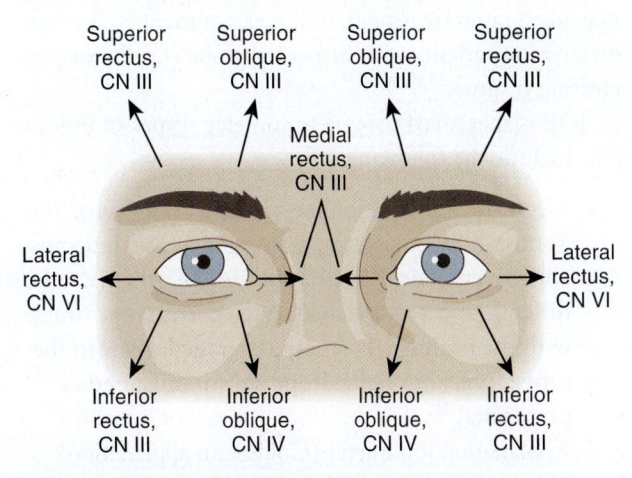

Figure 7-15 Innervation and movement of extraocular muscles.

retinal detachment, or prior injury; a teardrop-shaped pupil suggests a globe rupture.[50,69,82]

Pupils are tested using a penlight in a darkened room. The normal pupillary response is a brisk constriction, with both pupils constricting to the same size.[50]

Ophthalmoscope Examination

The ophthalmoscope is used to look at the fundus, optic nerve, disc, and the major blood vessels. If possible, dim the lights to enable the patient's pupil to dilate; alternatively, the provider may dilate the pupil with medication. Serial assessment of pupillary size and reactivity is an important part of neurologic assessment; therefore, dilation of the pupil in the setting of head injury is contraindicated.[50,82] If the patient is having a difficult time keeping their eyes open, topical anesthetics may be used. Note that these medications are *not* sent home with the patient—their use without medical supervision puts the patient at risk for inhibited corneal healing.[50] Additionally, the use of medications to dilate the pupil may blur vision for hours and make it unsafe for the patient to drive. This factor should be considered when preparing for patient discharge.

Intraocular Pressure Measurement

Intraocular pressure (IOP) is fairly stable; however, if the production of aqueous humor exceeds the outflow in cases such as glaucoma or hyphema, IOP is increased. The opposite condition, decreased IOP, results from a decrease in the production of fluid, severe dehydration, or a disruption in the globe. IOP measurement is routinely performed in patients who have loss of vision, suspected glaucoma, or blunt trauma. Normal pressure readings are 10–21 mm Hg (1.33–2.80 kPa). IOPs exceeding 21 mm Hg (2.80 kPa) may warrant consultation with an ophthalmologist, and pressure greater than 30 mm Hg (4.00 kPa) may need rapid treatment. IOP measurement is contraindicated for patients with suspected globe rupture or penetrating trauma.[38,50,64]

IOP is measured using a tonometer. Types of tonometry include the following:

- Electronic indentation tonometry (Tono-pen): The Tono-pen is an electronic device that uses a disposable cover (**Figure 7-16**). This device, which can be difficult to use, is touched to the cornea four times, with the findings then being averaged. Prior to the procedure, anesthetic drops are administered as prescribed.[38]
- Applanation tonometry (Goldmann applanation): This procedure is used by most ophthalmologists and optometrists and is usually found on the slit lamp.[38,58]

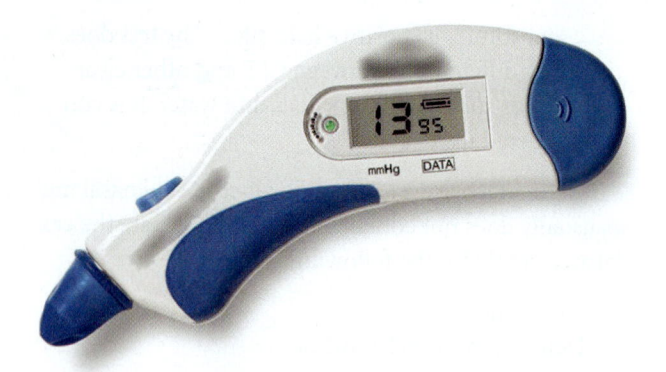

Figure 7-16 *Electronic indentation tonometry (Tono-pen).*

Selected Head Injuries

Selected head injuries discussed in this section include coup/contrecoup injury, focal brain injuries, diffuse injuries, penetrating injuries, and craniofacial fractures.

Coup/Contrecoup Injury

When the head strikes a solid object, the sudden deceleration force may result in bony deformity and injury to cranial contents. Within the cranial vault, a pressure wave is generated at the point of impact, which may tear tissue and cause injury at the site of impact (coup injury). As the pressure wave travels across the cranial contents and dissipates, injury may occur on the side opposite the impact (contrecoup injury). **Figure 7-17** shows both types of injury. It is possible to suffer this type of head injury without experiencing a direct blow to the head.[31] Assessment findings include the following:

- Altered level of consciousness
- Behavioral, motor, or speech deficits
- Abnormal motor posturing
- Signs of increased ICP

Focal Brain Injuries

Focal brain injuries occur in a localized area with identifiable brain lesions noted on diagnostic imaging. These lesions may expand, causing damage to other areas of the brain or resulting in secondary brain injury from increased ICP. Focal brain injuries include cerebral contusion, intracerebral hematoma, epidural hematoma, subdural hematoma, and herniation syndromes.[69]

Cerebral Contusion

A cerebral contusion is bruised or damaged brain tissue. It is usually caused by blunt trauma and is the most common type of brain injury.[10,69] Most cerebral contusions

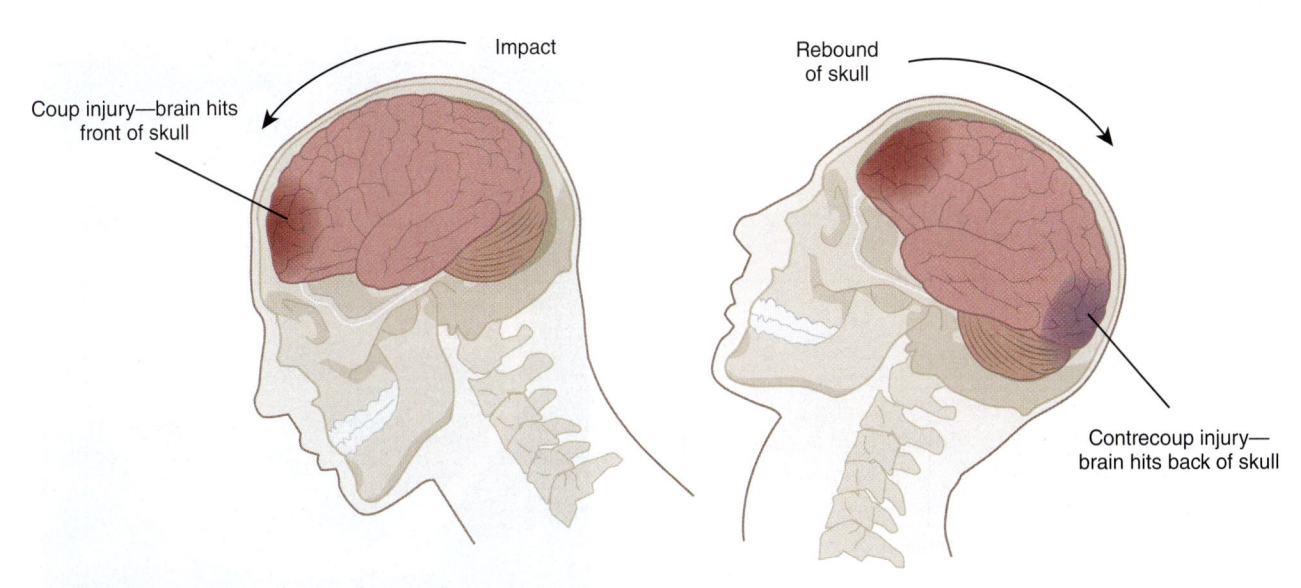

Figure 7-17 *Coup/contrecoup brain injury.*

are located in the frontal and temporal lobes, but they may also occur in tissue beneath a depressed skull fracture. Contusions begin when the capillaries within the brain tissue are damaged, resulting in hemorrhage, infarction, necrosis, and edema.[69] Significant contusions with swelling may cause a midline shift within the cranial vault and can continue to evolve over 2 to 3 days.[45] Delayed hemorrhage or formation of intracranial hematomas may occur.[4]

Intracerebral Hematoma

Similar to cerebral contusions, intracerebral hematomas occur in the frontal and temporal lobes, and less often deep within the brain tissue. These hematomas may be single or multiple and may be associated with skull fractures and cerebral contusions.[69] Intracerebral hematomas may create a significant mass effect, increase ICP, and result in neurologic deterioration. Assessment findings include the following[69]:

- Progressive and often rapid decline in level of consciousness
- Headache
- Signs of increasing ICP (Refer to Table 7-2)
- Pupil abnormalities
- Contralateral hemiparesis, hemiplegia, or abnormal motor posturing

Epidural Hematoma

An epidural hematoma occurs when a collection of blood forms between the dura mater and the skull. Such hematomas are frequently associated with fractures of the temporal bone that lacerate the middle meningeal artery (**Figure 7-18**). Because the source of bleeding is arterial, blood can accumulate rapidly, and the expanding hematoma may cause compression of underlying brain tissue, a rapid rise in ICP, decreased CBF, and secondary brain injury.[69] Large epidural hematomas require immediate surgical intervention, whereas small epidurals may be managed nonoperatively with frequent neurological assessment and repeat CTs.[10] The most common causes of epidural hematoma are MVCs and falls, but they can also result from sports-related injuries.

Assessment findings include the following[10,42,54,69]:

- Transient loss of consciousness followed by a lucid period lasting minutes to hours and then rapid deterioration in neurologic status. Although this is considered the "classic" presentation of a patient with an epidural hematoma, many patients do not present with this history or symptomatology.
- Headache and dizziness.
- Nausea and vomiting.
- Contralateral hemiparesis, hemiplegia, or abnormal motor posturing (flexion or extension).
    - Extension is associated with brain stem herniation and poor outcomes.
    - Ipsilateral unilateral fixed and dilated pupil may occur.

Subdural Hematoma

A subdural hematoma occurs when a collection of blood forms immediately beneath the dura mater, usually following impact involving acceleration, deceleration, or combination forces. Subdural hematomas are usually caused by tearing of the bridging veins and associated direct injury to the underlying brain tissue (refer to Figure 7-18). They may be acute, subacute, or chronic.[4]

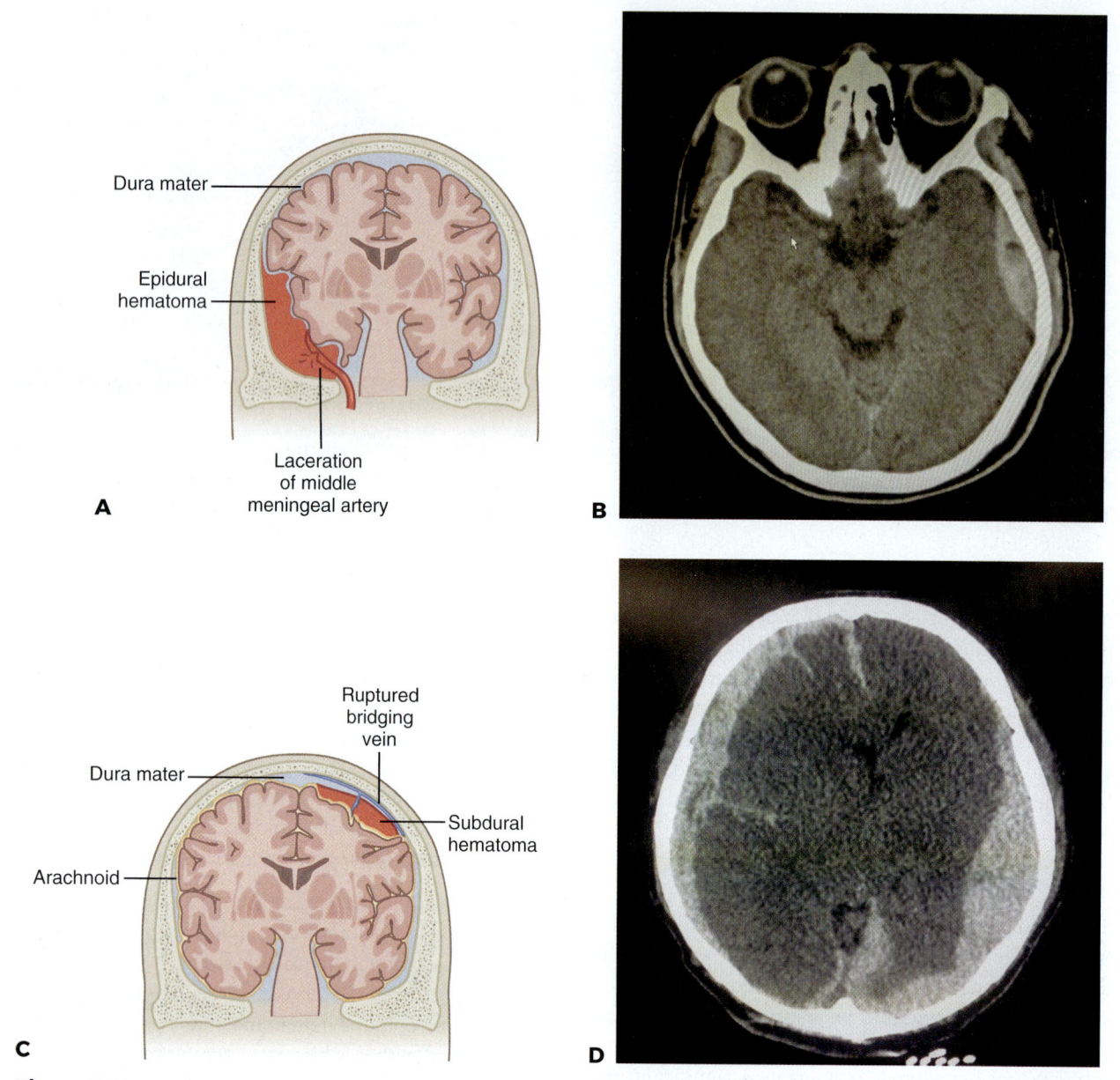

Figure 7-18 *Epidural and subdural hematomas.* **A.** *Diagram of epidural hematoma.* **B.** *Scan showing epidural hematoma.* **C.** *Diagram of subdural hematoma.* **D.** *Scan showing subdural hematoma.*
B, D. © O_Akira/ Shutterstock.

Acute Subdural Hematoma

Patients with acute subdural hematomas generally manifest signs and symptoms within 72 hours of the injury event. In patients taking anticoagulant/antiplatelet medications, the progression of an acute subdural can occur more rapidly.[42] The hematoma can cause a reduction in CBF. This type of bleed is commonly the result of a fall or assault, with a smaller percentage of acute subdural hematomas being caused by MVCs. Assessment findings in patients with such hematomas include the following[4]:

- Nausea, vomiting, and headache
- Changes in level of consciousness
- Ipsilateral dilated or nonreactive pupil
- Unilateral weakness or hemiparesis

Chronic Subdural Hematoma

Chronic subdural hematomas are frequently associated with repeated falls in older adults, patients taking anticoagulation medications, and patients with chronic alcohol use.[42] This increased incidence is due to brain atrophy, fragility of the bridging veins, and coagulation alterations. The onset of signs and symptoms and the effect on neurologic function vary depending on the size and rapidity of the hematoma formation. Signs and symptoms in patients with chronic subdural hematomas develop over time and may not be evident for weeks to months after the injury event.[4] Symptoms may be intermittent and may be confused with transient ischemic attacks or decline associated with aging. The symptoms may include the following[25,42,45,69]:

- Alterations in cognitive abilities or altered or steady decline in level of consciousness
- Headache—the most common symptom
- Loss of memory or altered reasoning
- Motor deficit—contralateral hemiparesis, hemiplegia, or abnormal motor posturing or ataxia
- Slurred speech, difficulty with word finding
- Ipsilateral unilateral fixed and dilated pupil
- Incontinence
- Seizures

Symptoms may progress and require surgical evacuation. In the older adult, this may result in other complications, and the subdural may reaccumulate. A procedure called middle meningeal embolization has begun to be used to treat chronic subdural hematomas. This procedure is done in interventional radiology suites and has far less risk than surgery. Additional studies are being done to provide further evidence for the safety and efficacy of this procedure.[12,35,37]

Herniation Syndrome

Herniation is a shifting of brain tissue with displacement into abnormal anatomic places as the result of bleeding or edema (**Figure 7-19**).[69] This shift compresses, tears, or shears the vasculature, decreasing perfusion. The most common trauma herniation syndrome is uncal herniation. Assessment findings may include the following[42,54,69]:

- Asymmetric pupillary reactivity
- Unilateral or bilateral pupillary dilation
- Abnormal motor posturing

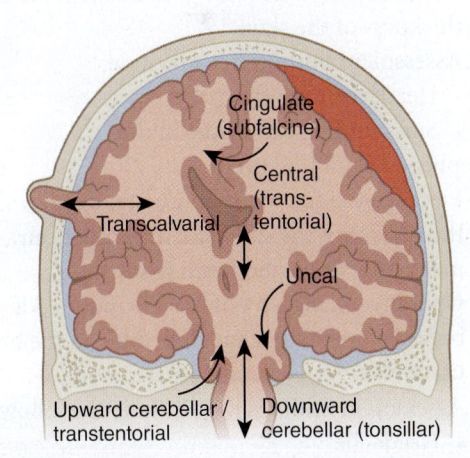

Figure 7-19 *Herniation syndromes.*

- Other evidence of neurologic deterioration (paralysis, change in level of consciousness, or loss of normal reflexes)

The two major types of supratentorial herniation are named by the site of herniation[69]:

- Uncal transtentorial herniation: The uncus of the temporal lobe is displaced unilaterally over the tentorium into the posterior fossa, causing a shift of the midbrain to the opposite side.
- Central or transtentorial herniation: The cerebral hemispheres are pushed downward through the tentorial notch, directly compressing the brain stem.

Diffuse Injuries

Diffuse TBIs occur over a widespread area. They may not always be identifiable on CT imaging because the damage involves contusions or shearing and stretching of the axons, rather than a localized hematoma, contusion, or laceration.[4,69,71] These injuries commonly follow a direct blow to the head and very often are sports related. Patients who sustain these injuries may have varying degrees of symptoms that range from lasting minutes to causing permanent injury or death.[69]

Mild Traumatic Brain Injury or Concussion

A mild form of diffuse injury is concussion, often called a mild TBI. The injury to the brain is caused by blunt injury to the head or neck. It can also be caused by acceleration/deceleration mechanisms, which result in the brain physically coming in contact with the bony skull.[10] Most concussions have no findings on CT. Pathophysiological changes occur at the cellular level with axonal disruption as well as neurochemical disruptions. Changes in neurologic status last for a very brief period (i.e., loss of consciousness < 30 minutes).[54,69,74] Patients may have mild TBI symptoms for several hours or days after injury. Assessment findings include the following[41,44]:

- GCS score of 13–15 (at least 30 minutes postinjury)
- Confusion and disorientation
- Headache, dizziness, and nausea and vomiting
- Poor concentration, anxiety, and irritability
- Posttraumatic amnesia for less than 24 hours
- Photophobia/phonophobia[4,10,54]

Postconcussive Syndrome

Patients who sustain a mild TBI may develop postconcussive syndrome. Typically, postconcussive syndrome manifests several days or months after the head trauma. Signs and symptoms usually resolve but may persist for long periods. These patients may require ongoing evaluation, treatment, and extended rehabilitation before they are able to return to their previous level of activities or athletic participation. Because it cannot be determined who will develop postconcussive syndrome, education related to this condition is included in patient discharge instructions, along with information regarding when to return for care. Those injured in organized sports should have guidance regarding return to play from a sports medicine trainer or medical provider. Physical and mental rest may be required while the patient remains symptomatic, followed by a gradual return to work/school.[10,54,69,74] Assessment findings may include the following[10,54,74]:

- Nausea
- Dizziness and persistent headache
- Memory and judgment impairment, as well as attention deficits
- Insomnia and sleep disturbance
- Loss of libido
- Anxiety, irritability, depression, and emotional lability
- Noise and light oversensitivity
- Attention or concentration problems

Diffuse Axonal Injury

DAI is widespread microscopic damage, primarily to the axons. DAI results from diffuse shearing, tearing, or compressive stresses from a rotational or acceleration/deceleration mechanism of injury.[45] Such damage may also occur following hypoxic or ischemic insults from the initial trauma.[4] DAI presents as diffuse, microscopic, hemorrhagic lesions and cerebral edema, which may be detected on magnetic resonance imaging. Deeper brain structures, the brain stem, and the reticular activating system (responsible for regulating wakefulness and sleep) are most at risk for injury, which commonly results in prolonged coma. The DAI is graded as Grades I through III based on the location of the lesion and severity of the injury. Severe DAI is associated with significant morbidity and mortality, and patient management is focused on preservation of basic vital functions, prevention of secondary injury, and support for the family.[10,45,54,69]

Assessment findings may include the following:

- Unconsciousness
- Increased ICP
- Abnormal motor posturing
- Hyperthermia with temperature between 40°C and 40.5°C (104°F and 105°F)
- Excessive sweating
- Mild to severe memory loss; cognitive, behavioral, and intellectual deficits

Penetrating Injuries

Penetrating injuries to the brain can be life-threatening, and it is essential to discover the site and extent of the injury. The most common cause of penetrating injuries of the brain is firearm-related injuries.[20] The decision to operate is based on CT findings and GCS. The presence of a large contusion, hemorrhage, or hematoma, especially when both hemispheres are involved, is associated with increased mortality.[4] Keep the following points in mind when dealing with penetrating injuries to the brain:

- Leave any protruding penetrating objects in place and stabilize them.[4]
- Prepare for emergent surgery or transfer to a trauma center with neurosurgical capabilities.
- Consider limiting resuscitation efforts in the presence of devastating injuries. The following variables are associated with mortality[47]:
  - Age greater than 50 years
  - Self-inflicted injury
  - Hypotension
  - Coagulopathy
  - Respiratory distress
  - Low GCS score
  - Fixed and dilated pupils
  - High ICP

Craniofacial Fractures

Craniofacial fractures include skull fractures, maxillofacial fractures, and mandibular fractures.

Skull Fractures

The significance of a skull fracture is the force it takes to cause the injury. Injuries may occur to the skull vault or the base.[4] Types of skull fractures include the following:

- Linear skull fracture
  - A nondisplaced fracture goes through the entire thickness of the skull[10,74]
  - Assessment findings may include:
    - Headache
    - Surrounding soft-tissue injury
- Depressed skull fracture
  - Pieces of the fractured bone extend below the surface of the skull and may cause dura mater laceration and brain tissue injury. Operative management may be required if bone fragments remain embedded in the brain tissue.[10,42]
  - Assessment findings may include the following[54]:
    - Headache
    - Surrounding soft-tissue injury

Selected Head Injuries

- Palpable depression of the skull over the fracture site (assess with care)
- Possible open fracture
- Possible decreased level of consciousness
- Basilar skull fracture (**Figure 7-20**)
- Fracture of any of the five bones in the base of the skull is associated with a considerable amount of force.
- The injury can result in punctures or lacerations to brain tissue or CNs and CSF leakage.
- It may also result in laceration of the dura mater, creating an open passage for CSF, which places the patient at risk for infections (meningitis, encephalitis, brain abscess).[69]
- Basilar skull fracture often occurs concurrently with facial fractures.

- Fractures may cross the carotid canals and injure the carotid arteries. CT angiography may be used to identify and manage the bleeding.[4]
- Assessment findings may include the following[4,10]:
  - Headache and dizziness
  - Hearing loss
  - Altered level of consciousness
  - CSF in rhinorrhea or otorrhea
  - Periorbital ecchymoses (raccoon eyes)
  - Mastoid ecchymoses (Battle sign)
  - Bleeding behind the tympanic membrane (hemotympanum)
  - Facial nerve palsy (CN VII injury)

Maxillary Fractures

The Le Fort classification system provides precise definitions of maxillary fractures (**Figure 7-21**).[17] These fractures occur as a result of blunt force to the midface and are commonly as a result of assaults and MVCs.[39] Of particular concern are the problems related to airway obstruction and bleeding; close observation is required to ensure the patency of the airway. Operative management is indicated in the case of bony displacement or when the fracture affects function or form of the face.[39]

The three types of Le Fort fracture are detailed in Figure 7-21.[72] A Le Fort I fracture is a transverse maxillary bone fracture that occurs above the level of the teeth and results in a separation of the teeth from the maxilla. Assessment findings include the following[19,56]:

- Independent movement of the maxilla from the rest of the face

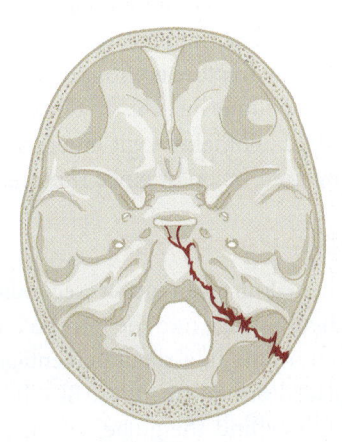

Figure 7-20 *Basilar skull fracture.*

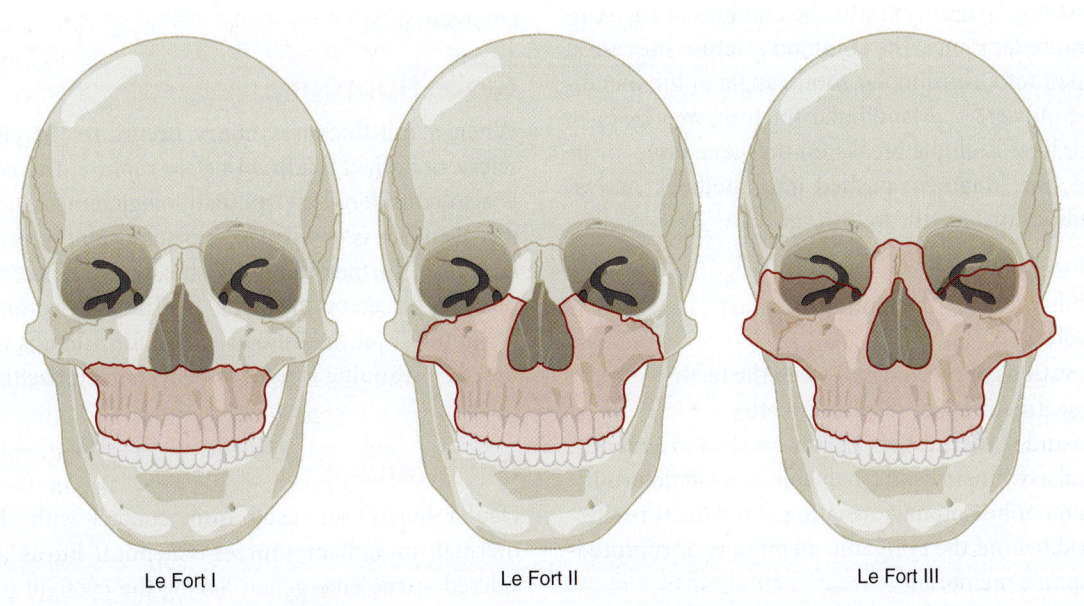

Figure 7-21 *Le Fort classification system.*

Le Fort I   Le Fort II   Le Fort III

- Slight swelling of the maxillary area
- Lip laceration or fractured teeth
- Malocclusion

A Le Fort II (Figure 7-21) fracture is a pyramidal maxillary bone fracture involving the midface area.[39] The apex of the fracture transverses the bridge of the nose. The two lateral fractures of the pyramid extend through the lacrimal bone of the face and ethmoid bone of the skull into the median portion of both orbits. The base of the fracture extends above the level of the upper teeth into the maxilla. Assessment findings include the following[19,56,65]:

- Massive facial edema
- Nasal swelling with obvious fracture of the nasal bones
- Epistaxis
- Malocclusion
- Possible CSF rhinorrhea

A Le Fort III (Figure 7-21) fracture is a complete craniofacial separation involving the maxilla, zygoma, orbits, and bones of the cranial base. This is the most severe type, and caregivers should also be concerned about injury to the eyes and optic nerve.[39] Assessment findings include the following[19,56]:

- Massive facial edema
- Mobility and depression of zygomatic bones
- Periorbital ecchymoses (raccoon eyes)
- Diplopia
- Open bite or malocclusion
- CSF in rhinorrhea or otorrhea

Mandibular Fractures

Mandibular fractures occur to the horseshoe-shaped lower jawbone that attaches to the cranium at the temporomandibular joints. The common fracture sites are at the canine tooth, third molar tooth, angle of the mandible, and condyles.[27,65] Mandibular fractures may be open or closed, have multiple breaks on the same bone, or be impacted (one fragment pushed into another). Assessment findings include the following[17,27,65]:

- Malocclusion
- Inability to open the mouth (trismus)
- Drooling
- Lacerations or bleeding between the teeth
- Loose, fractured, or displaced teeth
- Pain and tenderness, especially on jaw movement
- Facial asymmetry and a palpable step-off deformity
- Edema or hematoma formation at the fracture site
- Blood behind the tympanic membrane or ruptured tympanic membrane
- Anesthesia/paresthesia of the lower lip/chin

Selected Eye Injuries

Selected eye injuries discussed in this section include corneal injury, orbital fracture, retrobulbar hematoma, globe rupture, and ocular burns.

Corneal Injury

Traumatic injury to the cornea can result from abrasion, laceration, or foreign bodies. Corneal abrasions are commonly caused by fingernail injury or contact lens use. The corneal epithelium is highly innervated, so injury to it results in a great deal of pain. Staining of the eye with fluorescein can help identify the abrasion. A slit lamp is used to visualize lacerations and foreign bodies.[28,77]

Orbital Fracture

Orbital fractures are usually a result of a direct blow to the eye. The orbital floor and ethmoid bones are the weakest parts of the orbit and at high risk for fracture. A complication of this type of fracture is entrapment of the inferior rectus or inferior oblique muscle.[50,77] Orbital fractures are not considered an ophthalmologic emergency unless the patient has impaired vision or globe rupture.[50]

Retrobulbar Hematoma

Retrobulbar hematoma can occur secondary to blunt trauma. This hemorrhage into the retrobulbar space (behind the globe) occurs in a small percentage of patients with nondisplaced orbital fractures. Bleeding causes increased pressure behind the globe, which causes an elevation in intraocular pressure (IOP) that compresses the optic nerve and blood vessels. Early recognition is imperative to save vision. This is a true ophthalmologic emergency.[28,77]

Globe Rupture

When a full-thickness injury occurs to the cornea or sclera, or both, it is termed a *globe rupture*. This condition is also considered an ophthalmologic emergency. Once the diagnosis is confirmed, it is important to protect the area from further injury by shielding the eye, avoiding pressure placed on the globe.[28,77] The most common area of rupture is at the limbus, where the sclera is the thinnest. CT scanning is used to help characterize the injury further.[28]

Ocular Burns

Ocular burns can result from contact with chemical, thermal, or radiant sources. Chemical burns are considered a true emergency. Saving the eyesight in such a case requires immediate irrigation of the eye; this takes precedence over completion of a history, testing the pH of the eye, and thorough assessment.[24,50] Alkaline products cause liquefaction necrosis and produce burns that are deeper than acid burns. In general, acidic burns are less severe, causing immediate damage through coagulation necrosis, which ultimately forms a barrier to deeper penetration. The exceptions to this pattern are burns caused by hydrofluoric and sulfuric acids, which cause the same severity of burn as alkali substances.[28]

Assessment findings, treatment, and follow-up for eye injuries are summarized in **Table 7-6**.[24,28,64,77]

Interventions for the Patient with Head Trauma

For the patient with severe TBI (GCS score of 3–8) consider the following essential interventions[4,6,11,16,32,69,82]:

- Assist with early intubation and ventilation. Maintain oxygen saturation > 95%.
- Ensure that a focused neurologic examination has been performed before giving sedating medications.

TABLE 7-6 Summary of Assessment Findings, Treatment, and Follow-Up for Eye Injuries

Eye Injury	Assessment Findings	Treatment	Follow-Up
Corneal injury	Photophobia Pain Eye redness, tearing Lid swelling Foreign body sensation in the eye	Topical anesthesia Slit lamp evaluation Topical ophthalmic nonsteroidal anti-inflammatory drugs No eye patch For laceration, may need topical antibiotic prophylaxis Remove foreign body	Follow-up with ophthalmologist in 24–48 hours Ophthalmology consultation for large/partial corneal lacerations, deep and large foreign bodies
Orbital fracture	Periorbital ecchymosis Facial swelling Double vision Enophthalmos (posterior displacement of eyeball within the orbit) Ptosis	Nasal decongestant Ice packs to the orbit for 48 hours Oral antibiotics Analgesics (acetaminophen, ibuprofen)	Large fractures of orbital floor may require urgent surgery Patients with visual changes, impaired ocular motion, or concern for ruptured globe should have immediate ophthalmology consult; otherwise, outpatient follow-up within 1 to 2 weeks Discharge instructions: Avoid blowing nose, sneezing, coughing, and/or performing Valsalva maneuver
Retrobulbar hematoma	Severe pain Decreased vision or loss of vision Reduced eye movement Double vision Proptosis Increased intraocular pressure	Administer medications to decrease IOP Emergency decompression via lateral canthotomy	Emergent consultation with ophthalmology

(continues)

TABLE 7-6 Summary of Assessment Findings, Treatment, and Follow-Up for Eye Injuries (*continued*)

Eye Injury	Assessment Findings	Treatment	Follow-Up
Globe rupture	Irregular or teardrop-shaped pupils Periorbital ecchymosis Decreased visual acuity and EOM Severe subconjunctival hemorrhage Deep eye pain Nausea	Avoid any pressure on the globe Apply a rigid shield to protect the affected eye Consider tetanus vaccine Keep patient NPO Assess and treat pain Administer antiemetics to decrease risk of vomiting (which may increase IOP) Elevate the head of bed (to decrease IOP) Avoid ophthalmic drops or medications Administer systemic antibiotics	Emergent consultation with ophthalmology Prepare patient for CT scan, operating room
Ocular burns	Swelling of the sclera Conjunctival irritation Corneal clouding (may be indicative of severe burn) Pain	Determine baseline pH of both eyes Topical anesthesia Immediate copious irrigation until the pH returns to normal range (pH = 7.4); stop irrigation for 5 minutes and retest pH. If pH has changed, may need to continue irrigation. Remove particulate matter Visual acuity reassessment	Ophthalmology consultation and close follow-up

IOP = intraocular pressure; EOM = extraocular eye movement; NPO = nothing by mouth; CT = computed tomography; pH = negative log of hydrogen ion concentration.

Data from Guluma, K., & Lee, J. E. (2018). Ophthalmology. In R. M. Walls, R. S. Hockberger, & M. Gaushe-Hill (Eds.), *Rosen's emergency medicine: Concepts and clinical practice* (9th ed., pp. 790–819). Elsevier; Nolan-Kelley, L. (2022). Ocular emergencies. In V. Sweet & A. Foley (Eds.), *Sheehy's emergency nursing: Principles and practice* (7th ed., pp. 365–376). Elsevier; Toldi, J. P., & Thomas, J. L. (2020). Evaluation and management of sports-related eye injuries. *Current Sports Medicine Reports, 19*(1), 29–34.

- Obtain an ABG early in the care of the patient so that PaO_2 and $PaCO_2$ targets can be obtained (refer to Table 7-3). Monitor $ETCO_2$ continuously and maintain 35–40 mm Hg (4.67–5.33 kPa).[43,82]
- Hyperventilation may be used temporarily for signs of herniation only ($ETCO_2$ 30–35 mm Hg [4.00–4.67 kPa] or respiratory rate = 20 breaths/min).
- Monitor BP frequently (maintain SBP ≥ 100–110 mm Hg). Avoid hypotension. Assist with arterial line insertion to aid in BP monitoring.
- Administer blood products or warmed isotonic crystalloid intravenous fluid as ordered to treat hypotension.[69]
- Obtain blood sample for laboratory testing. Use point of care testing if available.
  - Glucose
  - Type and crossmatch
  - Coagulation studies
  - Electrolytes
- Administer reversal agents as ordered (for patients on anticoagulant/antiplatelet medications).

- Evaluate for other injuries.
- Accompany the patient to CT imaging, and monitor vital signs closely during the transport.
- Assist with communication to neurosurgery or with emergent transfer to a trauma center with neurosurgical capabilities as needed.
- Once cervical spine injury has been ruled out, elevation of the patient's head of bed by 30–45 degrees is recommended to decrease ICP.[18] Position the head midline to facilitate venous drainage. Ensure that the cervical collar is not too tight.
- Prepare for insertion of an ICP monitor device, and then monitor and treat the ICP according to institutional protocols. A brain tissue oxygenation monitoring device can be inserted at the same time as ICP monitor placement. ICP monitoring should be considered for the following patients[82]:
    - Patients with severe TBI (GCS score of 3–8) with an abnormal CT scan
    - Patients with GCS score greater than 8 with abnormal CT scan with high risk of progression (large hematomas or coagulopathy)
    - Patients who have worsening CT results or deterioration on neurologic examination
- Administer hypertonic saline, as prescribed.
    - This treatment may be used to decrease ICP and has less effect on SBP than mannitol.[4,18]
    - Administer hypertonic saline as a bolus rather than via continuous infusion. Various concentrations may be used depending on the patient's condition and provider preference. Monitor serum sodium levels.[4,16,18,32]
- Administer mannitol, as prescribed:
    - Rule out other injuries before administering this medication.
    - Administer mannitol via bolus rather than via continuous infusion with a dosage of 0.25 to 1 g/kg rapidly over 5 minutes (20% solution). Other dosage amounts may be used to control elevated ICP.[4,11]
    - Indications for mannitol include acute neurologic deterioration indicated by[4]:
        - Dilated pupils
        - Loss of consciousness
        - Hemiparesis while the patient is being monitored
    - Mannitol is *not* used in patients with active intracranial bleeding.[57]
        - Mannitol is *contraindicated for use in hypotensive patients* because it will not lower ICP in hypovolemia and is a potent osmotic diuretic.[4]
- Administer anticonvulsant medication, as prescribed.[4]
- Early posttraumatic seizures, defined as those that occur within the first 7 days after injury, occur in 12–25% of patients with severe head injuries.[11] Prolonged seizures can contribute to secondary brain injury. Seizure activity is associated with higher incidence of pneumonia and acute respiratory distress syndrome as well. Seizure prophylaxis is usually administered to patients at risk for early posttraumatic seizure,[40] which include those with the following conditions:
    - Linear or depressed skull fracture
    - Seizure at the time of injury
    - History of seizures
    - Penetrating brain injury
    - Severe head injury
    - Acute subdural hematoma
    - Acute epidural hematoma
    - Age 65 years or younger
    - Chronic alcoholism[11,54,69]
- Maintain normal body temperature. Use external warming/cooling devices to achieve normal body temperature as appropriate. When treating fever in patients with head trauma, consider the following[10,69]:
    - Hyperthermia increases ICP and the cerebral metabolic rate.
    - Shivering increases the cerebral metabolic rate and may precipitate a rise in ICP, so causing shivering with the cooling process should be avoided.
- Do not pack the ears or nose if a CSF leak is suspected.[10]
- Administer tetanus prophylaxis, as needed.[10]
- Assist with wound repair, as indicated.[10]
- Ensure adequate pain management first followed by sedation for ventilated patients. Use short-acting agents.[10,82]
- Administer other medications, as prescribed.
- If the change in mental status is suspected to be the result of an overdose, naloxone may be given for opioid use, and flumazenil for benzodiazepine use. Use caution when giving either of these medications; abrupt withdrawal from long-term opioid use or reversal of benzodiazepine use as an anticonvulsant may precipitate seizures or vomiting, causing further deterioration.
- Administer antibiotics, as prescribed.[4]
- When handing off care to another nurse, perform neurologic assessment together at bedside to assist with continuity and trending.

Diagnostics and Interventions for Head Trauma

Reevaluation adjuncts include radiographic and laboratory studies.

Radiographic Studies

Radiographic studies include the following[4,10]:

- CT scans
  - Patient movement may produce artifact and result in an inaccurate or suboptimal CT result. Patient movement may be a result of seizures, inability to cooperate based on mental status changes, or inappropriate flexion or extension.
  - Sedation may be administered as prescribed.
    - Closely monitor patients who have received sedation or neuromuscular-blocking medications during a CT procedure.
    - Be judicious with the use of sedation because of change in the ability to do neurologic assessment.
- Magnetic resonance imaging
  - Magnetic resonance imaging is not typically used in the acute resuscitation phase. It may be indicated to provide better delineation of a patient's injury and prognosis at a later time.
- Angiography
  - Angiography may be indicated if vascular injury is known or suspected.
  - CT angiography is common in the initial evaluation of the patient with suspected vascular injury and can be done much more quickly (less than 5 minutes) using less contrast than traditional angiography.
- Skull series
  - Radiographs of the skull are generally not needed and have largely been replaced by CT of the head.[69]

If the patient is being emergently transferred, the transfer should not be delayed to perform radiologic testing.[4] If time permits while awaiting helicopter or ground transport, CT imaging can be obtained. Ensure that images are sent with the patient or can be retrieved by the tertiary center.

Laboratory Studies

Laboratory studies may include the following:

- Arterial blood gas: Obtain an ABG measurement early in the care of the patient so that PaO_2 and $PaCO_2$ targets can be obtained (refer to Table 7-3); serial ABG measurements may need to be drawn to trend when making changes to ventilator settings.[61]
- Blood glucose: Hypoglycemia may play a role in the patient's altered neurologic status. Hyperglycemia has been identified as one of many secondary insults that can impact neurologic recovery. Both hypo- and hyperglycemia should be avoided.[23]
- Coagulation studies
  - Analysis of coagulation status may be helpful in directing the management for those patients taking anticoagulants or antiplatelet medications.[69]
- Blood alcohol and urine toxicology screens
  - These studies may be helpful to determine the presence or absence of alcohol or other substances that may contribute to an altered mental status.[4,10,54]

Reevaluation and Post-Resuscitation Care

Reevaluation of the patient with head trauma includes the following steps:

- Serial scoring of the GCS or FOUR score—this is crucial for early detection of patient deterioration[4]
- Frequent reassessment of pupils
- ABG trending, plus ensuring that appropriate adjustments are made to prevent hypoxia
- Trends in vital signs, especially BP, respiratory rate and pattern, temperature, SpO_2, and $ETCO_2$
- Reevaluation for development of the following:
  - Headache
  - Nausea
  - Vomiting
  - Seizure activity
  - Changes in motor or sensory function
  - Response to interventions such as fluid administration and diuretic therapy

Continuous ICP Monitoring

Continuous ICP monitoring is important for assessing brain injury and the response of the patient to treatment.[59] The addition of a brain tissue oxygenation monitoring device can provide early detection of secondary brain injury, such as cerebral hypoxia and possible ischemia. Such an oxygenation device determines the level of oxygen delivery to the cerebral tissues and monitors the temperature of the brain tissue. Any change in brain tissue can alter cerebral metabolism and affect CBF and ICP. The monitoring system detects poor oxygenation to the brain tissue before ICP changes can be detected. In combination with this early detection, early intervention and management can result in a better patient outcome.[66]

Definitive Care or Transport

Consider early the need to transport the patient to a trauma center and/or prepare the patient for operative intervention, hospital admission, or transfer, as indicated.

Emerging Trends

As the science and evidence of trauma care continue to evolve, tools and procedures to improve patient outcomes continue to be trialed and refined. Evidence is tested and replicated, and new standards of care are transitioned into practice. This section on trauma care considerations explores some of the evidence and the potential significance for trauma patient care.

Point of Care Ocular Ultrasonography

Point of care ocular ultrasonography is emerging as a diagnostic tool for the evaluation of traumatic eye injuries.[52] This technology can facilitate the evaluation of altered vision, pain, trauma to the eye, and head injury. It is not used in cases involving globe rupture due to the risk of vitreous extrusion.[52] Certain foreign bodies, such as wood, glass, or organic foreign matter, can be better visualized with ultrasound.

Middle Meningeal Artery Embolization

Middle meningeal artery embolization is emerging as a procedural treatment of chronic subdural hematomas. Chronic subdural hematoma can last for some time and contribute to a process of chronic inflammation. Immature blood vessels develop and may continually leak blood into the area. Middle meningeal artery embolization is performed in interventional radiology; it obliterates flow to the immature blood vessels and decreases the chance for recurrence. This procedure has greatly decreased the need for craniotomy.[9,12,25,30,78]

Summary

Approximately 69 million people worldwide suffer a TBI each year.[22] Early intervention and appropriate resuscitation are crucial to prevent or minimize the effects of secondary brain injury that can result from a hypoxic event, cerebral edema, hypotension, or increased ICP. Facilitating oxygenation and ventilation and maintaining BP are priorities in treating patients with TBI. Frequently reassessing the patient's neurologic status and communication with trauma providers helps to ensure that interventions are implemented in a timely fashion.

References

1. Afifi, A. M., Sanchez, R, J., & Djohen, R, S. (2018). Anatomy of the head and the neck. In P. C. Neligan & E. D. Rodrigues (Eds.), *Craniofacial, head and neck surgery and pediatric plastic surgery* (4th ed., Vol. 3, pp. 2–20). Elsevier.
2. Almojuela, A., Hasen, M., & Zeiler, F. A. (2019). The Full Outline of UnResponsiveness (FOUR) score and its use in outcome prediction: A scoping systematic review of the adult literature. *Neurocritical Care, 31*(1), 162–175. https://doi.org/10.1007/s12028-018-0630-9
3. American College of Surgeons. (2018). Airway and ventilatory management. In *Advanced trauma life support: Student course manual* (10th ed., pp. 22–41).
4. American College of Surgeons. (2018). Head trauma. In *Advanced trauma life support: Student course manual* (10th ed., pp. 103–126).
5. American College of Surgeons. (2018). Initial assessment and management. In *Advanced trauma life support: Student course manual* (10th ed., pp. 2–21).
6. American College of Surgeons Committee on Trauma. (2015). *ACS TQIP best practices in the management of traumatic brain injury.* ACS Trauma Quality Improvement Program. American College of Surgeons. https://www.facs.org/media/mkej5u3b/tbi_guidelines.pdf
7. Anestis, D. M., Tsitsopoulos, P. P., Tsonidis, C. A., & Foroglou, N. (2020). The current significance of the FOUR score: A systematic review and critical analysis of the literature. *Journal of the Neurological Sciences, 409*, Article 116600. https://doi.org/10.1016/j.jns.2019.116600
8. Balakrishnan, S., Harsini, S., Reddy, S., Tofighi, S., & Gholamrezanezhad, A. (2020). Imaging review of ocular and optic nerve trauma. *Emergency Radiology, 27*(1), 75–85. https://doi.org/10.1007/s10140-019-01730-y
9. Ban, S. P., Hwang, G., Byoun, H. S., Kim, T., Lee, S. U., Bang, J. S., Han, J. H., Kim, C. Y., Kwon, O. K., & Oh, C. W. (2018). Middle meningeal artery embolization for chronic subdural hematoma. *Radiology, 286*, 992–999. https://doi.org/10.1148/radiol.2017170053
10. Broering, B. (2020) Head trauma. In V. Sweet & A. Foley (Eds.), *Sheehy's emergency nursing: Principles and practice* (pp. 401–418). Elsevier.
11. Carney, N., Totten, A. M., O'Reilly, C., Ullman, J. S., Hawryluk, G. W. J., Bell, M. J., Bratton, S. L., Chesnut, R., Harris, O. A., Kissoon, N., Rubiano, A. M, Shutter, L., Tasker, R. C., Vavilala, M. S., Wilberger, J., Wright, D. W., & Ghajar, J. (2016). *Guidelines for the management of severe traumatic brain injury* (4th ed.). Brain Trauma Foundation. https://braintrauma.org/uploads/03/12/Guidelines_for_Management_of_Severe_TBI_4th_Edition.pdf
12. Catapano, J. S., Nguyen, C. L., Wakim, A. A., Albuquerque, F. C., & Ducruet, A. F. (2020). Middle meningeal artery embolization for chronic subdural hematoma. *Frontiers in Neurology, 11*, Article 557233. https://doi.org/10.3389/fneur.2020.557233

13. Centers for Disease Control and Prevention. (n.d.) *Traumatic brain injury & concussion: Get the facts about TBI.* https://www.cdc.gov/traumaticbraininjury/get_the_facts.html
14. Centers for Disease Control and Prevention. (n.d.). *Traumatic brain injury & concussion: TBI Data.* https://www.cdc.gov/traumaticbraininjury/data/index.html#:~:text=Based%20on%20the%20most%20recent,TBI%2Drelated%20deaths%20in%202020.&text=This%20represents%20more%20than%20611,TBI%2Drelated%20deaths%20per%20day
15. Chapman, K., & Dragan, K. E. (2022, July 4). Hypercarbia. *StatPearls.* StatPearls Publishing. https://www.ncbi.nlm.nih.gov/books/NBK559154/
16. Chesnut, R. M., Temkin, N., Videtta, W., Petroni, G., Lujan, S., Pridgeon, J., Dikmen, S., Chaddock, K., Barber, J., Machamer, J., Guadagnoli, N., Hendrickson, P., Aguilera, S., Alanis, V., Bello Quezada, M. E., Bautista Coronel, E., Bustamante, L. A., Cacciatori, A. C., Carricondo, C. J., Carvajal, F., . . . Urbina, Z. (2020). Consensus-based management protocol (CREVICE Protocol) for the treatment of severe traumatic brain injury based on imaging and clinical examination for use when intracranial pressure monitoring is not employed. *Journal of Neurotrauma, 37*(11), 1291–1299. https://doi.org/10.1089/neu.2017.5599
17. Chukwulebe, S., & Hogrefe, C. (2019). The diagnosis and management of facial bone fractures. *Emergency Medicine Clinics of North America, 37*(1), 137–151. https://doi.org/10.1016/j.emc.2018.09.012
18. Cook, A., Jones, G., Hawryluk, G., Mailloux, P., McLaughlin, D., Papangelou, A., Samuel, S., Tokumaru, S., Venkatasubramanian, C., Zacko, C., & Zimmermann, L. L. (2020). Guidelines for the acute treatment of cerebral edema in neurocritical care patients. *Neurocritical Care, 32,* 647–666. doi:10.1007/s12028-020-00959-7
19. Dağaşan, V. Ç., Burdurlu, M. C., & Baysal, E. (2020). Diagnosis and management of midfacial fractures. In C. Evereklioğlu (Ed.), *Academic studies in health sciences-II* (Vol. 2, pp. 155–166). Gece. https://www.gecekitapligi.com/Webkontrol/uploads/Fck/health2yayin_6.pdf
20. D'Agostino, R., Kursinskis, A., Parikh, P., Letarte, P., Harmon, L., & Semon, G. (2020). Management of penetrating traumatic brain injury: Operative versus non-operative intervention. *The Journal of Surgical Research, 257,* 101–106. https://doi.org/10.1016/j.jss.2020.07.046
21. DeMers, D., & Wachs, D. (2022, April 14). Physiology, mean arterial pressure. *StatPearls.* StatPearls Publishing. https://www.ncbi.nlm.nih.gov/books/NBK538226/
22. Dewan, M. C., Rattani, A., Gupta, S., Baticulon, R. E., Hung, Y. C., Punchak, M., Agrawal, A., Adeleye, A. O., Shrime, M. G., Rubiano, A. M., Rosenfeld, J. V., & Park, K. B. (2019). Estimating the global incidence of traumatic brain injury. *Journal of Neurosurgery, 130*(4), 1080–1097. https://doi.org/10.3171/2017.10.jns17352
23. Dietrich, W., & Bramlett, H. (2022). *Bradley and Daroff's neurology in clinical practice* (8th ed., pp. 897–906). Elsevier.
24. Dua, H. S., Ting, D., Al Saadi, A., & Said, D. G. (2020). Chemical eye injury: Pathophysiology, assessment and management. *Eye, 34*(11), 2001–2019. https://doi.org/10.1038/s41433-020-1026-6
25. Fiorella, D., & Arthur, A. (2019). Middle meningeal artery embolization for the management of chronic subdural hematoma. *Journal of Neurointerventional Surgery, 11*(9), 912–915. https://doi.org/10.1136/neurintsurg-2019-014730
26. Georges, A., & Das, J. M. (2022, January 5). Traumatic brain injury. *StatPearls.* StatPearls Publishing. https://www.ncbi.nlm.nih.gov/books/NBK459300/
27. Gisness, C. M. (2020). Maxillofacial trauma. In V. Sweet & A. Foley (Eds.), *Sheehy's emergency nursing: Principles and practice* (7th ed., pp. 419–430). Elsevier.
28. Gordon, A. A., Tran, L. T., & Phelps, P. O. (2020). Eyelid and orbital trauma for the primary care physician. *Disease-a-Month, 66*(10), Article 101045. https://doi.org/10.1016/j.disamonth.2020.101045
29. Guluma, K., & Lee, J. E. (2018). Ophthalmology. In R. M. Walls, R. S. Hockberger, & M. Gaushe-Hill (Eds.), *Rosen's emergency medicine: Concepts and clinical practice* (9th ed., pp. 790–819). Elsevier.
30. Haldrup, M., Ketharanathan, B., Debrabant, B., Schwartz, O. S., Mikkelsen, R., Fugleholm, K., Poulsen, F. R., Jensen, T., Thaarup, L. V., & Bergholt, B. (2020). Embolization of the middle meningeal artery in patients with chronic subdural hematoma-a systematic review and meta-analysis. *Acta Neurochirurgica, 162*(4), 777–784. https://doi.org/10.1007/s00701-020-04266-0
31. Hall, J., & Hall, M. (2021). Cerebral blood flow, cerebrospinal fluid, and brain metabolism. In *Guyton and Hall textbook of medical physiology* (14th ed., pp. 777–784). Elsevier.
32. Hawryluk, G., Aguilera, S., Buki, A., Bulger, E., Citerio, G., Cooper, D. J., Arrastia, R. D., Diringer, M., Figaji, A., Gao, G., Geocadin, R., Ghajar, J., Harris, O., Hoffer, A., Hutchinson, P., Joseph, M., Kitagawa, R., Manley, G., Mayer, S., Menon, D. K., . . . Chesnut, R. M. (2019). A management algorithm for patients with intracranial pressure monitoring: The Seattle International Severe Traumatic Brain Injury Consensus Conference (SIBICC). *Intensive Care Medicine, 45*(12), 1783–1794. https://doi.org/10.1007/s00134-019-05805-9
33. Hötte, G. J., & De Keizer, R. (2021). Ocular injury and emergencies around the globe. *Atlas of the Oral and Maxillofacial Surgery Clinics of North America, 29*(1), 19–28. https://doi.org/10.1016/j.cxom.2020.11.002
34. Institute of Neurological Sciences NHS Greater Glasgow and Clyde. (2015). *Glasgow Coma Scale: Do it this way.* https://www.glasgowcomascale.org/downloads/GCS-Assessment-Aid-English.pdf?v=3
35. Ironside, N., Nguyen, C., Do, Q., Ugiliweneza, B., Chen, C. J., Sieg, E. P., James, R. F., & Ding, D. (2021). Middle meningeal artery embolization for chronic subdural hematoma: A systematic review and meta-analysis. *Journal of NeuroInterventional Surgery, 13*(10), 951–957. https://doi.org/10.1136/neurintsurg-2021-017352
36. Jain, S., & Iverson, L. M. (2021, June 20). Glasgow Coma Scale. *StatPearls.* StatPearls Publishing. https://www.ncbi.nlm.nih.gov/books/NBK513298/

37. Kan, P., Maragkos, G. A., Srivatsan, A., Srinivasan, V., Johnson, J., Burkhardt, J. K., Robinson, T. M., Salem, M. M., Chen, S., Riina, H. A., Tanweer, O., Levy, E. I., Spiotta, A. M., Kasab, S. A., Lena, J., Gross, B. A., Cherian, J., Cawley, C. M., Howard, B. M., Khalessi, A. A., ... Thomas, A. J. (2021). Middle meningeal artery embolization for chronic subdural hematoma: A multi-center experience of 154 consecutive embolizations. *Neurosurgery, 88*(2), 268–277. https://doi.org/10.1093/neuros/nyaa379

38. Knoop, K. J., & Dennis, W. R. (2019). Ophthalmologic procedures. In J. R. Roberts (Ed.), *Roberts and Hedges' clinical procedures in emergency medicine and acute care* (7th ed., pp. 1295–1337). Elsevier.

39. Larrabee, K., Kao, A., Barbetta, B., & Jones, L. (2021). Midface including Le Fort level injuries. *Facial Plastic Surgery Clinics of North America, 30*(1), 63–70. https://doi.org/10.1016/j.fsc.2021.08.005

40. Majidi, S., Makke, Y., Ewida, A., Sianati, B., Qureshi, A. I., & Koubeissi, M. Z. (2017). Prevalence and risk factors for early seizure in patients with traumatic brain injury: Analysis from National Trauma Data Bank. *Neurocritical Care, 27*(1), 90–95. https://doi.org/10.1007/s12028-016-0363-6

41. McCrea, M. A., Nelson, L. D., & Guskiewicz, K. (2017). Diagnosis and management of acute concussion. *Physical Medicine and Rehabilitation Clinics of North America, 28*(2), 271–286. https://doi.org/10.1016/j.pmr.2016.12.005

42. March, K. (2018). Head injury and dysfunction. In V. Good & P. Kirkwood (Eds.), *Advanced critical care nursing* (2nd ed., pp. 218–252). Elsevier.

43. Marehbian, J. S. M., Edlow, B. L., Hinson, H. E., & Hwang, D. Y. (2017). Medical management of the severe traumatic brain injury patient. *Neurocritical Care, 27*, 430–446.

44. Misch, M. R., & Raukar, N. P. (2020). Sports medicine update: Concussion. *Emergency Medicine Clinics of North America, 38*(1), 207–222. https://doi.org/10.1016/j.emc.2019.09.010

45. Mondor, E. (2022). Trauma. In L. Urden, K. Stacy, & L. Mary (Eds.), *Critical care nursing* (9th ed., pp. 791–830). Elsevier.

46. Mount, C. A., & Das, J. M. (2022, April 5). Cerebral perfusion pressure. *StatPearls*. StatPearls Publishing. https://www.ncbi.nlm.nih.gov/books/NBK537271/

47. Mueller, K., Cirivello, M. J., Bell, R. S., & Armonda, R. A. (2018). Penetrating brain injury. In R. G. Ellenbogen, L. N. Sekhar, & N. D. Kitchen (Eds.), *Principles of neurological surgery* (4th ed., pp. 420–444). Elsevier.

48. Newgard, C., Fischer, P. E., Michaels, H., Jurkovich, G. J., Lerner, B. E., Fallat, M. E., Delbridge, T. R., Brown, J. B., & Bulger, E. M. (2022). National guideline for the field triage of injured patients: Recommendations of the National Expert Panel of Field Triage, 2021. *The Journal of Trauma and Acute Care Surgery, 93*(2), e49–e60. https://doi.org/10.1097/TA.0000000000003627

49. Newton, E., & Taira, T. (2022). Head trauma. In K. Bakes, J. Buchanan, M. Moreira, R. Byyny, & P. Pons (Eds.), *Emergency medicine secrets* (7th ed., pp. 491–495). Elsevier.

50. Nolan-Kelley, L. (2022). Ocular emergencies. In V. Sweet & A. Foley (Eds.), *Sheehy's emergency nursing: Principles and practice* (7th ed., pp. 365–376). Elsevier.

51. Nyam, T. E., Hung, S., Shen, M., Yu, T., & Kuo, J. (2017). FOUR score predicts early outcome in patients after traumatic brain injury. *Neurocritical Care, 26*(2), 225–231. https://doi.org/10.1007/s12028-016-0326-y

52. Ojaghihaghighi, S., Lombardi, K. M., Davis, S., Vahdati, S. S., Sorkhabi, R., & Pourmand, A. (2019). Diagnosis of traumatic eye injuries with point-of-care ocular ultrasonography in the emergency department. *Annals of Emergency Medicine, 74*(3), 365–371. https://doi.org/10.1016/j.annemergmed.2019.02.001

53. Okasha, A. S., Fayed, A. M., & Saleh, A. S. (2014). The FOUR score predicts mortality, endotracheal intubation and ICU length of stay after traumatic brain injury. *Neurocritical Care, 21*(3), 496–504. https://doi.org/10.1007/s12028-014-9995-6

54. Papa, L., & Goldberg, S. A. (2018). Head trauma. In R. M. Walls, R. S. Hockberger, & M. Gaushe-Hill (Eds.), *Rosen's emergency medicine: Concepts and clinical practice* (9th ed., pp. 301–329). Elsevier.

55. Patton, K. T., & Thibodeau, G. A. (2018). Nervous system. In *The human body in health and disease* (7th ed., pp. 248–289). Elsevier.

56. Phillips, B. J., Turco, L. M. (2017). Le Fort fractures: A collective review. *Bulletin of Emergency & Trauma, 5*(4), 221–230. https://beat.sums.ac.ir/article_44391_b1e8b9bad595103fbbf5404ea65f9ef5.pdf

57. Phillips, N., & Hornacky, A. (2021). Neurosurgery of the brain and peripheral nerves. In *Berry and Kohn's operating room technique* (14th ed., pp. 770–787). Elsevier.

58. Phillips, N., & Hornacky, A. (2021). Ophthalmic surgery. In *Berry and Kohn's operating room technique* (14th ed., pp. 806–825). Elsevier.

59. Picetti, E., Rossi, S., Abu-Zidan, F. M., Ansaloni, L., Armonda, R., Baiocchi, G. L., Bala, M., Balogh, Z. J., Berardino, M., Biffl, W. L., Bouzat, P., Buki, A., Ceresoli, M., Chesnut, R. M., Chiara, O., Citerio, G., Coccolini, F., Coimbra, R., Di Saverio, S., Fraga, G. P., ... Catena, F. (2019). WSES consensus conference guidelines: Monitoring and management of severe adult traumatic brain injury patients with polytrauma in the first 24 hours. *World Journal of Emergency Surgery, 14*, Article 53. https://doi.org/10.1186/s13017-019-0270-1

60. Rabinstein, A., & Braksick, S. (2022). Neurointensive care. In J. Jankovic, M. John, S. Pomeroy, & N. Newman (Eds.), *Bradley and Daroff's neurology in clinical practice* (8th ed., pp. 776–792). Elsevier.

61. Rakhit, S., Nordness, M. F., Lombardo, S. R., Cook, M., Smith, L., & Patel, M. B. (2021). Management and challenges of severe traumatic brain injury. *Seminars in Respiratory and Critical Care Medicine, 42*(1), 127–144.

62. Reid, L. D., & Fingar, K. R. (2020). Inpatient stays and emergency department visits involving traumatic brain injury, 2017 (Statistical Brief #255). In *Healthcare Cost and Utilization Project (HCUP) statistical briefs*. Agency for Healthcare Research and Quality. https://www.ncbi.nlm.nih.gov/books/NBK556732/

63. Reith, F., Lingsma, H. F., Gabbe, B. J., Lecky, F. E., Roberts, I., & Maas, A. (2017). Differential effects of the Glasgow Coma Scale score and its components: An analysis of 54,069 patients

with traumatic brain injury. *Injury, 48*(9), 1932–1943. https://doi.org/10.1016/j.injury.2017.05.038

64. Rockafellow, A., Busby E., WuDunn D., Grover, S., & Salman, S. O. (2021). Evidence-based protocol for ophthalmology consult for orbital fractures. *Journal of Oral and Maxillofacial Surgery, 79*(7), 1507–1513. https://doi.org/10.1016/j.joms.2021.02.026

65. Rodriguez, E. D., Dorafshar, A. H., & Manson, P. N. (2018). Facial injuries. In P. C. Neligan (Ed.), *Craniofacial, head and neck surgery and pediatric plastic surgery* (Vol. 3, 4th ed., pp. 47–81). Elsevier.

66. Rosenthal, G., & Le Roux, P. D. (2023). Invasive physiologic monitoring for traumatic brain injury. In H. R. Winn (Ed.), *Youmans and Winn neurological surgery* (8th ed., pp. 3027–3040). Elsevier.

67. Sasser, S. M., Hunt, R. C., Faul, M., Sugarman, D., Pearson, W. S., Dulski, T., Wald, M. M., Jurkovich, G. J., Newgard, C. D., Brooke Lerner, E., Cooper, A., Wang, S. C., Henry, M. C., Salomone, J. P., & Galli, R. L. (2012). Guidelines for field triage of injured patients: Recommendations of the National Expert Panel on Field Triage, 2011. *MMWR Recommendations and Reports, 61*(RR-1), 1–20. https://www.cdc.gov/mmwr/preview/mmwrhtml/rr6101a1.htm

68. Scarboro, M., & McQuillan, K. A. (2021). Traumatic brain injury update. *AACN Advanced Critical Care, 32*(1), 29–50.

69. Scarboro, M., Massetti, J., & Aresco, C. (2020). Traumatic brain injury. In K. McQuillan & M. Makic, *Trauma nursing: From resuscitation through rehabilitation* (5th ed., pp. 332–409). Elsevier.

70. Schizodimos, T., Soulountsi, V., Iasonidou, C., & Kapravelos, N. (2020). An overview of management of intracranial hypertension in the intensive care unit. *Journal of Anesthesia, 34*(5), 741–757. https://doi.org/10.1007/s00540-020-02795-7

71. Shahlaie, K., Zwienenberg-Lee, M., & Muizelaar, J. (2017). Clinical pathophysiology of traumatic brain injury. In H. Winn (Ed.), *Youmans and Winn Neurological Surgery* (7th ed., pp. 2834–2859). Elsevier.

72. Solheim, J. (2013). Facial, ocular, ENT, and dental trauma. In B. B. Hammond & P. G. Zimmerman (Eds.), *Sheehy's manual of emergency care* (7th ed., 439–452). Mosby Elsevier.

73. Stacy, K. M. (2022). Neurologic anatomy and physiology. In L. D. Urden & M. E. Lough (Eds.), *Critical care nursing: Diagnosis and management* (9th ed., pp. 534–564). Elsevier.

74. Stippler, M., & Mahavadi, A. (2022). Craniocerebral trauma. In J. Jankovic, J. Mazziotta, S. Pomeroy, & N. Newman (Eds.), *Bradley and Daroff's neurology in clinical practice* (8th ed., pp. 914–928). Elsevier.

75. Teasdale, G., & Jennett, B. (1974). Assessment of coma and impaired consciousness: A practical scale. *The Lancet, 304*, 81–84.

76. Teasdale, G., Maas, A., Lecky, F., Manle G., Stocchetti, N., & Murray, G. (2014). The Glasgow Coma Scale at 40 years: Standing the test of time. *The Lancet Neurology, 13*(8), 844–854. https://doi.org/10.1016/S1474-4422(14)70120-6

77. Toldi, J. P., & Thomas, J. L. (2020). Evaluation and management of sports-related eye injuries. *Current Sports Medicine Reports, 19*(1), 29–34. https://doi.org/10.1249/JSR.0000000000000677

78. Waqas, M., Vakhari, K., Weimer, P., Hashmi, E., Davies, J., & Siddiqui, A. (2019). Safety and effectiveness of embolization for chronic subdural hematoma: Systematic review and case series. *World Neurosurgery, 126*, 228–236. https://doi.org/10.1016/j.wneu.2019.02.208

79. Watson, V. L., Louis, N., Seminara, B. V., Muizelaar, J. P., & Alberico, A. (2017). Proposal for the rapid reversal of coagulopathy in patients with non-operative head injuries on anticoagulant and/or antiplatelet agents: A case study and literature review. *Neurosurgery, 81*(6), 899–909. https://doi.org/10.1093/neuros/nyx072

80. Wijdicks, E. F., Bamlet, W. R., Maramottom, B. V., Manno, E. M., & McClelland, R. L. (2005). Validation of a new coma scale: The FOUR score. *Annals of Neurology, 58*, 585–593. https://doi.org/10.1002/ana.20611

81. Wolters Kluwer. (2021). Glasgow coma scale and pediatric Glasgow coma scale. UpToDate. Retrieved January 22, 2022, from https://www.uptodate.com/contents/image?imageKey=PEDS%2F59662

82. Zimmerman, L., Tran, D., Lovett, M., Mangat, H. (2019). *Emergency neurological life support traumatic brain injury protocol version 4.0.* Neurocritical Care Society. https://higherlogicdownload.s3.amazonaws.com/NEUROCRITICALCARE/fdc4bb32-6722-417b-8839-f68ac1ef3794/UploadedImages/ENLS_Documents/ENLS_V4.0_protocol%20files/ENLS_V_4_0_Protocol_TBI_FINAL.pdf

CHAPTER 8

Thoracic and Neck Trauma

Roger M. Casey, MSN, RN, CEN, TCRN, FAEN

OBJECTIVES

Upon completion of this chapter, the learner will be able to:
1. Describe mechanisms of injury associated with head trauma.
2. Describe pathophysiologic changes as a basis for assessment of the patient with head trauma.
3. Demonstrate the nursing assessment of the patient with head trauma.
4. Plan appropriate interventions for the patient with head trauma.
5. Evaluate effectiveness of nursing interventions for the patient with head trauma.

Knowledge of normal anatomy and physiology serves as the foundation for understanding anatomic derangements and pathophysiologic processes that may result from trauma. Before reading this chapter, it is strongly suggested that the learner review the following material. Anatomy is not emphasized in the classroom but is the basis of skill evaluation and the foundation of questions for testing purposes.

Anatomy and Physiology of the Thoracic Cavity and Neck

The anatomy and physiology of the thoracic cavity and neck involve a number of systems and structures, including the respiratory system, heart and thoracic great vessels, and the neck.

Respiratory System

Three processes transfer oxygen from the atmosphere to the lungs and bloodstream: ventilation, diffusion, and perfusion. See Chapter 5, "Airway and Ventilation," for a detailed description of the physiology of ventilation.

The upper airway consists of the nose, oropharynx, larynx, and trachea. The lower airway consists of the bronchi, bronchioles, and alveoli with their associated capillaries found within the lungs.[37]

The thoracic cavity extends from the top of the sternum to the diaphragm and is enclosed by the sternum, ribs, and costal cartilage. The main thoracic structures are the lungs and the mediastinum. The mediastinum is the space between the sternum, thoracic vertebrae, and diaphragm. The heart, pericardium, esophagus, thoracic aorta, superior and inferior vena cava, phrenic and vagus nerves, and other vascular structures are found within the mediastinum.[37]

The correlation of thoracic surface landmarks and the underlying structures is important in the physical assessment of the chest (**Figure 8-1**).[12,21,37]

Heart and Thoracic Great Vessels

The heart is enclosed within the mediastinum, with the right ventricle located behind the sternum and the left ventricle anterior to the thoracic vertebrae. The heart is surrounded by the pericardium. The two layers of the pericardium consist of a tough, outer layer (parietal) and a thinner, serous layer (visceral) closely adhering to the heart.[21] The space between the two layers contains approximately 25 mL of lubricating pericardial fluid, which allows the heart to expand and contract without causing friction against surrounding structures.

Cardiac output (CO) is a product of heart rate (HR) and stroke volume (SV): CO = HR × SV. CO is defined as the volume of blood ejected from the heart in 1 minute.[37] (See Chapter 6, "Shock," for more information.) Stroke volume, in turn, is affected by the factors identified in **Table 8-1**. Injury to the myocardium can affect

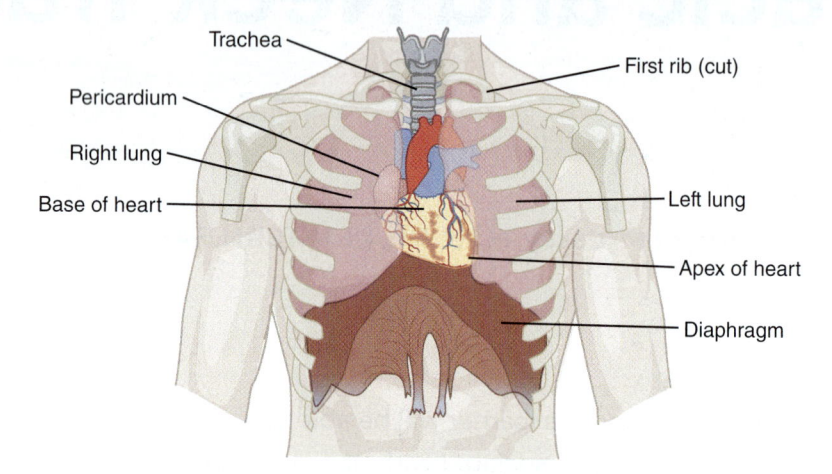

Figure 8-1 *Chest and anatomic landmarks.*

TABLE 8-1	Factors Influencing Cardiac Output
Factor	**Description**
Preload	The volume of blood in the left ventricle at the end of diastole.
	Preload is directly related to the amount of blood volume that is returned to the heart.
	If there is less volume, the ventricles will not have much stretch, decreasing preload.
	A bleeding trauma patient may have reduced preload as the total blood volume decreases.
Afterload	The resistance of the system (either systemic or pulmonary) that the ventricles must overcome to eject blood.
	Intrathoracic pressure affects right ventricular pressure as it contracts against the pulmonary system.
	The patient's blood pressure and elasticity of the peripheral vasculature affect left ventricular pressure.
	A hypotensive trauma patient may have reduced afterload because the pressure within the vasculature system is lower than that in the ventricles.
Contractility	The heart's contractile strength also known as inotropy.
	Factors affecting myocardial contractility include preload and sympathetic nervous system stimulation.

Data from Hartjes, T. M. (Ed.). (2018). *AACN core curriculum for high acuity, progressive, and critical care nursing* (7th ed.). Elsevier; Lough, M. E. (2022). Cardiovascular anatomy and physiology. In L. D. Urden, K. M. Stacy, & M. K. Lough (Eds.), *Critical care nursing: Diagnosis and management* (9th ed., pp. 167–189). Elsevier; Stacy, K. M. (2022). Pulmonary anatomy and physiology. In L. D. Urden, K. M. Stacy, & M. K. Lough (Eds.), *Critical care nursing: Diagnosis and management* (9th ed., pp. 421–440). Elsevier.

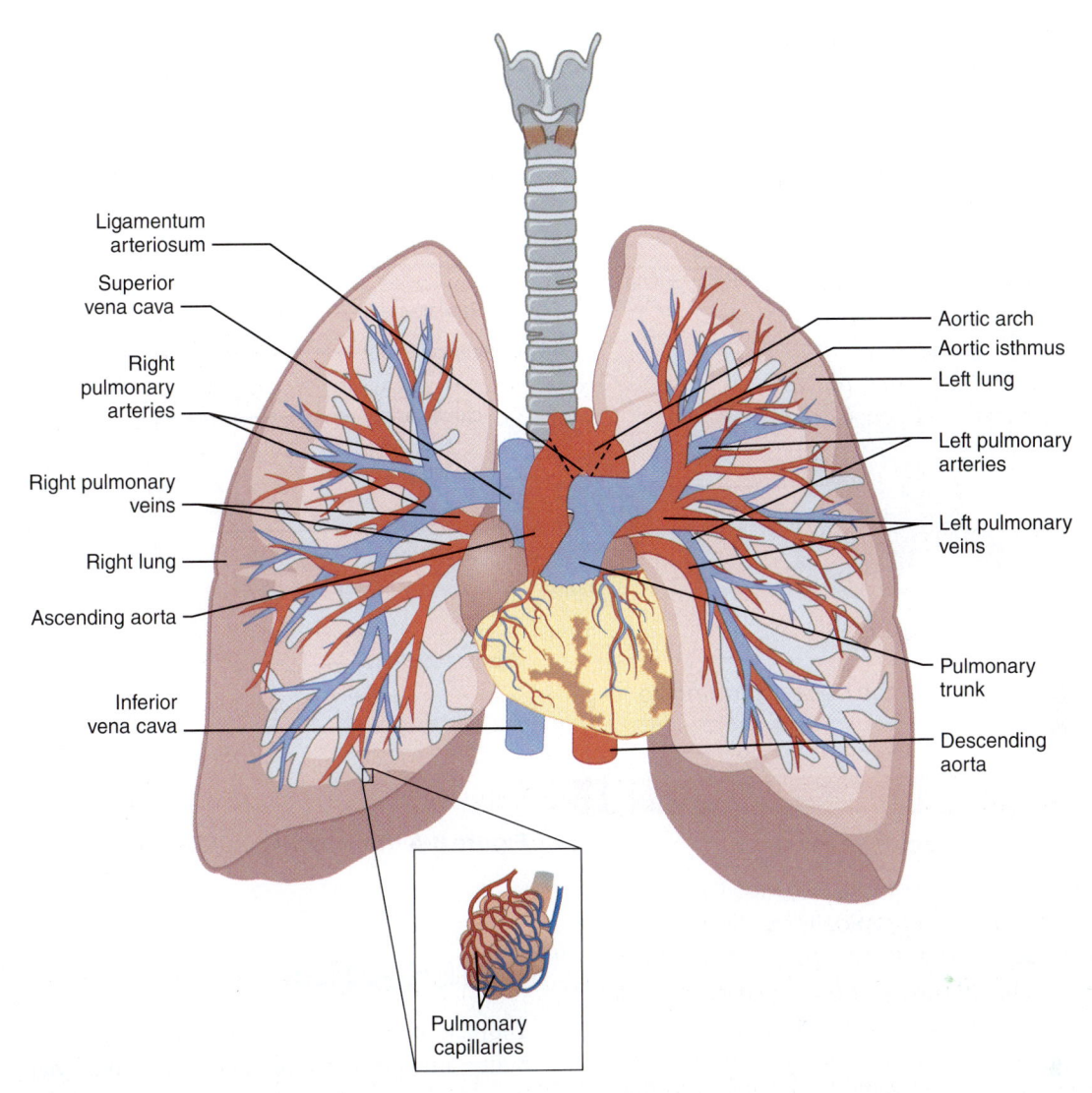

Figure 8-2 *Thoracic vasculature.*

any one of these functions, resulting in decreased cardiac output and the ability to perfuse oxygenated blood to the tissues.

The thoracic aorta carries oxygenated blood from the heart to the body and is located in the mediastinum. The three segments of the thoracic aorta are the ascending aorta, the aortic arch, and the descending aorta (**Figure 8-2**). The ascending aorta is the portion located most proximal to the heart. The aortic arch extends from the ascending thoracic aorta to the descending thoracic aorta and is the source for both the carotid and subclavian arteries. The descending aorta continues distally from the aortic arch and constricts slightly at the aortic isthmus, where it is held in place by the ligamentum arteriosum, the left mainstem bronchus, and the paired intercostal arteries. The aortic isthmus is the transition from the relatively fixed aortic arch to the more free and mobile descending aorta. The aortic isthmus is less able to tolerate rapid acceleration/deceleration forces than the rest of the aorta. It is most often the site of aortic injury.[27]

Neck

The neck contains several important anatomic structures relative to its size (**Figure 8-3**). It is commonly divided into three zones, based on bony and superficial landmarks.[13,15]

- Zone I landmarks: thoracic outlet to the cricoid cartilage
- Zone II landmarks: the cricoid cartilage to the angle of the mandible
- Zone III landmarks: angle of the mandible to the base of the skull

The neck's anatomic structures are contained within two fascial layers. The superficial fascia contains the platysma muscle, which protects the underlying structures. If the platysma is damaged, injury to the structures beneath is suspected. The deep cervical fascia supports the muscles, vessels, and organs of the neck. The compartments

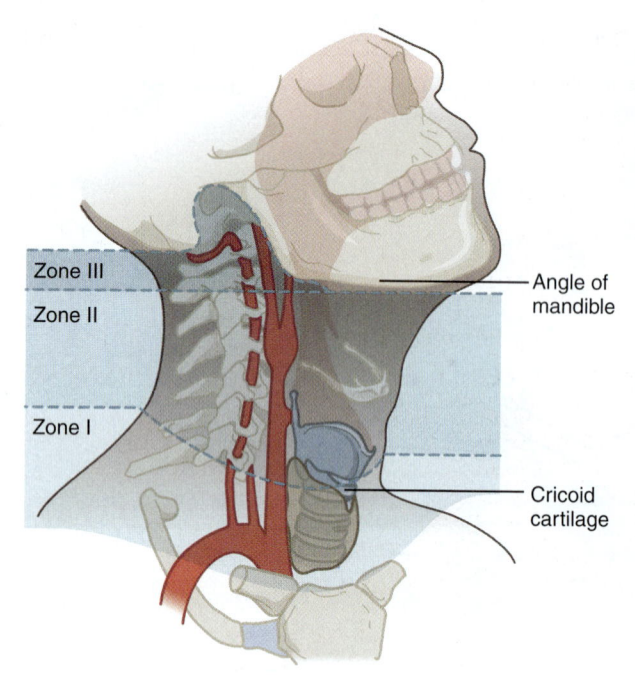

Figure 8-3 Anatomy of the neck (including zones).

> ### CLINICAL PEARL
> #### Mortality and Neck Injuries
> Mortality is the highest with injuries to Zone I in the neck because they typically involve major vessels, the trachea, the esophagus, and the lungs.[13] The most frequently injured is Zone II, which contains vital airway and vascular structures.[13,22] The trauma nurse will have a high degree of suspicion of a more serious underlying injury in patients who have dysphonia (vocal changes/difficulty), dysphagia, subcutaneous emphysema, or hematomas to the neck region; these indicate vascular trauma, airway injuries, or esophageal injuries that may not be diagnosed on imaging studies.[13,14]

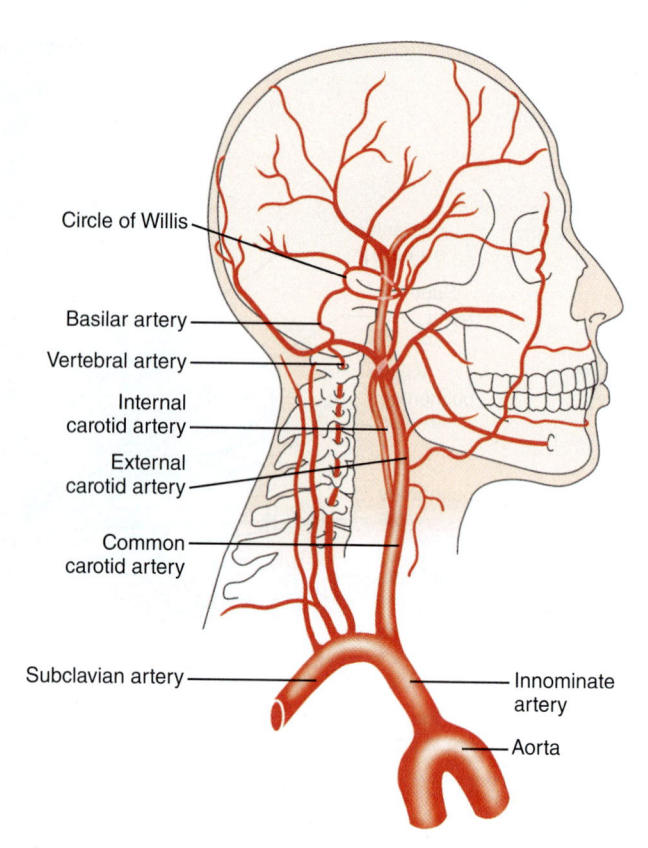

Figure 8-4 The vascular supply to the brain.

formed by the fascia may limit external bleeding but may also allow a hematoma to form, which may compromise the airway.[14]

The vascular supply for the brain and the brain stem arises from the vertebral and internal carotid arteries (**Figure 8-4**).

Nerve roots from C5 through T1 merge, forming the brachial plexus (**Figure 8-5**). This structure then subdivides and merges to form the multiple nerves, such as the axillary, musculocutaneous, median, radial, and ulnar nerves, that are responsible for arm and hand function.[13,37]

Introduction

Thoracic and neck trauma are a significant cause of morbidity and mortality in trauma patients. Many of the injuries that occur in this anatomic region are severely life threatening if not identified and treated in a rapid manner. Motor vehicle collisions (MVCs) are the most common cause of blunt trauma to the neck and thoracic regions, while gunshot wounds and stabbings are the most common cause of penetrating trauma. Identifying these injuries through a thorough assessment process is key to increasing the chances of patient survival.[1,35,37]

Epidemiology

Thoracic and neck trauma can cause significant life-threatening injuries that necessitate emergent intervention. In the United States, MVCs involving automobiles, motorcycles, and pedestrians account for more than half of all blunt injuries to the neck and chest.[1,35,37] Thoracic injuries are present in 20% of trauma patients presenting for care.[20] Penetrating injuries to the neck have a mortality rate of up to 10% in adults and are most commonly caused by personal assaults with firearms and stabbing instruments.[28] Interpersonal violence is increasingly a more common cause of thoracic trauma.[1,37]

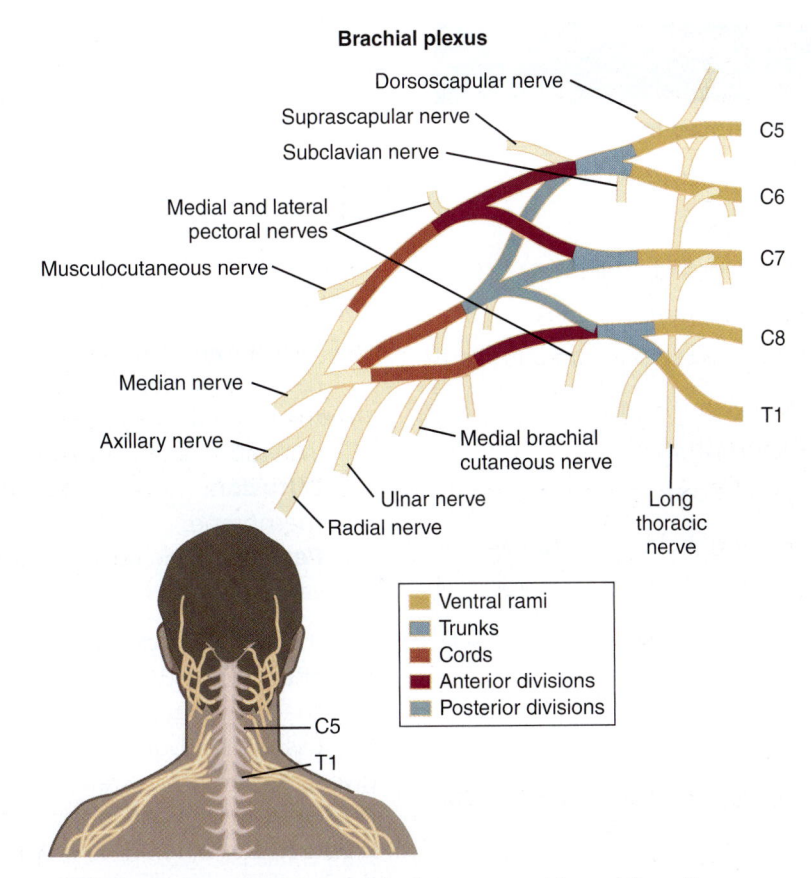

Figure 8-5 *Nerves responsible for arm and hand functions.*

Biomechanics and Mechanisms of Injury

While MVCs are the most common cause of thoracic trauma, other mechanisms of injury (MOIs) include falls, crush injuries, assaults, gunshot and stabbing wounds, and pedestrian-versus-vehicle collisions.[1,31,35,37] Additional considerations include the following:

- The energy forces associated with acceleration and deceleration can result in devastating injury to the major vessels as the body makes impact and the internal organs stay in motion. The descending aorta is at increased risk of being torn because it is fixed in place by the ligamentum arteriosum.[1,11]
- Mechanical energy forces applied to the thorax can cause rib fractures, pulmonary contusion, pneumothorax, hemothorax, and blunt cardiac injury. The sternum and first and second ribs are relatively more resistant to energy forces because they are protected.[1] First rib fractures are an indicator of life-threatening injuries in trauma patients.[33] Because more force is required to damage these structures, there is increased risk of injury to the underlying structures, as well as an increased risk of death.[1,33]
- Direct blunt injury to the myocardium may result in ventricular perforation or rupture and can often be fatal.
- Penetrating injury to the heart commonly injures the right ventricle because of its anterior position in the thoracic cavity.

Usual Concurrent Injuries

Thoracic injuries are often associated with life-threatening conditions such as airway disruption, impaired breathing, or impaired circulation. Thoracic trauma is most often associated with concurrent head, spine, extremity, and abdominal injuries. Thoracic skeletal injuries are often linked with specific injuries (**Table 8-2**).[7,9,25]

CLINICAL PEARL

Penetrating Thoracic Wound Below the Fourth Intercostal Space

If a penetrating thoracic wound is found below the fourth intercostal space, penetration into the abdominal cavity is suspected until proved otherwise.[1]

TABLE 8-2 Thoracic Skeletal Fractures and Associated Injuries

Fractures	Associated Injuries
Sternal fractures	Blunt cardiac injury
	Pneumothorax
First and second rib fractures	Great vessel injuries
	Brachial plexus injuries
	Head and spinal cord injuries
Multiple rib fractures and flail chest	Pulmonary contusion
	Pneumothorax
	Hemothorax
Lower rib fractures (7–12)	Liver (right-sided fractures)
	Spleen (left-sided fractures)

Data from Dennis, D. M., Bellister, S. A., & Guillamondegui, O. D. (2017). Thoracic trauma. *Surgical Clinics of North America*, 97, 1047–1064. https://doi.org/10.1016/j.suc.2017.06.009; Fallouh, H., Dattani-Patel, R., & Rathinam, D. (2017). Blunt thoracic trauma. *Surgery*, 35(5), 262–268; Mondor, E. E. (2022). Trauma. In L. D. Urden, K. M. Stacy, & M. K. Lough (Eds.), *Critical care nursing: Diagnosis and management* (9th ed., pp. 791–830). Elsevier.

Penetrating thoracic trauma can occur with penetrating abdominal trauma as a result of the movement of the diaphragm in and out of the thoracic cavity.

Neck injuries may be isolated, but they may also be associated with head, cervical spine, or upper thoracic injuries. Determining the specific zone of neck injury is helpful in identifying the structures that may be injured, the need for diagnostic studies, and the approach to surgical management. An emerging trend is to use advanced imaging techniques, such as computed tomography (CT) angiography or MRI, in patients with stable penetrating neck injuries to determine if surgical intervention is required. Regardless of the zone of injury, physical examination should guide providers as to whether imaging is used or if the patient should be prepared for exploratory neck surgery.[5,14,15]

Injuries to the neck may occlude the airway, interrupt blood flow to the brain, or cause cervical spinal cord injury. Because of the risk of concurrent cervical spinal injuries, the motion of patients with neck injuries is restricted, and they are assessed for cervical spinal injury.[13]

Pathophysiology as a Basis for Assessment Findings

An understanding of the physiological processes associated with organs likely affected in certain types of injuries will help the trauma nurse anticipate potential problems, interventions, monitoring, and management for the trauma patient.

CLINICAL PEARL

Ventilation, Diffusion, and Perfusion

Definitions for each term follow:

- **Ventilation:** The active, mechanical movement of air into and out of the lungs during the respiratory cycle, which consists of both inspiration and expiration.
- **Diffusion:** The exchange of gases across a membrane.
- **Perfusion:** The flow of blood through the vasculature to the body tissues.

Ventilation brings oxygen into the lungs. Gas is exchanged in the alveolar capillaries and enters the bloodstream. Blood delivers oxygen to the tissues. Carbon dioxide (CO_2) results from glycolysis and the Krebs cycle at the cellular level and is brought back to the lungs by the blood to be exhaled as a waste product. End-tidal carbon dioxide ($ETCO_2$) monitoring can be used to determine whether ventilation is effective; it is more sensitive than monitoring pulse oximetry. An increase in $ETCO_2$ can indicate airway obstruction, embolism, or other clinical changes affecting ventilation, diffusion, or perfusion.[11,23,37]

Ineffective Ventilation

Trauma to the thoracic cavity, the neck, and the structures within these areas can result in ineffective ventilation. Any loss of integrity to the lungs or diaphragm may compromise normal respiration and ventilation.[11,25,37]

A pneumothorax, pulmonary bleeding, pulmonary contusions, and sternal or rib fractures may interfere with the mechanics of breathing, owing to both increased intrathoracic pressure and pain. Sternal and rib fractures can also result in damage to underlying organs. Pulmonary contusions may cause interstitial and alveolar edema. Lacerations to the lung allow for the accumulation of blood in the interstitial and alveolar spaces. Oxygen (O_2) and carbon dioxide (CO_2) diffusion across the alveolar membrane is impaired by interstitial and alveolar edema or blood. Damaged alveoli and capillary injuries produce abnormalities in the ventilation-to-perfusion ratio.[23,37]

Penetrating injury to the chest wall and lacerated lung tissue can cause the loss of normal negative intrapleural pressure. The collection of air or blood in the pleural space may cause lung collapse. The degree of collapse depends on the extent of the air or blood that collects in the pleural space and the severity of the underlying lung injury.[1]

The airway can be easily compromised or occluded as a result of neck trauma. Edema or hematomas from disrupted blood vessels following a neck injury may narrow or completely obstruct the upper airway. Tears or lacerations of the tracheobronchial tree can disrupt the integrity of the upper and lower airway. Patients with these injuries initially present with dramatic symptoms, including airway obstruction, hemoptysis, cyanosis, and subcutaneous emphysema from massive air leaks into the tissues of the face, neck, and chest.[1,13]

Ineffective Circulation

Air or blood that continues to accumulate in the thoracic cavity can cause an increase in intrapleural pressure on the side of the chest that is injured. If this pressure is allowed to expand without intervention, a tension pneumothorax results; this causes a mediastinal shift that compresses the heart and great vessels, resulting in a decrease in venous return (preload) and subsequent decrease in cardiac output. The increased pressure can also compress the opposite lung, further decreasing ventilation. In such a case, the patient usually exhibits signs of increased work of breathing, tachypnea, shortness of breath, tachycardia, hypotension, and a unilateral decrease in breath sounds on the injured side. Neck vein distention from the increased intrathoracic pressure and tracheal deviation caused by the mediastinal shift are late signs. Neck vein distention and may not be evident because of hypovolemia.[1,31]

Injury to the heart or great vessels that results in immediate uncontrolled hemorrhage can be fatal. Direct injury to the heart may cause damage to the tissue, reduce myocardial contractility, and ultimately lead to a reduction in cardiac output. The rapid accumulation of even small amounts of blood in the pericardial sac may result in compression of the heart (pericardial tamponade), making it difficult for the heart to fill during diastole, and in turn resulting in decreased cardiac output. Assessment findings include hypotension, tachycardia, muffled heart sounds, and neck vein distention.[1,11,31] Jugular venous distention may not be evident in significantly hypovolemic patients.[11,31]

Injury to the arteries in the neck may cause decreased blood flow to the brain, subsequently producing cerebral hypoxia and neurologic deficits. Penetrating injuries to certain neck vessels (carotid or vertebral arteries or vertebral, brachiocephalic, and jugular veins) may cause rapid exsanguination.[13,15]

Nursing Care of the Patient with Thoracic or Neck Trauma

Refer to Chapter 4, "Initial Assessment," for information on the systematic approach to the nursing care of the trauma patient. The following assessment parameters are specific to patients with thoracic or neck trauma.

Primary Survey

If there is no uncontrolled, life-threatening external hemorrhage resulting in the need to reprioritize to C-ABC, the primary survey begins with alertness and airway.

A: Alertness and Airway

Assess the patient's alertness and airway.

Assessment

Inspect for the following:

- Injuries to the neck that may indicate edema or blood in the airway
- Signs of injury that may obstruct or impede the patient's ability to maintain a patent airway:
  - Foreign objects
  - Loose or missing teeth
  - Blood, vomitus, or secretions
  - Edema
  - Burns or evidence of inhalation injury
  - Tongue swelling
  - Hematoma (underlying blunt trauma)
  - Subcutaneous emphysema (from a pneumothorax or a tracheal or esophageal laceration)
  - Impaled objects
  - Lacerations
  - Bleeding
  - Tracheal deviation (from a tension pneumothorax)

Auscultate for restrictive airway sounds. Hoarseness and stridor may be signs of tracheal injury and airway narrowing.

Interventions

Interventions include the following:

- Apply direct pressure to bleeding sites.
  - Take care to ensure that pressure to control bleeding does not impede airway patency.

- Suction the oropharynx.
- Stabilize any impaled objects.
- Insert airway adjuncts as needed to maintain patency.
- Prepare to assist with a definitive airway as indicated.

Cervical Spinal Stabilization/Spinal Motion Restriction

Neck trauma carries a risk for concurrent cervical spinal injury. Whenever trauma to the neck occurs, take care to restrict spinal motion until injury can be ruled out.[13,37]

B: Breathing and Ventilation

Breathing and ventilation assessment and interventions come next.

Assessment

Inspect for the following:

- Chest wall injuries that may severely impair the adequacy of breathing, such as open chest wounds or flail segments
- Breathing effectiveness, to include rate and depth of respirations (if present) and work of breathing
- Symmetrical or paradoxical chest wall movement
- Evidence of blunt or penetrating trauma to the thorax or upper abdomen

Auscultate for the following:

- Equality of bilateral breath sounds
- Unilateral or generalized diminished breath sounds (pneumothorax or hemothorax)

Percuss for the following:

- Dullness or hyperresonance of the chest (presence of blood or air)

Palpate for the following:

- Tenderness (contusions, rib fractures)
- Edema (hematomas, contusions)
- Hematoma/ecchymosis (contusions, rib fractures)
- Subcutaneous emphysema (pneumothorax, tension pneumothorax, tracheal or esophageal laceration)
- Bony crepitus (possible fractured ribs or sternum)
- The trachea at the level of the suprasternal notch to assess for tracheal deviation (tension pneumothorax)

Interventions

Interventions include the following:

- Administer supplemental oxygen as indicated.
- Prepare to monitor and titrate oxygen delivery after the patient is stabilized. See Chapter 5, "Airway and Ventilation," for information regarding hyperoxia.
- Implement selected interventions described later in this chapter based on assessment findings.

C: Circulation and Control of Hemorrhage

If there is a high degree of suspicion of cardiac injury, auscultate for muffled heart sounds or murmurs. Palpate for the following:

- Central pulses
- Compare the quality of pulses between the left and right and the lower and upper extremities
- External jugular veins for distention
- Extremities for motor and sensory function
  - Lower extremity paresis or paralysis may indicate an aortic injury or thoracic spinal injury.[31]
  - Upper extremity paresis or paralysis may indicate a brachial plexus injury.

Reevaluation

If the assessment findings provoke a suspicion of uncontrolled internal bleeding, a chest radiograph or focused assessment with sonography for trauma (FAST) examination (**Figure 8-6**) may be indicated. Determine whether the patient needs immediate definitive operative intervention or transport.[1]

Chest Radiograph

A supine chest radiograph will likely identify any significant pneumothorax. If a hemothorax is suspected, the position of the patient during the test directly influences the reading. If the patient is supine, blood will likely spread throughout the affected side, creating general opacification. If the patient is upright, the air–fluid boundary will appear horizontally. If a potential spinal cord injury has been ruled out, an upright chest radiograph can be used to evaluate a hemothorax. Chest radiographs may suggest an aortic injury but cannot confirm or rule out the diagnosis; mediastinal widening can also be caused by venous bleeding from clavicular, sternal, or thoracic spine fractures as well as other abnormalities.[31]

Focused Assessment with Sonography for Trauma

A FAST examination may be indicated to detect the presence of pericardial blood and heart wall motion. Extended examination (eFAST) may reveal the presence of sternal fractures as well as the presence of pneumothorax

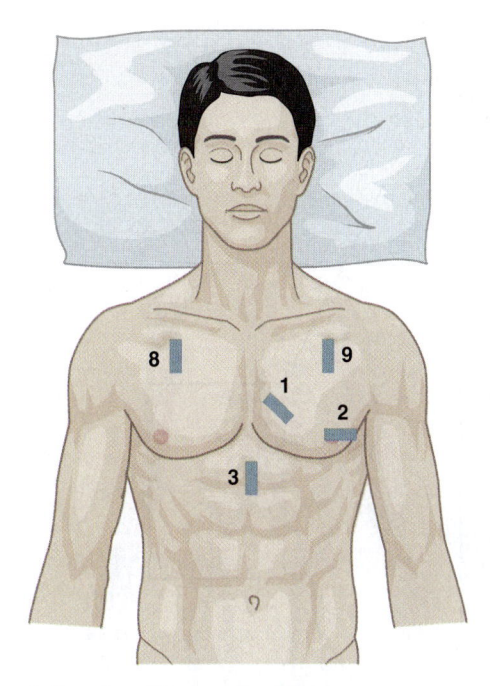

1. Parasternal long cardiac view
2. Apical four-chamber cardiac view
3. Inferior vena cava view
8. Pulmonary view
9. Pulmonary view

Figure 8-6 *FAST exam in thoracic trauma.*

the thoracotomy and cardiac tamponade has been diagnosed or is highly suspected, a decompressive needle pericardiocentesis may be performed, preferably under ultrasound guidance.[1(p70)]

Resuscitative thoracotomy is rarely successful in patients with blunt chest trauma and cardiac arrest.[1,31]

CLINICAL PEARL

Internal Defibrillation

When defibrillation is required following a resuscitative thoracotomy, the internal paddles are placed on opposite sides of the myocardium. (A saline-soaked gauze dressing may be placed between the myocardium and the paddles to improve conduction and decrease injury to the myocardium.) Lower energy settings are used for internal defibrillation because the paddles are placed directly on the myocardium. For adults, 30 to 50 joules should be used. Internal paddles are programmed to deliver a maximum of 50 joules.[10]

or cardiac tamponade.[1,31] See Chapter 9, "Abdominal and Pelvic Trauma," for more information on performing the FAST examination.

Resuscitative Thoracotomy

Resuscitative thoracotomy may be necessary when a patient with penetrating chest trauma arrives with unstable vital signs, impending arrest, or sudden loss of vital signs. Indications for performing this invasive procedure in the resuscitation room include:

- Relief of cardiac tamponade
- Support cardiac output (with internal massage)
- Cross-clamp the descending aorta (to preserve blood flow to the brain and thoracic organs)
- Defibrillate the heart internally (more effective than external defibrillation)
- Limit hemorrhage from the heart or great vessels

In regard to the need for or success of resuscitative thoracotomy in the emergency department (ED), the American College of Surgeons notes that

[with] the availability of a surgical team skilled in repair of such injuries, a resuscitative thoracotomy may be required if there is no return of spontaneous circulation. If no surgeon is available to perform

Resuscitative Endovascular Balloon Occlusion of Aorta

An emerging option is the resuscitative endovascular balloon occlusion of the aorta (REBOA). With REBOA, a catheter enters via the femoral artery into the aorta in specified zones to provide an endovascular block, similar to cross-clamping the aorta during a thoracotomy (**Figure 8-7**).[17,19] REBOA may achieve occlusion more rapidly than thoracotomy in the hands of a skilled practitioner. Indications for REBOA include the following:

- Traumatic life-threatening hemorrhage below the diaphragm in the presence of hemorrhagic shock with transient responders or nonresponders to resuscitation
- Patients arriving at the ED in arrest from injury due to presumed life-threatening hemorrhage below the diaphragm
- Inflation of the balloon in the distal thoracic aorta (Zone I) for intra-abdominal or retroperitoneal hemorrhage or traumatic arrest, or the distal abdominal aorta (Zone III) for severe pelvic, junctional, or proximal lower extremity hemorrhage

Note that REBOA is an emerging procedure, so the evidence supporting its use, as well as evidence of complications arising from its use, is limited, but it can be

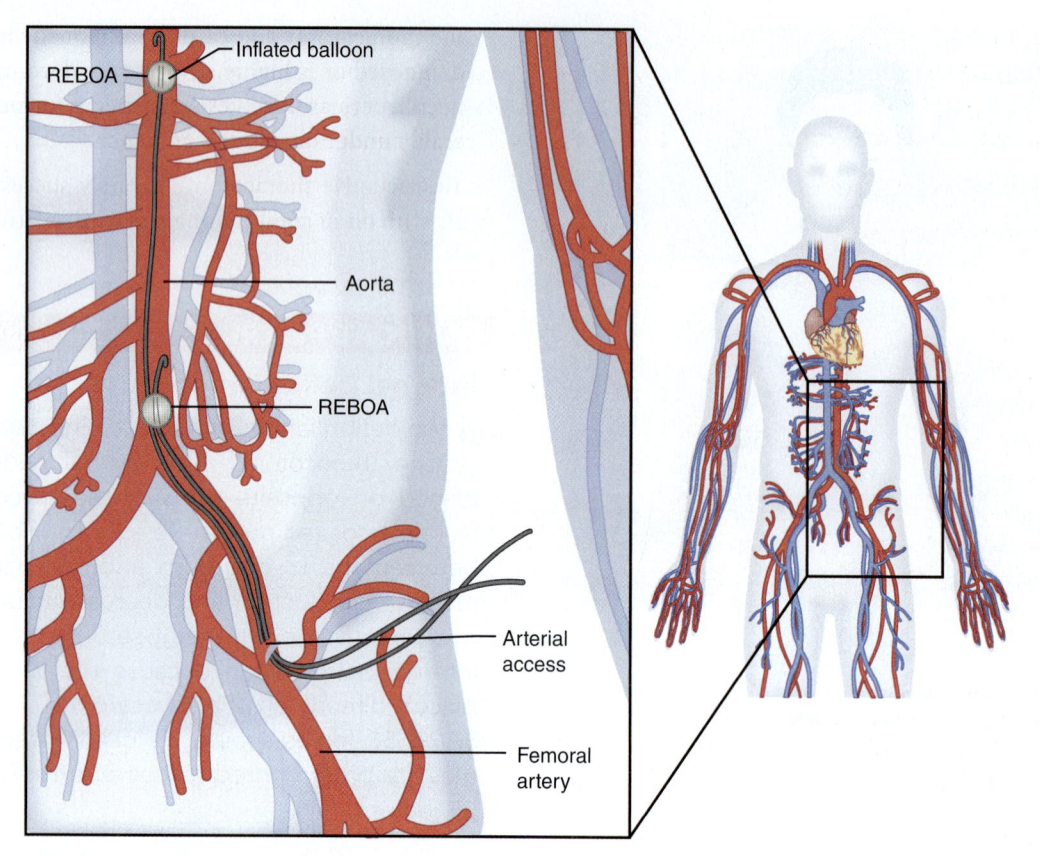

Figure 8-7 *Resuscitative endovascular balloon occlusion of aorta (REBOA).*
Reproduced from King, D. R. (2019). Initial care of the severely injured patient. *The New England Journal of Medicine, 380*(8), 763–770. https://doi.org/10.1056/NEJMra1609326

effective with experienced providers.[8,29,32] The American College of Surgeons and the American College of Emergency Physicians have provided a joint statement with recommendations for REBOA use, guidelines, and recommendations for implementation; "REBOA is contraindicated in the setting of major thoracic hemorrhage or pericardial tamponade."[3(p3)]

Secondary Survey

The secondary survey begins after all life-threatening injuries have been identified and treated and starts with the history and head-to-toe assessment.

H: History

Questions specific to patients with thoracic or neck injuries include:

- Is the MOI blunt or penetrating?
- Is the patient complaining in a way that would indicate that one or more of the following conditions is present?
    - Dyspnea
    - Dysphagia
    - Dysphonia
- Was there a cardiac event prior to the injury?

If cardiopulmonary resuscitation is being performed, when was it started and why? This information is important in determining the indications for performing an emergency thoracotomy or when to consider withdrawal of support.

Selected Neck and Thoracic Injuries

This section covers selected neck and thoracic injuries.

Tracheobronchial Injury

Although rare, tracheobronchial trauma can be the result of blunt or penetrating trauma to the chest or neck.[31] The majority of penetrating injuries occur in the proximal trachea. Direct blows to the neck or "clothesline"-type injuries are common mechanisms for blunt tracheobronchial trauma. Diagnosis is based on assessment findings and confirmed with bronchoscopy or CT for large disruptions. Bronchoscopy can be used to help advance an endotracheal tube (ETT) past the injury to ensure adequate ventilation.[22,28,31]

Assessment Findings

Assessment findings include the following:

- Dyspnea or tachypnea
- Hoarseness
- Subcutaneous emphysema in the neck, face, or upper thorax
- Pneumothorax, possibly tension pneumothorax
- Hemoptysis
- Decreased or absent breath sounds
- Signs and symptoms of airway obstruction

Interventions

Attempts at endotracheal intubation may cause further injury or contribute to airway occlusion. Anesthesiology, if available, may reduce the risk of intubation injury. Other approaches that may minimize trauma to the airway include use of flexible endoscopy, a smaller endotracheal tube, or an emergent cricothyrotomy, if indicated.[1,22,28]

Esophageal Injury

Injury to the esophagus is most commonly caused by penetrating trauma; injury due to blunt trauma is rare.[41]

Assessment Findings

Assessment findings include the following[1,31,39]:

- Air in the mediastinum with possible widening
- Concurrent left pneumothorax or hemothorax
- Esophageal matter in a chest tube
- Subcutaneous emphysema
- Hemoptysis
- Hoarseness
- Dysphagia
- Neck tenderness or hematoma
- Pleuritic pain that worsens with swallowing or flexion of the neck
- Pain may be located in the back, epigastric area, or substernal and becomes progressively worse over time

Interventions

The only intervention in this case is to prepare for surgery.

Neck Trauma

Neck trauma may result in injuries to the airway structures (trachea or larynx), blood vessels (subclavian, jugular, carotid, and vertebral), esophagus, endocrine glands (thyroid and parathyroid), thoracic duct, and brachial plexus. MOIs may be either blunt or penetrating. Examples of blunt trauma include direct blows or clothesline-type injury to the neck region. Penetrating trauma may be caused by either sharp instruments or missile injuries (gunshot wounds). Neck trauma may damage significant airway or vascular structures or the spinal column.

Assessment Findings

Assessment findings include the following:

- Dyspnea or tachypnea
- Hemoptysis
- Subcutaneous emphysema
- Decreased or absent breath sounds
- Penetrating wounds or impaled objects
- Bruits, which may indicate potential carotid artery injury
- Active external bleeding
- Expanding hematoma
- Neurologic deficits (aphasia or loss of extremity movement or sensation)
- Dysphonia
- Dysphagia

Interventions

Interventions include the following:

- Stabilize any impaled objects.
- Control external bleeding with direct pressure.
- Continuously monitor for continued bleeding or expanding hematomas.
- Prepare for definitive airway if indicated.
- Prepare for surgery if unstable.
- Prepare for diagnostic imaging (e.g., CT angiography).

Diagnostic imaging will apply primarily to the stable patient. Patients with neck injury can be categorized as whether or not they will require emergent or urgent surgical intervention. These patients can generally be divided into four categories: (1) hemodynamically unstable, (2) hard signs of injury with or without hemodynamic instability, (3) hemodynamically stable with soft signs of injury, and (4) asymptomatic. Patients in either of the first two categories will most likely go to the operating room emergently. Soft and hard signs of neck trauma are listed in **Table 8-3**.[28] If a patient displays hard signs of injury but remains hemodynamically stable, they may go directly to surgery or undergo evaluation and imaging and then be taken to the operating room for surgical exploration.[28]

TABLE 8-3 Soft versus Hard Signs of Penetrating Neck Trauma

Soft Signs	Hard Signs
Minor hemoptysis	Rapidly expanding/pulsatile hematoma
Minor hematemesis	Massive hemoptysis
Dysphonia, dysphagia	Air bubbling from wound
Subcutaneous or mediastinal air	Severe hemorrhage
Nonexpanding hematoma	Shock not responding to fluids
	Unilateral decreased or absent radial pulse
	Vascular bruit or thrill
	Stridor/hoarseness or airway compromise
	Strokelike neurological deficits
	Massive subcutaneous emphysema

Modified from Newton, K., & Claudius, I. (2023). Neck trauma. In R. M. Walls, R. S. Hockberger, M. Gausche-Hill, T. B. Erickson, & S. R. Wilcox (Eds.), *Rosen's emergency medicine: Concepts and clinical practice* (10th ed., pp. 368–375, e3). Elsevier.

Rib and Sternal Fractures

Rib fractures are found in approximately 43% of patients presenting with thoracic trauma; fractures of the first and second ribs are associated with great vessel injuries.[20] More than 90% of patients with multiple rib fractures have associated injuries, most commonly involving the head, neck, abdomen, and/or extremities.[1] If the patient has fractures of the right lower ribs, suspect the possibility of underlying injury to the liver.[1] In contrast, fractures of the left lower ribs are suggestive of injuries to the spleen.[1] With any displaced rib fracture, lung contusion or laceration is possible. Patients 65 years or older with multiple rib fractures have a greater risk of pneumonia and a higher mortality compared with younger people.[1,30,31]

Sternal fractures are usually caused by a blow to the anterior chest and may be associated with pulmonary contusion.[1] Because of the force required to fracture the sternum, most of these fractures are not isolated; they may be associated with multiple rib or thoracic spine fractures. A severely displaced sternal fracture may indicate serious cardiac injury.[1,6,37]

Assessment Findings

Assessment findings include the following:

- Dyspnea
- Localized pain on movement, palpation, or inspiration
- Patient assumes a position of comfort, which splints the chest wall to reduce pain
- Paradoxical chest wall movement (flail)
- Chest wall contusions
- Bony crepitus or deformity

Interventions

Interventions include the following:

- Administer supplemental oxygen as needed.
- Administer analgesia to promote adequate chest expansion and depth of respiration.
- Prepare for intubation and ventilatory support if severe respiratory distress is present.

Flail Chest

A flail chest injury is defined as the fracture of two or more sequential ribs in two or more locations that results in a flail section (**Figure 8-8**).[20,31,42] This flail segment creates an unstable chest wall that moves paradoxically, drawing in with chest expansion and pushing out with exhalation.[6,11,31] In the mechanics of breathing, inspiration is generated by negative intrapleural pressure that draws air in from the outside. This type of negative pressure cannot be generated with a flail segment because of its paradoxical motion.[11,31] This paradoxical, or asynchronous, movement of the chest may be limited by the surrounding musculature, making it generally more easily detected with palpation than with inspection. Ineffective ventilation in flail chest is caused by several factors:

- Pain that causes the patient to splint, with rapid, shallow breathing
- Deformity of the chest wall that results in loss of tidal volume, atelectasis, and the ability to clear secretions[6,31]
- Underlying injury to thoracic organs, including parenchymal laceration, pulmonary contusion, pneumothorax, or hemothorax[20,31,42]

Assessment Findings

Assessment findings include the following:

- Dyspnea
- Diminished breath sounds
- Chest wall pain
- Chest wall contusions
- Paradoxical movement of the chest
  - If the patient is splinting as a response to pain, this movement may be difficult to visualize.
  - Administration of analgesia may reduce the splinting response due to pain, improve visibility of the flail chest, and improve ventilation.

Interventions

Interventions include the following:

- Support adequate oxygenation and ventilation.
- Administer analgesia to the patient.
- Prepare for intubation and mechanical ventilation.
- Anticipate possible surgical intervention.[20]

Simple Pneumothorax

A simple (closed) pneumothorax can be caused by either blunt or penetrating trauma (**Figure 8-9**). With such an injury, air escapes from the injured lung into the pleural space, and negative intrapleural pressure is lost, resulting in a partial or complete collapse of the lung.[1,33]

> **CLINICAL PEARL**
>
> **Pneumothorax with Positive-Pressure Ventilation**
>
> Mechanically ventilated patients with even a relatively small pneumothorax are at a higher risk for expansion of the pneumothorax or development of a tension pneumothorax because of positive-pressure ventilation. Maintain a high index of suspicion for this condition with ventilated patients who have a pneumothorax and no thoracostomy tube.

Assessment Findings

Assessment findings include the following:

- Dyspnea or tachypnea
- Tachycardia
- Decreased or absent breath sounds on the injured side
- Chest pain

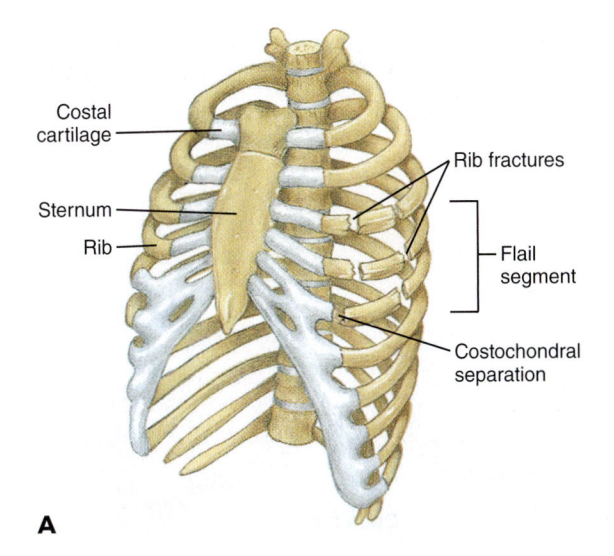

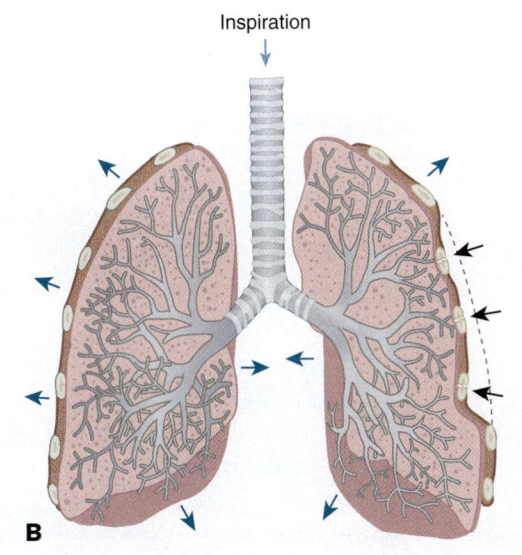

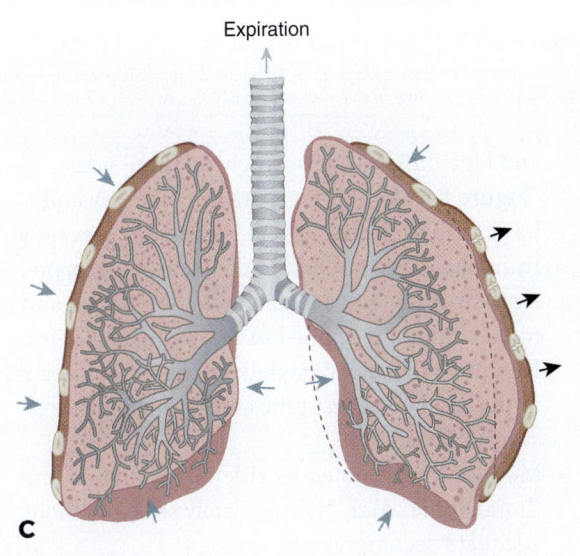

Figure 8-8 Flail chest. **A.** Flail chest injury. **B.** Paradoxical movement inward on inspiration. **C.** Paradoxical movement outward on expiration.

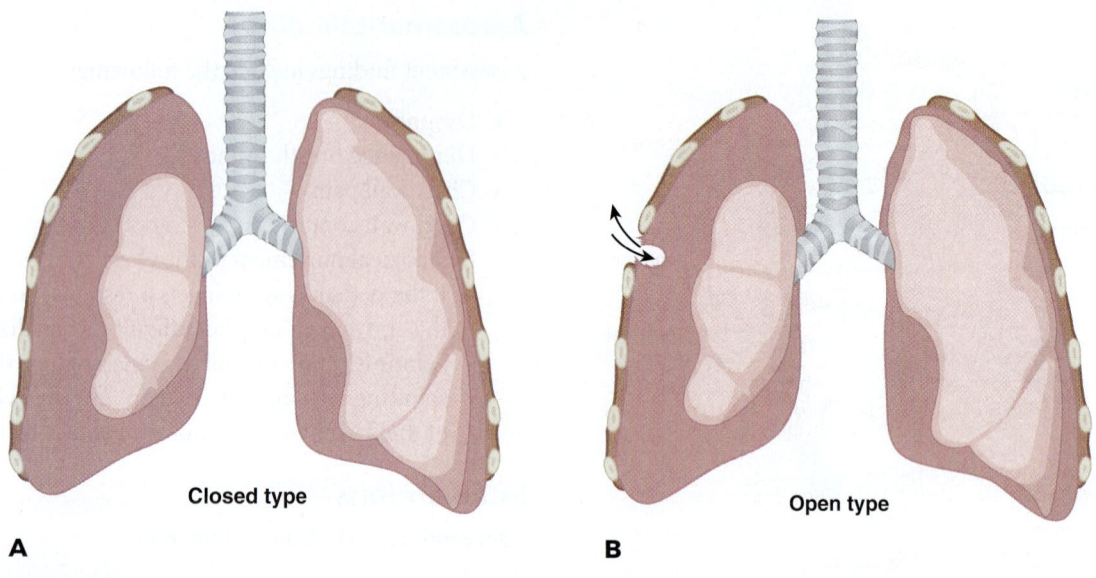

Figure 8-9 *Types of trauma-related pneumothorax.* **A.** *Closed type.* **B.** *Open type.*

Interventions

A simple pneumothorax is treated based on the size, presence of symptoms, and stability of the patient. For those patients who are asymptomatic and stable, observation, with or without oxygen therapy, is often adequate. Supplemental oxygen promotes reabsorption of pleural air. For patients with a larger pneumothorax and those who are unstable or likely to deteriorate, a chest tube is placed to evacuate the pleural air and maintain the lung expansion.[11,34] Pain assessment and appropriate administration of analgesia is also important.[11]

Open Pneumothorax

An open (complex or communicating) pneumothorax can be the result of a penetrating wound through the chest wall that causes air to become trapped in the intrapleural space[31] (see Figure 8-8B). During inspiration, air enters the pleural space through the wound and through the trachea.

Assessment Findings

In addition to the assessment findings of a simple pneumothorax, the following may be present:

- Subcutaneous emphysema (air escaping from the lung into the subcutaneous tissue)
- Chest wound that creates a sucking or sonorous sound on inspiration[31]

Interventions

Interventions include the following:

- Completely cover open chest wounds with a nonporous dressing (plastic wrap, petroleum gauze)

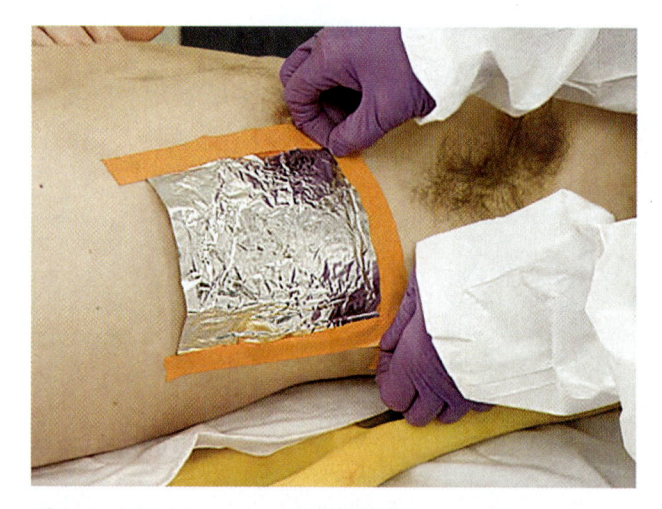

Figure 8-10 *Three-sided dressing.*
Reproduced from American College of Surgeons. (2018). *Advanced trauma life support: Student course manual* (10th ed., pp. 62–81).

and tape the dressing securely on three sides (**Figure 8-10**).[1] This measure is temporary and has variable effectiveness; it is meant to prevent air from becoming trapped in the pleural space, potentially leading to a tension pneumothorax, and is more commonly applied in the prehospital setting. Definitive repair is completed as quickly as possible in the form of a chest tube and wound closure or surgical repair.[1]

- Monitor for the potential risk of tension pneumothorax if the wound is completely sealed without adequate decompression.
- If signs and symptoms of a tension pneumothorax develop after the application of the dressing, immediately remove the dressing and reevaluate the patient.

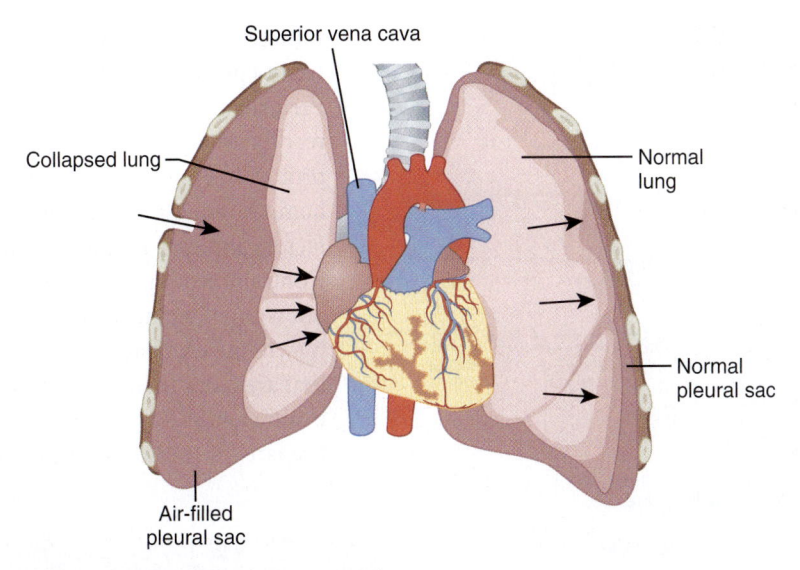

Figure 8-11 *Tension pneumothorax.*

Tension Pneumothorax

A tension pneumothorax occurs when air enters the pleural space but cannot escape on expiration. The increasing intrathoracic pressure causes the lung on the injured side to collapse (**Figure 8-11**). If the pressure is not relieved, the mediastinum can shift toward the uninjured side, compressing the heart, the great vessels, and, ultimately, the opposite lung. An alert, responsive patient may be able to compensate for a short time by increasing the respiratory rate, tidal volume, and chest expansion; a sedated and intubated patient may not be able to mount this response. As the intrathoracic pressure rises, venous return is hampered, cardiac output decreases, and hypotension occurs.[1,31]

Assessment Findings

Assessment findings include the following[1]:

- Anxiety or severe restlessness
- Chest pain
- Severe respiratory distress
- Significantly diminished or absent breath sounds on the injured side
- Tachycardia
- Hypotension
- Distended neck, head, and upper extremity veins (may not be evident if the patient has experienced significant blood loss)
- Tracheal deviation or a shift toward the uninjured side (late sign)
- Symptoms such as jugular venous distention, tracheal shift, and cyanosis may not be present unless the patient's condition has deteriorated; thus, they are considered late signs of tension pneumothorax.[31]
- Cyanosis

Interventions

Interventions include the following:

- Immediate decompression is indicated for patients who exhibit the assessment findings of a tension pneumothorax. If the patient is relatively stable, an immediate and rapid chest radiograph may confirm the diagnosis.[34,43] However, an e-FAST examination may be faster than a chest radiograph.[31]
- Do not delay interventions in the deteriorating patient to perform chest radiography.
- If chest tube placement is not readily available, immediately prepare for needle decompression.
    - A 14-gauge needle is inserted into the second intercostal space in the midclavicular line *or* the fifth intercostal space at the anterior axillary line, depending on the patient's habitus. The American College of Surgeons recommends a needle length of 5 cm for smaller adults and 8 cm for a large adult.[1]
    - The needle should be placed over the top of the third or sixth rib to avoid the neurovascular bundle that runs under each rib (**Figure 8-12**).[1,34]
- Prepare for chest tube placement, which is the definitive treatment.

A rush of air and improvement in the patient's condition is both diagnostic (confirming the condition) and therapeutic (removing the threat) and should be noted immediately.[43]

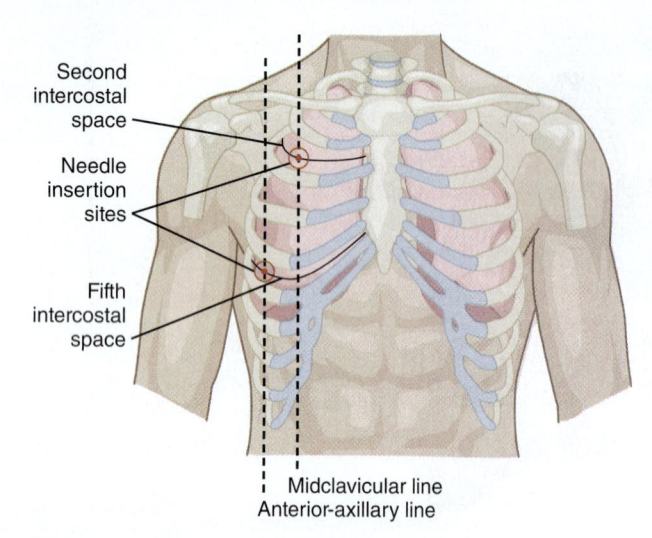

Figure 8-12 *Insertion sites for needle decompression.*

Hemothorax

A hemothorax is caused by blood accumulating in the pleural space. It results from injury to multiple structures, including the lung, costal blood vessels, great vessels, and other structures. Hemothorax may also result from laceration to the liver or spleen, combined with an injury to the diaphragm. A massive hemothorax is defined as the rapid accumulation of more than 1,500 mL of blood in the pleural space.[1,11,31]

Assessment Findings

Assessment findings include the following:

- Anxiety or restlessness
- Dyspnea or tachypnea
- Chest pain
- Signs of shock, such as tachycardia, cyanosis, diaphoresis, and hypotension
- Decreased breath sounds on the injured side

Interventions

Interventions include the following:

- Prepare for chest tube insertion.
- Ensure that two large-caliber intravenous (IV) catheters are patent and blood is available if needed to treat large-volume blood loss. If immediate open thoracotomy is performed, chest tube insertion is deferred.
- The large-bore chest tube is inserted at the fifth intercostal space at the anterior or midaxillary line (Figure 8-12). After the chest tube is inserted, it is connected to a chest drainage system.
- Initiate massive transfusion protocol according to facility protocols and policies.
- Perform autotransfusion if banked blood is not readily available according to facility policy and protocols. Autotransfused blood from a massive hemothorax may have low levels of coagulation factors and may require plasma and platelets.[1] Contraindications to autotransfusion include known malignancy; contamination caused by injury to the esophagus, bowel, or stomach; wounds that are older than 3 hours; and hepatic or renal insufficiency.[11]
- Prepare for transfer to the operating room/suite.

> **CLINICAL PEARL**
>
> **Hemothorax Management: Large-Bore Chest Tube**
>
> Blood is thick and has the capability to clot off smaller-diameter tubes. The largest-bore chest tube for the size of the patient should be considered to avoid unnecessary tube obstruction events.

Pulmonary Contusion

Pulmonary contusions most commonly occur as a result of absorption of energy across the pulmonary structures and chest wall from forces such as those experienced in MVCs and falls.[11,31] A contusion develops when capillary blood leaks into the lung parenchyma, leading to edema and inflammation. The contusion may be localized or diffuse. The degree of respiratory insufficiency is related to the size of the contusion, the severity of the injury to the alveolar–capillary membrane, and the development of subsequent atelectasis. The subtle assessment findings associated with pulmonary contusions usually develop over time rather than immediately after injury.[31] Pulmonary contusions are not always identified on a plain radiograph but may be more apparent on CT imaging; however, this rarely changes management. Potentially significant complications include pneumonia and acute respiratory distress syndrome. Severe pulmonary contusions can occur without the presence of rib fractures.[31]

Assessment Findings

Assessment findings include the following:

- Dyspnea
- Ineffective cough
- Increased work of breathing

- Hypoxia
- Chest pain
- Chest wall, bruises, contusions, or abrasions
- Hemoptysis

Interventions

Interventions include the following:

- Maintain SpO$_2$ between 94% and 98% for adequate oxygenation and to avoid hyperoxia. See Chapter 5 for additional information.
- Minimize or use IV fluids judiciously.
- Prepare for possible intubation and ventilatory support.

> **CLINICAL PEARL**
>
> **Pulmonary Contusion**
>
> Pulmonary contusions may produce only vague symptoms[7] and begin to progress at 4-6 hours following the trauma; they can take as long as 24-48 hours to fully develop. Care of a pulmonary contusion is generally supportive in nature—maximizing oxygenation and pain management. Judicious use of fluids should be considered to prevent increase in intraparenchymal hemorrhage, atelectasis, or consolidation by infusing fluids into the injured region of the lung.[31]

Blunt Cardiac Injury

Blunt cardiac injury includes myocardial contusion and, less commonly, injury to the ventricular septum, coronary arteries, or cardiac valves. This type of injury usually occurs from a direct impact or compression of the thoracic cavity. The majority of blunt cardiac injuries are caused by MVCs, with motorcycle collisions, falls, and blast injuries being other common mechanisms.[31] Maintain a high index of suspicion for blunt cardiac injury in a patient with an abnormally poor cardiovascular response to his or her injuries.[1,34]

Complications of blunt cardiac injury include the following[31]:

- Congestive heart failure
- Hemopericardium with cardiac tamponade
- Cardiac rupture
- Valvular rupture
- Intraventricular thrombi
- Coronary artery occlusion
- Ventricular aneurysms, life-threatening dysrhythmias
- Conduction abnormalities

Assessment Findings

Assessment findings include the following:

- Electrocardiogram abnormalities, including persistent sinus tachycardia, premature ventricular contractions, atrial fibrillation, ST segment changes, ischemia, or atrioventricular block[31]
- Elevated cardiac enzymes, (e.g., troponin, CK)
- Hematomas/ecchymosis (chest wall contusion)
- Chest pain

Interventions

Interventions include the following:

- Monitor the heart rate and rhythm.
- Administer IV fluid judiciously.[31]
- Treat dysrhythmias.
  - Monitor the patient continuously because the signs and symptoms may not be immediately evident.
  - Administer analgesics.
  - Perform an echocardiogram.
  - Monitor cardiac biomarkers (CK-MB [creatine kinase–muscle/brain], troponin).
  - Elevated cardiac troponin levels in a patient with suspected blunt cardiac injury can be a result of skeletal muscle injury and may not necessarily stem from cardiac ischemia.[31]

Cardiac Tamponade

Cardiac tamponade is a collection of blood in the pericardial sac. Typically, the MOI for cardiac tamponade is penetrating trauma, and it is rare in blunt trauma.[31] Blood that collects between the heart and nondistensible pericardial sac, even as little as 50 mL, compresses the heart and decreases the ability of the ventricles to fill, subsequently causing decreased stroke volume and cardiac output. The decrease in cardiac output is related to both the amount of blood in the pericardial sac and its rate of accumulation.[1]

Assessment Findings

Assessment findings include the following:

- Beck's triad[38]
  - Hypotension
  - Distended neck veins
  - Muffled heart sounds (may be difficult to assess or may be absent)

- Chest pain
- Tachycardia or pulseless electrical activity
- Dyspnea
- Cyanosis
- Inspiratory drop in systolic blood pressure by at least 10 mm Hg (1.33 kPa) (pulsus paradoxus)[16]

The classic symptoms known as Beck's triad rarely present in unison; hypovolemia may prevent distention of the neck veins, and the often-loud trauma bay may disallow identifying muffled heart tones.[25,31]

Interventions

Prepare for pericardial decompression:

- A surgical pericardectomy can be done that removes part of the pericardium to create a "window." This pericardial window will prevent blood from accumulating in the pericardial sac.
- Needle pericardiocentesis may also be used to relieve the symptoms of cardiac tamponade, but it is only a temporary solution (**Figure 8-13**). For any patient experiencing a pericardial tamponade and needing pericardiocentesis, surgical evaluation of the heart is required.[1,25,34]

Aortic Disruption

Injuries to the thoracic aorta are usually caused by blunt trauma but may also be caused by penetrating trauma. The most frequently injured site of the aorta is distal to the left subclavian artery and adjacent to the ligamentum arteriosum. Deaths from aortic injury most commonly occur at the scene; aortic disruption has a mortality rate of up to 90%.[26,31] Of those patients who survive to hospitalization, there is an in-hospital mortality rate of 46%.[26]

Assessment Findings

Assessment findings include the following:

- Fractures of the sternum, first or second rib, or scapula
- Cardiac murmurs
- Back or chest pain
- Unequal extremity pulse strength or blood pressure (significantly greater in the upper extremities)
- Hypotension
- Tachycardia
- Skin changes
  - Diaphoresis
  - Pallor
  - Cyanosis
- Paraplegia (due to disruption of spinal perfusion from aortic injury)
- Radiographic findings:
  - Widened mediastinum
  - Right-sided tracheal deviation
  - Left hemothorax

Interventions

Interventions include the following:

- Prepare for angiography or surgery.
- Consider a massive transfusion protocol (see Chapter 6, "Shock," for more information).
- Consider permissive hypotension.

Ruptured Diaphragm

A ruptured diaphragm is a potentially life-threatening injury. It can be the result of blunt or penetrating trauma, but it most commonly occurs from high-speed MVCs. The left hemidiaphragm is more likely to be affected because the right hemidiaphragm is protected by the solid mass of the liver (**Figure 8-14**).[1] When the diaphragm is ruptured, the abdominal contents can herniate into the thoracic cavity, compressing the lung and obstructing the patient's ability to take a breath. If left untreated, this condition may lead to respiratory compromise.[1]

Penetrating trauma below the fourth intercostal space indicates a potential for ruptured diaphragm and concurrent abdominal injury. Without increased awareness and a thorough assessment, this injury may go unrecognized. Penetrating trauma to the lateral chest walls and flanks is also associated with diaphragmatic injuries because of the close proximity, steep slope, and large surface area of the diaphragm.[1]

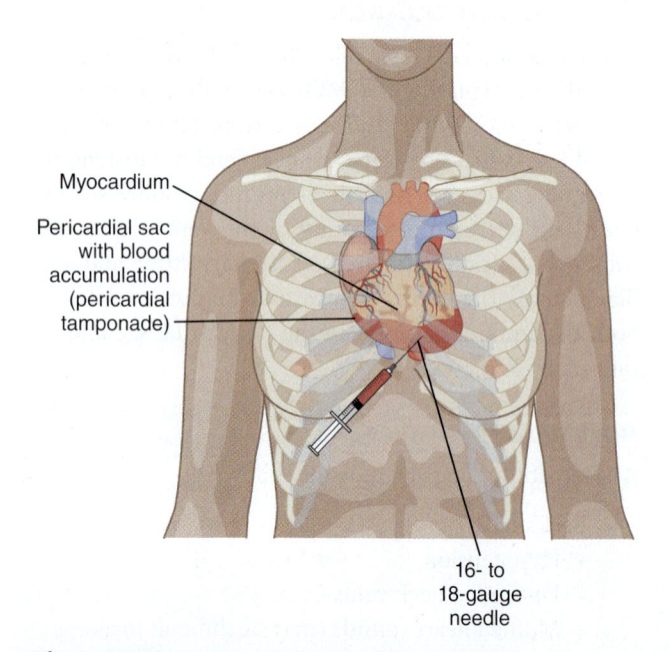

Figure 8-13 *Pericardiocentesis.*

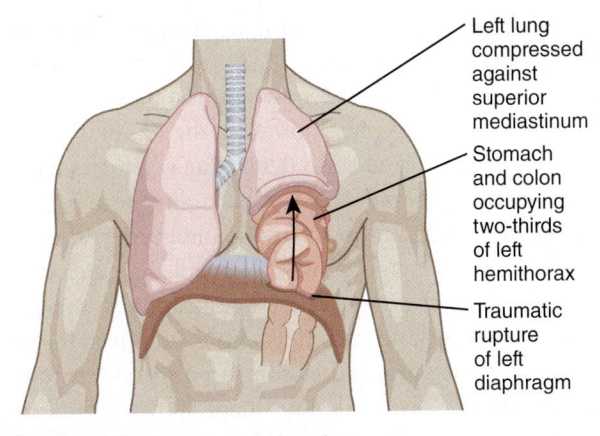

Figure 8-14 Ruptured diaphragm.

Assessment Findings

Assessment findings include the following:

- Dyspnea or orthopnea
- Dysphagia
- Abdominal pain
- Pain in the shoulder indicating intraperitoneal bleeding. Left shoulder pain is a classic sign of splenic injury (Kehr's sign) but stems from diaphragmatic irritation.
- Bowel sounds auscultated in the lung fields on the injured side
- Decreased breath sounds on the injured side

Interventions

The intervention is to prepare for surgery.

Reevaluation

Reevaluation begins with imaging studies.

Imaging Studies

Imaging studies include the following:

- A thoracic CT scan can reveal injuries to the thoracic skeletal structure, pulmonary parenchyma, and the aorta.
- Bronchoscopy, laryngoscopy, or esophagoscopy may be indicated in certain neck injuries.
- CT angiography may be used to evaluate suspected vascular injuries in the chest.
- Ultrasound may identify pericardial effusion, hemothorax, pneumothorax, and even rib fractures.

Other Studies

Other studies may include the following:

- Electrocardiogram may identify possible injury to the myocardium.
- An elevated central venous pressure may be noted in patients with tension pneumothorax or cardiac tamponade. Patients with hypovolemia may have a low central venous pressure.
- Echocardiography provides an accurate assessment of the cardiac function (wall motion, valvular function, estimated cardiac output) and can identify the presence of pericardial fluid. Transesophageal echocardiography is the most accurate form of this technology.
- Lab studies may also be performed:
  - Arterial blood gases
  - Troponin
  - Amylase
  - Lipase

Chest Drainage Systems

Consider the following points when managing a chest drainage system:

- Be familiar with the facility's equipment and policies and procedures because of variations across products.
- Cover the insertion site securely with tape. Tape all tubing connections between the patient and the chest drainage system to prevent inadvertent disconnection.
- Obtain a chest radiograph to verify improvement in the hemothorax or pneumothorax.
- Maintain the chest drainage system below the level of the chest to facilitate the flow of drainage and prevent reflux back into the pleural space. For systems that use a water seal, keep the collection chamber upright to prevent loss of the water seal.
- Coil the tubing gently on the bed without any dependent loops or kinks, maintaining the collection chamber below the level of the heart.
- Use the FOCA mnemonic for assessment and documentation (see **Table 8-4**).

TABLE 8-4 Assessing and Troubleshooting Chest Drainage Systems

Assessing: FOCA	Troubleshooting: DOPE
Fluctuation in the water seal chamber	**D**isplaced tube
	Obstruction
Output	**P**neumothorax
Color of the drainage	**E**quipment failure
Air leak present	

Note. Fluctuation in the water seal chamber with inspiration and expiration is normal.

- Follow the DOPE mnemonic to troubleshoot for problems (see Table 8-4).
- Notify the physician of the following and anticipate the need for surgery[1]:
  - If the initial chest drainage is greater than 1,500 mL
  - If there is a continuing blood loss of more than 200 mL per hour for 2–4 hours
- During patient transport, clamping of the chest tube is contraindicated because it may cause the development of a tension pneumothorax.

Reevaluation and Post-Resuscitation Care

Reevaluation of the patient with thoracic or neck trauma includes monitoring the following:

- Airway patency, respiratory effort, and ventilation adequacy
- Signs of developing tension pneumothorax following the application of an occlusive dressing
- Neck hematomas for signs of expansion
- Heart sounds
- Vital signs indicating a shock syndrome
- Chest tube drainage systems for the amount of drainage and any change in drainage characteristics
- Arterial blood gases for respiratory and/or metabolic acidosis

Definitive Care or Transport

Prepare for surgery, admission, or transport to a trauma center.

Emerging Trends

For years, the standard treatment for immediate relief of tension pneumothorax has been needle decompression on the affected side of the chest. In recent years, there has been some promising investigation into using a finger thoracostomy to relive a tension pneumothorax in lieu of the needle decompression,[1] especially in the prehospital setting. A finger thoracostomy is performed in the same manner as a thoracostomy to place a chest tube, but a chest tube is not immediately introduced into the pleural cavity. This is a relatively quick means to relieve a tension pneumothorax.[4,36] The American College of Surgeons notes that needle decompression can fail, and a finger thoracostomy can ensure adequate decompression of the chest and eliminate tension pneumothorax as the cause of decompensation.[1] Additional research is needed to prove the efficacy of this technique when used by qualified healthcare providers.

In the care of patients requiring chest tubes for treating hemothorax and pneumothorax, the size of the chest tube has been researched to determine whether smaller tubes will provide adequate chest drainage to resolve the underlying hemothorax or pneumothorax. The evidence is promising; it shows that small-diameter chest tubes (20–22 Fr) do not differ significantly in the efficacy of drainage, rate of complications, and need for additional invasive procedures compared with large tubes (28–30 Fr).[24,40,44] Some studies have shown promising results in using even smaller chest tubes (14 Fr).[18] Additional research has been recommended to further bolster the evidence for use of small-diameter chest tubes.

> **CLINICAL PEARL**
>
> **Notify the Physician**
>
> Notify the physician of the following and anticipate the need for surgery:
>
> - If the initial chest drainage is greater than 1,500 mL
> - If there is a continuing blood loss of more than 200 mL per hour for 2–4 hours

> **CLINICAL PEARL**
>
> **Do Not Clamp the Chest Tube!**
>
> During patient transport, clamping of the chest tube is contraindicated because it may cause the development of a tension pneumothorax.

Summary

Thoracic and neck trauma both have the potential to cause immediate life-threating alterations in airway, breathing, and circulation. Understanding the anatomy, MOI, and pathophysiology related to these injuries can prepare the trauma nurse to accurately and rapidly assess for and proactively and effectively intervene with life-threatening injuries to effect optimal patient outcomes.

References

1. American College of Surgeons. (2018). Airway and ventilatory management. In *Advanced trauma life support: Student course manual* (10th ed., 22–41).
2. American College of Surgeons. (2018). Thoracic trauma. In *Advanced trauma life support: Student course manual* (10th ed., 62–81).

3. Bulger, E. M., Perina, D. G., Qasim, Z., Beldowicz, B., Brenner, M., Guyette, F., Rowe, D., Kang, C., Gurney, J., DuBose, J., Joseph, B., Lyon, R., Kaups, K., Friedman, V. E., Eastridge, B., & Stewart, R. (2019). Clinical use of resuscitative endovascular balloon occlusion of the aorta (REBOA) in civilian trauma systems in the USA, 2019: A joint statement from the American College of Surgeons Committee on Trauma, the American College of Emergency Physicians, the National Association of Emergency Medical Services Physicians and the National Association of Emergency Medical Technicians. *Trauma Surgery & Acute Care Open*, 4(1), e000376. https://doi.org/10.1136/tsaco-2019-000376

4. Butler, F. K., Holcomb, J. B., Shackelford, S. A., Montgomery, H. R., Anderson, S., Cain, J. S., Champion, H. R., Cunningham, C. W., Dorlac, W. C., Drew, B., Edwards, K., Gandy, J. V., Glassberg, E., Gurney, J., Harcke, T., Jenkins, D. A., Johannigman, J., Kheirabadi, B. S., Kotwal, R. S., ... Zietlow, S. P. (2018). Management of suspected tension pneumothorax in tactical combat casualty care: TCCC guidelines change 17-02. *Journal of Special Operations Medicine*, 18(2), 19–35. https://doi.org/10.55460/xb1z-3bju

5. Coleman, K., Hudnall, A., Grabo, D. J., Pillai, L., Borgstrom, D. C., Wilson, A., & Bardes, J. M. (2021). Penetrating trauma to the neck: Using your vascular toolkit. *Journal of Trauma and Acute Care Surgery*, 91(2), e51–e54. https://doi.org/10.1097/ta.0000000000003159

6. Dehghan, N., Mah, J. M., Schemitsch, E. H., Nauth, A., Vicente, M., & McKee, M. D. (2018). Operative stabilization of flail chest injuries reduces mortality to that of stable chest wall injuries. *Journal of Orthopaedic Trauma*, 32(1), 15–21. https://doi.org/10.1097/bot.0000000000000992

7. Dennis, D. M., Bellister, S. A., & Guillamondegui, O. D. (2017). Thoracic trauma. *Surgical Clinics of North America*, 97, 1047–1064. https://doi.org/10.1016/j.suc.2017.06.009

8. Engberg, M., Lönn, L., Konge, L., Mikkelsen, S., Hörer, T., Lindgren, H., Søvik, E., Svendsen, M., Frendø, M., Taudorf, M., & Russell, L. (2021). Reliable and valid assessment of procedural skills in resuscitative endovascular balloon occlusion of the aorta. *Journal of Trauma and Acute Care Surgery*, 91(4), 663–671. https://doi.org/10.1097/ta.0000000000003338

9. Fallouh, H., Dattani-Patel, R., & Rathinam, D. (2017). Blunt thoracic trauma. *Surgery*, 35(5), 262–268. https://doi.org/10.1016/j.mpsur.2017.02.005

10. Foley, A., & Sweet, V. (2020). Cardiovascular emergencies. In *Sheehy's emergency nursing: Principles and practice* (7th ed., pp. 227–248). Elsevier.

11. Gaasch, S., & Andersen, K. (2020). Thoracic trauma. In K. A. McQuillan & M. B. Makic (Eds.), *Trauma nursing: From resuscitation to rehabilitation* (5th ed., pp. 503–552). Elsevier.

12. Hartjes, T. M. (Ed.). (2018). *AACN core curriculum for high acuity, progressive, and critical care nursing* (7th ed.). Elsevier.

13. Hom, D. B., Harmon, J. J., Jr., & Maisel, R. H. (2020). Penetrating and blunt trauma to the neck. In P. W. Flint, B. H. Haughey, V. J. Lund, K. T. Robbins, R. Thomas, M. M. Lesper, & H. W. Francis (Eds.), *Cummings otolaryngology: Head and neck surgery* (7th ed., pp. 1840–1851). Elsevier.

14. Ibraheem, K., Khan, M., Rhee, P., Azim, A., O'Keeffe, T., Tang, A., Kulvatunyou, N., & Joseph, B. (2018). "No zone" approach in penetrating neck trauma reduces unnecessary computed tomography angiography and negative explorations. *Journal of Surgical Research*, 221, 113–120. https://doi.org/10.1016/j.jss.2017.08.033

15. Ibraheem, K., Wong, S., Smith, A., Guidry, C., McGrew, P., McGinness, C., Duchesne, J., Taghavi, S., Harris, C., & Schroll, R. (2020). Computed tomography angiography in the "no-zone" approach era for penetrating neck trauma: A systematic review. *Journal of Trauma and Acute Care Surgery*, 89(6), 1233–1238. https://doi.org/10.1097/ta.0000000000002919

16. Imazio, M., & De Ferrari, G. (2020). Cardiac tamponade: An educational review. *European Heart Journal. Acute Cardiovascular Care*, 10(1), 102–109. https://doi.org/10.1177/2048872620939341

17. King, D. R. (2019). Initial care of the severely injured patient. *The New England Journal of Medicine*, 380(8), 763–770. https://doi.org/10.1056/NEJMra1609326

18. Kulvatunyou, N., Bauman, Z. M., Zein Edine, S., de Moya, M., Krause, C., Mukherjee, K., Gries, L., Tang, A. L., Joseph, B., & Rhee, P. (2021). The small (14 Fr) percutaneous catheter (P-CAT) versus large (28–32 Fr) open chest tube for traumatic hemothorax: A multicenter randomized clinical trial. *Journal of Trauma and Acute Care Surgery*, 91(5), 809–813. https://doi.org/10.1097/ta.0000000000003180

19. Lee, L. O., Potnuru, P., Stephens, C. T., & Pivalizza, E. G. (2021). Current approaches to resuscitative endovascular balloon occlusion of the aorta use in trauma and obstetrics. *Advances in Anesthesia*, 39, 17–33. https://doi.org/10.1016/j.aan.2021.07.002

20. Lodhia, J., Konstantinidis, K., & Papagiannopoulos, K. (2019). Surgical management of multiple rib fractures/flail chest. *Journal of Thoracic Disease*, 11(4), 1668–1675. https://doi.org/10.21037/jtd.2019.03.54

21. Lough, M. E. (2022). Cardiovascular anatomy and physiology. In L. D. Urden, K. M. Stacy, & M. K. Lough (Eds.), *Critical care nursing: Diagnosis and management* (9th ed., pp. 167–189). Elsevier.

22. Louro, J., & Varon, A. J. (2021). Airway management in trauma. *International Anesthesiology Clinics*, 59(2), 10–16. https://doi.org/10.1097/AIA.0000000000000316

23. Luehrs, P. (2017). Continuous end-tidal carbon dioxide monitoring. In D. L. Wiegand (Ed.), *AACN procedure manual for high acuity, progressive, and critical care* (7th ed., pp. 103–110). Elsevier.

24. Maezawa, T., Yanai, M., Huh, J., & Ariyoshi, K. (2020). Effectiveness and safety of small-bore tube thoracostomy (≤ 20 Fr) for chest trauma patients: A retrospective observational study. *The American Journal of Emergency Medicine*, 38(12), 2658–2660. https://doi.org/10.1016/j.ajem.2020.09.028

25. Mondor, E. E. (2022). Trauma. In L. D. Urden, K. M. Stacy, & M. K. Lough (Eds.), *Critical care nursing: Diagnosis and management* (9th ed., pp. 791–830). Elsevier.

26. Mouawad, N. J., Paulisin, J., Hofmeister, S., & Thomas, M. B. (2020). Blunt thoracic aortic injury—Concepts and

management. *Journal of Cardiothoracic Surgery, 15*(1). https://doi.org/10.1186/s13019-020-01101-6

27. Neschis, D. G., Vignon, P., & Lang, R. M. (2022). Clinical features and diagnosis of blunt thoracic aortic injury. *UpToDate*. Retrieved September 5, 2022, from https://www.uptodate.com/contents/clinical-features-and-diagnosis-of-blunt-thoracic-aortic-injury

28. Newton, K., & Claudius, I. (2023). Neck trauma. In R. M. Walls, R. S. Hockberger, M. Gausche-Hill, T. B. Erickson, & S. R. Wilcox (Eds.), *Rosen's emergency medicine: Concepts and clinical practice* (10th ed., pp. 368–375, e3). Elsevier.

29. Osborn, L. A., Brenner, M. L., Prater, S. J., & Moore, L. J. (2019). Resuscitative end-vascular balloon occlusion of the aorta: Current evidence. *Open Access Emergency Medicine, 11*, 29–38. https://doi.org/10.2147/OAEM.S166087

30. Plummer, E. (2020). Trauma in the elderly. In K. A. McQuillan & M. B. Makic (Eds.), *Trauma nursing: From resuscitation to rehabilitation* (5th ed., pp. 704–718). Elsevier.

31. Raja, A. S. (2023). Thoracic trauma. In R. M. Walls, R. S. Hockberger, M. Gausche-Hill, T. B. Erickson, & S. R. Wilcox (Eds.), *Rosen's emergency medicine: Concepts and clinical practice* (10th ed., pp. 376–397, e2). Elsevier.

32. Ribeiro Junior, M. F., Feng, C. D., Nguyen, A. M., Rodrigues, V. C., Bechara, G. K., de-Moura, R., & Brenner, M. (2018). The complications associated with resuscitative endovascular balloon occlusion of the aorta (REBOA). *World Journal of Emergency Surgery, 13*(1). https://doi.org/10.1186/s13017-018-0181-6

33. Sammy, I. A., Chatha, H., Lecky, F., Bouamra, O., Fragoso-Iñiguez, M., Sattout, A., Hickey, M., & Edwards, J. E. (2017). Are first rib fractures a marker for other life-threatening injuries in patients with major trauma? A cohort study of patients on the UK Trauma Audit and Research Network database. *Emergency Medicine Journal, 34*(4), 205–211. https://doi.org/10.1136/emermed-2016-206077

34. Schellenberg, M., & Inaba, K. (2018). Critical decisions in the management of thoracic trauma. *Emergency Medicine Clinics of North America, 36*(1), 135–147. https://doi.org/10.1016/j.emc.2017.08.008

35. Sharp, A. C., & Simon, L. V. (2023). Multiple trauma. In R. M. Walls, R. S. Hockberger, M. Gausche-Hill, T. B. Erickson, & S. R. Wilcox (Eds.), *Rosen's emergency medicine: Concepts and clinical practice* (10th ed., pp. 280–293, e2). Elsevier.

36. Sharrock, M., Shannon, B., Garcia Gonzalez, C., Clair, T., Mitra, B., Noonan, M., Fitzgerald, P., & Olaussen, A. (2021). Prehospital paramedic pleural decompression: A systematic review. *Injury, 52*(10), 2778–2786. https://doi.org/10.1016/j.injury.2021.08.008

37. Stacy, K. M. (2022). Pulmonary anatomy and physiology. In L. D. Urden, K. M. Stacy, & M. K. Lough (Eds.), *Critical care nursing: Diagnosis and management* (9th ed., pp. 421–440). Elsevier.

38. Stolz, L., Valenzuela, J., Situ-LaCasse, E., Stolz, U., Hawbaker, N., Thompson, M., & Adhikari, S. (2017). Clinical and historical features of emergency department patients with pericardial effusions. *World Journal of Emergency Medicine, 8*(1), 29–33. https://doi.org/10.5847/wjem.j.1920-8642.2017.01.005

39. Sudarsham, M., & Cassivi, S. (2019). Management of traumatic esophageal injuries. *Journal of Thoracic Disease, 11*(Suppl. 2), S172–S176. https://doi.org/10.21037/jtd.2018.10.86

40. Tanizaki, S., Maeda, S., Sera, M., Nagai, H., Hayashi, M., Azuma, H., Kano, K., Watanabe, H., & Ishida, H. (2017). Small tube thoracostomy (20–22 Fr) in emergent management of chest trauma. *Injury, 48*(9), 1884–1887. https://doi.org/10.1016/j.injury.2017.06.021

41. Thurman, P. (2020). Abdominal injuries. In K. A. McQuillan & M. B. Makic (Eds.), *Trauma nursing: From resuscitation through rehabilitation* (5th ed., pp. 553–574). Elsevier.

42. Udekwu, P., Roy, S., McIntyre, S., & Farrell, M. (2018). Flail chest: Influence on length of stay and mortality in blunt chest injury. *The American Surgeon, 84*(9), 1406–1409. https://doi.org/10.1177/000313481808400940

43. Waters, J. (2017). Chest tube placement (assist). In D. L. Wiegand (Ed.), *AACN procedure manual for high acuity, progressive, and critical care* (7th ed., pp. 178–183). Elsevier.

44. Yoshioka, Y., & Ishikura, H. (2020). Chest trauma management with small-bore chest tube. *Journal of Emergencies, Trauma, and Shock, 13*(4), 318–319. https://doi.org/10.4103/jets.jets_57_20

CHAPTER 9

Abdominal and Pelvic Trauma

Steven Talbot, MSN, RN, CEN, TCRN

OBJECTIVES

Upon completion of this chapter, the learner will be able to:
1. Describe mechanisms of injury associated with abdominal and pelvic trauma.
2. Describe pathophysiologic changes as a basis for the assessment of the trauma patient with abdominal and pelvic injuries.
3. Demonstrate the nursing assessment of the trauma patient with abdominal and pelvic injuries.
4. Plan appropriate interventions for the trauma patient with abdominal and pelvic injuries.
5. Evaluate the effectiveness of nursing interventions for the trauma patient with abdominal and pelvic injuries.

Knowledge of normal anatomy and physiology of the abdominal and pelvic cavity is required to understand the pathophysiologic changes that may occur as a result of trauma; these changes are critical elements in the assessment and care of the trauma patient.[2] Anatomy is not emphasized in the classroom but is the basis of physical assessment and skill evaluation and the foundation of questions for testing purposes.

Anatomy and Physiology of the Abdominal and Pelvic Cavity

The material in this section begins with a discussion of the abdominal and pelvic cavity itself and then turns to the organs, structures, and vasculature within it (**Figure 9-1**).[1]

Abdominal and Pelvic Cavity

The abdominal and pelvic cavity extends from the diaphragm to the groin and is enclosed by the abdominal wall and the bones and muscles of the pelvis; the abdominal cavity contains the stomach, spleen, liver, gallbladder, small bowel, and some of the large bowel.[69] It is lined with a serous membrane, the peritoneum, which forms a protective cover for many of the abdominal structures. The peritoneum is a single layer in part of the abdomen, in double layers over the stomach, and fan shaped over the small bowel to anchor it to the abdominal wall, where the peritoneum is called the mesentery.[71]

The esophagus begins at the hypopharynx and enters the stomach in the upper abdominal cavity, just below the diaphragm. The stomach lies transversely in the upper abdominal cavity and distally connects to the small

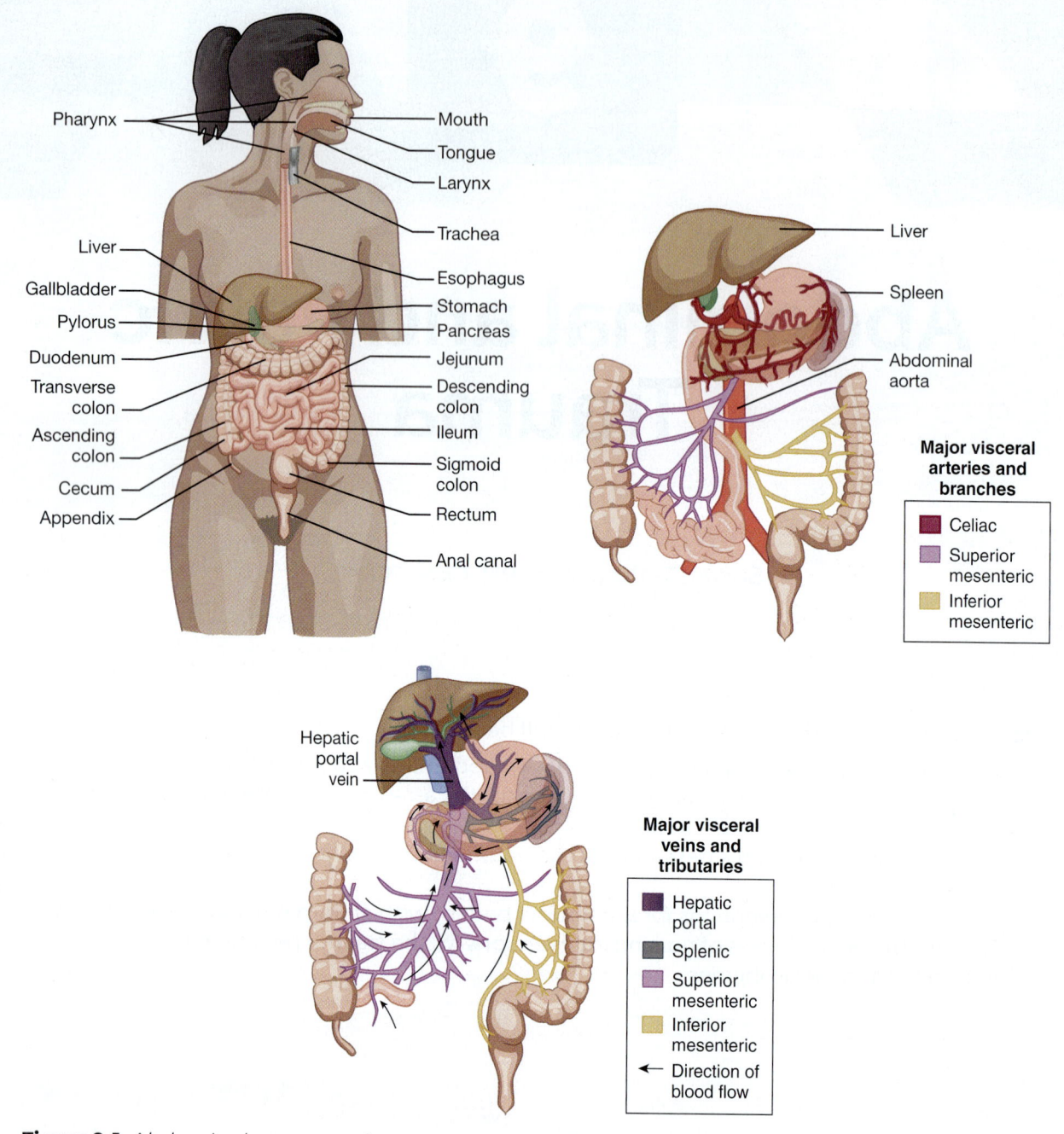

Figure 9-1 *Abdominal organs and structures.*

bowel. The small bowel is divided into three sections: the duodenum, jejunum, and ileum. It attaches to the pylorus and coils in the abdominal cavity, connecting to the large bowel at the ileocecal valve, which prevents the backward flow of fecal material. The large bowel starts at the ileocecal sphincter and extends to the anus; it includes the cecum, colon, rectum, and anal canal.[71]

The right upper quadrant of the abdominal cavity contains the liver, the gallbladder, the right kidney, and the hepatic flexure of the colon. The pancreas lies behind and beneath the stomach, and the spleen is in the left upper quadrant, above the left kidney and below the diaphragm.[69]

The pelvic cavity is the area surrounded by the pelvic bones, encompassing the lower part of the retroperitoneal and intraperitoneal spaces.[2] The pelvis contains portions of the large bowel and rectum, the urinary bladder, the internal female reproductive organs, and iliac vessels.[2,69]

The flank and back encompass the retroperitoneal space posterior to the peritoneal lining of the abdomen.

This area contains the abdominal aorta, inferior vena cava, most of the duodenum, pancreas, kidneys, and ureters.[2]

Abdominal Solid Organs

The abdominal solid organs include the liver, spleen, kidneys, and pancreas. The kidneys and pancreas are discussed later in the section "Retroperitoneal Organs."

Liver

The liver is the heaviest organ of the body, weighing about 3 pounds in an adult.[71] It is divided into two main lobes, right and left, by the falciform ligament, which also serves to attach the liver to the abdominal wall and surface of the diaphragm.[28,71] The margin of the larger right lobe lies at the 6th–10th ribs.[67]

The liver is highly vascular and has a rich blood supply from both the hepatic artery and the portal vein. The hepatic artery provides oxygenated blood at the rate of 400–500 mL/minute, which is approximately 5–7% of cardiac output.[38] The hepatic vein receives deoxygenated blood from multiple sources, including the inferior and superior mesenteric veins, the splenic vein, and the gastric vein, and it delivers 1,000–1,500 mL/min of blood to the liver.[38,70] The liver can store a large volume of blood that can be released to maintain systemic volume in the presence of hemorrhage.

Metabolism of carbohydrates, fats, and proteins, as well as glucose conversion and release, is regulated by the liver. The liver also synthesizes fats from carbohydrates and proteins that have been broken down to amino acids. Bile is secreted to assist in the emulsification and absorption of fats. The liver also synthesizes prothrombin, fibrinogen, and clotting factors. Vitamin K absorption is dependent on the liver producing adequate amounts of bile.

Spleen

The spleen, a fist-sized organ that is the largest of the lymphoid organs, is located in the left upper quadrant of the abdominal cavity. It filters and cleans the blood and serves as a blood reservoir—it can store more than 300 mL of blood.[39] A drop in blood pressure causes the sympathetic nervous system to stimulate constriction of the splenic sinuses, triggering the spleen to expel as much as 200 mL of blood into the venous circulation in an effort to restore blood volume and venous pressure; this process can elevate the hematocrit by 4%. Bloodborne antigens encounter lymphocytes in the spleen, stimulating the body's immune response.

High levels of circulating leukocytes often occur after splenectomy. In addition, iron levels decrease, immune function is diminished, and the blood contains more defective blood cells when the spleen has been removed.[39]

Abdominal Hollow Organs

The abdominal hollow organs include the gallbladder, stomach, small bowel, and large bowel.

Gallbladder

The gallbladder is a pear-shaped sac located in the right upper quadrant of the abdomen, anteriorly on the surface of the inferior liver. The gallbladder stores approximately 90 mL of bile between meals. Within 30 minutes of eating, the gallbladder starts contracting, forcing bile into the duodenum, and prevents duodenal contents from entering the pancreato-biliary system.[38] The gallbladder mucosa absorbs water and electrolytes, leaving behind a high concentration of bile salts, bile pigments, and cholesterol.

Stomach

The stomach is located inferior to the diaphragm in the epigastric, umbilical, and left hypochondriac regions of the abdomen.[71] This J-shaped organ connects the esophagus to the duodenum and has four main regions: the cardia, fundus, body, and pylorus. The superior opening of the stomach is surrounded by the cardia, while the fundus is found to the left of the cardia. The largest central portion is called the body. The pylorus connects the stomach to the duodenum. The position and size of the stomach depend on diaphragmatic movement, with the diaphragm moving it inferiorly with inhalation, and exhalation pulling it up superiorly. The blood supply to the stomach comes from a branch of the celiac artery; this organ is highly vascular.[71]

Small Bowel

The small bowel is divided into three regions.[71] The shortest region, the duodenum, starts at the pyloric sphincter and extends until it joins the jejunum; it is approximately 25 cm long.[71] The jejunum is approximately 1 m long and extends to the ileum.[71] The ileum is the largest portion, measuring about 2 m long, and joins the large bowel at the ileocecal sphincter. The wall of the small bowel is composed of four layers: mucosa, submucosa, muscularis, and serosa.[71] The superior mesenteric artery supplies blood to the small bowel and proximal colon, as much as 800 mL of blood per minute.[38]

Large Bowel

The large bowel begins at the ileum and extends to the anus.[71] The three regions of the large bowel are the cecum, colon, and rectum. The cecum is a 6 cm pouch that merges with the tube-shaped colon. The colon is divided into the ascending, transverse, descending, and sigmoid sections. The ascending and descending colon lie in the retroperitoneal portion of the abdominopelvic cavity. The ascending colon is found on the right side of the abdomen; it meets the inferior surface of the liver and then turns at the right colic (hepatic) flexure. The colon crosses the abdomen to the left side as the transverse colon and passes inferior to the iliac crest as the descending colon. The sigmoid colon begins near the left iliac crest and ends at the rectum near the third sacral vertebra. The end of the rectum forms the anal canal. The inferior mesenteric artery supplies the distal colon and rectum with approximately 480 mL of blood per minute.[38]

Pelvic Structures

The pelvic girdle consists of a ring formed by the sacrum, the coccyx, and two innominate bones.[5] Each innominate bone is formed by the fusion of the ilium, ischium, and pubic bones.[73] The bones are connected posteriorly to the sacrum at the sacroiliac joints and are joined anteriorly at the symphysis pubis. The bony pelvis functions as a stable support for the vertebral column and pelvic organs, serving as a link between the axial skeleton and the lower extremities. The pelvic girdle connects the bones of the lower limbs to the axial skeleton.

Pelvic Organs

The pelvic organs include the bladder, ureters, and urethra, and the male and female reproductive organs.[2]

Bladder, Ureters, and Urethra

The ureters are two narrow tubes that lie between the renal pelvis and the urinary bladder in the retroperitoneal cavity and connect to the base of the urinary bladder on the posterior aspect.[74] In males, the urinary bladder is found in the pelvic cavity posterior to the pubic symphysis and anterior to the rectum; in females, it is anterior to the vagina and inferior to the uterus. This distensible organ collapses when it is empty and becomes pear-shaped and rises into the abdominal cavity as urine volume increases. The average urinary bladder capacity is 700–800 mL.

The urethra is the terminal portion of the urinary system, leading from the floor of the urinary bladder as the outlet of urine from the body. The male urethra passes through the prostate, then through the deep muscles of the perineum, and to the exterior orifice through the penis.[74]

Reproductive Organs

The internal female reproductive organs include the ovaries, fallopian tubes, uterus, and vagina; the external reproductive organs consist of the vulva and the perineum.[5,72] The floor of the pelvis is formed by the perineal fascia, levator ani, and the coccygeus muscles.

The male reproductive organs include the testes, epididymis, ductus deferens, ejaculatory ducts, urethra, seminal vesicles, prostate, scrotum, and penis.[6] The testes are located in the scrotum, and the penis contains the urethra. The penis is attached to the inferior surface of the perineum at the ischial and inferior pubic rami, where this organ is surrounded by muscle. The weight is supported by the fundiform ligament on the inferior part and the suspensory ligament from the pubic symphysis; these ligaments are continuous with the fascia of the penis.

Abdomen and Pelvic Vasculature

Abdominal and pelvic trauma may result in vascular injury, causing life-threatening hemorrhage from major abdominal vessels and pelvic vasculature.[51] Blood loss within the pelvis can result from bony fractures and/or from lacerations or tearing of the vascular structures.[2,5] Unstable pelvic fractures have a great potential for blood loss and associated mortality due to increased radius and loss of the tamponade affect in the pelvis.[51] Pelvic fractures alone may result in significant blood loss that leads to shock and can potentiate shock from other injuries.[2]

Hemorrhage may occur from injury to major vessels such as the external iliac arteries or the hypogastric vascular distribution, a network of small arterial branches that supply blood to the pelvic structures. The midline retroperitoneum, the upper lateral retroperitoneum, the pelvic retroperitoneum, and the portal hepatic/retrohepatic inferior vena cava areas are the four major zones in which bleeding occurs. **Table 9-1** identifies the vessels located in these four zones.[25]

Retroperitoneal Organs

The main retroperitoneal organs are the kidneys and pancreas.

Kidneys

The kidneys are located in the retroperitoneal area between the last thoracic and third lumbar vertebrae, where they are partially protected by the 11th and 12th ribs. The right kidney is slightly lower than the left kidney because the liver occupies space superior to the right kidney. The average kidney is 10–12 cm wide and 5–7 cm long.[74] The border of each kidney faces the

TABLE 9-1 Major Vessels Resulting in Hemorrhage in Abdomen and Pelvic Trauma
Zone 1: Midline Retroperitoneum
Proximal superior mesenteric artery
Proximal renal artery
Superior mesenteric vein
Infrarenal abdominal aorta
Infrahepatic inferior vena cava
Zone 2: Upper Lateral Retroperitoneum
Renal artery
Renal vein
Zone 3: Pelvic Retroperitoneum
Iliac artery
Iliac vein
Zone 4: Portal Hepatic/Retrohepatic Inferior Vena Cava
Portal vein
Hepatic artery
Retrohepatic vena cava

Data from Feliciano, D. V., & Asensio, J. A. (2021). Abdominal vessels. In E. E. Moore, D. V. Feliciano, & K. L. Mattox (Eds.), *Trauma* (9th ed., pp. 747–769). McGraw Hill.

vertebral column near the renal hilum, where the ureter emerges with blood vessels, lymphatic vessels, and nerves.

The kidneys regulate the concentrations of sodium, potassium, calcium, chloride, and phosphate in the blood. In addition, they regulate blood pH and blood volume by adjusting the conservation or elimination of water in urine.[74] Blood pressure is adjusted through the kidneys' secretion of renin. These organs also produce hormones that stimulate the production of red blood cells. The kidneys can use amino acids to help maintain glucose levels, and they function to excrete waste from the body.

The kidneys receive 1,000–1,200 mL of blood per minute, which accounts for as much as 25% of the cardiac output.[40] Approximately 600–700 mL of plasma flows through the kidney each minute (known as the renal plasma flow) in the presence of a normal hematocrit. The plasma moves over the glomerulus capillaries and into the Bowman space, where its filtration results in secretion of wastes and reabsorption of essential electrolytes and organic molecules. The plasma filtration occurs at a rate of approximately 120–140 mL/minute, called the glomerular filtrate rate. The glomerular filtrate rate affects renal blood flow, and if mean arterial pressure decreases or vascular resistance increases, renal blood flow will decrease. Severe hypoxia and hemorrhage result in sympathetic stimulation and vasoconstriction, such that both glomerular filtrate rate and renal blood flow are reduced, resulting in decreased organ perfusion.[40,74]

Pancreas

The pancreas is approximately 12–15 cm long and 2.5 cm thick and lies posterior to the stomach.[71] It functions as both an endocrine gland and an exocrine gland. The pancreas consists of a head, a body, and a tail; two ducts connect it to the duodenum. This gland receives its arterial blood supply from branches of the celiac and superior mesenteric arteries. Venous blood leaves the head of the pancreas via the portal vein, and the body and tail are drained by the splenic vein into the portal vein.[40]

The pancreas exocrine cells excrete digestive enzymes called pancreatic juices that enter the small bowel via two ducts. The 1,200–1,500 mL of pancreatic juice produced by the pancreas each day contains water, salt, sodium bicarbonate, and enzymes.[71] The enzymes buffer acidic gastric fluids, stop the action of pepsin in the stomach, and create the proper pH of digestive enzymes in the small intestine.[40,71]

The pancreas endocrine cells, called pancreatic islets, secrete glucagon, insulin, somatostatin, and pancreatic polypetide.[38] When blood glucose is too low, glucagon is released, and insulin release is inhibited; conversely, insulin release is stimulated when the glucose level is too high.[11]

Introduction

Abdominal and pelvic trauma can lead to significant blood loss resulting in hypovolemic shock but often is not clinically apparent on patient arrival.[2] Physical exam findings and knowledge of injury patterns can alert the trauma nurse to patients who are at high risk of hemorrhage and will need aggressive treatment to achieve homeostasis and prevent shock. The absence of abdominal pain or tenderness does not exclude injury because injured intestinal structures may produce minimal hemorrhage. Unexplained hypotension may be the only clinical indicator of a pelvic fracture with hemorrhage; when hypotension develops, its cause must be identified rapidly, and prompt intervention is required. It is important to remember that the presence of distracting injuries or intoxication increases the difficulty of the assessment.

Unrecognized intra-abdominal or pelvic injury can lead to hemorrhage and early death. Movement of the trauma patient, particularly logrolling, can cause life-threatening hemorrhage; logrolling should be avoided in patients with suspected spine or pelvic fractures before imaging to rule out these injuries.[55,59] Logrolling may be indicated if there is suspicion of a penetrating injury causing hemodynamic instability or airway compromise, such as vomiting that cannot be cleared with suction.[55,59] Alternative methods to move the patient include air-assisted-mattresses and the 6-plus lift-and-slide.[24,59] If imaging is deferred or confirms the presence of an unstable spine or pelvis, consideration of risk and benefit is used with any patient movement, and extreme care must be taken. The healthcare team uses the safest technique possible with available staff and handling devices. A thorough initial assessment accompanied by ongoing or frequent reassessments, including vital signs, is essential for a patient who has sustained abdominal and/or pelvic trauma.

Epidemiology

Abdominal and pelvic trauma is associated with significant morbidity and mortality. An estimated 85% of all abdomen and pelvic injuries are caused by blunt trauma; these injuries are the seventh leading cause of death in the world, and the third most common injury sustained in trauma patients.[62] Penetrating abdominopelvic trauma occurs less frequently than blunt trauma but has a higher mortality rate; gunshot wounds (GSWs) have a mortality rate eight times higher than that for stab wounds.[10,33]

Mechanisms of Injury

The mechanism of injury (MOI) for abdominal and pelvic trauma is classified as blunt or penetrating. The injuries sustained during such trauma will be determined by the energy and type of force, and the density and strength of the structure receiving the energy. **Table 9-2** summarizes common MOIs and potential resulting injuries.[2]

TABLE 9-2 Abdominal and Pelvic Mechanism of Injury History with Implications for Injury

Type of Mechanism	History Questions	Implication for Injury
Motor vehicle collision	What was the type of crash? › Lateral impact (T-bone) › Rear end › Frontal	Provide further clues regarding suspected concurrent injuries.
	Was the patient restrained? What type of restraint? › Lap belt › Lap belt and shoulder harness › Air bag deployment	The locations of restraints can provide further clues regarding suspected injuries.
	Was it properly positioned?	Improper placement may cause compression and rupture of hollow organs and vasculature, as well as laceration of solid organs. This is difficult to determine.
	Was the patient ejected?	Ejection from a compartment may cause penetrating injury in addition to blunt injury. Rapid deceleration can cause vessels to stretch and shear, causing tears, dissection, rupture, or aneurysm formation.
	What was the speed of the vehicle?	Acceleration injuries can result in a hyperextension of the neck, producing "whiplash"-type injuries. Speed will influence the severity of injuries.

Type of Mechanism	History Questions	Implication for Injury
	What was the extent of vehicular damage? How long did extrication take?	The extent of damage and length of the extrication process give an indication of the amount of energy transferred into the passenger compartment and, ultimately, the patient's body.
	What was the patient's location within the vehicle?	Location, together with extent and type of crash, gives clues for body position and areas possibly injured.
Falls	How far did the patient fall?	Falls from heights from more than 20 feet are associated with increased injury severity (for pediatric patients, height and length of fall are important).
	On what type of surface did the patient land?	Type of surface gives an indication of the severity of energy impact.
	Which body part was the point of impact?	The body part impacted will be the focal point of assessment. If the patient landed on their feet, energy will be transferred from the feet through the body to the head.
Assault/struck by an object	Where on the body was the patient struck?	The location of the point of impact will be the focus of the assessment.
	Has the patient undergone bariatric or other abdominal/pelvic surgery?	Previous surgery to the abdomen may have weakened the musculature and the protection it provides.
Penetrating trauma	What type of weapon or object was used?	Stab wounds traverse adjacent structures.
	In the case of GSWs, what was the distance from the assailant? What was the caliber and velocity of the weapon? Was special ammunition used, such as exploding bullets, armor-piercing bullets, or buckshot?	GSWs may cause additional injuries based on their trajectory, cavitation effect, and bullet fragmentation.
	What was the estimated blood loss at the scene?	

GSW = gunshot wound.
Data from American College of Surgeons. (2018). Abdominal and pelvic trauma. In *Advanced trauma life support: Student course manual* (10th ed., pp. 83–101).

Blunt Trauma

Blunt injuries caused by a direct blow result in compression or crush injuries to the abdominal and pelvic viscera and pelvic bones.[2] Blunt trauma is most often caused by motor vehicle collisions (MVCs), assaults, and falls; less commonly, it occurs in conjunction with blast injuries.[2,10] Blunt trauma can cause injuries to both solid and hollow organs, resulting in hemorrhage or peritonitis; the spleen, liver, and bowel are the organs most commonly injured, but injuries may also occur in the retroperitoneal cavity to the duodenum, kidneys, pancreas, ureters, bladder, and internal reproductive organs in females.[2,23] The liver, spleen, and kidneys may sustain injury when the anterior abdominal wall is compressed against the thoracic cage or vertebral column, with these organs being lacerated or rupturing.[23] In addition, the following considerations apply in case of blunt trauma:

- Hollow organs are susceptible to blunt trauma injuries, and restrained occupants of motor vehicles are at higher risk for hollow viscus injuries.[2,48] The stomach, small bowel, large bowel, uterus, and bladder can rupture when a sudden increase in intra-abdominal pressure occurs.[23] Hollow viscus injuries are more difficult to identify because of their slow leakage of contents; as a result, diagnosis is often being delayed until the patient develops fever, unexplained leukocytosis, and increasing abdominal pain.[41,48]

- Deceleration or shearing injuries occur when movable organs sustain trauma between nonfixed anatomy and fixed anatomy. Organs with fixed sites susceptible to sudden deceleration include the small bowel, the large bowel, abdominal vasculature, and pelvic vasculature.[2] Fractures of the pelvis can occur secondary to MVCs, pedestrian injuries, and falls.

Penetrating Trauma

Penetrating trauma occurs as the result of GSWs, stab wounds, or impaled objects.[10] GSWs penetrate the peritoneum 80% of the time, causing vascular or visceral injuries.[33] High-energy GSWs transfer more kinetic energy, and increased damage surrounding the missile track is caused by temporary cavitation; by comparison, low-energy GSWs and stab wounds cause tissue damage by lacerating and tearing structures.[2] Penetrating trauma caused by GSWs most often results in injury to the small bowel, colon, liver, and abdominal vascular structures.[2] Nearly all GSWs with incursion into the peritoneum will require an emergency laparotomy, although occasionally, an isolated injury to the liver may be managed medically.[33]

Stab wounds most commonly result in injury to the liver, small bowel, diaphragm, and colon; stab wounds penetrate the peritoneum 66% of the time.[2,33] Abdominal stab wounds require surgical intervention in the presence of hemodynamic instability, impalement, or evisceration, or when peritonitis develops. Penetrating injuries can be more difficult to identify when hidden in the skin folds of obese patients.[2] Patients who are hemodynamically stable and without signs of peritonitis may be candidates to be managed medically.[2]

Usual Concurrent Injuries

Trauma to the abdomen or pelvis can result in injuries to more than one body system. The mechanism of injury will raise suspicion for specific injuries. The trauma nurse is alert to concurrent injuries that may include the following:

- Thoracic injuries may include hemothorax, pneumothorax, or lung contusions.[43]
- Lower rib fractures are associated with liver and spleen injuries.[67]
- Lower posterior rib fractures are associated with a higher incidence of renal injuries.[64]
- Pelvic fractures are associated with bladder, urethral, rectal, and vaginal injuries.[76]
- Lumbar spine fractures are associated with a higher incidence of retroperitoneal hemorrhage.[53]
- Fractures of ribs 11 or 12 or the transverse process of a lumbar vertebra may be associated with a renal or ureteral injury.[64]

Pathophysiology as a Basis for Assessment Findings

The two main pathophysiological bases for assessment findings are hemorrhage and pain.

Hemorrhage

Trauma to the abdominal and pelvic cavity can lead to significant hemorrhage from the organs and the bony pelvis; significant blood loss can be present without changes in the appearance of the abdominal or pelvic cavity.[2] Rapid identification of abdominal and pelvic injury can reduce the risk of death due to hemorrhage; control of hemorrhage is a priority, and interventions include early administration of blood products and judicious use of isotonic crystalloids. The patient who has profound hemodynamic instability and who has sustained trauma to the torso without other identifiable injuries is assumed to have visceral, vascular, or pelvic injury. See Chapter 6, "Shock," for details on hemorrhage management.

Pain

The trauma nurse's assessment of the abdomen and pelvis includes the subjective complaint of pain. Pain, rigidity, and involuntary guarding can be signs of abdominal and pelvic injury.[2] Palpation of the abdomen can elicit signs of peritoneal irritation; rebound tenderness is demonstrated when the sudden release of the palpation elicits movement of the peritoneum and internal organs and results in pain.[4] Involuntary muscle guarding is a sign of peritoneal irritation; voluntary guarding can result in an unreliable examination.[2] Peritoneal irritation can be caused by the following conditions:

- Hemorrhage
- Leakage of gastric contents
- Leakage of bowel contents

Referred pain can result from abdominal and pelvic trauma, as pain travels along nerve pathways and is referred to a different body part.[16] Examples include the following:

- Left shoulder pain may occur with splenic injury (Kehr's sign).
- Right shoulder pain may occur with liver injury.[67]
- Palpation in one quadrant may elicit pain in another quadrant.
- Peritonitis can cause pain to be referred to the scrotum.[16]

Nursing Care of the Patient with Abdominal and Pelvic Trauma

Nursing care of the patient with abdominal and pelvic trauma begins with the primary survey.

Primary Survey

The primary survey may reveal signs of uncontrolled abdominal and/or pelvic hemorrhage that requires immediate treatment, such as application of a pelvic binder, pelvic imaging, or focused assessment with sonography for trauma (FAST) examination.

Chapter 4, "Initial Assessment," describes the systematic approach to the nursing assessment of the trauma patient. The following information is specific to injuries that affect the abdominal and pelvic regions.

Laboratory Monitoring

Laboratory values to monitor include the following:

- Serial laboratory tests are required to evaluate the stability of the patient, and a decrease in hemoglobin (Hgb) and hematocrit (Hct) will be noted in the presence of continued bleeding. Alteration in electrolytes and coagulopathy may occur with the administration of crystalloids and blood products.[24]
- Potassium level may increase with blood transfusions because of the high concentration of potassium in banked blood.
- Calcium levels may drop as calcium citrate in banked blood binds with free calcium in the patient's body.
- Blood urea nitrogen (BUN) and creatinine will rise in patients with poor renal perfusion.[2]

Secondary Survey

The secondary survey begins with a head-to-toe assessment after all life-threatening injuries have been identified and treated.

CLINICAL PEARL

Signs and Symptoms

Be aware of these signs during the secondary survey:

- *Kehr's sign*: Pain in the shoulder indicating intraperitoneal bleeding. Left shoulder pain is a classic sign of splenic injury.
- *Cullen's sign*: Periumbilical ecchymosis indicating intraperitoneal bleeding.
- *Grey Turner's sign*: Bruising to the flank indicating retroperitoneal bleeding.

H: Head-to-Toe Assessment

Inspect for the following:

- Note any asymmetry, abdominal contour, and abdominal distention.
- Abrasions and contusions from restraint devices can provide clinical indication of injuries. Visible seat belt ecchymosis across the lower abdomen is associated with abdominal wall disruption, hollow viscus injury, and lumbar vertebral fracture (Chance fracture).[67]
- Periumbilical ecchymosis (Cullen's sign) and flank ecchymosis (Grey Turner's sign) may occur several hours after injury; frequent reassessments are crucial.[67]

Perineal bleeding, rectal bleeding, or the presence of blood at the urinary meatus may indicate urethral injury in males and unstable fractures in females.[2] Auscultate for the presence, hypoactivity, or absence of bowel sounds:

- Bowel sounds may be absent when ileus occurs secondary to trauma.
- Bowel sounds may be decreased or absent when blood or fluid is present in the peritoneum.

Percuss for dullness over solid organs and over hollow organs. Abnormal findings include the following:

- Dullness in the hollow organs, which may indicate fluid or a solid mass
- Hyperresonance, which indicates air over solid organs

Palpate:

- For femoral pulses
- All four quadrants of the abdominal area for tenderness, rebound tenderness, rigidity, and voluntary and involuntary guarding

- For pelvic stability (defer for obvious or reported pelvic fractures)
  - Gently apply pressure to both iliac crests downward and medially, assessing for instability.
  - Apply pressure only once to decrease the risk of disrupting early clot formation, which could cause further hemorrhage.[2,65]
- The iliac crest, lightly applying pressure on it, which can cause inferior displacement of the leg that indicates vertical instability[2]
- Flanks for tenderness (without turning the patient if pelvic fracture is suspected)

General Interventions for All Patients with Abdominal and Pelvic Trauma

Hemodynamic monitoring for patients with suspected abdominal and pelvic trauma begins in the secondary assessment.

- Initiate goal-directed therapy for shock, including administration of warmed blood products and/or crystalloids. (See Chapter 6 for more information.)
- Insertion of a urinary catheter is contraindicated if there is blood at the urethral meatus. Stop catheter insertion if any difficulty is encountered when advancing the catheter, which could indicate a urethral injury.[2]
- The abdominal exam that identifies rebound tenderness with palpation does not proceed with additional assessment if the patient has signs of peritoneal irritation, as it may induce avoidable pain.[2]

Selected Abdominal Injuries

Selected abdominal injuries are described in the following sections. **Table 9-3** summarizes the assessment, diagnosis, and management of abdominal injuries.

Liver Injuries

The liver is the organ most commonly injured as the result of trauma. The posterior superior section of the right lobe is the largest section and most often the site of injury because of its proximity to the ribs and the spine. Suspect liver injury with right-side rib fractures. The liver can have a laceration or hematoma, and even low-grade hepatic trauma can cause hemodynamic instability. The hematoma or laceration is defined by a grading system, with grade I as minor and grade VI as most severe (**Table 9-4**).[13,66]

Assessment Findings

Assessment findings include the following:

- Tenderness, guarding, or rigidity in the upper right quadrant[66]
- Elevated liver function tests without history of liver disease
- Ecchymosis in the right upper quadrant or around the umbilicus (Cullen's sign)[56]

TABLE 9-3 Selected Abdominal Injuries: Assessment, Diagnostics, and Definitive Care

	Liver	Spleen	Pancreas	Small Bowel	Large Bowel and Rectum	Stomach and Esophagus
Assessment						
Inspection	Nipple line to mid-abdomen, right side Lacerations Abrasions Contusions Open wounds	LUQ Lacerations Abrasions Contusions Open wounds	Epigastric area radiating to the back, extending to the LUQ Pain initially minimal, becoming increasingly worse	Left side of the abdomen Lacerations Abrasions Contusions Open wounds	Pelvic and abdominal areas Lacerations Abrasions Contusions Open wounds	Neck, chest, and epigastric area Lacerations Abrasions Contusions Open wounds
Auscultation	Hypoactive or absent	Hypoactive or absent	Hypoactive or absent	Hypoactive or absent	Hypoactive or absent	Hypoactive or absent

Selected Abdominal Injuries

	Liver	Spleen	Pancreas	Small Bowel	Large Bowel and Rectum	Stomach and Esophagus
Palpation	RUQ tenderness Muscle rigidity Spasm Involuntary guarding	LUQ tenderness Left shoulder pain Muscle rigidity Spasm Involuntary guarding	Abdominal or LUQ tenderness with deep palpation	Peritoneal irritation, including rebound tenderness and guarding	Abdominal tenderness or rebound tenderness	Esophageal: neck, chest, shoulders, or abdomen Gastric: Pain in epigastric area
Percussion	Dullness	Dullness	Dullness	Dullness	Dullness	Dullness
Reevaluation Adjuncts (Diagnostics)						
Radiographs and Other Diagnostic Tests	Abdominal radiographs CT	Repeat CT imaging to assess for ongoing bleeding	CT: 80% sensitive; missed diagnosis may occur	CT DPL/DPA FAST (least sensitive)	CT with oral, IV, and rectal contrast DPL Sigmoidoscopy	Abdominal radiographs CT DPL FAST (least sensitive)
Laboratory Studies	LFTs Serial H&H Coagulation profile	Serial H&H	Amylase elevated, but not definitive to diagnose	—	—	—
Definitive Care	Nonoperative management Operative management Angioembolization	Nonoperative management Operative management Angioembolization	Nonoperative management Operative management	Operative management	Operative management	Operative management

LUQ = left upper quadrant; RUQ = right upper quadrant; CT = computed tomography; DPL/DPA = diagnostic peritoneal lavage/diagnostic peritoneal aspirate; FAST = focused assessment sonography in trauma; LFTs = liver function tests; H&H = hemoglobin and hematocrit.

Definitive Care

Definitive care includes the following:

- Nonoperative management (NOM) is for patients who are hemodynamically stable and have isolated liver injuries, no other intra-abdominal surgical requirements, and no peritoneal signs, and for whom CT scan and intensive care unit beds are available.[66]
- Operative management is considered in hemodynamically unstable patients or those who require other intra-abdominal surgical intervention.
- Angiography—to assess injury and to provide hemorrhage control or need for embolization—is used for high-grade liver injuries in patients who are hemodynamically stable.[68]

Spleen Injuries

The spleen is highly vascular, with minimal elasticity and flexibility, and can lacerate under sudden abdominal pressure caused by blunt trauma; the vascularity makes this organ susceptible to hemorrhage. Splenic injuries occur in patients who have trauma to the left side of the

TABLE 9-4 Liver Injury Grading

Grade	Injury Description
I	Hematomas: Subcapsular and nonexpanding; affects less than 10% of surface area Lacerations: Less than 1 cm parenchymal depth and nonbleeding
II	Hematomas: 10–50% of subcapsular surface; less than 1 cm intraparenchymal hematoma Lacerations: Capsular tear with active bleeding; 1–3 cm in length
III	Hematomas: More than 50% surface area or actively bleeding; ruptured subcapsular or parenchymal hematoma; intraparenchymal hematoma more than 10 cm or expanding Lacerations: Less than 3 cm deep into parenchyma
IV	Ruptured parenchymal hematomas with active bleeding or parenchymal disruption; affects 25–75% of a hepatic lobe
V	Parenchymal disruption involving more than 75% of hepatic lobe Vascular injury involving retrohepatic cava or juxtahepatic venous injury
VI	Hepatic avulsion with avulsion from vascular structures

Data from Bruns, R. B., & Kozar, R. A. (2021). Liver and biliary tract. In E. E. Moore, D. V. Feliciano, & K. L. Mattox (Eds.), *Trauma* (9th ed., pp. 657–678). McGraw Hill.

body. Splenic injuries are classified in severity from grade I through grade V (**Table 9-5**).[18]

Assessment Findings

Assessment findings include the following[2,23,50]:

- Abdominal distention, asymmetry, abnormal contour, or abdominal rigidity
- Abrasions, contusions, ecchymosis, lacerations, or open wounds in the left upper quadrant
- Tenderness or guarding with palpation of the left upper quadrant
- Left shoulder pain that worsens with inspiration (Kehr's sign)
- Ecchymosis of the left flank (Grey Turner's sign)
- Contrast extravasation on CT scan

TABLE 9-5 Splenic Injury Grading

Grade	Injury	Description
I	Hematoma	Subcapsular, less than 10% surface area
	Laceration	Capsular tear, less than 1 cm parenchymal depth
II	Hematoma	Subcapsular, 10–50% surface area
	Laceration	Intraparenchymal, less than 5 cm diameter
		1–3 cm parenchymal depth not involving a parenchymal vessel
III	Hematoma	Subcapsular, more than 50% surface area or expanding
	Laceration	Ruptured subcapsular or parenchymal hematoma
		Intraparenchymal hematoma of 5 cm or greater
		More than 3 cm parenchymal depth or involving trabecular vessels
IV	Laceration	Laceration of segmental or hilar vessels producing major devascularization (more than 25% of spleen)
V	Laceration	Completely shatters spleen
	Vascular	Hilar vascular injury which devascularized spleen

Reproduced from Coccolini, F., Montori, G., Catena, F., Kluger, Y., Biffl, W., Moore, E. E., Reva, V., Bing, C., Bala, M., Fugazzola, P., Bahouth, H., Marzi, I., Velmahos, G., Ivatury, R., Soreide, K., Horer, T., Ten Broek, R., Pereira, B. M., Fraga, G. P., Inaba, K., . . . Ansaloni, L. (2017). Splenic trauma: WSES classification and guidelines for adult and pediatric patients. *World Journal of Emergency Surgery, 12*, 40. https://doi.org/10.1186/s13017-017-0151-4

Definitive Care

The goal of spleen injury care is NOM to preserve the immunologic function of the spleen; angiography and embolization may be performed when the patient is hemodynamically stable and has moderate to severe lacerations.[18]

NOM is recommended in patients with the following characteristics:

- Hemodynamically stable
- Age less than 55 years[18]
- Absence of peritoneal signs

NOM includes the following care:

- Serial hemoglobin and hematocrit measurements
- Serial abdominal exams
- Serial FAST exams
- Admission by a surgeon at a trauma center

Operative management is highly likely when the patient has the following characteristics:

- Age greater than 55 years[18]
- Hemodynamic instability
- Massive transfusion requirements
- Presence of other intra-abdominal injuries requiring laparotomy
- Severe traumatic brain injury that limits the patient's ability to participate in ongoing abdominal exams[18]

Postoperative Considerations

Patients who have undergone splenectomy have permanent immunologic impairment and are at highest risk for infection in the first two years post-splenectomy. These patients will need education on the importance of meningococcal, pneumococcal, and influenza vaccines, as recommended by the Centers for Disease Control and Prevention (CDC); the first doses are given within 14 days of splenectomy. The patient is cautioned to seek medical care for minor animal bites, unexplained fever, and before traveling to regions with endemic malaria.[18]

Pancreatic Injuries

Pancreatic injuries are rare.[21] However, they are frequently accompanied by injury to other structures, including the liver, stomach, spleen, and vasculature.[67] Pancreatic injuries can occur with blunt trauma when the pancreas sustains sudden pressure against the bony spinal column; however, pancreatic trauma occurs more frequently in penetrating trauma.[2,21] Pancreatic injuries are associated with major morbidity and mortality caused by hemorrhage, pancreatic leaks, abscesses, infection, fistula, pancreatitis, and endocrine and/or exocrine insufficiency.[21]

Assessment Findings

Assessment findings include the following[21,23]:

- Serial abdominal examinations: Abdominal pain may become increasingly worse.
- Epigastric pain radiating to the back.
- The patient has increased rigidity and involuntary guarding.
- Serial amylase and lipase may help confirm pancreatic injury. Amylase and lipase may be elevated, but a normal amylase level does not rule out a pancreatic injury; up to 35% of patients with a pancreatic injury have a normal amylase level.[21]
- Symptoms may not manifest for 24–72 hours because of the retroperitoneal location of the pancreas.[67]

Definitive Care

NOM of pancreatic trauma may be appropriate for patients who are hemodynamically stable. Laparotomy or surgical drainage is indicated for patients with hemodynamic instability or other injuries associated with pancreatic trauma.[8]

Small and Large Bowel Injuries

Small bowel injuries most often occur as a result of penetrating trauma.[67] Injury from blunt trauma occurs when the bowel is crushed between the abdominal wall (external force) and the spine, leading to perforation, hematoma, or edema that increases the risk of intestinal obstruction. Small bowel injuries occur frequently in the presence of solid-organ and spinal injuries.[17]

Injuries to the large bowel can occur as the result of blunt or penetrating trauma. Blunt trauma can cause a perforation from increased pressure. Penetrating trauma can result in hemorrhage and intraperitoneal injury.[2]

Bowel injuries may be difficult to identify because they may not be associated with hemorrhage or exhibit signs or symptoms on the initial or secondary survey. Failure to identify injuries to the bowel that results in a treatment delay of as little as 60–90 minutes is associated with greater mortality.[46]

Assessment Findings

Assessment findings include the following:

- Involuntary guarding and rebound tenderness
- Increasing abdominal pain[48]
- Open abdominal wounds with or without evisceration
- CT scan that shows the presence of free fluid, air, mesenteric hematoma, or intravenous (IV) contrast extravasation in the abdominal cavity[46]
- Hemodynamic instability, persistently elevated white blood cell count, increased amylase, and rising lactic acid[48]

Definitive Care

NMO includes the following care:

- Serial abdominal examinations
- Serial FAST exams
- Repeat CT scans
- Reassessment

Operative management is required when the peritoneum is penetrated, the patient is hemodynamically unstable, or peritonitis develops.[20] Initial surgical management may result in exploratory laparotomy to control hemorrhage and visceral contamination, with delayed fascial closure performed in some instances.

Rectal Injuries

Rectal injuries are more common with penetrating trauma but can occur with blunt trauma often associated with pelvic fractures.[47] Proximal injuries to the rectum are treated as colon or intraperitoneal injuries. The presence of perineal lacerations increases the risk of rectal injuries.

Assessment Findings

Assessment findings include the following:

- External lacerations or hematomas
- Scrotal hematoma
- Foreign objects

Definitive Care

A flexible sigmoidoscope or proctoscope, along with a computed tomography (CT) scan, may be used to visualize the rectal mucosa in order to determine the presence of injury. Partial-thickness lacerations can extend to full-thickness wounds.[47] Extraperitoneal rectal injuries are managed with repair or diversion colostomy.

Stomach Injuries

Most injuries to the stomach are due to penetrating trauma; blunt injuries are rare.[67] Injuries to the aorta and thoracic spine raise suspicion for stomach injuries, even though these injuries rarely pose an immediate threat to life.[15] Stomach injuries may include hematomas, superficial tears, or full-thickness perforations; such injuries are less common but carry a high mortality rate.[52]

Assessment Findings

Assessment findings include the following:

- Epigastric tenderness or rigidity
- Involuntarily guarding
- Hematemesis or occult blood from a nasogastric (NG) tube[2]

Definitive Care

Operative management is the primary choice for patients with stomach injuries.[51]

Selected Pelvic Cavity Injuries

This section presents selected pelvic cavity injuries.

Reproductive Organs

Injuries to the pelvis and perineum from blunt or penetrating trauma can result in injuries to the reproductive organs. Straddle injuries may occur from straddle-type falls and motorcycle crashes, resulting in injury to the external genitalia.[64] Injuries involving the genitalia and reproductive organs are not usually life-threatening. However, they can have life-altering consequences and resultant loss for the patient and their significant other(s).

Male and Female Genitalia

Males sustain genitalia injury most frequently from blunt trauma. Common injuries are testicular contusion or rupture and/or penile fracture, which often involves injury to the urethra.[64] Injury to the male genitalia may warrant ultrasound to determine the presence of injuries.

Females may sustain injury to reproductive organs from pelvic fractures, straddle injuries, or sexual assaults. Such injuries can result in vaginal and perineal lacerations that can cause acute blood loss and hypovolemic shock.[64] Penetrating trauma may involve the uterus, ovaries, or fallopian tubes. The trauma nurse assesses for the possibility of sexual assault for any patient who presents with vaginal, perineal, or rectal lacerations in the absence of other trauma.

Assessment Findings

Assessment findings include the following[64]:

- Penile swelling, ecchymosis, and tenderness
- Scrotal and testicular swelling, ecchymosis, and tenderness
- Lacerations or penetrating injuries of the genitalia
- Labial swelling, ecchymosis, and tenderness
- Blood at the vaginal introitus
- Blood at the urinary meatus

Definitive Care

Operative management depends on the location, extent, and the presence of contamination of the wounds. Vaginal wounds may require operative management; penile fractures will require operative management.[64] Wound care management follows standard wound care guidelines.

Bladder and Urethral Injuries

Bladder and urethral injuries are common with pelvic fractures.[64] The bladder is generally protected by its position in the true pelvis, but rupture may cause extravasation of urine into the peritoneal cavity. Intraperitoneal bladder rupture is caused by a rapid increase in pressure that causes the structure to burst, allowing extravasation of urine into the peritoneum; this can result in a chemical peritonitis.[3] Extraperitoneal bladder rupture occurs more commonly, especially with pelvic fracture, and will result in urine extravasation remaining outside the peritoneum.[60]

The urethral position close to the pubic arc in the pelvis renders the urethra highly susceptible to injury when fractures disrupt the pelvic ring[64] (**Table 9-6**).[32] Pelvic fractures can result in urethral injuries that can cause urinary obstruction, strictures, urinary incontinence, and erectile dysfunction.[51,64] Such injuries are suspected with penile fracture or penetrating trauma to the penis that is accompanied by gross hematuria, inability to urinate, or the presence of blood at the urethral meatus.

Assessment Findings

Assessment findings include the following[2,51,64]:

- Blood at the urethral meatus
- Inability to urinate
- Suprapubic hematoma
- Palpable bladder
- Abdominal distention
- Hematuria
- Rising creatinine/BUN
- Pelvic instability

Definitive Care

Extraperitoneal bladder rupture is managed nonoperatively with a urinary catheter and follow-up cystogram. Intraperitoneal bladder rupture requires operative management because of the high risk of peritonitis and inadequate healing without surgical intervention.[64] Suprapubic catheters and delayed reconstruction are frequently required in the presence of hemodynamic instability and with severe urethral injuries, whereas partial urethral tears may be treated with gentle insertion of a urinary catheter during a urethrogram.

Pelvic Fractures

Four patterns of injury may result in pelvic fractures. Three of these patterns are depicted in **Table 9-7**[2,54]; the fourth is a combined mechanism of injury that demonstrates multiple fracture patterns. The most common patterns involve lateral compression and vertical shear fractures.[27]

Pelvic fractures may cause hemorrhage from lacerated veins, arteries, or the fractures themselves.[54,78] Anterior–posterior compression and vertical shear fractures have higher incidence of vascular injury and hemorrhage; hemorrhage may be severe and cause hemodynamic instability, requiring multiple resources for stabilization.[54]

Assessment Findings

Assessment considerations include the following[2,51,77]:

- Palpable motion, pain, or bony crepitus on palpation of the pelvis
- Swelling, tenderness, bruising to the pubis, iliac bones, hips, or sacrum
- Hypovolemic shock—may or may not be present
- Shortening or abnormal rotation of the leg on the affected side
- Blood at the urinary meatus, hematuria, or intra-abdominal injury
- Rectal bleeding

Definitive Care

Definitive care includes the following measures[2]:

- Early consideration for transfer to a trauma center is essential and is not delayed by obtaining imaging studies.

TABLE 9-6 Simplified Tile Classification of Pelvic Ring Injuries

Type	Stability	Examples
A	Stable	Iliac wing fractures
		Avulsions or fractures of the iliac spines or ischial tuberosity
		Nondisplaced pelvic ring fractures
B	Rotationally unstable, vertically stable	Open book fractures
		Lateral compression fractures
		Bucket-handle fractures
C	Rotationally unstable, vertically unstable	Vertical shear injuries

Modified from Halawi, M. J. (2015). Pelvic ring injuries: Emergency assessment and management. *Journal of Clinical Orthopaedics & Trauma*, 6(4), 252–258. https://doi.org//10.1016/j.jcot.2015.08.002

TABLE 9-7 Classification of Pelvic Fractures

Anterior–Posterior Compression Fracture	Lateral Compression Fracture	Vertical Shear Fracture
Produces external rotation of the hemipelvis	Lateral force is directed into the pelvis	Occurs secondary to falls when the sacroiliac joint is vertically displaced
Separation of the symphysis pubis that tears the posterior ligaments	Hemipelvis rotates internally, reducing the pelvic volume and injuring the pelvic vascular structure, resulting in hemorrhage	Iliac vasculature is disrupted and may result in severe hemorrhage
Disrupted pelvic ring tears the posterior venous plexus and branches of the iliac arterial system	Most common type of fracture	High incidence of vascular injury and hemorrhage
High incidence of vascular injury and hemorrhage		

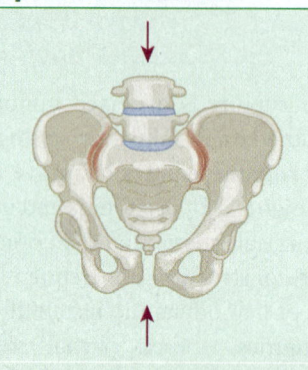

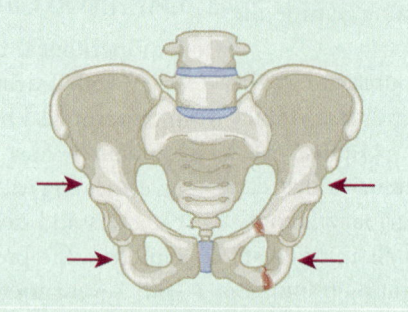

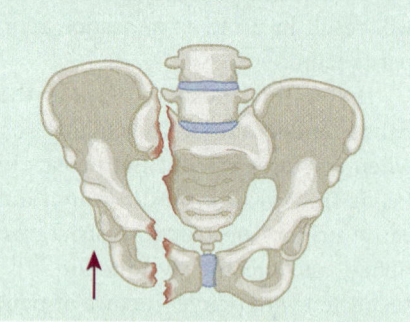

Data from American College of Surgeons. (2018). Abdominal and pelvic trauma. In *Advanced trauma life support: Student course manual* (10th ed., pp. 82–101); Nassar, A., Knowlton, L., & Spain, D. A. (2021). Pelvis. In D. V. Feliciano, K. L. Mattox, & E. E. Moore (Eds.), *Trauma* (9th ed., pp. 773–788). McGraw Hill.

- Pelvic binder application will help attain stabilization and control hemorrhage by exerting external pressure (**Figure 9-2**). A folded sheet tied around the pelvis at the level of the greater trochanters (**Figure 9-3**) can be utilized if a pelvic binder is unavailable.[51] Internal rotation of the lower extremities after the binder or sheet is applied prevents movement that can potentially worsen the hemorrhage.[2] If hemorrhage is suspected and hemodynamic instability is present, consider placing the pelvic binder during the primary survey.
- Longitudinal skeletal traction through the skin may be indicated for vertical shear injuries.[2]
- Hemodynamically stable patients may be managed with angioembolization.
- Hemodynamically unstable patients are managed with one or a combination of modalities:
  - Pre-peritoneal packing
  - Pelvic external fixation

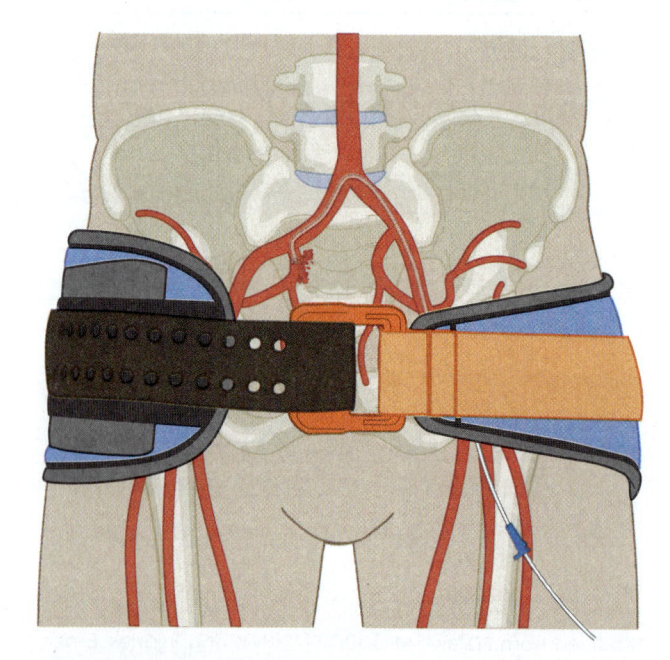

Figure 9-2 *Pelvic binder.*

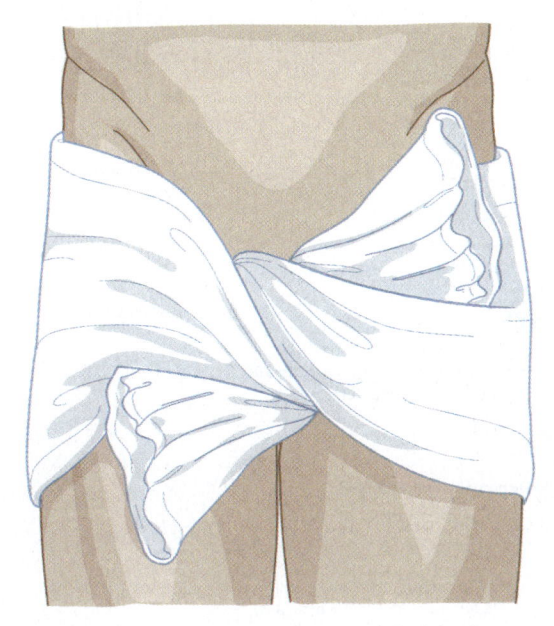

Figure 9-3 *A folded sheet as a pelvic binder.*

TABLE 9-8	Renal Injury Scale
Grade	Description of Injury
1	Contusion of subcapsular hematoma
2	Cortical laceration less than 1 cm deep
3	Cortical laceration more than 1 cm without urinary extravasation
4	Laceration into collecting system, segmental vascular injury
5	Shattered kidney, renal pedicle injury or avulsion

Reproduced from Bryk, D. J., & Zhao, L. C. (2016). Guideline of guidelines: A review of urological trauma guidelines. *BJU International, 117*(2), 226–234. https://doi.org/10.1111/bju.13040

Renal Injuries

Renal injuries are classified with a grading system in which grade 1 is the least severe and grade 5 is the most severe (**Table 9-8**).[14] The kidney is the most commonly injured genitourinary organ and is highly susceptible to deceleration injuries because of its fixed position within the renal pelvis and vascular pedicle; isolated injuries to the renal artery and vein are uncommon except in the multisystem-injured patient.[64]

Assessment Findings

Assessment findings include the following[2,44,64]:

- Hematuria—microscopic in minor injuries and gross hematuria in severe injuries
- Flank tenderness, abdominal rigidity, costovertebral-angle tenderness, or palpable flank mass
- Ecchymosis over the flank
- Rising BUN and creatinine

Definitive Care

NOM is recommended in hemodynamically stable patients unless other abdominal organs are injured.[64] Grade 5 and vascular injuries may require operative management. Renal angioembolization is also used to manage arterial hemorrhage as an alternative to operative management.[9]

Diagnostics and Interventions for Abdominal and Pelvic Trauma

Reevaluation adjuncts for abdominal and pelvic trauma includes laboratory studies and imaging studies.

Laboratory Studies

Lab studies that aid in diagnosis and management of abdominal and pelvic trauma include the following:

- Type and crossmatch
- Complete blood count
- Coagulation studies to assess clotting function and for monitoring for the development of disseminated intravascular coagulopathy
- Baseline BUN and creatinine
- Urine pregnancy test in all females of reproductive age
- Urinalysis for the evaluation of hematuria
- Gastric contents for occult blood
- Serial Hgb and Hct

Imaging Studies

Imaging studies are often done initially and repeated as care is ongoing.[31,42]

- Plain films can be done at the bedside to evaluate the patient for free air, free fluid, fractures, and foreign bodies.
- Retrograde urethrograms are done before insertion of a urinary catheter when a urethral injury is suspected.[30,64] A cystogram is performed to evaluate the bladder and urethra.

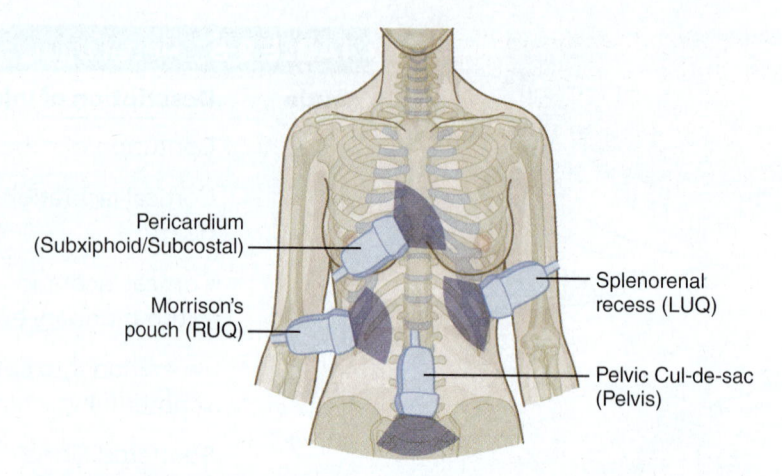

Figure 9-4 Focused assessment with sonography for trauma: The four scanning windows of the E-FAST abdominal examination.

From Ferreira, F., Barbosa, E.T., Silva, A.R. (2014). Abdominal views: Technique, anatomy, abnormal images, scanning tips, and tricks. In M. Zago (Ed.), *Essential US for Trauma: E-FAST* (pp. 19–37). Springer. https://doi.org/10.1007/978-88-470-5274-1

FAST Examination

- A FAST exam is done at the bedside to identify pathological fluid in the abdominal and pelvic cavities (**Figure 9-4**).[26] The sensitivity and accuracy of this exam depend on the location and quantity of fluid and the provider performing and interpreting the exam. At least 150–200 mL of fluid must be present to be identified. Free fluid in the right upper quadrant is identified 66% of the time, and fluid originating from injuries to the left upper lobe of the liver is identified more than 93% of the time with a FAST exam.[58] FAST exams reduce the use of more invasive diagnostic peritoneal lavage and can be repeated if clinical changes or hemodynamic changes occur.[61]
- A negative FAST study does not rule out injury and may warrant a follow-up CT scan.
- Serial FAST exams can identify increasing abdominal fluid collections from hemorrhage.
- Positive FAST exams in hemodynamically unstable patients indicate the need for emergent operative management.[61]

Computed Tomography

CT scan with IV contrast is the most widely used imaging modality for patients who sustain abdominal and pelvic trauma. Multidetector CT scan has become the standard in trauma centers and is highly reliable in identifying solid organ and intestinal injuries.[34,79] Only hemodynamically stable patients should undergo CT scanning. A relative contraindication to use of contrast is preexisting renal function abnormality.

- CT scan with contrast is used to identify abdominal and pelvic injuries.
- CT has high reliability in identifying solid-organ injuries and pelvic fractures.[79]
- CT will reveal free air in the abdomen, which is indicative of injury to hollow viscus organs.[2]
- CT will show free fluid, which is a sign of injury that can help identify the extent of organ injury.
- CT may show extravasation of contrast, which is indicative of vascular injury.
- CT can show bowel wall or mesenteric thickening, which can occur with hematoma formation or in the presence of ischemia caused by mesenteric vascular injury.[7]

Angiography

Angiography is provided by interventional radiologists, who deploy a catheter to identify the site of active bleeding of vessels. Embolization places microcoils, absorbable gelatin (i.e., gel foam), or small occlusion balloons in the vessel to interrupt blood flow and thereby stop hemorrhage.[54] Patients who may benefit from angioembolization are hemodynamically stable and have identified injuries on CT scan. The spleen is the organ most commonly treated with angioembolization, but this technique is also widely used for hemorrhage control in patients with pelvic fractures.[49,63] Angiography and embolization are being used more frequently for hemorrhage control and have allowed for increased NOM of trauma patients.[54]

Contrast-induced nephropathy may occur with angiography and CT scans with contrast, and the risk of this complication increases with advanced age, preexisting renal disease, diabetes, and hypotension. Nephropathy secondary to contrast has been reduced with changes in contrast osmolality.[49]

Angiography is not limited to the abdominal organs and can be utilized for other anatomic areas of bleeding.

Resuscitative Endovascular Balloon Occlusion of the Aorta

Resuscitative endovascular balloon occlusion of the aorta (REBOA) is used for hemorrhage control at noncompressible torso sites below the diaphragm.[12,29] REBOA is performed at trauma centers where surgeons are immediately available when life-threatening hemorrhage is unresponsive to resuscitation.[12]

During REBOA, the femoral artery is cannulated with a balloon catheter, and the balloon is inflated to occlude blood flow distally, stopping the life-threatening hemorrhage (see Chapter 5, "Airway and Ventilation").[12,35,36,37] See **Table 9-9** for indications and contraindications of REBOA.

Nonoperative Management of Penetrating Abdominal Wounds

Historically, patients with injuries penetrating the abdominal fascia have been treated with surgical exploration and repair as indicated. Today, however, there is a growing trend toward NOM of penetrating abdominal trauma in stab wounds and selective GSWs.[19,22,57] Patients who would meet the criteria for selective NOM of penetrating abdominal trauma include those who are hemodynamically stable and do not have any peritoneal signs. Observation includes 12 hours of nothing by mouth, with abdominal exams by the trauma surgeon occurring every 2 hours for the first 12 hours. If the patient remains stable, the diet is advanced, and monitoring continues for 12–24 additional hours. Following 24–48 hours of observation, the patient can be discharged.

Diagnostic Peritoneal Lavage/ Diagnostic Peritoneal Aspiration

Diagnostic peritoneal lavage (DPL)/diagnostic peritoneal aspiration (DPA) is performed by the surgical team to rapidly identify the presence of hemorrhage in patients who are hemodynamically unstable after experiencing blunt or penetrating trauma.[2] This procedure can also be utilized if FAST and CT are not available, and there is suspicion of bleeding in a hemodynamically stable patient. Contraindications to DPL/DPA include previous abdominal surgeries, morbid obesity, known coagulopathy, and advanced cirrhosis. Retroperitoneal injuries will not be identified with DPL/DPA.

Positive DPL/DPA findings will require operative interventions and include the following results[2]:

- Aspiration of gastrointestinal contents, bile, or vegetable fibers
- Aspiration of greater than 10 mL of blood or greater than 100,000 RBCs/mm³ on Gram stain
- Aspiration of greater than 500 WBCs/mm³, food fibers, or bacteria on Gram stain

Procedure

A nasogastric tube and urinary catheter are placed for gastric and urinary decompression before the procedure. The DPL is done by either open or closed technique. Sterile technique is maintained by the surgeon performing the procedure. Aspiration of blood is attempted with an 18-gauge needle. If gross blood is aspirated, operative management is indicated. The absence of gross blood is followed with the instillation of 1 L of warmed isotonic crystalloid solution into the peritoneal cavity through IV blood tubing attached to a catheter. The fluid is spread through the abdomen by gentle agitation. The fluid is drained to a container placed below the level of insertion, and specimens are sent to the lab to evaluate for the presence of RBCs, white blood cells, and bacteria.[2]

Blood tubing is used when infusing isotonic fluid into the abdominal cavity because traditional IV tubing has a one-way check valve that will prohibit the return of the fluid after the lavage of the abdomen. Blood tubing typically does not include a one-way check valve.

Fluid return from DPL is considered adequate if greater than 20% of the instilled volume is returned. Complications may include hemorrhage, peritonitis from the procedure, laceration of the urinary bladder, injury

TABLE 9-9 REBOA Indications and Contraindications

Indications	Contraindications
Hemorrhage control	Traumatic aortic injury
Ruptured aortic aneurysm	Hemorrhage proximal to zones of occlusion
Postpartum bleeding	PEA greater than 10 minutes
Hypotension from hemorrhagic shock	Terminal illness

to other structures that requires operative management, and wound infection at the lavage site.[2]

Selected Nursing Considerations for the Trauma Patient Undergoing Radiologic Evaluation

Remove clothing and metal piercings before imaging. Continuous hemodynamic monitoring with the trauma nurse present during imaging is maintained while the patient is out of the emergency department or trauma unit.

Specific nursing considerations include the following:

- CT scan
  - IV contrast is widely used, following institutional policy.
  - Ensure that the patient is monitored continuously during transport and while in the imaging area.
- FAST examination
  - Transducer gel will be required for the exam.
  - FAST exams have higher reliability when the patient has a full bladder.[2]
- Angiography
  - Ensure that the patient is monitored continuously during transport and while in the interventional radiology suite.

Reevaluation and Post-Resuscitation Care

Reassessment is required because patients who sustain abdominal and pelvic trauma can present with subtle clinical indicators of life-threatening injury. The trauma nurse will perform ongoing assessments to identify injuries sustained and provide appropriate interventions. Systematic reassessments are required to identify subtle changes in patient condition. Ongoing reassessments may include the following:

- Serial primary survey assessments
- Continuous hemodynamic monitoring
- Serial abdominal examinations
- Frequent reassessment of identified injuries for clinical changes
- Serial lab studies to trend changes

Emerging Trends

As the science and evidence of trauma care continue to evolve, new therapies are being trialed and refined. This section on emerging trends explores resources that have the potential to alter care of patients with abdominal and pelvic trauma.

Abdominal Aortic Junctional Tourniquet: Go for the Green

The Abdominal Aortic Junctional Tourniquet (AAJT) was developed by the U.S. Special Operations Forces and received Federal Drug Administration approval in 2012. The indication for the use of this junctional tourniquet is hemorrhage in the upper extremities, lower extremities, or pelvis, in areas that are otherwise noncompressible.[57,75] This device provides point pressure that can be used to compress the abdominal aorta, axillary vessels, or inguinal vessels. The wider area of compression lowers the risk of the device moving from the required position or tissue injury occurring from compression; the junctional tourniquet can be placed by prehospital providers.

Summary

Abdominal and pelvic trauma can result in high morbidity and mortality in injured patients. The liver and spleen are the most commonly injured solid organs following blunt trauma, whereas penetrating injuries most frequently affect the large and small bowel, liver, and vasculature.[45] Observation of patients with blunt abdominal trauma includes serial abdominal exams, repeat FAST exams, and repeat lab exams to identify abdominal and pelvic injury and improve outcomes.

Patients with severe pelvic fractures may sustain hemorrhage that will require rapid intervention by the trauma team, frequent assessments by the trauma nurse, and transfer to a trauma center. Hemorrhagic shock can occur from severe injuries to the abdominal and pelvic region, and these injuries can potentiate shock states from other injuries. Interventions to stabilize the patient with abdominal and pelvic injuries include the administration of blood products, application of the pelvic binder, and preparing the patient for operative management. For some patients with abdominal and pelvic trauma, care has transitioned to nonoperative management. The trauma nurse is essential in providing ongoing assessments to identify changes in patients who have sustained abdominal and pelvic trauma.

References

1. Agur, M. R., & Dalley, A. F. (2019). Abdomen. In *Moore's essential clinical anatomy* (6th ed., pp. 253–338). Wolters Kluwer.
2. American College of Surgeons. (2018). Abdominal and pelvic trauma. In *Advanced trauma life support: Student course manual* (10th ed., pp. 82–101).
3. Arumugam, P. K. (2017). Isolated intraperitoneal rupture of the urinary bladder following blunt trauma abdomen.

International Surgery Journal, 4(5), 1822–1824. https://doi.org/10.18203/2349-2902.isj20171649

4. Ball, J. W., Dains, J. E., Flynn, J. A., Solomon, B. S., & Stewart, R. W. (2023). Abdomen. In *Seidel's guide to physical examination* (10th ed., pp. 403–407). Elsevier.

5. Ball, J. W., Dains, J. E., Flynn, J. A., Solomon, B. S., & Stewart, R. W. (2023). Female genitalia. In *Seidel's guide to physical examination* (10th ed., pp. 448–498). Elsevier.

6. Ball, J. W., Dains, J. E., Flynn, J. A., Solomon, B. S., & Stewart, R. W. (2023). Male genitalia. In *Seidel's guide to physical examination* (10th ed., pp. 448–498). Elsevier.

7. Bhakta, A., Magee, D. S., Peterson, M. S., & O'Mara, M. S. (2017). Angioembolization is necessary with any volume of contrast extravasation in blunt trauma. *International Journal of Critical Illness and Injury Science, 7*(1), 18–22. https://doi.org/10.4103/IJCIIS.IJCIIS_125_16

8. Biffl, W. L., Ball, C. G., Moore, E. E., Lees, J., Todd, S. R., Wydo, S., Privette, A., Weaver, J. L., Koenig, S. M., Meagher, A., Dultz, L., Udekwu, P. O., Harrell, K., Chen, A. K., Callcut, R., Kornblith, L., Jurkovich, G. J., Castelo, M., Schaffer, K. B., & WTA Multicenter Trials Group on Pancreatic Injuries. (2021). Don't mess with the pancreas! A multicenter analysis of the management of low-grade pancreatic injuries. *The Journal of Trauma and Acute Care Surgery, 91*(5), 820–828. https://doi.org/10.1097/TA.0000000000003293

9. Bloom, B. A., & Gibbons, R. C. (2017, December 18). Trauma, focused assessment with sonography for trauma (FAST). *StatPearls.* StatPearls Publishing. https://www.ncbi.nlm.nih.gov/books/NBK470479/

10. Bordoni, P. H. C., Santos, D. M. M. D., Teixeria, J. S., & Bordoni, L. S. (2017). Deaths from abdominal trauma: Analysis of 1888 forensic autopsies. *Revista do Colégio Brasileiro de Cirurgiões, 44*(6), 582–595. https://doi.org/10.1590/0100-69912017006006

11. Brashers, V. L., & Huether, S. E. (2019). Mechanisms of hormonal regulation. In S. E. Huether, K. L. McCance, & V. L. Brashers (Eds.), *Understanding pathophysiology* (7th ed., pp. 429–447). Elsevier.

12. Brenner, M., Bulger, E. M., Perina, D. G., Henry, S., Kang, C. S., Rotondo, M. F., Chang, M. C., Weireter, L. J., Coburn, M., Winchell, R. J., & Stewart, R. M. (2018). Joint statement from the American College of Surgeons Committee on Trauma (ACS COT) and the American College of Emergency Physicians (ACEP) regarding the clinical use of resuscitative endovascular balloon occlusion of the aorta (REBOA). *Trauma Surgery & Acute Care Open, 3*(1), Article e000154. https://doi.org/10.1136/tsaco-2017-000154

13. Bruns, R. B., & Kozar, R. A. (2021). Liver and biliary tract. In D. V. Feliciano, K. L. Mattox, & E. E. Moore (Eds.), *Trauma* (9th ed., pp. 657–678). McGraw Hill.

14. Bryk, D. J., & Zhao, L. C. (2016). Guideline of guidelines: A review of urological trauma guidelines. *BJU International, 117*(2), 226–234. https://doi.org/10.1111/bju.13040

15. Burlew, C. C., & Moore, E. E. (2017). Abdominal esophagus and stomach. In G. C. Velmahos, E. Degiannis, & D. Doll (Eds.), *Penetrating trauma* (pp. 351–356). Springer.

16. Calixte, N., Brahmbhatt, J., & Parekattil, S. (2017). Genital pain: Algorithm for management. *Translational Andrology and Urology, 6*(2), 252–257. https://doi.org/10.21037/tau.2017.03.03

17. Chereau, N., Wagner, M., Tresallet, C., Lucidarme, O., Raux, M., & Menegaux, F. (2016). CT scan and diagnostic peritoneal lavage: Towards a better diagnosis in the area of nonoperative management of blunt abdominal trauma. *Injury, 47*(9), 2006–2011. https://doi.org/10.1016/j.injury.2016.04.034

18. Coccolini, F., Montori, G., Catena, F., Kluger, Y., Biffl, W., Moore, E. E., Reva, V., Bing, C., Bala, M., Fugazzola, P., Bahouth, H., Marzi, I., Velmahos, G., Ivatury, R., Soreide, K., Horer, T., Ten Broek, R., Pereira, B. M., Fraga, G. P., Inaba, K., . . . Ansaloni, L. (2017). Splenic trauma: WSES classification and guidelines for adult and pediatric patients. *World Journal of Emergency Surgery, 12*, 40–66. https://doi.org/10.1186/s13017-017-0151-4

19. Como, J. J., Bokhari, F., Chiu, W. C., Duane, T. M., Holevar, M. R., Tandoh, M. A., Ivatury, R. R., & Scalea, T. M. (2010). Practice management guidelines for selective non-operative management of penetrating abdominal trauma. *Journal of Trauma, 68*(3), 721–733. https://doi.org/10.1097/TA.0b013e3181cf7d07

20. Croce, M. A., & Fabian, T. C. (2021). Colon and rectum. In D. V. Feliciano, K. L. Mattox, & E. E. Moore (Eds.), *Trauma* (9th ed., pp. 737–746). McGraw Hill.

21. Dave, S., Toy, F. K., London, S. (2022). Pancreatic trauma. *StatPearls.* StatPearls Publishing. https://www.ncbi.nlm.nih.gov/books/NBK459365/

22. Dayananda, K., Kong, V., Bruch, J., Oosthuizen, G., Laing, G., & Clarke, D. (2017). Selective non-operative management of abdominal stab wounds is a safe and cost-effective strategy: A South Africa experience. *Annals of the Royal College of Surgeons of England, 99*, 490–496. https://doi.org/10.1308/rcsann.2017.0075

23. Diercks, D. B., & Clarke, S. (2021). Initial evaluation and management of blunt abdominal trauma in adults. *UpToDate.* Retrieved April 16, 2018, from https://www.uptodate.com/contents/initial-evaluation-and-management-of-blunt-abdominal-trauma-in-adults

24. Emergency Nurses Association. (2016). *Avoiding the log roll maneuver: Alternative methods for safe patient handling* [Topic brief]. https://enau.ena.org/Users/LearningActivity/LearningActivityDetail.aspx?LearningActivityID=LJMRSp85WwPew%2bHMK6%2b5YQ%3d%3d

25. Feliciano, D. V., & Asensio, J. A. (2021). Abdominal vessels. In D. V. Feliciano, K. L. Mattox, & E. E. Moore (Eds.), *Trauma* (9th ed., pp. 747–769). McGraw Hill.

26. Ferreira, F., Barbosa, E. T., & Silva, A. R. (2014). Abdominal views: Technique, anatomy, abnormal images, scanning tips, and tricks. In M. Zago (Ed.), *Essential US for trauma: E-FAST* (pp. 19–37). Springer. https://doi.org/10.1007/978-88-470-5274-1

27. Fitzgerald, M., Esser, M., Russ, M., Mathew, J., Varma, D., Wilkinson, A., Mannambeth, R. V., Smit, D., Bernard, S., & Mitra, B. (2017). Pelvic trauma mortality reduced by integrated

trauma care. *Emergency Medicine Australia, 29*(4), 444–449. https://doi.org/10.1111/1742-6723.12820

28. Garber, V., & Newton, B. W. (2021, July 26). Anatomy, abdomen and pelvis, falciform ligament. *StatPearls.* StatPearls Publishing. https://www.ncbi.nlm.nih.gov/books/NBK539858/#:~:text=The%20falciform%20ligament%20is%20the,inside%20the%20abdomen%20during%20surgery

29. Goin, G., Massalou, D., Bege, T., Contargyris, C., Avaro, J.-P., Pauleau, G., & Balandraud, P. (2017). Feasibility of selective non-operative management for penetrating abdominal trauma in France. *Journal of Visceral Surgery, 154,* 167–174. https://doi.org/10.1016/j.jviscsurg.2016.08.006

30. Gómez, R. G., Mundy, T., Dubey, D., El-Kassaby, A. W., Kodama, R., & Santucci, R. (2014). SIU/ICUD consultation on urethral strictures: Pelvic fracture urethral injuries. *Urology, 83*(Suppl. 3), S48–S58. https://doi.org/10.1016/j.urology.2013.09.023

31. Grünherz, L., Jensen, K. O., Neuhaus, V., Mica, L., Werner, C. M. L., Ciritsis, B., Michelitsch, C., Osterhoff, G., Simmen, H.-P., & Sprengel, K. (2018). Early computed tomography or focused assessment with sonography in abdominal trauma: What are the leading opinions? *European Journal of Trauma & Emergency Surgery, 44*(1), 3–8. https://doi.org/10.1007/s00068-017-0816-4

32. Halawi, M. J. (2015). Pelvic ring injuries: Emergency assessment and management. *Journal of Clinical Orthopaedics & Trauma, 6*(4), 252–258. https://doi.org/10.1016/j.jcot.2015.08.002

33. Hamm, A. D., Burlew, C. C., & Moore, E. E. (2018). Penetrating abdominal trauma. In A. H. Harken & E. E. Moore (Eds.), *Abernathy's surgical secrets* (7th ed., pp. 115–120). Elsevier.

34. Haroon, S. A., Rahimi, H., Merritt, A., Baghdanian, A., Baghdanian, A., & LeBedis, C. A. (2019). Computed tomography (CT) in the evaluation of bladder and ureteral trauma: Indications, technique, and diagnosis. *Abdominal Radiology, 44*(12), 3962–3977. https://doi.org/10.1007/s00261-019-02161-6

35. Hoehn, M. R., Hansraj, N. Z., Pasley, A. M., Brenner, M., Cox, S. R., Pasley, J. D., Diaz, J. J., & Scalea, T. (2019). Resuscitative endovascular balloon occlusion of the aorta for non-traumatic intra-abdominal hemorrhage. *European Journal of Trauma & Emergency Surgery, 45*(4), 713–718. https://doi.org/10.1007/s00068-018-0973-0

36. Hörer, T. M., Cajander, P., Jans, A., & Nilsson, K. F. (2016). A case of partial aortic balloon occlusion in an unstable multi-trauma patient. *Trauma, 18*(2), 150–154. https://doi.org/10.1177/1460408615624727

37. Howie, W. (2019). Resuscitative endovascular balloon occlusion of the aorta (REBOA) as an option for uncontrolled hemorrhagic shock: Current best practices and anesthetic implications. *AANA Journal, 87*(1), 19–25.

38. Huether, S. E. (2020). Structure and function of the digestive system. In S. E. Huether, K. L. McCance, & V. L. Brashers (Eds.), *Understanding pathophysiology* (7th ed., pp. 858–878). Elsevier.

39. Huether, S. E. (2020). Structure and function of the hematologic system. In S. E. Huether, K. L. McCance, & V. L. Brashers (Eds.), *Understanding pathophysiology* (7th ed., pp. 484–504). Elsevier.

40. Huether, S. E. (2020). Structure and function of the renal and urologic systems. In S. E. Huether, K. L. McCance, & V. L. Brashers (Eds.), *Understanding pathophysiology* (7th ed., pp. 712–727). Elsevier

41. Jones, E. L., Stovall, R. T., Jones, T. S., Bensard, D. D., Burlew, C. C., Johnson, J. L., Jurkovich, G. J., Barnett, C. C., Pieracci, F. M., Biffl, W. L., & Moore, E. E. (2014). Intra-abdominal injury following blunt trauma becomes clinically apparent within 9 hours. *Journal of Trauma and Acute Care Surgery, 76*(4), 1020–1023. https://doi.org/10.1097/TA.0000000000000131

42. Khurana, B., Sheehan, S. E., Sodickson, A. D., & Weaver, M. J. (2014). Pelvic ring fractures: What the orthopedic surgeon wants to know. *Radiographics, 34*(5), 1317–1333. https://doi.org/10.1148/rg.345135113

43. Lee, K., & Lee, J. G. (2016). Management of thoracic aortic injury after blunt trauma: Nine cases at a single medical center. *Journal of Trauma and Injury, 29*(4), 146–150. http://doi.org/10.20408/jti.2016.29.4.146

44. Loffroy, R., Chevallier, O., Gehin, S., Midulla, M., Berthod, P. E., Galland, C., Briche, P., Duperron, C., Majbri, N., Mousson, C., & Falvo, N. (2017). Endovascular management of arterial injuries after blunt or iatrogenic renal trauma. *Quantitative Imaging in Medicine and Surgery, 7*(4), 434–442. https://doi.org/10.21037/qims.2017.08.04

45. Lotfollahzadeh, S., & Burns, B. (2022, June 3). Penetrating abdominal trauma. *StatPearls.* StatPearls Publishing. https://www.ncbi.nlm.nih.gov/books/NBK459123/

46. McMahon, K. R., & Balasubramanya, R. (2022, June 26). Intestinal trauma. *StatPearls.* StatPearls Publishing. https://www.ncbi.nlm.nih.gov/books/NBK557624/

47. Mahan, M. E., & Toy, F. K. (2022, July 4). Rectal trauma. *StatPearls.* StatPearls Publishing. https://www.ncbi.nlm.nih.gov/books/NBK551636/

48. Matsumoto, S., Sekine, K., Funaoka, H., Funabiki, T., Shimizu, M., Hayashida, K., & Kitano, M. (2017). Early diagnosis of hollow viscus injury using intestinal fatty acid–binding protein in blunt trauma patients. *Medicine, 96*(10), Article e6187. http://doi.org/10.1097/MD.0000000000006187

49. Matsushima, K., Piccinini, A., Schellenberg, M., Cheng, V., Heindel, P., Strumwasser, A., Benjamin, E., Inaba, K., & Demetriades, D. (2018). Effect of door-to-angioembolization time on mortality in pelvic fracture: Every hour of delay counts. *Journal of Trauma and Acute Care Surgery, 84*(5), 685–692. https://doi.org/10.1097/TA.0000000000001803

50. Maung, A. A., & Kaplan, L. J. (2021). Management of splenic injury in the adult trauma patient. *UpToDate.* Retrieved October 6, 2022, from https://www.uptodate.com/contents/management-of-splenic-injury-in-the-adult-trauma-patient?search=Management%20of%20splenic%20injury%20in%20the%20adult%20trauma%20patient.&

source=search_result&selectedTitle=1~100&usage_type=default&display_rank=1

51. Mondor, E. E. (2022). Trauma. In L. D. Urden, K. M. Stacy, & M. E. Lough (Eds.), *Critical care nursing: Diagnosis and management* (9th ed., pp. 791–830). Elsevier.

52. Naiem, A. A., Taqi, K. M., Al-Kendi, B. H., & Al-Qadhi, H. (2016). Missed gastric injuries in blunt abdominal trauma: Case report with review of literature. *Sultan Qaboos University Medical Journal, 16*(4), Article e508. https://doi.org/10.18295/squmj.2016.16.04.019

53. Nakao, S., Ishikawa, K., Ono, H., Kusakabe, K., Fujimura, I., Ueno, M., Idoguchi, K., Mizushima, Y., & Matsuoka, T. (2018). Radiological classification of retroperitoneal hematoma resulting from lumbar vertebral fracture. *European Journal of Trauma and Emergency Surgery, 45*, 353–363. https://doi.org/10.1007/s00068-018-0907-x

54. Nassar, A., Knowlton, L., & Spain, D. A. (2021). Pelvis. In D. V. Feliciano, K. L. Mattox, & E. E. Moore (Eds.), *Trauma* (9th ed., pp. 773–788). McGraw Hill.

55. National Institute for Health and Care Excellence. (2017). *Fractures (complex): Assessment and management.* https://www.nice.org.uk/guidance/ng37/chapter/Recommendations#hospital-settings

56. Pannu, A. K., Saroch, A., & Sharma, N. (2017). Cullen's sign & acute pancreatitis. *QJM, 110*(5), 315. https://doi.org/10.1093/qjmed/hcx047

57. Rall, J. M., Redman, T. T., Ross, E. M., Morrison, J. J., & Maddry, J. K. (2018). Comparison of zone 3 resuscitative endovascular balloon occlusion of the aorta and the abdominal aortic and junctional tourniquet in a model of junctional hemorrhage in swine. *Journal of Surgical Research, 26*, 31–39. https://doi.org/10.1016/j.jss.2017.12.039

58. Richards, J. R., & McGahan, J. P. (2017). Focused assessment with sonography in trauma (FAST) in 2017: What radiologists can learn. *Radiology, 283*(1), 30–48. https://doi.org/10.1148/radiol.2017160107

59. Rodrigues, I. F. (2017). To log-roll or not to log-roll—That is the question! A review of the use of the log-roll for patients with pelvic fractures. *International Journal of Orthopaedic and Trauma Nursing, 27*, 36–40. https://doi.org/10.1016/j.ijotn.2017.05.001

60. Shafi, H., Darzi, A., Ahangar, S. K., & Asghari, Y. (2017). Non-operative management of intraperitoneal bladder rupture due to blunt abdominal trauma. *Trauma Monthly, 22*(5), Article e38079. https://doi:10.5812/traumamon.38079

61. Shah, S., & Pendor, A. (2018). Role of MDCT scanner in evaluation of solid organ injuries in significant blunt abdominal trauma. *International Journal of Scientific Research, 6*(9), 29–30. https://www.worldwidejournals.com/international-journal-of-scientific-research-(IJSR)/fileview.php?val=September_2017_1504181019__11.pdf

62. Sharma, R. S., Kumar, S., Damole, S., Vivekbhaskar, D., & Gandhi, A. (2017). Clinical study of hollow viscus and solid organ injury in blunt abdominal trauma and its management. *International Journal of Information Research and Review, 4*(4), 3963–3966. https://www.ijirr.com/sites/default/files/issues-pdf/1940.pdf

63. Simon, M. A., Russo, R. M., Davidson, A. J., Faulconer, E. R., DeSoucy, E., Loja, M. N., Johnson, M. A., Williams, T, DuBose, J. J., & Dawson, D. D. (2017). A case of resuscitative endovascular balloon occlusion of the aorta (REBOA) use in penetrating abdominal aortic injury. *Journal of Endovascular Resuscitation and Trauma Management, 1*(1), 53–57. doi:10.26676/jevtm.v1i1.12

64. Snyder, K. A. (2020). Genitourinary injuries and renal management. In K. A. McQuillan & M. B. Flynn Makic (Eds.), *Trauma nursing: From resuscitation through rehabilitation* (5th ed., pp. 575–598). Elsevier.

65. Storch, B. (2017, August 22). *Pelvic vertical shear fractures.* Core EM. https://coreem.net/core/pelvic-vertical-shear-fractures/

66. Taha, A. M., Abdallah, A. M., Sayed, M. M., Mohamed, S. I., & Hamad, M. (2017). Nonoperative management of isolated blunt liver trauma: A task of high skilled surgeons. *Journal of Surgery, 5*(6), 118–123. https://doi.org/10.11648/j.js.20170506.16

67. Thurman, P. (2020). Abdominal injuries. In K. A. McQuillan & M. B. Flynn Makic (Eds.), *Trauma nursing: From resuscitation through rehabilitation* (5th ed., pp. 553–574). Elsevier.

68. Tignanelli, C. J., Joseph, B., Jakubus, J. L., Iskander, G. A., Napolitano, L. M., & Hemmila, M. R. (2018). Variability in management of blunt liver trauma and contribution of level of American College of Surgeons Committee on Trauma verification status on mortality. *Journal of Trauma and Acute Care Surgery, 84*(2), 273–279. https://doi.org/10.1097/TA.0000000000001743

69. Tortora, G. J., & Derrickson, B. H. (2021). An introduction to the human body. In *Principles of anatomy and physiology* (16th ed., pp. 1–28). Wiley.

70. Tortora, G. J., & Derrickson, B. H. (2021). The cardiovascular system: Blood vessels and hemodynamics. In *Principles of anatomy and physiology* (16th ed., pp. 771–845). Wiley.

71. Tortora, G. J., & Derrickson, B. H. (2021). The digestive system. In *Principles of anatomy and physiology* (16th ed., pp. 941–999). Wiley.

72. Tortora, G. J., & Derrickson, B. H. (2021). The genital system. In *Principles of anatomy and physiology* (16th ed., pp. 1106–1159). Wiley.

73. Tortora, G. J., & Derrickson, B. H. (2021). The skeletal system: The appendicular skeleton. In *Principles of anatomy and physiology* (16th ed., pp. 242–268). Wiley.

74. Tortora, G. J., & Derrickson, B. H. (2021). The urinary system. In *Principles of anatomy and physiology* (16th ed., pp. 1042–1087). Wiley.

75. Trauma News. (2019, August 16). Combat-tested abdominal/junctional tourniquet proven equivalent to REBOA. *Trauma System News.* https://trauma-news.com/2019/08/combat-tested-abdominal-junctional-tourniquet-proven-equivalent-to-reboa/

76. Tullington, J. E., & Blecker, N. (2022, May 8). Pelvic trauma. *StatPearls.* StatPearls Publishing. https://www.ncbi.nlm.nih.gov/books/NBK556070/

77. Walsh, C. (2020). Genitourinary injuries and renal management. In K. A. McQuillan & M. B. Flynn Makic (Eds.), *Trauma nursing: From resuscitation through rehabilitation* (5th ed., pp. 599–638). Elsevier.
78. Wu, K., Posluszny, J. A., Branch, J., Dray, E., Blackwell, R., Hannick, J., & Luchette, F. A. (2015). Trauma to the pelvis: Injuries to the rectum and genitourinary organs. *Current Trauma Reports*, *1*(1), 8–15. https://doi.org/10.1007/s40719-014-0006-3
79. Yang, X. Y., Wei, M. T., Jin, C. W., Wang, M., & Wang, Z. Q. (2016). Unenhanced computed tomography to visualize hollow viscera and/or mesenteric injury after blunt abdominal trauma: A single-institution experience. *Medicine*, *95*(9), Article e2884. https://doi.org/10.1097/MD.0000000000002884

CHAPTER 10

Spinal and Musculoskeletal Trauma

Carolyn Dixon, DNP, MS, RN, FNP-BC, CEN, TCRN

OBJECTIVES

Upon completion of this chapter, the learner will be able to:
1. Describe mechanisms of injury associated with spinal and musculoskeletal trauma.
2. Describe pathophysiologic changes as a basis for assessment for spinal cord and/or musculoskeletal injuries.
3. Demonstrate the nursing assessment and appropriate interventions for the trauma patient with spinal and/or musculoskeletal injuries.

Knowledge of normal anatomy and physiology serves as a foundation for understanding the anatomic derangements and pathophysiologic processes that may result from trauma. Anatomy is not emphasized in the classroom, but it is the basis of physical assessment and skill evaluation and the foundation of questions for testing purposes.

Anatomy and Physiology of the Spinal Cord and Vertebral Column

This section serves as a review of the anatomy and physiology of the spinal cord and vertebral column.

Spinal Cord

The spinal cord provides two-way communication between the brain and the peripheral nervous system. It occupies the upper two-thirds of the vertebral canal and is wider in the cervical and lumbar areas to accommodate the nerve cells that supply the extremities. The spinal cord usually ends at the level of the first lumbar vertebra in adults, with the sacral nerve roots descending from this point to their appropriate exit points through the intervertebral foramina. Two consecutive rows of nerve roots, the dorsal and ventral roots, emerge from each side of the spinal cord. These nerve roots join distally to form 31 pairs of spinal nerves. The end of the spinal cord, the conus medullaris, is cone shaped. Spinal nerves continue outward from the conus medullaris, forming a nerve bundle known as the cauda equina.[56,61]

The spinal cord and column are divided into the cervical, thoracic, lumbar, and sacral regions. In a cross-section view, the spinal cord has a butterfly- or H-shaped core (**Figure 10-1**). It contains a central mass of gray matter that is divided into three paired horns:

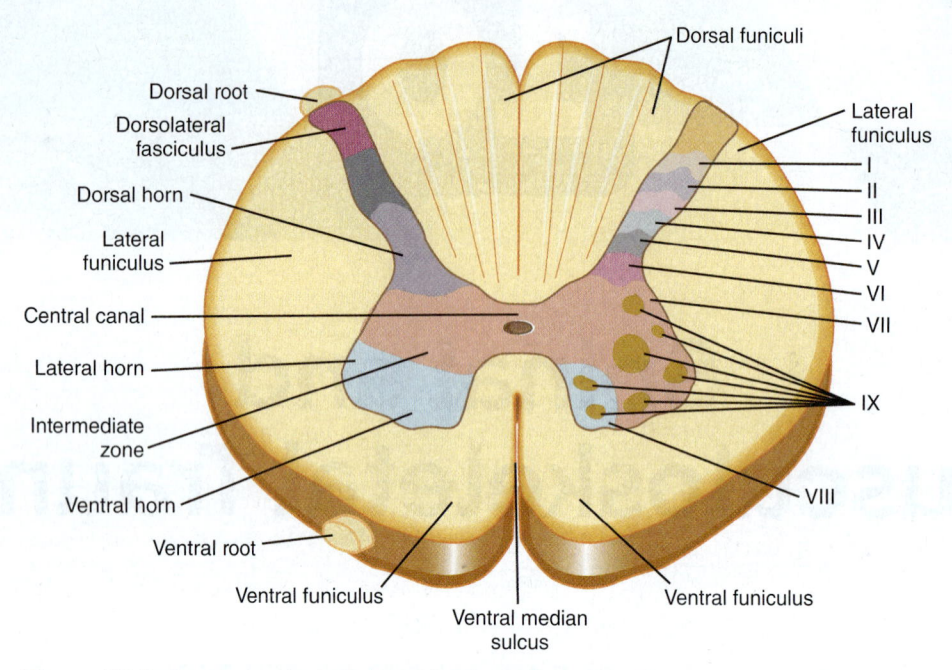

Figure 10-1 Cross-section of the spinal cord.

ventral (anterior), intermediolateral, and dorsal (posterior). The horns of the spinal cord are responsible for voluntary motor activity. The ventral horn provides the motor components of the spinal nerves. The intermediolateral horn contains the preganglionic sympathetic fibers of the thoracic, lumbar, and sacral spine. The dorsal horn contains the peripheral sensory neurons.[56,61,68] The gray matter is surrounded by the white matter, which consists of myelinated nerve fibers that form the anterior, lateral, and posterior columns. Each column contains ascending sensory tracts that transmit impulses to the brain, while the descending tracts transmit impulses down the spinal cord.[56,61,68]

Motor Function

Impulses are conducted between the brain and the spinal cord through the upper motor neurons.[25] The upper motor neurons form the corticospinal tract (**Figure 10-2**), which is responsible for fine motor skills, and the extra-corticospinal tract, which is responsible for gross motor movement (**Table 10-1**).[25,34,61,68] Upper motor neurons cross at the medulla of the brain stem to the opposite side and descend down the corticospinal tract, hence the loss of movement observed in the contralateral side after a head injury. Some fibers descend through the white matter on the same side and cross at specific spinal cord segments, resulting in ipsilateral loss of movement when they are damaged.[61] Impulses that originate in the upper motor neurons are conducted to the lower motor neurons by the spinal cord and innervate the skeletal muscle

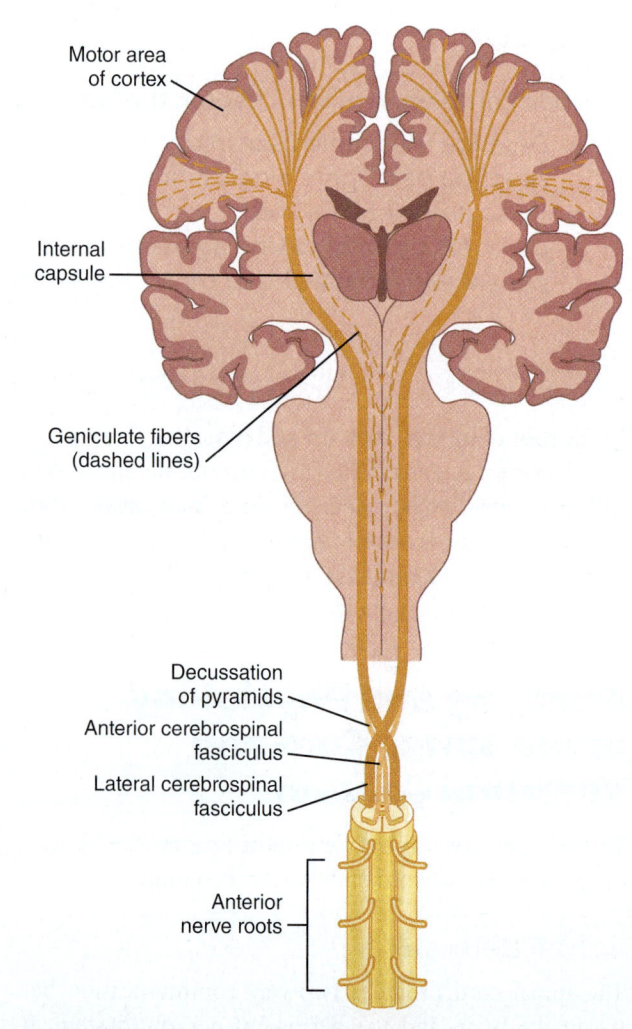

Figure 10-2 Corticospinal tracts.

TABLE 10-1	Motor and Sensory Spinal Nerve Tracts		
Nerve Tracts	**Origin**	**Function**	**Location in Spinal Cord**
Descending tracts: corticospinal (pyramidal)	Cerebral cortex	Voluntary motor	Anterolateral
Ascending tracts: spinothalamic	Sensory receptors located throughout the body	Pain Temperature Crude touch	Anterolateral
Posterior (dorsal) tracts	Sensory receptors located throughout the body	Proprioception Fine touch Two-point discrimination	Posterior (dorsal)

Data from Harrow-Mortelliti, M., Reddy, V., & Jimsheleishvili, G. (2022). Physiology, spinal cord. *StatPearls*. StatPearls Publishing. https://www.ncbi.nlm.nih.gov/books/NBK544267/; Stacy, K. M. (2022). Neurologic anatomy and physiology. In L. D. Urden, K. M. Stacy, & M. E. Lough (Eds.), *Critical care nursing: Diagnosis and management* (9th ed., pp. 534–564). Elsevier.

groups. The cervical nerve fibers from the corticospinal tract, located in the central portion of the ventral horn, innervate the upper extremities. The sacral fibers from the corticospinal tract, located in the peripheral portion of the ventral horn, innervate the lower extremities.[56,61,68]

Sensory Function

Sensory pathways include impulse routes that are combined into spinal reflex arcs (sensory) or those that are transmitted to higher centers in the brain to be interpreted (cortical).

Reflex Arc

The reflex arc is a stimulus-response mechanism that does not require ascending or descending spinal cord pathways to function. Examples of reflex arcs include deep tendon reflexes (e.g., patellar reflex) and the withdrawal reflex (e.g., withdrawal from a hot surface or catching oneself from falling). The reflex arc is the only part of the neural path with withdrawal responses. The stimulus that triggers the withdrawal response continues to travel up the spinothalamic tract to the cortex, registering pain or imbalance.[61,68]

The essential structures of the reflex arc include the following[58]:

- Receptor (sense organ, cutaneous end organ, or neuromuscular spindle)
- Afferent (sensory) neuron
- Association (interneuron) neuron
- Efferent (motor) neuron
- Effector neuron (muscle, tendon, or gland that produces response)

An anatomically and physiologically intact reflex arc will function even if there is a disruption of spinal cord function above the level of the reflex.[61,68]

Cortical Sensation

Cortical sensation includes both simple and deep sensation. Pain, touch, and temperature are known as simple sensations because their detection is carried out by discrete sensory organs, such as the skin. Information from general somatic receptors in the skin is conducted over the small-diameter fibers of the spinal nerves into the dorsal horn of the spinal cord's gray matter. Pain and temperature fibers enter the spinal cord and travel within one to two spinal segments and then cross before ascending in the spinothalamic tract.[56,61,68] Light touch sensation fibers cross immediately upon entering the spinal cord and then ascend in the spinothalamic tract.[43]

Deep sensation includes proprioception, vibration sensation, and deep muscle pain. These afferent (ascending) impulses are transmitted by fibers entering the spinal cord via the dorsal roots and ascend via a spinal tract. Proprioception and vibration fibers ascend via the posterior column and cross in the medulla. These sensations are referred to as cortical because an intact cerebral hemisphere is required to interpret the impulses.[56,61,68]

Spinal Nerves

There are 31 pairs of spinal nerves: 8 cervical pairs, 12 thoracic pairs, 5 lumbar pairs, 5 sacral pairs, and 1 coccygeal pair. Each pair of spinal nerves exits the spinal cord bilaterally and contains a dorsal and ventral root.

The dorsal root transmits sensory impulses, innervating specific dermatomes (**Figure 10-3**) in the body, and the ventral root transmits motor impulses.[61,68]

The cervical nerves innervate the head, diaphragm, neck, shoulders, and upper arms. The thoracic nerves innervate the thorax and abdomen, and portions of the buttocks and upper arm. The intercostal muscles are innervated by spinal nerves T1 through T12. The lumbar nerves innervate the groin region and lower extremities. The sacral nerves S3 to S5 supply the perianal muscles, which control voluntary contraction of the external bladder sphincter and the external anal sphincter (**Table 10-2**).[6,56,61,68]

Nerve Plexuses

A plexus is an area where the nerves converge in groups. These nerve clusters connect the peripheral and central nervous systems, enabling signals to travel from the brain and spinal cord to the rest of the body. Without these connections, the brain would not be able to communicate with the rest of the body. There are four major nerve plexuses[56,61,68]:

- The *cervical* plexus is formed by the first four cervical nerves, which innervate the muscles of the neck and shoulders. In addition, the phrenic nerve arises from C3, C4, and C5 and innervates the diaphragm.

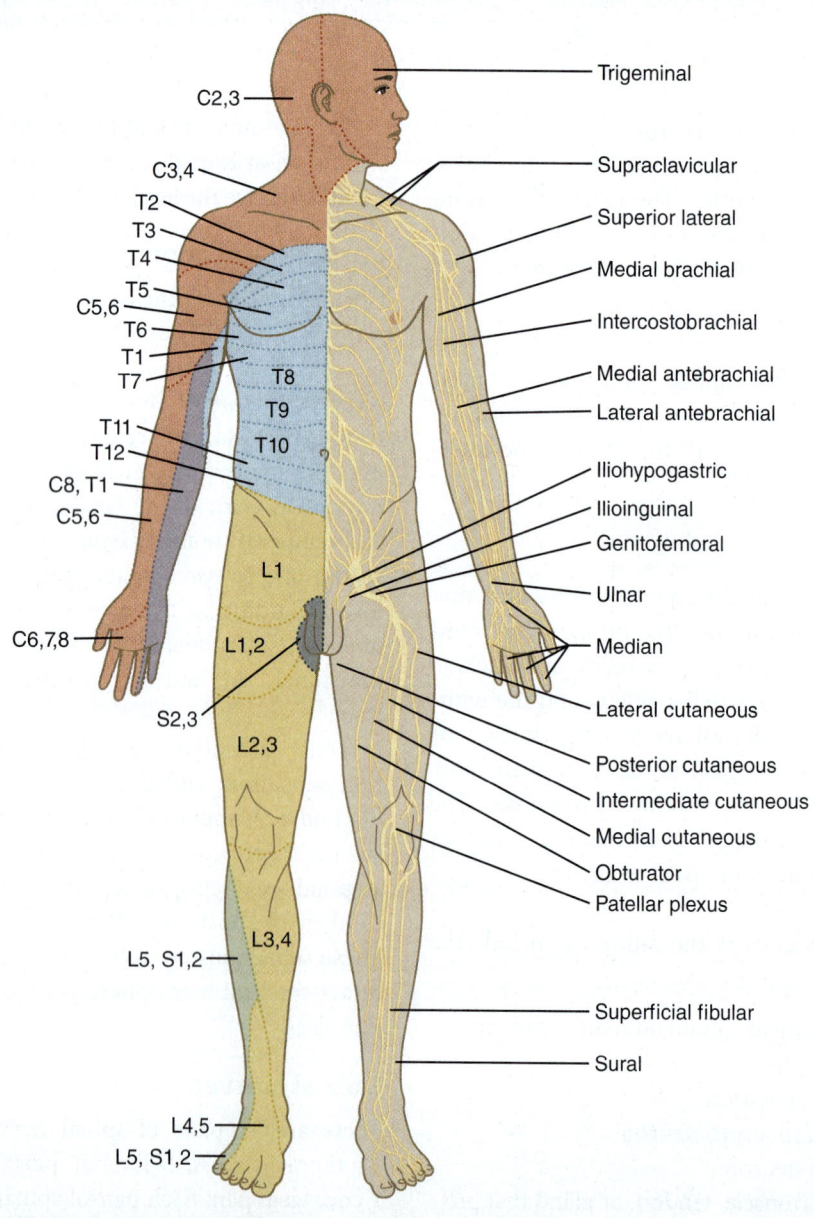

Figure 10-3 *Dermatomes.*

TABLE 10-2 Spinal Nerve Segments and Areas of Innervation

Spinal Nerve Segment	Area Innervated
C5	Area over the deltoid
C6	Thumb
C7	Middle finger
C8	Little finger
T4	Nipple
T8	Xiphisternum
T10	Umbilicus
T12	Symphysis pubis
L4	Medial aspect of the calf
L5	Web space between the first and second toes
S1	Lateral border of the foot
S3	Ischial tuberosity area
S4 and S5	Perianal region

Data from American College of Surgeons. (2018). Spine and spinal cord trauma. In *Advanced trauma life support: Student course manual* (10th ed., p. 132).

- The *brachial* plexus is formed by spinal nerves C5 to C8 and T1 and supplies motor control and sensation to the arm, wrist, and hand. The brachial plexus branches include the ulnar and radial nerves.
- The *lumbar* plexus is formed by spinal nerves L1 to L4, which give rise to the femoral nerve and innervate the anterior portion of the lower body.
- The *sacral* plexus is formed by spinal nerves L5 to S4, which are the origin of the sciatic nerve and innervate the posterior portion of the lower body.

Autonomic Nervous System

The autonomic nervous system (ANS) fibers innervate smooth muscle, cardiac muscle, and glands, controlling involuntary vital functions such as blood pressure (BP), heart rate, body temperature, appetite, fluid balance, gastrointestinal motility, and sexual function.[56,67] The ANS has two subdivisions: the parasympathetic nervous system and the sympathetic nervous system. The parasympathetic nervous system originates from nerves in the craniosacral regions of the central nervous system, whereas the sympathetic nervous system originates from the thoracolumbar region of the spinal cord. The parasympathetic division regulates bodily functions under normal body conditions. In contrast, sympathetic system activity increases during periods of physiologic and psychological stress. Specific responses from autonomic stimulation depend on the type and number of receptors located within a tissue, organ, or system. The generalized responses that result from stimulation of both systems are listed in **Table 10-3**.[56,61,67]

Vertebral Column

The vertebral column is stabilized by ligaments and contains 33 vertebrae: 7 cervical, 12 thoracic, 5 lumbar, 5 sacral, and 4 coccygeal vertebrae (**Figure 10-4**).[56] The typical vertebra is composed of a weight-bearing anterior body and a posterior vertebral arch. The arch consists of two pedicles (right and left), two laminae, four articular processes (facets), two transverse processes, and one spinous process (**Figure 10-5**). The spinous process can be felt when palpating the back. Together, the arch and the body form an enclosure called the *vertebral foramen*, which encircles and protects the spinal cord.[56,61,70]

Cervical Vertebrae

The cervical vertebrae are the smallest and most mobile of the vertebrae. The first cervical vertebra, the *atlas*, supports the weight of the head and articulates with the occipital condyles of the skull. The atlas differs from the other vertebrae in that it has no spinous process or vertebral body. In addition, the foramen opening for the spinal cord is larger than in the other vertebrae. The *axis*, C2, has a perpendicular projection called the odontoid process, or *dens*. The atlas articulates with the axis on the odontoid process.[56,61,70]

Thoracic Vertebrae

The thoracic vertebrae, T1 through T12, attach to the ribs, which limits flexion and extension. It permits more rotation than the lumbar region but less than the cervical region. The vertebrae in this region are strong, with added support provided by the ribs.[56,61,70]

Lumbar, Sacral, and Coccygeal Vertebrae

The five lumbar vertebrae (L1–L5) are the largest and strongest of the vertebral column. This area of the spine has some freedom of movement and rotation. The five sacral vertebrae (S1–S5) fuse together to form the sacrum. The final four coccygeal vertebrae are fused, forming the coccyx.[56,61,70]

TABLE 10-3 Effects of Sympathetic and Parasympathetic Stimulation

Target Tissue, Organ, or System	Result of Sympathetic Stimulation	Result of Parasympathetic Stimulation
Skin	↑ Secretions from sweat glands Piloerection	N/A
Cardiac	↑ Heart rate, conduction, and contractility	↓ Heart rate, conduction, and contractility
Vascular	Peripheral vasoconstriction	Dilatation of blood vessels causing an erection
Respiratory	↑ Respiratory rate Bronchial dilation Pulmonary vascular constriction	Bronchial constriction
Hepatic	↑ Glycogen breakdown and synthesis of new glucose	Promotes glycogen synthesis
Stomach and intestines	↓ GI motility and tone Sphincter contraction ↓ Gastric secretions and mesenteric blood flow	↑ GI motility and tone Sphincter relaxation ↑ Gastric secretions
Renal	↑ Renin secretion Vascular constriction causes urinary output	N/A
Adrenal medulla	Catecholamines, norepinephrine, and epinephrine released from adrenal glands	N/A

Data from Stacy, K. M. (2022). Neurologic anatomy and physiology. In L. D. Urden, K. M. Stacy, & M. E. Lough (Eds.), *Critical care nursing: Diagnosis and management* (9th ed., pp. 534–564). Elsevier; Tortora, G. J., & Derrickson, B. H. (2021). The autonomic nervous system. In *Principles of anatomy and physiology* (16th ed., pp. 546–568). Wiley.

Ligaments and Intervertebral Discs

The vertebral bodies are connected by a series of ligaments that provide support and stability for the vertebral column. The anterior and posterior longitudinal ligaments run the length of the vertebral column and stabilize the discs and vertebral bodies to prevent excessive flexion and extension. The spinous and transverse processes act as points of attachment for muscles and other ligaments. Fibrocartilaginous discs are located between the vertebral bodies and act as shock absorbers during weight bearing and as articulating surfaces for the subsequent vertebral bodies. The more flexible cervical and lumbar regions contain thicker intervertebral discs.[56,67]

Vascular Supply

Blood is supplied to the spinal cord by the vertebral arteries and the aorta. The cord is primarily perfused by the anterior and posterior spinal arteries, which branch off from the vertebral artery at the cranial base. Injuries to the spinal cord or surrounding area can lacerate these arteries, resulting in hematoma formation, which may compress the cord. Injury to the vessels can be devastating because collateral circulation does not develop in this area.[56,61]

Anatomy and Physiology of Musculoskeletal System

The musculoskeletal system provides support, protection, and functional movement to the human body. This system includes bones, joints, tendons, ligaments, cartilage, vessels, nerves, and muscle.

Bones and Supporting Structures

Bones are composed of several different types of tissue: cartilage, dense connective tissue, epithelium, adipose tissue, and nervous tissue[69,71]:

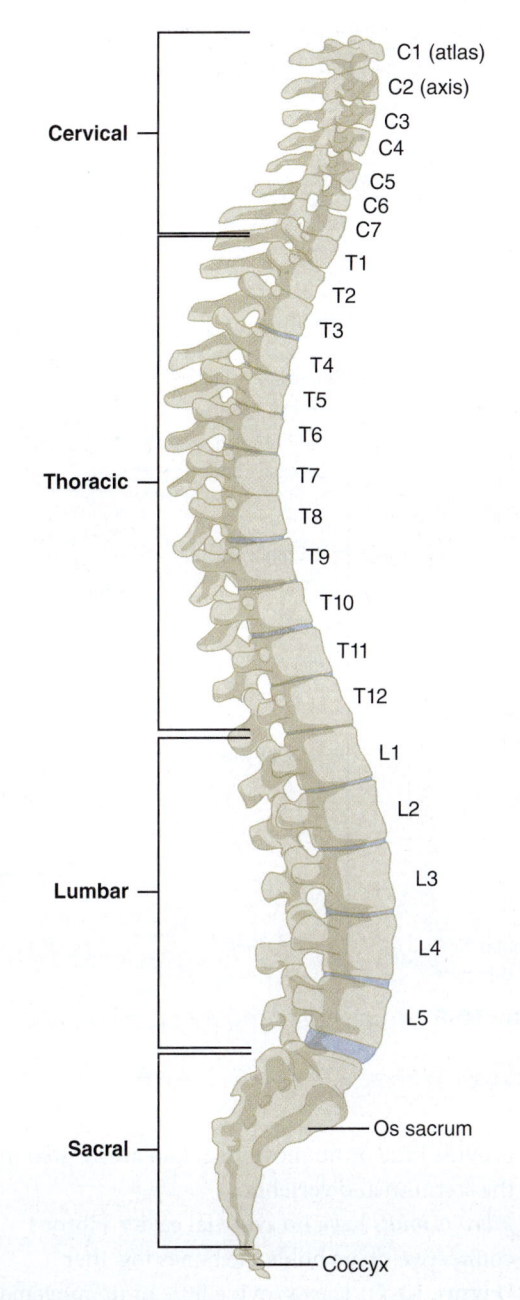

Figure 10-4 *The spine.*

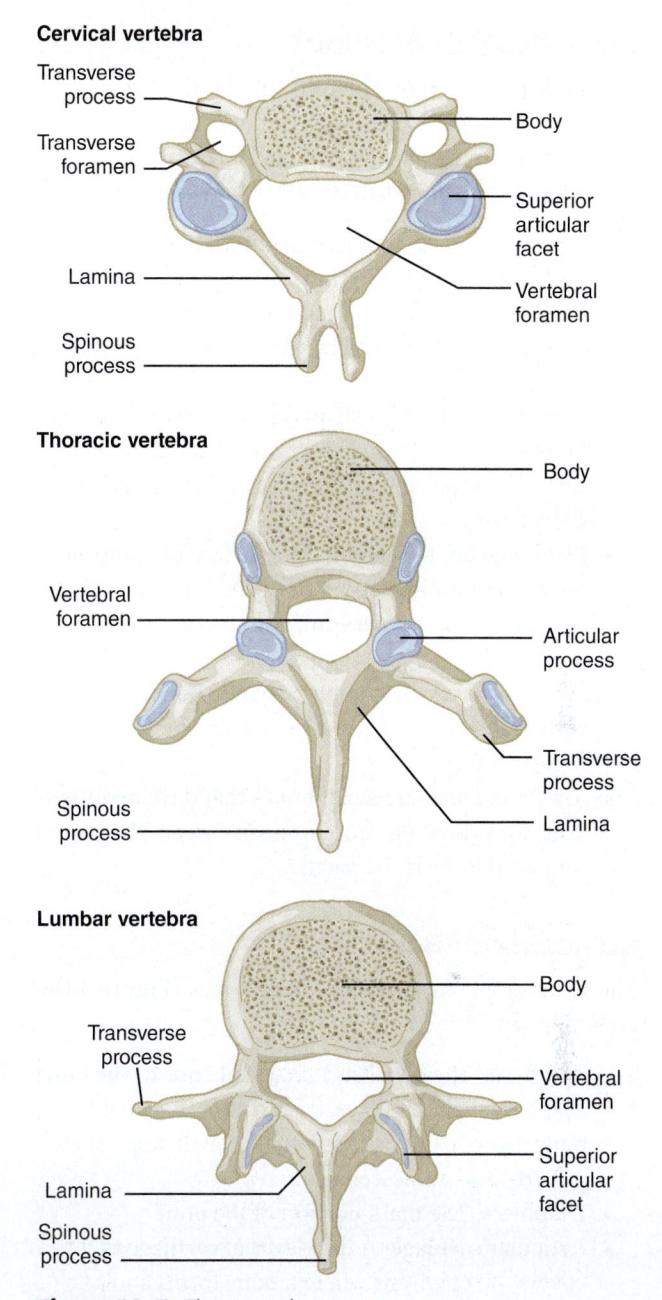

Figure 10-5 *The vertebrae.*

- *Cartilage* is a matrix of cells capable of retaining water. This enables the cartilage to rebound after compression. After bone, cartilage is the firmest structure in the body.
- *Dense connective tissue* includes protein fibers that form thick bundles of collagen fibers for structures such as tendons and ligaments. Tendons connect muscles to bones, and ligaments connect bones to bones.
- *Epithelial tissue* covers and protects deeper tissue surfaces.
- *Adipose tissue* contains lipids and functions to insulate, store energy, and protect against injury.
- *Nervous tissue* is characterized by its ability to conduct electrical signals.

The two primary types of bone tissues are compact tissue and spongy tissue (cancellous). Compact bone is the strongest bone tissue. It forms the shaft of long bones and the exterior covering of other bones. Cancellous bone is located in the bone's interior, along stress lines, and aids in the bone's resistance to stress without breaking. The cancellous tissue found in the hips, vertebrae, ribs, sternum, and ends of long bones stores red marrow and is the site of blood cell production in adults.[69]

Classification of Bones

The adult human body contains 206 bones; infants and children have more bones because some fuse together as the body develops. Most bones can be classified into five categories: long, short, flat, irregular, and sesamoid[69]:

- *Long bones* have a greater length than width, with a slight curvature for strength. Compact bone tissue comprises the shaft of long bones. Examples of long bones are the femur, tibia, fibula, humerus, radius, and ulna.
- *Short bones* are cube-shaped and consist of cancellous bone with a thin layer of compact bone on its surface. Carpal and tarsal bones are classified as short bones.
- *Flat bones* are thin and have a surface of compact bone surrounding a layer of cancellous bone. The cranial bones, the sternum, and the ribs are flat bones.
- *Irregular bones* are complex-shaped bones. The vertebrae, hip bones, and some facial bones are irregular bones.
- *Sesamoid bones* are small bones that develop in tendons for protection from excessive wear. The largest sesamoid bone is the patella.[74]

Structure of Bone

The structural components of long bones (**Figure 10-6**) are as follows[69,71]:

- Epiphysis: The distal and proximal ends of the bone
- Epiphyseal plate: A layer of cartilage that enables bone growth and ossifies when growth stops after puberty and adolescence
- Diaphysis: The main portion of the bone
- Articular cartilage: A thin layer of cartilage that covers the epiphysis where a bone forms a joint with another bone
- Periosteum: The connective tissue that covers the bone, except at articular surfaces
- Medullary cavity: The space within the diaphysis that contains yellow bone marrow in adults

Joints, Tendons, and Ligaments

Joints are classified into three types: synovial, cartilaginous, and fibrous.

- *Synovial joints* are a fluid-filled cavity. The bones are held together with connective tissue and ligaments. Synovial joints enable free movement and are located at the knee, elbow, and hip.
- *Cartilaginous joints* have no synovial cavity. Cartilage holds the bones together. Cartilaginous joints provide little or no movement and are located in the sternum and vertebra.
- *Fibrous joints* have no synovial cavity. Fibrous connective tissue holds the bones together (**Figure 10-7**). They provide little or no movement and are found in the skull, tibia, and fibula.

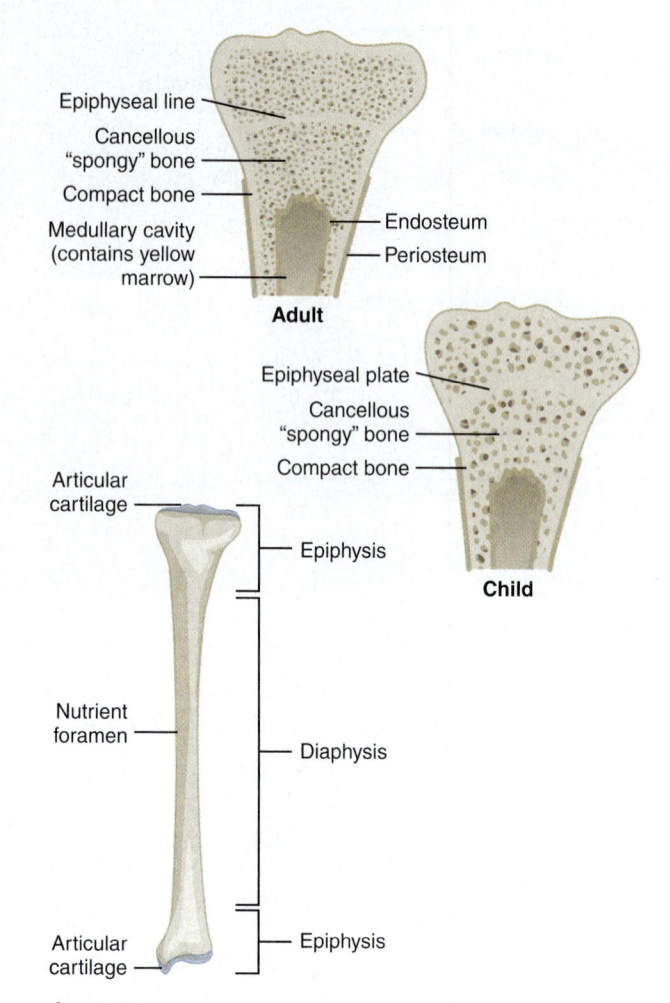

Figure 10-6 *Structural components of long bones.*

Other supportive structures in the musculoskeletal system include tendons, ligaments, and skeletal muscle.

- *Tendons* are cords of dense tissue that attach muscles to bones and control movement of the extremity by extension or flexion of the muscle groups.
- *Ligaments* are fibrous capsules that are arranged in parallel bundles of dense connective tissue and are highly resistant to strains. Ligaments hold the bones together in the joints.
- *Skeletal muscle* has striations of dark and light bands containing connective tissues that surround muscle fibers, blood vessels, and nerves. Skeletal muscle is attached to bone by fibrous connective tissue or tendons.

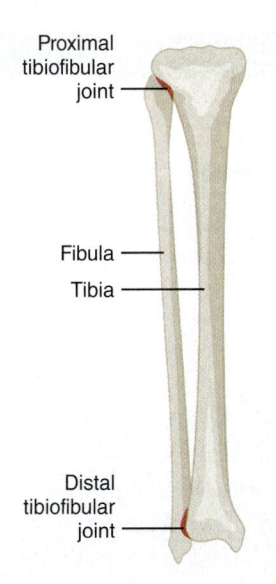

Figure 10-7 *The tibiofibular joint: An example of a fibrous joint.*

Blood and Nerve Supply

Bone is highly vascular. Periosteal arteries supply blood to the periosteum and outer part of compact bones. Metaphyseal arteries supply blood to the bone marrow of long bones. Veins are located in the diaphysis, epiphysis, and the periosteum. The metaphyseal and epiphyseal arteries supply blood to red bone marrow and bone tissue.[69,71] Bone is also highly innervated. The periosteum contains many sensory nerves that conduct pain sensation—hence, the pain experienced with a fracture.

Introduction

All trauma patients with multiple injuries are at risk for spinal cord injury (SCI), regardless of the presence or absence of neurologic deficit. Given the significant impact of a SCI on the patient's health and abilities, it is essential that trauma nurses who care for these patients maintain adequate spinal motion restriction to avoid any excessive manipulation of the spine until injury can be ruled out. In patients with a high index of suspicion for an unstable spine, it is recommended that logrolling be avoided if at all possible. However, logrolling may be indicated if there is suspicion of a penetrating injury causing hemodynamic instability or airway compromise, such as vomiting that cannot be cleared with suction.[45,55] Musculoskeletal trauma can cause single-system or multisystem injuries, which may result in hemodynamic or neurovascular compromise. MOIs include falls, motor vehicle collisions (MVCs), assaults, sports activities, and home- or work-related incidents. Falls are the leading cause of musculoskeletal injury in all age groups, with the exception of teens and young adults, and they are the leading cause of injury-related death in the older adult[4] (see Chapter 15, "The Older Trauma Patient," for additional information).

Epidemiology

Worldwide, the incidence of SCI ranges from 250,000 to 500,000 cases each year.[14,21] In the United States, there are approximately 17,000 new cases each year.[14] Men and older adults have the highest incidences of SCI worldwide.[21] Musculoskeletal system diagnoses account for 7.6% of all conditions treated in United States. Of these complaints, fractures, sprains, and strains are the most common reason for seeking emergency care.[15]

Mechanisms of Injury and Biomechanics

Spinal injuries may occur as a result of penetrating or blunt trauma.[14] Mechanisms of injury (MOIs) include the following:

- Vehicular collisions (including autos, motorcycles, bicycles, all-terrain vehicles, and boats): 38%
- Falls: 30%
- Violence (includes gunshot wounds, person-to-person wounds, or other penetrating wounds): 13%
- Sports and recreational activities: 9%
- Other causes (medical and surgical etiologies): 5%

Most injuries to the spinal cord or vertebral column are the result of blunt injuries from acceleration or deceleration forces. These rapid energy forces push the spinal column and supporting structures beyond their usual range of motion.[44,56] Four distinct types of forces can be applied to the vertebral column: hyperextension, hyperflexion, rotation, or axial loading forces. **Table 10-4** summarizes those forces and their associated injuries.[38,44,56]

Penetrating injuries from gunshot wounds may cause disruption in the integrity of the vertebral column. Stab wounds do not usually cause instability of the vertebral column. However, the wounding object may damage the spinal cord and blood vessels or nerve roots.

Fall Risk

Comorbidities increase the risk of complications from falls. Specific medications, such as antiplatelet agents and anticoagulants, may be associated with a higher incidence of traumatic brain injury. Therefore, it is important to evaluate the event that may have precipitated the fall. Consider if the fall was the result of the following:

- A mechanical event (trip or slip)
- A comorbid event (stroke, hypoglycemia, orthostatic hypotension, syncope, myocardial infarction)
- Medication use
- Alcohol use

TABLE 10-4 Mechanisms of Injury to the Vertebral Column

Mechanism of Injury	Etiology of Injury (Cause)	Result of Injury (Effect)	Example	Common Location of Injury
Hyperextension	Backward thrust of the head beyond the anatomic capacity of the cervical vertebral column	Damage to anterior ligaments ranging from stretching to ligament tears Bony dislocations	Rear-end MVC resulting in whiplash	Cervical spine
Hyperflexion	Forceful forward flexion of the cervical spine with the head striking an immovable object	Wedge fractures Facet dislocations Subluxation (due to ligament rupture) Teardrop, odontoid, or transverse process fractures	Head-on MVC with head striking the windshield, creating a starburst effect	Cervical spine
Rotational	A combination of forceful forward flexion with lateral displacement of the cervical spine	Rupture of the posterior ligament and/or anterior fracture Dislocation of the vertebral body	MVC to front or rear lateral area of the vehicle, resulting in conversion of forward motion to a spinning-type motion	Cervical spine
Axial loading (compression)	Direct force transmitted along the length of the vertebral column	Burst and laminar fractures Secondary edema of the spinal cord, resulting in neurologic deficits	Diver striking the head on the bottom of the pool or landing on the feet after a long fall	Cervical, thoracic, and lumbar spine

Data from Kaji, A., & Hockberger, R. S. (2022). Spinal column injuries in adults: Definitions, mechanisms, and radiographs. *UpToDate*. Retrieved October 19, 2022, from https://www.uptodate.com/contents/spinal-column-injuries-in-adults-definitions-mechanisms-and-radiographs; Mondor, E. E. (2022). Trauma. In L. D. Urden, K. M. Stacy, & M. E. Lough (Eds.), *Critical care nursing: Diagnosis and management* (9th ed., pp. 791–830). Elsevier; Russo McCourt, T. (2020). Spinal cord injuries. In K. A. McQuillan & M. B. Flynn Makic (Eds.), *Trauma nursing: From resuscitation through rehabilitation* (5th ed., pp. 454–502). Elsevier.

Types of Injuries

The cervical spine is the most common site for spinal injury because it is the area with the most mobility and exposure.[6] An estimated 50% of spinal injuries occur at the cervical level of the spinal cord, 35% of injuries occur in the thoracic level, and 11% of injuries occur to the lumbar area.[1] The most common location of SCI is the fifth cervical vertebral area.[1] Extreme forces are required to produce fractures and dislocations in the thoracic region; injuries to the thoracic vertebrae are frequently accompanied by a SCI.

The extremities are the most common site of traumatic skeletal injuries. Injuries may involve bone, soft tissue, muscles, nerves, tendons, blood vessels, and joint spaces. Musculoskeletal injuries include fractures, dislocations, amputations, sprains, strains, penetrating injuries, ligament tears, tendon lacerations, and neurovascular compromise. **Table 10-5** provides definitions of these injuries.

Common mechanisms and their associated musculoskeletal injuries include the following:

- Falling onto outstretched hands (FOOSH)
  - Colles fracture (distal radius)
  - Scaphoid fracture

TABLE 10-5 Classification of Musculoskeletal Injuries

Injury Type	Description
Fracture	Disruption in the continuity of a bone
Dislocation	Ends of two or more bones that make up a joint are forced from their normal position
Amputation	Removal of all or part of a limb
Sprain	Stretch or tear to a ligament
Strain	Stretch or tear to a tendon or muscle
Subluxation	Partial dislocation of two or more bones that make up a joint
Contusion	Area of broken capillaries or venules beneath the skin with extravasation of blood
Avulsion	Tissue is torn away or separated
Crush	Tissue is compressed between two hard surfaces and damaged
Mangled	Injury to three or more systems in a limb (soft tissue, bone, nerve, vascular)

- Monteggia fracture: Dislocation (ulnar shaft fracture with radial head dislocation)
- Galeazzi fracture: Dislocation (distal radial fracture with a distal ulnar epiphyseal fracture)
- Jumps/falls with a feet-first landing involve axial loading forces that diffuse upward
  - Thoracolumbar vertebral compression fractures
  - Calcaneus fractures (can distract from other injuries because of intense pain)
  - Pelvic/acetabular fractures
  - Tibial plateau fractures
  - Wrist/forearm fractures
- High-impact trauma (passenger compartment intrusion or when unrestrained occupant is thrown forward into the dashboard of the vehicle)
  - Patella fractures
  - Femur fractures, hip fractures, dislocations, and popliteal artery damage—commonly associated with knee trauma
- Pedestrian-versus-vehicle injuries
  - Bilateral tibia–fibula fractures
  - If the pedestrian is struck by a larger vehicle (sport-utility vehicle, van, or truck), suspect pelvic injuries

Usual Concurrent Injuries

Concurrent musculoskeletal and spinal injuries may include closed head injuries, thoracic injuries, and abdominal injuries.[62] Approximately 5% of patients with a brain injury have an associated spinal injury, and 25% of patients with a spinal injury have a mild brain injury.[6] When a patient incurs a cervical spinal fracture, a second noncontiguous vertebral column fracture occurs 10% of the time.[6] Thoracic injuries may be associated with injuries to the thoracic vertebrae, whereas pelvic fractures are frequently associated with injuries to the lumbar spine. A fall from a height that results in a calcaneus fracture is an additional pattern of injury associated with compression fractures of the lumbar spine.[6] Patients with SCIs often have decreased or altered sensation and/or proprioception, making it difficult to identify other potentially serious injuries.

Seat belts applied incorrectly may be associated with concurrent injuries. Serious injury to the anterior neck may be associated with the use of diagonal torso belts alone. Lumbar vertebral fractures or dislocations may result from the use of a lap belt only.[5] Musculoskeletal injuries can be predictors of concurrent spinal injuries, so knowledge of concurrent injury patterns can help the trauma nurse identify and properly assess for primary and concurrent injuries. In the presence of an open fracture, there is a 70% incidence of an associated nonskeletal injury.[5] Table 10-5 describes injuries associated with musculoskeletal trauma.

Pathophysiology as a Basis for Assessment Findings

Before assessing for a SCI, the mechanisms associated with these injuries must be understood. When blunt force is applied to spinal tissues and the supporting structures, the effects shown in **Figure 10-8** should be anticipated. Primary and secondary mechanisms of injury may result in an acute SCI with resulting neurologic dysfunction.

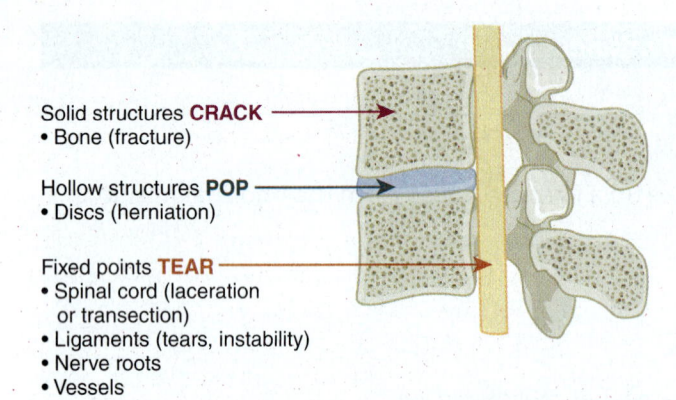

Figure 10-8 *The effects of force on spinal structures.*

Solid structures **CRACK**
- Bone (fracture)

Hollow structures **POP**
- Discs (herniation)

Fixed points **TEAR**
- Spinal cord (laceration or transection)
- Ligaments (tears, instability)
- Nerve roots
- Vessels

Primary Spinal Cord Injury

Primary SCI refers to the initial mechanical damage to the spinal cord and includes the following conditions[6,44,56]:

- Laceration or puncture of the cord from displaced or jagged bone fragments
- Crushed or contused disc material
- Stretching or crushing of the spinal cord
- Torn or strained ligaments
- Bleeding into the vertebral column or edema that compresses the spinal cord
- Direct injury to the cord, including the following:
  - Cord concussion: A transient dysfunction of the spinal cord that lasts for 24–48 hours. This injury may be observed in patients with preexisting degenerative disease and resultant narrowing of the vertebral foramen.
  - Cord contusion: Bruising of the neural tissue causing edema, ischemia, and possible infarction of tissue from cord compression. The degree of neurologic deficit depends on the size, location, and local physiologic changes related to the bleeding.
  - Cord transection: Complete disruption of the neural elements. With cord transections, all cord-mediated functions below the level of the injury are permanently lost.
  - Incomplete cord transection: An interruption in the vascular perfusion to the spinal cord may result in cord ischemia or necrosis. Ischemia results in temporary deficits; prolonged ischemia results in necrosis of the spinal cord, with permanent neurologic deficits.

Healthcare providers' adoption of the "time is spine" concept has been shown to improve long-term outcomes for patients with acute SCI.[31] This is an approach intended to ensure rapid identification of patients who sustain acute SCI, to include early transfer to specialized centers, early decompressive surgery, and early delivery of additional supportive treatments (e.g., BP augmentation).

> **NOTE**
>
> **Spinal Cord Injury without Radiographic Abnormality**
>
> In addition to primary injuries, SCI without radiographic abnormality (SCIWORA) may occur. Pathophysiological characteristics include the following:
> - Generally caused by stretching or shearing of the spinal cord
> - Most frequently seen in young children because of the immature development of their spinal structures[17]
>
> Data from Criddle, L. M. (Ed.). (2022). Spine and spinal cord injuries. In *TCAR trauma care after resuscitation* (11th ed., pp. 147–161). TCAR Education Programs.

Secondary Spinal Cord Injury

Patients with SCI are susceptible to the same secondary injuries found in patients with traumatic brain injury. Secondary injuries result from biochemical and cellular reactions that cause inflammation of tissues, which can lead to permanent loss of function without proper interventions (**Figure 10-9**).

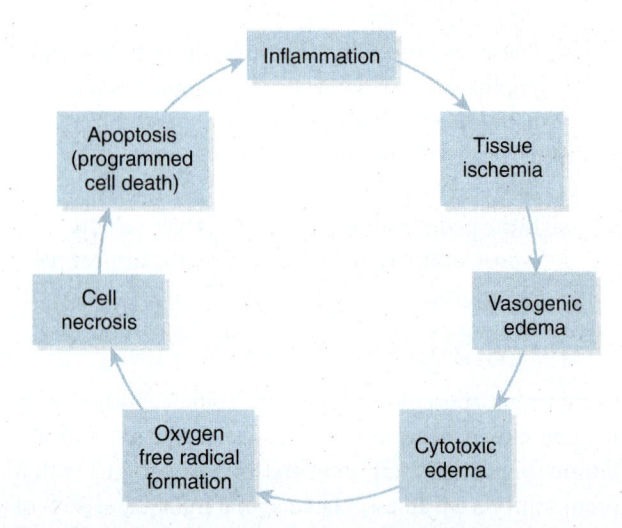

Figure 10-9 *Secondary injury cycle.*

Understanding the pathophysiology related to secondary injury is essential to reducing cell loss and optimizing the patient's functional outcome.

Vascular System Response

Neurogenic shock occurs when high thoracic or cervical damage to the spinal cord results in an abrupt disruption of sympathetic innervation and the regulation of vasomotor and vagal tone, producing a loss of vascular resistance and vasodilation (**Table 10-6**).[6,27,56] The loss of vascular tone results in peripheral vasodilation, reduced systemic vascular resistance, decreased venous return, decreased cardiac output, and lowered BP.[6,30,56] Although the patient experiences hypotension, it is not the result of a change in blood volume. It is a form of distributive shock that causes the circulating blood volume to pool in the peripheral vasculature. See Chapter 6, "Shock," for additional information.

Assessment findings include the following[6,30,56]:

- Bradycardia
  - Because of the loss of sympathetic innervation to the heart, the body is unable to respond to hypovolemia with a tachycardic response, resulting in an unopposed parasympathetic response
- Hypotension due to decreased cardiac output and bradycardia
  - Loss of sympathetic innervation results in decreased catecholamine (epinephrine) production, which limits vasoconstriction
  - Vasodilation yields a widened pulse pressure, with resulting hypovolemia
- Warm, normal skin color due to peripheral vasodilation
  - Core temperature instability due to the loss of sympathetic response and inability to vasodilate and vasoconstrict

Hypotension in SCI results in decreased blood supply to the spinal cord, further exacerbating tissue injury. This results in loss of function, which may be either temporary (hours to days) or permanent. With appropriate supportive measures, neurogenic shock usually resolves over days to weeks.[6,30,56] Hypotension in patients with musculoskeletal trauma is a result of hemorrhage from the disruption of musculoskeletal integrity. Musculoskeletal trauma can result in large-volume hemorrhage, which is the leading cause of preventable death in trauma.[5]

Nervous System Response

Spinal shock occurs when normal activity in the spinal cord at and below the level of injury ceases because of a disruption or inhibition of impulses in the spinal cord (Table 10-6).[56] When the spinal cord is injured, a cascade of events takes place:

- Blood supply to the cord may be disrupted.
- Axons are severed or damaged.
- Conduction of electrical activity of neurons and axons is compromised.
- All of the above result in loss of function, which can last from several hours to several days. When patients sustain an incomplete SCI, the presence of spinal shock can delay assessment of the full extent of injury; once spinal shock has resolved, a full assessment can be performed.[17]

TABLE 10-6 Neurogenic and Spinal Shock

	Neurogenic Shock	**Spinal Shock**
Precipitating injury	High thoracic or cervical cord injury	SCI at any level
Pathophysiology	Temporary loss of vasomotor tone and sympathetic innervation	Transient loss of reflex (flaccidity) below the level of injury
Duration	Temporary, often lasting less than 72 hours	Variable
Signs/symptoms	Hypotension	Flaccidity
	Bradycardia	Loss of reflexes
	Loss of ability to sweat below level of injury	Bowel and bladder dysfunction

Data from American College of Surgeons. (2018). Spine and spinal cord trauma. In *Advanced trauma life support: Student course manual* (10th ed., pp. 128–147); Fox, A. D. (2014). Spinal shock: Assessment and treatment of spinal cord injuries and neurogenic shock. *Journal of Emergency Medical Services, 39*(11), 64–67.

Spinal shock results in a complete loss of reflex function below the level of the injury.[6,56,75] A transient hypotensive period resulting from poor venous circulation may also occur. Disruption in the thermal control centers results in sweating and lack of ability to regulate body temperature. Onset of spinal shock is usually immediate. The timing of resolution of spinal shock is not well established, and the intensity and duration of spinal shock vary with the severity and level of the lesion. The changes are most prominent at the level of the injury and in two cord segments above and below. Additional assessment findings include the following[56,75]:

- Transient loss of muscle tone (flaccidity) and complete or incomplete paralysis may occur with loss of reflexes and sensation at or below the level of the injury.
- Bowel and bladder dysfunction may occur.
- The return of sacral reflexes, bladder tone, and the presence of hyperreflexia indicates the resolution of spinal shock.
- The presence of rectal tone and perineal sensation indicate sacral sparing.

Immune (Inflammatory) Response

Once the spinal cord is damaged, the immune system is activated. The function of immune cells once they enter the damaged spinal cord is not well established.[38] Nevertheless, it is understood that the immune response includes the following[1,28,40,44]:

- Within minutes of the injury, endothelial cells that line the blood vessels in the spinal cord become edematous.
- The combination of leaking, swelling, and sluggish blood flow prevents the normal delivery of oxygen and nutrients to neurons.
- Edema in the white matter impairs cord circulation and leads to the development of ischemia.
- The resulting cellular ischemia may cause a temporary loss of function.

Spinal cord neurons do not regenerate. Therefore, severe injury and cellular death may result in the following assessment findings:

- Temporary or permanent loss of function
- Flaccidity
- Loss of reflexes

Alterations in Neurovascular Exam

Musculoskeletal injuries disrupt capillaries and cellular membranes. Hemorrhage in the area surrounding the injury may be visible or occult. As arterial blood flow becomes obstructed, tissue oxygenation decreases, resulting in tissue ischemia and cellular death. During this progression, pain increases, and pulses may become more difficult to palpate. The extremity becomes pale, cyanotic, and cool, and capillary refill time increases.

Bone or joint displacement can compress surrounding nerves, causing pathophysiologic changes distal to the injury. Compressed or lacerated nerves may interrupt conduction pathways, blocking or delaying nerve impulses. The nerve injury can result in alterations in pain sensation and partial or complete loss of motor and sensory function distal to the injured nerve. Increased pain, even when pulses remain present, is a sign of worsening cellular hypoxia and is often the first sign of increased compartment pressures.[13] However, patients who are unresponsive or intubated will not be able to report this pain. In these patients, it is important to have a high index of suspicion based on the mechanism of injury (MOI). Such patients will need frequent reevaluation to detect subtle changes that are indicative of compartment syndrome.

Other Related Pathophysiologic Changes

Other pathophysiologic changes are respiratory and related to pain.

Respiratory System

Respiratory system changes include the following:

- Respiratory arrest: Injury to the cord at the C3–C5 level can cause loss of phrenic nerve function, resulting in a paralyzed diaphragm and inability to breathe.
- Hypoventilation: Injury to the spinal cord between T1 and T11 may result in the loss of intercostal muscles and decreased respiratory effort. Loss of innervation from T7 to T12 may result in loss of the use of abdominal muscles for support of breathing.

Pain

The ability to perceive pain may be disrupted and result in an inadequate physical assessment.

Selected Vertebral Column and Spinal Cord Injuries

This section covers selected vertebral column and SCIs.

Spinal Cord Injuries

SCIs are classified based on the following characteristics[6,30,56]:

- Level of injury
- Severity of neurologic deficit
- Spinal cord syndromes

Level of Injury

The vertebral level is the level of vertebrae where the injury occurred; the neurologic injury level is determined by clinical assessment and is the lowest level that has positive sensory and motor function.

The vertebral level may not be the same as the neurologic level because the spinal cord tracts are not exactly synonymous with the level of vertebrae. Level of injury usually refers to the neurologic level.

The sensory level is the point of demarcation where there is no or decreased sensation below and normal sensation above.

Severity of Neurologic Deficit

SCI can be characterized as an incomplete or complete lesion.

Incomplete Spinal Cord Lesion

Incomplete lesions are referred to as specific incomplete spinal cord syndromes (**Figure 10-10** and **Table 10-7**).[51] Comparison of motor and sensory function of bilateral upper and lower extremities is important to discerning the exact cord syndrome[14,44,56]:

- **Anterior cord syndrome**
  - Also known as anterior spinal artery syndrome.
  - MOI often involves extreme hyperflexion.
  - Caused by an injury or disruption of the anterior spinal artery (**Figure 10-11**), which supplies the anterior two-thirds of the spinal cord.
  - Complete motor loss of function below the level of the injury is caused by injury of the spinothalamic tract.
  - Loss of pain and temperature sensation occurs below the level of injury.
  - Urinary retention is present.

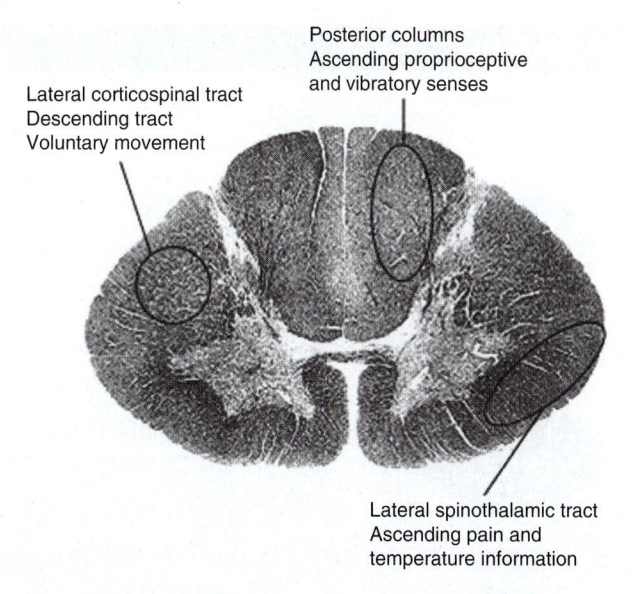

Figure 10-10 *Incomplete spinal cord syndromes.*
Courtesy of John Sundsten, Digital Anatomist Project, University of Washington.

  - Outcomes are usually poor, with minimal recovery of function.
  - The dorsal columns remain intact, so the patient retains proprioception and vibratory sensation.
- **Posterior cord syndrome (rare injury)**
  - Also known as dorsal column syndrome.
  - MOI is cervical hyperextension.
  - Caused by an injury or ischemia to the posterior one-third of the spinal cord, which is usually well perfused by the posterior spinal arteries (Figure 10-11).
  - Deficits include loss of deep touch, vibration, and proprioception senses.
  - Motor and most sensory functions are generally spared.
  - Outcomes are variable, with many patients experiencing difficulty walking that is due to the loss of proprioception.
- **Central cord syndrome**
  - MOI can be from hyperextension or hyperflexion. It most frequently occurs as a result of hyperextension.
  - Common in older adults because of chronic cervical spondylosis and often associated with a low-energy fall (e.g., fall from standing).
  - Caused by edema or contusion near the center of the spinal cord that essentially squeezes the cord.
  - Characterized by loss of motor and sensory function in the upper extremities that is greater than that of the lower extremities. As an example, a patient with a central cord injury might

TABLE 10-7 Spinal Cord Syndromes

Syndrome	Sensory	Motor	Sphincter Involvement
Central cord syndrome	Variable	Upper-extremity weakness, distal > proximal	Variable
Brown-Sequard syndrome	Ipsilateral position and vibration sense loss Contralateral pain and temperature sensation loss	Motor loss Ipsilateral to cord lesion	Variable
Anterior cord syndrome	Loss of pain and touch sensation Vibration, position sense preserved	Motor loss or weakness below cord level	Variable
Transverse cord syndrome—complete	Loss of sensation below level of cord injury	Loss of voluntary motor function below cord level	Sphincter control lost

Reproduced from Perron, A. D., & Huff, J. S. (2018). Spinal cord disorders. In R. M. Walls, R. S. Hockberger, & M. Gausche-Hill (Eds.), *Rosen's emergency medicine* (9th ed., pp. 1298–1306). Elsevier.

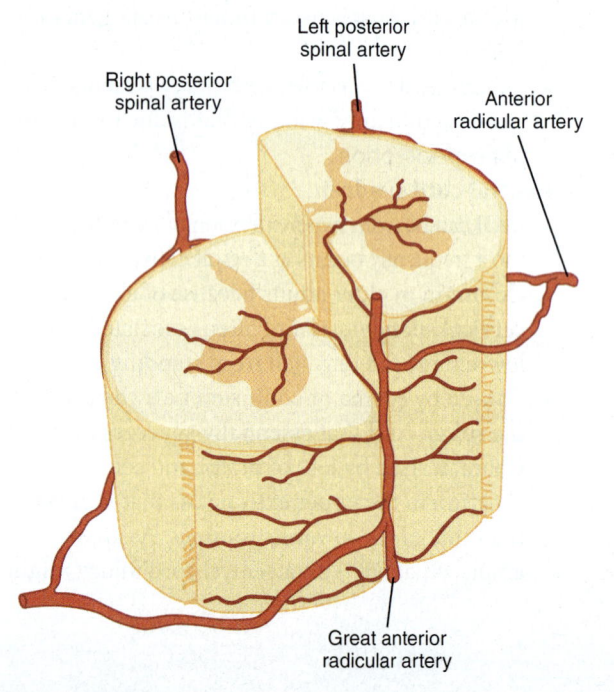

Figure 10-11 *Arterial circulation of the spinal cord.*

be able to walk but would not be able to use their hands or arms to open the door.
- Fine motor control in the hands is the most common loss of function.
- Outcomes can be positive for return of function as inflammation decreases around the injured cord, but the capacity to regain full function decreases with patient age.
- **Brown-Sequard syndrome**
  - Also known as hemicord syndrome.
  - MOI is from penetrating trauma to the spinal cord but can be from hyperextension or disc herniation.
  - Deficits are caused by a partial transection of the spinal cord.
  - Classic assessment findings are intact motor function and decreased sensation on one side of the body and decreased motor function and intact sensation on the opposite side. An example is the patient who can pick up

a hot pan with his hand but cannot feel his hand burning.
- Outcomes are mixed, but patients can experience some improvement of functioning with time and therapy.

A patient with an incomplete SCI has some sensory and/or motor function below the level of the injury. Sacral sparing is characterized by some structural integrity of the lowest sacral segments of the spinal cord at S4 and S5. Sacral sparing is identified by the following findings[1,32]:

- Intact perianal sensation
- Voluntary anal sphincter tone
- Voluntary great toe flexor function

Note that a patient with an incomplete lesion may not exhibit sacral sparing in the presence of spinal shock. As spinal shock resolves, sacral sparing may become evident.

Complete Spinal Cord Lesion

Patients with a complete SCI lesion (transection) lose all motor and sensory function at and below the level of the lesion. Assessment findings include the following[6,44,56]:

- Absent motor function below the level of the injury
- Flaccid paralysis and bilateral external rotation of the legs at the hips
- Absent sensory function below the level of the injury, such as loss of pain, touch, temperature, pressure, vibration, and proprioception
- Loss of all reflexes below the level of the injury
- Loss of ANS function
  - Hypotension, resulting in venous pooling in the extremities
  - Bradycardia
  - Poikilothermia, which causes the patient to assume the temperature of the surroundings below the level of the lesion—primarily related to the absence of sympathetic tone and the inability of the patient to shiver or sweat to regulate body temperature
  - Loss of voluntary bowel and bladder function
- Paralytic ileus with abdominal distention
- Priapism
- Respiratory depression

Vertebral Injuries

Vertebral injuries are described as fractures, subluxations, dislocations, or penetrating injuries and are classified as stable or unstable.[9,73]

Atlas and Axis Fractures

The atlas (C1) and the axis (C2) vertebrae enable the majority of head and neck movement because of their relationship to the occiput.[56] **Table 10-8** describes four fractures and dislocations involving this region.[6,39,73] Although rare, most fatalities related to SCI occur at the craniocervical junction, with associated subluxation or dislocation.[56,73] The risk of neurologic injury secondary to SCI increases with age-related degenerative changes such as rheumatoid arthritis, ankylosing spondylitis, osteoporosis, and spinal stenosis; specific mechanisms of injury; and specific locations of injury.[37,73]

Vertebral Fracture Stability

Vertebral fractures are frequently classified as stable or unstable. Spinal stability is defined as the ability of the spine to maintain its alignment and protect the neural structures during normal physiologic loads.[37]

The integrity of ligamentous and bony structures will dictate the stability of the vertebral column. The loss of ligamentous integrity can result in an unstable spinal injury and subsequent damage to the spinal cord or nerve roots.[37] During resuscitation, treat patients with potential SCI as though they have an unstable injury, and maintain spinal motion restriction until SCI can be ruled out (**Table 10-9**).[6,9,56]

Subluxation or Dislocation

Injuries to the anterior and posterior ligaments may produce unilateral or bilateral facet dislocation, resulting in dislocation of the vertebrae. If the vertebrae are not completely dislocated, the injury is termed a subluxation. Dislocations and subluxations may occur simultaneously with a fracture. The presence of vertebral displacement (spondylolisthesis) or dislocation (traumatic spondyloptosis) places the patient at a significant risk for further damage until the injury is fully evaluated. For this reason, patients presenting with pain or evidence of a high-energy acceleration/deceleration MOI should remain in spinal motion restriction until clinically or radiologically cleared by the emergency care provider.[6,9,56,73]

Vertebral Body Fractures

Vertebral fractures most often occur in the vertebral body itself or in combination with an injury to another part of the vertebrae. The mobility of the cervical and lumbar regions results in greater frequency of these injuries.[6,9]

Fractures of the transverse or spinous processes of the vertebrae are considered minor vertebral fractures because they do not typically result in associated neurologic

TABLE 10-8 C1 and C2 Fractures and Dislocations

Fracture/Dislocation	Mechanism of Injury	Description	Clinical Considerations
(C1) Atlanto-occipital dislocation	Hyperflexion with distracting injury	Dislocation of atlas from the occipital bone	Commonly fatal Common cause of death in abusive head trauma
(C1) Atlas fracture, burst fracture, or Jefferson fracture	Axial loading forces transmitted from occiput to spine	Disrupts anterior and posterior rings of C1 Lateral displacement of lateral masses Spinal cord involvement rare	Treat as unstable until definitive evaluation
(C1) Rotary: subluxation	May occur spontaneously or with minor trauma	Persistent rotation of the head (torticollis)	Most often seen in children Stabilize in the rotated position
Axis (C2) fractures Odontoid fracture: Type I Type II Type III Posterior element fracture (hangman's fracture)	Hyperextension	Occur in about 18% of axis fractures Approximately 60% of C2 fractures involve the odontoid process Involve tip of the odontoid and are relatively uncommon Occur through base of dens and are most common Occur at base of dens and extend obliquely into the body of the axis C2 posterior elements are affected	Consider transverse ligament injury Maintain cervical collar until definitive evaluation is complete

Data from American College of Surgeons. (2018). Spine and spinal cord trauma. In *Advanced trauma life support: Student course manual* (10th ed., pp. 128–147); Lei, F., Ou, D., Huang, X., Pang, M., Chen, X., Yang, B., & Wang, Q. (2019). Surgery versus conservative treatment for type II and III odontoid fractures in a geriatric population. A meta-analysis. *Medicine*, *98*(44), Article e10281. https://doi.org/10.1097/MD.0000000000010281; Whitney, E., & Alastra, A. J. (2022, May 23). Vertebral fracture. *StatPearls*. StatPearls Publishing. https://www.ncbi.nlm.nih.gov/books/NBK547673/

compromise and are considered mechanically stable. However, significant forces are required to cause these fractures, so they may be associated with other injuries.[6,9,56]

Vertebral fractures of the thoracic and lumbar spine are typically caused by high-energy trauma and can result in spinal cord damage with neurologic deficits. However, osteoporosis can place the older adult at risk for such fractures, even with low-energy trauma.

The unique anatomic and functional features of each vertebral region result in specific injuries. Greater force is required to fracture the thoracic vertebrae because of the support provided by the sternum and the ribs. However, the relative immobility of the thoracic spine, as compared with the flexibility of the lumbar spine, can result in a fracture at the thoracolumbar junction (T11–L1); this injury is most often the result of acute hyperflexion and rotation.[47] These injuries result in unstable fractures that are vulnerable to rotational movement, so great care is required when logrolling these patients.[47] See Table 10-9 for more information.[6,56]

Selected Musculoskeletal Injuries

This section presents selected musculoskeletal injuries.

Selected Fractures

A fracture is a complete or incomplete interruption in the continuity of the bone cortex. **Table 10-10** outlines the classification of fractures. **Figure 10-12** illustrates each type of fracture.

Femur Fractures

Major trauma is often the cause of femoral shaft fractures, which can occur in the proximal, distal, or midshaft

Selected Musculoskeletal Injuries

TABLE 10-9 Thoracic Vertebral Fractures

Fracture	Mechanism of Injury	Description
Anterior compression (wedge)	Axial loading Flexion	Anterior portion is rarely more than 25% shorter than the posterior body Most are stable
Burst (comminuted)	Vertical axial compression	Comminuted fracture of vertebral body May result in SCI Unstable
Chance fracture (seat belt fracture)	Hyperflexion	Horizontal fracture lines with injury to bone and ligaments Suspect injuries to organs in the peritoneal cavity Certain types are unstable
Fracture–dislocation	Extreme flexion	Disruption of the pedicles, facets, and lamina of the thoracic or lumbar vertebrae Subluxation can result in complete neurologic deficit Unstable Relatively uncommon

Data from American College of Surgeons. (2018). Spine and spinal cord trauma. In *Advanced trauma life support: Student course manual* (10th ed., pp. 128–147); Anandasivam, N. S., Ondeck, N. T., Bagi, P. S., Galivanche, A. R., Samule, A. M., Bohl, D. D., & Grauer, J. N. (2021). Spinal fractures and/or spinal cord injuries are associated with orthopedic and internal organ injuries in proximity to the spinal injury. *North American Spine Society Journal, 6*, Article 10057. https://www.sciencedirect.com/science/article/pii/S2666548421000093; Russo McCourt, T. (2020). Spinal cord injuries. In K. A. McQuillan & M. B. Flynn Makic (Eds.), *Trauma nursing: From resuscitation through rehabilitation* (5th ed., pp. 454–502). Elsevier.

TABLE 10-10 Classification of Fractures

Fracture	Description
Open	Fracture site is accompanied by compromised skin integrity near or over the fracture.
Closed	Skin is intact over or near the fracture site.
Complete	Bony cortex is completely interrupted.
Incomplete	Bony cortex is not completely interrupted.
Comminuted	Bone is splintered into fragments.
Greenstick	Bone bends or is buckled.
Impacted	Bone is wedged into distal and proximal fracture sites.
Displaced	Bone fracture sites are not aligned.

femur. Fractures of the femoral shaft resulting from high-energy forces are often associated with other injuries. Femur fractures can result in significant blood loss because of the rich blood supply they receive. Patients can lose 1.5 liters or more of blood, which can be life threatening. Thus, long bone fractures have the potential to cause shock, especially when these injuries are combined with comorbid factors.[5,20,71] Assessment findings with femur fractures may include the following:

- Pain and the inability to bear weight
- Internal or external rotation with shortening
- Edema
- Deformity of the thigh
- Evidence of hypovolemic shock
- Evidence of neurovascular compromise in distal extremity

Fat Embolism Syndrome

Fat from within the medullary cavity is released into the bloodstream when long bones are fractured; fat emboli can be detected in the lungs in as many as 90% of patients

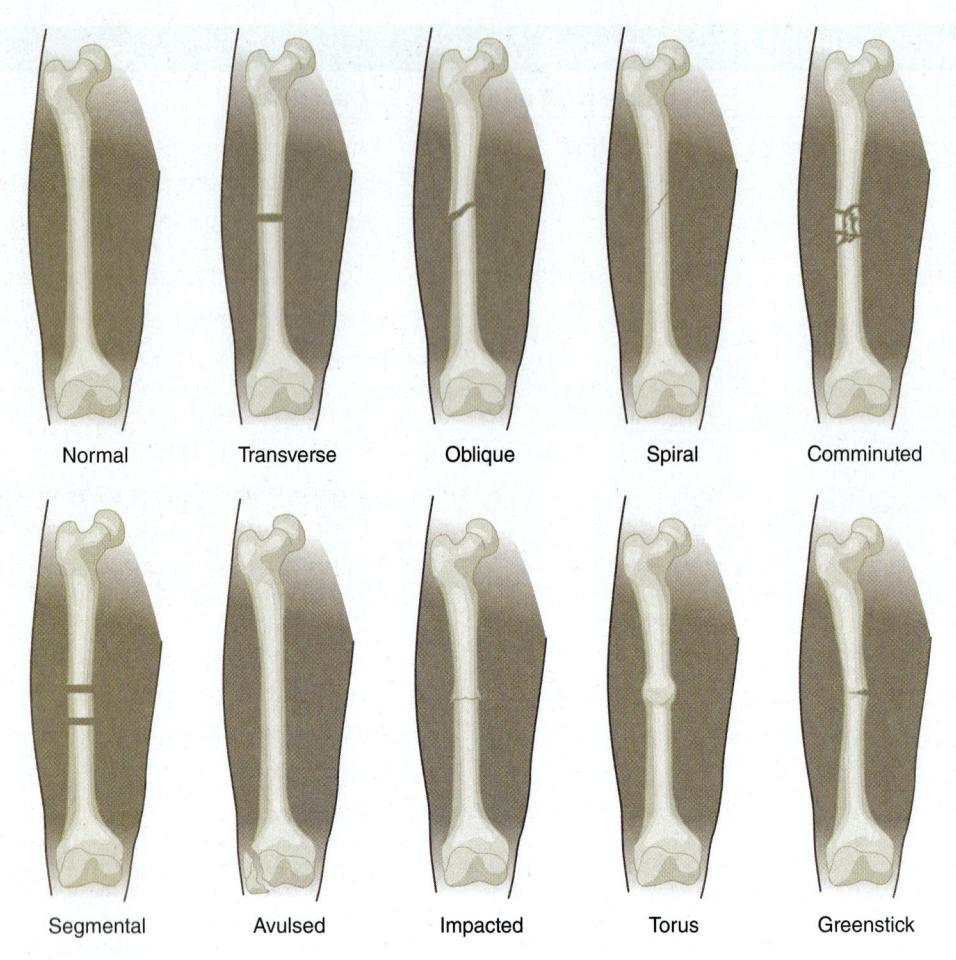

Figure 10-12 *Types of fractures.*

with long bone fractures on computed tomography (CT). Most patients do not experience significant symptoms because of the microscopic nature of the majority of fat emboli. Subclinical fat emboli are often found during autopsy of patients with major trauma and other injuries that were incompatible with life.

Of those patients who survive their initial traumatic injuries, 0.9% to 11.2% develop fat embolism syndrome (FES) from long bone fractures.[2] FES typically occurs between 24 and 72 hours post-injury.[71] Fat embolism is a clinical diagnosis, and its assessment findings may include the following[2,71]:

- Presence of a long bone fracture (usually femur)
- Sudden mental status change or focal neurologic findings (when other causes have been ruled out)
- Respiratory distress and hypoxemic respiratory failure
- Tachycardia
- Pyrexia
- Petechial rash (conjunctiva, anterior chest, axilla)
- Visual changes
- Oliguria/anuria
- Thrombocytopenia
- Anemia

Open Fractures

Open fractures are commonly associated with high-energy transfer mechanisms, and patients will frequently have other life-threatening injuries.[60] All open fractures are considered contaminated because of their exposure to the environment, and patients are at risk for infection. Hence, early administration of antibiotics is necessary. These sites of injury exhibit poor wound healing, with a risk of osteomyelitis and sepsis.

Open wounds near a joint may indicate joint space involvement, and some open fractures with neurologic injury, prolonged ischemia, and muscle damage may require amputation. Assessment findings for open fractures include the following:

- Open wound over or near a fracture
- Open wound with protrusion of bone
- Pain
- Neurovascular compromise
- Bleeding (may be controlled or severe)

Amputations

Traumatic amputations are rare, occurring in 1% of trauma patients, but they have serious morbidities and a high mortality rate of approximately 15%.[53] Amputations often have a dramatic presentation and may be distracting to both the patient and the trauma team. The priority of care is to focus on the overall assessment and resuscitation of the patient to establish and maintain hemodynamic stability, including control of hemorrhage.

Assessment findings in an amputation include the following[53]:

- Obvious tissue loss
- Pain
- Bleeding (may be uncontrolled and severe)
- Complete amputation: Transected vasculature will retract and spasm, which results in decreased hemorrhage.
- Partial amputation: Vasculature remains connected to the distal body part with blood flow remaining intact, increasing the risk of uncontrolled hemorrhage and exsanguination.
- Hypovolemic shock (may or may not be present)

Crush Injury

A crush injury is caused by prolonged compression to an area of the body, resulting in ischemia to nerves, soft tissues, and muscles.[29] Examples of mechanisms of injury that may cause this type of injury include being trapped under a vehicle, industrial or construction accidents, or falls. Direct muscle injury may lead to muscle ischemia and, ultimately, cell death, with subsequent release of myoglobin and other cellular components such as potassium and proteolytic enzymes.[29] Crush injuries can result in severe complications, including compartment syndrome, hyperkalemia and other acute metabolic derangements (hypocalcemia and hyponatremia), acute kidney injury, and rhabdomyolysis.

Crush injuries can also cause hemorrhage from the damaged tissue, destruction of muscle and bone tissue, fluid loss due to inflammation, and third spacing that results in hypovolemic shock and infection. The manifestation of cell death and the release of intracellular contents into systemic circulation following massive crush injuries is known as crush syndrome. Patients who develop crush syndrome can quickly develop life-threatening arrhythmias, shock and hypotension, and, eventually, renal failure, acute respiratory distress syndrome, disseminated intravascular coagulation, and death.[29,71]

Mangled Extremity

A severe variant of a crush injury is the mangled extremity.[12,29] These injuries typically result from devastating injury mechanisms that are rarely encountered in civilian trauma care but can occur with high-caliber ballistic injuries, injuries from pedestrian-versus-train accidents, or injuries that involve machinery or farm equipment. The mangled extremity has extensive injury to bones, soft tissue, muscles, nerves, and vasculature, but remains technically attached to the body.[10,50] A limb may be mangled and partially amputated.[10] These injuries are often isolated but can also be found in conjunction with multisystem trauma and are, by definition, distracting injuries. Hemorrhage control remains the primary priority for these patients, and wound management is similar to the care of an amputated part.

Devastating ischemia can occur in a matter of hours, so it is vital to manage these injuries quickly to preserve limb function.[41,50] The Mangled Extremity Severity Score (MESS) is a decision tool that was developed to assist providers in determining which limbs have a likelihood of successful salvage and which require amputation (**Table 10-11**).[10,41,50] Limb salvage often results in prolonged hospitalization, infection, and increased mortality. It is essential that potentially salvageable limbs be identified immediately, as well as limbs that cannot be salvaged. This ensures that the patient will receive the appropriate interventions, resulting in optimal long-term functioning and recovery.[10,50]

With the advent of aggressive treatment modalities such as fasciotomy, microvascular surgery, tourniquets, vascular shunts, and damage control surgery, mangled limb salvage is increasingly successful.[10,29,50] However, the success rate varies and is dependent on available resources and specialties. Hemostasis remains the priority of care and can be difficult to achieve with the widespread tissue damage that occurs with a mangled extremity. Mangled extremities involve ripped tissue and vasculature that can bleed more briskly than injuries from a guillotine or clean-cut mechanism.

Compartment Syndrome

Compartment syndrome is a serious complication of musculoskeletal injury that involves increased pressure inside a fascial compartment (**Figure 10-13**).[42] These compartments are nondistensible, so increased pressure is not well tolerated or accommodated.

Increased compartment pressures can inhibit blood flow, leading to muscle and nerve damage or destruction. Elevated compartment pressures are commonly caused by hematoma formation secondary to fractures, leading to increased pressure or decreased space.[71,72] Increased pressure may occur from internal or external sources. Internal sources of pressure include hemorrhage or edema from fractures or crush injuries; external sources

TABLE 10-11 Mangled Extremity Severity Score

	Characteristics	Details	Points
Tissue Injury			
1	Low energy	Stab wound, simple closed fracture, small-caliber bullet	1
2	Medium energy	Open fracture, dislocated, moderate crush	2
3	High energy	Short gun, high velocity	3
4	Massive crush	Logging, railroad	4
Shock			
1	Normotensive	Blood pressure stable	0
2	Transient hypotension	Blood pressure unstable, systolic blood pressure < 90 mm Hg	1
3	Hypotension	In operating room	2
Ischemia			
1	None	No signs of ischemia	0
2	Mild	Diminished pulses	1
3	Moderate	Paresthesia, diminished motor activity	2
4	Advanced	Pulseless, paralysis	3
Age			
1	< 30 years		0
2	> 30 to < 50 years		1
3	> 50 years		2

Data from Asif, S., Thaiban, M. A., Alghamdi, A., Alqahtani, M., Suliman, A. A., Alanazi, W., Alharthi, Y., Almatrafi, S., Alshammari, S., Alghamdi, F., & Alsharyah, S. (2021). Management of mangled extremities: Upper versus lower limb differences. *Journal of Healthcare Sciences*, Article JOHS2021000224. http://doi.org/10.52533/JOHS.2021.1104; Loja, M. N., Sammann, A., DuBose, J., Li, C.-S., Liu, Y., Savage, S., Scalea, T., Holcomb, J. B., Rasmussen, T. E., Knudson, M. M., & AAST PROOVIT Study Group. (2017). The mangled extremity score and amputation: Time for a revision. *Journal of Trauma and Acute Care Surgery*, 82(3), 518–523. https://doi.org/10.1097/TA.0000000000001339; Okereke, I., & Abdelfatah, E. (2022). Limb salvage versus amputation for the mangled extremity: Factors affecting decision-making and outcomes. *Cureus*, 14(8), Article e28153. https://doi.org/10.7759/cureus.28153

of pressure include casts, dressings, traction splints, air splints, clothing, or jewelry. Patients with a coagulopathy are at increased risk for developing compartment syndrome. The increased pressure compromises blood flow to nerves, blood vessels, and muscles, resulting in cellular ischemia.

The muscles of the lower leg or forearm are the most frequent sites of compartment syndrome, but this condition can occur in any fascial compartment, including the back, buttocks, thigh, abdomen, and foot.[71,72] The degree of damage depends on the amount of pressure and the length of time perfusion is compromised within the compartment.[5] Muscle necrosis can occur within hours, resulting in permanent loss of function, which may require amputation.[71,72] Tissue is less able to tolerate ischemia as compartment pressure increases. Measured compartment pressure elevation confirms compartment syndrome. Basing the diagnosis on the loss of palpable pulse may result in tissue damage, because this is often a late sign.[71] Frequent reassessment and identification of neurovascular compromise can improve patient outcomes.

Assessment Findings

Initial findings in compartment syndrome are a feeling of tightness or severe pain when the muscle is stretched, and rigidity on palpation. The Ps associated with compartment syndrome or any serious neurovascular compromise to an extremity can be useful in identifying this condition; however, aside from pain and pressure, they are late signs, and damage may already be irreversible.

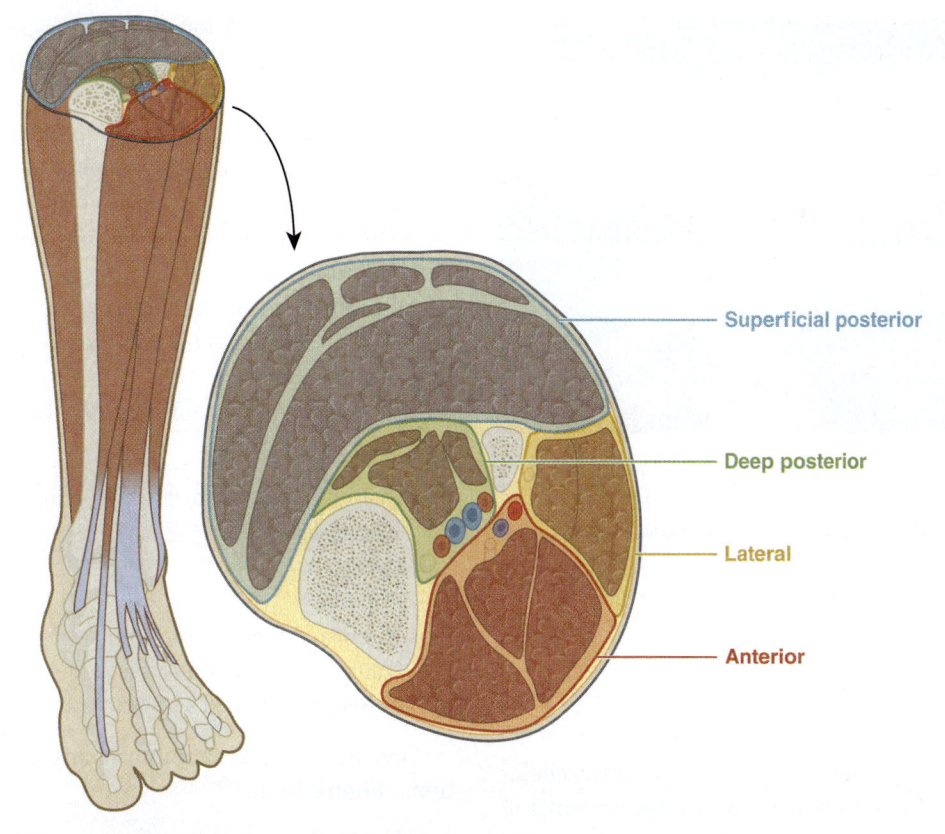

Figure 10-13 *Compartments of the lower leg.*
Data from Mayo Clinic. (n.d.). *Chronic exertional compartment syndrome.* http://www.mayoclinic.com/health/medical/IM00124

Any combination of these (or none at all) may be present in the patient with compartment syndrome. Following are the Ps[66,71,72]:

- **Pain:** A hallmark sign of compartment syndrome is pain out of proportion to the extent of the injury. Ischemic pain is often described as "burning" and is typically intense and severe. Pain with passive range of motion of the affected compartment can indicate development of, or existing, compartment syndrome.
- **Pressure:** The compartment or limb will feel tight or tense upon palpation. The skin may appear taut and shiny as the skin stretches.
- **Pulses:** Pulses can remain normal in the presence of compartment syndrome. Once compartment pressures are equal to or exceed the diastolic pressure within the arteries, weak or absent pulses may be noted—this is an ominous finding.
- **Paresthesia:** Numbness, tingling, or loss of sensation may occur as nerves and blood vessels are compressed. With loss of sensation, there may be relief of pain. This is indicative of a worsening perfusion, not an improvement.
- **Paralysis:** Motor dysfunction signifies injury to the nervous system.
- **Pallor:** Poor skin color and delayed capillary refill may indicate decreased perfusion.
- **Poikilothermia:** The limb may feel cool or assume the ambient temperature of the environment as a result of stagnation of blood in the limb.

When a patient is unconscious or unable to be clinically assessed at regular intervals, the affected extremity should be frequently assessed for the presence of tautness or tension. If possible, continuous measurement of the intramuscular pressure may be of benefit. Continuous pressure monitoring uses a prescribed perfusion pressure as a threshold for fasciotomy. Perfusion pressure is calculated as diastolic BP minus compartment pressure. Perfusion pressure sustained at less than 30 mm Hg (4 kPa) for 2 hours has a 93% positive predictive value for the diagnosis of acute compartment syndrome.[57] Fasciotomy may be safely avoided as long as the perfusion pressure remains greater than 30 mm Hg (4 kPa). Typically, the anterior compartment of the limb is monitored because the pressures within this compartment tend to be higher. When this method is used to assess compartment pressure, emergent fasciotomy may be avoided. **Figure 10-14** illustrates the measurement of compartment pressure in the posterior lower leg.[65]

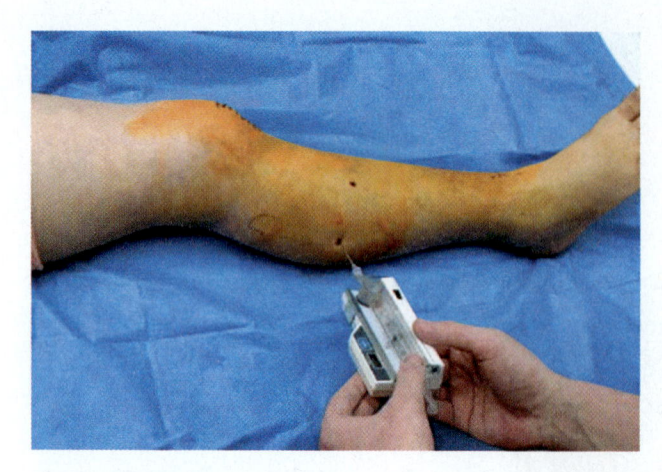

Figure 10-14 Compartment pressure measurement tool.

Reproduced from Tepordei, R. T., Stefan, G. T., Cozma, T., Nedelcu, A. H., Ovidiu, A., & Carmen, Z. L. (2014). A comparison of pressure measurement devices used in the acute compartment syndrome of the limbs. *Romanian Journal of Functional and Clinical, Macro- and Microscopical Anatomy and of Anthropology*, XIII(3), 369-372. http://revanatomie.ro/en/abstract.php?an_rev=2014&nr_rev=3&nr_art=23

Hyperkalemia

Potassium exists predominantly in the intracellular space, so cellular destruction releases large amounts of potassium into the serum, resulting in hyperkalemia and placing the patient at risk for cardiac dysrhythmias.[29] Elevation of potassium levels may be seen in the initial resuscitation period following a prolonged extraction or delayed transport. See Chapter 21, "Post-Resuscitation Care Considerations," for more information.

Rhabdomyolysis

Significant muscle damage and cellular destruction also release myoglobin, a muscle protein, into the bloodstream. Because myoglobin is excreted in the kidneys, the risk of acute kidney injury is high in patients with crush injury. The large myoglobin molecules can become trapped in the renal tubules, causing both prerenal and intrarenal failure. Patients with rhabdomyolysis are often profoundly hypovolemic because of the mechanism of muscle injury and vasoconstriction, and the third spacing caused by free radicals released during cellular lysis. This intravascular dehydration can exacerbate kidney injuries.[48] Assessment findings associated with rhabdomyolysis include the following:

- Muscle pain, numbness, or changes in sensation
- Muscle weakness or paralysis
- Dark red or brown urine (myoglobinuria)
- Extensive soft-tissue edema and bruising
- General weakness or malaise
- Evidence of hypovolemic shock, which may or may not be present
- Elevated creatine kinase levels

Treatment of rhabdomyolysis focuses on early intervention with aggressive fluid resuscitation to flush out myoglobin in order to prevent renal failure. It is recommended that the patient's urinary output be maintained at 100 mL per hour until the myoglobinuria is resolved.[5,48]

Joint Dislocations

Dislocations occur when the articulating surfaces of the joint become separated. Prolonged separation can cause nerve injury because of the anatomic proximity of nerves to the affected joint.

Assessment findings of joint dislocations include the following[5,19]:

- Inability to move the affected joint
- Joint deformity
- Pain
- Edema
- Abnormal range of motion
- Neurovascular compromise—diminished or absent pulses; diminished sensory function

Specific joint dislocations can have unique manifestations (**Figure 10-15**)[23]:

- Hip dislocations[11,19]
  - Often associated with significant trauma
  - 90% are posterior dislocations.
  - Complications of a hip dislocation:
    - Avascular necrosis of the femoral head
    - Sciatic nerve compression
    - Permanent disability
  - Reduction of the dislocated hip is a priority as soon as the patient is stabilized.

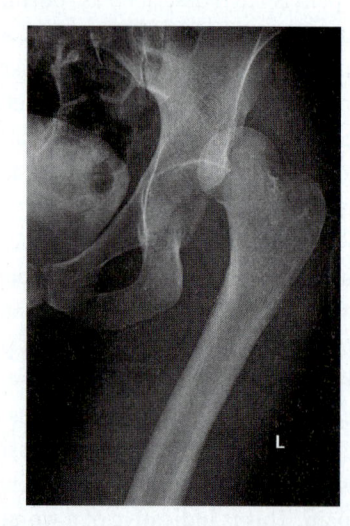

Figure 10-15 Radiograph of a posterior hip dislocation.

© 2022 Dr. Hani Makky Al Salam. Image courtesy of Dr. Hani Makky Al Salam and Radiopaedia.org.

- Ankle dislocations
  - May require immediate realignment to restore circulation
  - May occur in conjunction with open or closed fractures of the tibia/fibula
- Knee dislocations[33]
  - May result in peroneal nerve injury and damage to the popliteal artery and/or vein

Nursing Care of the Patient with Spinal and Musculoskeletal Trauma

Nursing care of the patient with spinal, vertebral column, and musculoskeletal injuries begins with preparation and triage.

Preparation and Triage

Preparation and triage include safe practice combined with safe care.

Safe Practice, Safe Care

A vital aspect of nursing care for patients with spinal and musculoskeletal trauma is the recognition that a vague history may indicate the presence of a serious injury. For example, an unwitnessed near-drowning may have sustained a SCI, an unconscious patient may have fallen, or the unresponsive infant arriving with seizures may have suffered abusive head trauma. When the mechanism is unclear, treat these patients as though they have a SCI until proven otherwise.

Triage

A patient with a spinal or musculoskeletal injury may meet the criteria for a higher triage acuity level in the case of a variety of findings, including hemodynamic instability, diminished respiratory effort from loss of innervation of the muscles of ventilation or thoracic injuries, changes in sensory and/or motor function, and alterations in level of consciousness.

Primary Survey and Resuscitation Adjuncts

Refer to Chapter 4, "Initial Assessment," for a systematic approach to the nursing care of the trauma patient. Because musculoskeletal injuries may have a dramatic presentation, they pose a significant risk of distraction to the trauma team. It is imperative that the systematic approach proceed as usual for every trauma patient regardless of readily apparent injuries.

A: Alertness and Airway

Cervical spinal motion restriction *is always* a part of the alertness and airway assessment and is particularly important in the patient with a significant MOI or suspected spinal injury. Patients with distracting musculoskeletal injuries (significant blood loss, open fractures) and those with possible intoxication or altered mental status are presumed to have sustained a SCI until proven otherwise.[6,62]

Assessment

Assess for an actual or suspected cervical spine injury.

Intervention

Place and maintain a cervical collar as indicated. Assess for correct placement and proper fit. Once motion restriction is verified, additional assessment of spinal cord integrity may be deferred until the completion of the primary survey. Apply manual stabilization as necessary throughout the primary and secondary surveys.

B: Breathing and Ventilation

Breathing and ventilation are assessed, and interventions are implemented as indicated.

Assessment

Shallow respirations or evidence of increased work of breathing may indicate a cervical or thoracic SCI. Cervical injuries may impair the patient's ability to breathe because of loss of phrenic nerve innervation, whereas thoracic injuries can result in loss of function of the muscles of respiration (intercostals).

Intervention

Be prepared to support a patient with an inadequate respiratory effort with bag-mask ventilation.

C: Circulation and Control of Hemorrhage

Identify the type of shock.

Assessment

Differentiate signs of hypovolemic/hemorrhagic shock from signs of neurogenic shock:

- Neurogenic shock presents with assessment findings of impaired cardiac output accompanied by bradycardia, a normal or strong pulse, and warm or flushed skin appearance.
- Hypovolemic/hemorrhagic shock is characterized by tachycardia, a weak peripheral pulse, and cool or pale skin. See Chapter 6, "Shock," for additional information.

Intervention

Intervention considerations include the following points:

- Use care when administering intravenous fluids to the patient in neurogenic shock to avoid development of pulmonary edema.
- Take measures to control hemorrhage.
- If there is no improvement in hypotension with fluid resuscitation, consider vasoactive support.[6]

D: Disability (Neurologic Status) Assessment

Disability or neurologic status assessment involves the following:

- The Glasgow Coma Scale (GCS) motor response score may not be reliable in the patient with a spinal or musculoskeletal injury. Score the patient's GCS as their highest level of motor response.
- Ineffective breathing, pain, or other causes may result in anxiety.

E: Exposure and Environmental Control

Identify exposure and environmental control considerations:

- Anticipate temperature instability with neurogenic shock that is due to peripheral vasodilation.
- External warming measures should be used. Continue to closely monitor temperature to avoid hypothermia or hyperthermia, given the potential for poikilothermia (inability to maintain body temperature).

G: Get Monitoring Devices and Give Comfort

Resuscitation adjuncts may include laboratory studies, monitoring, nasogastric or orogastric tubes, and oxygenation and ventilation management.

- **L: Laboratory studies.** Obtain arterial blood gas measurements to determine respiratory status and presence of ineffective gas exchange and cellular perfusion.
- **M: Monitoring.** Monitor cardiac rate/rhythm.
- **N: Nasogastric or orogastric tube.** Consider insertion of an orogastric tube for gastric decompression to prevent vomiting and potential aspiration of gastric contents in patients who must remain supine because of the need for spinal stabilization.
- **O: Oxygenation and ventilation.** Consider weaning oxygen based on oximetry to avoid hyperoxia. Monitor the effectiveness of oxygenation and ventilation with continuous pulse oximetry and capnography. Use capnography for early identification of inadequate ventilation, which may be masked because of the patient's inability to increase work of breathing.
- **P: Pain assessment and management.** Lack of pain may be a significant finding if SCI is suspected based on MOI or identified injuries.

Reevaluation

For known SCIs, early evaluation for interfacility transfer is recommended. If transfer is indicated, delegate or begin preparation before continuing to the secondary assessment. The American College of Surgeons supports transferring the patient with a known or suspected SCI to a specialized center or trauma center.[4,8] Spinal motion restriction during transport must be ensured.

Secondary Survey

The secondary survey involves the history, head-to-toe assessment, and inspection of posterior surfaces.

H: History

Questions specific to patients with spinal or musculoskeletal injuries include the following:

- Was there an MOI that is strongly associated with SCI?
- What symptoms were noted in the field, such as pain in the head or neck, numbness, tingling, loss of motor activity of the extremities, or loss of bladder or bowel control? Have the symptoms changed since the patient's arrival at the emergency department (ED)?
- What medications are currently used? Will any affect the assessment parameters in the patient (changes in heart rate and BP)?
- Is the patient's past medical history significant? Does the patient have diabetic neuropathy, which may affect the central nervous system examination? Is there a history of spinal injury, stenosis, arthritis, or osteoporosis that may increase the suspicion of injury despite a minor MOI?
- The MOI can reveal clues to specific trauma patterns. It is useful to know where the energy force was applied and where the pain is located. Attempt to reconstruct the event to determine the extent of injury and any potential injuries that may not be apparent. Utilize prehospital personnel to ensure complete understanding of the events surrounding the trauma, position of the patient, length of

extrication, and other pertinent factors. See Chapter 3, "Biomechanics and Mechanisms of Injury," for additional information.

Additional components of the history may include the following:

- MVCs
  - Extent of damage to the vehicle
  - Photographs of the vehicle/scene may be available from prehospital personnel or law enforcement.
  - Point of impact on the vehicle
  - Patient location within the vehicle and location at scene
  - Ejection from the vehicle
  - Air bag deployment
  - Use of a seat belt/restraint
  - Speed of the vehicle
  - Pedestrian struck by vehicle
  - Speed of the vehicle upon impact
  - Height or size/make of the vehicle
  - Vehicle points of impact
  - Patient point of impact
  - Dragged/thrown by vehicle
- Falls
  - Height of the fall
  - Landing surface: concrete, gravel, sand, grass, and so on
  - Point of impact: feet, head, back, and so on
- Crush injuries
  - Weight of crushing object
  - Length of time compressed/entrapped:
    - Longer periods of compression increase the risk of rhabdomyolysis and hyperkalemia and their speed of onset.
    - Body part or parts affected
- Blast injuries
  - Distance between the patient and the point of blast
  - Flying debris
  - Patient thrown by blast

Documentation that reflects an accurate and thorough initial assessment and history will facilitate trending of signs and symptoms. The absence of these symptoms with subsequent development later may indicate expansion of a hematoma or edema formation.

H: Head-to-Toe Assessment

Head-to-toe assessment covers the neck and cervical spine, pelvis/perineum, and extremities.

Neck and Cervical Spine

Palpate for the following:

- Use a second person to maintain manual stabilization of the cervical spine while opening the collar for palpation.[6] Close the collar after assessment, and confirm its proper placement.
- Gently palpate the neck for pain, tenderness, crepitus, subcutaneous emphysema, or step-off deformities between vertebrae.
- Frequently remind the patient to remain still during palpation and examination, and to avoid shaking or nodding the head; instead, the patient should verbalize areas that are painful on examination.

Cervical Spine Clearance

The prevalence of cervical spinal injury is approximately 2% following trauma, and accurate, timely diagnosis is imperative for avoiding catastrophic consequences.[7,35] The American College of Surgeons *Best Practices Guidelines: Spine Injury*[7] provides direction for clearing the cervical spine and recommended methodologies for diagnosing spinal injuries.

Two clinical decision tools to assess the patient's need for cervical spine imaging following trauma are the Canadian C-Spine Rule (**Appendix 10-1**)[16] and the National Emergency X-Radiography Utilization Study (NEXUS; **Appendix 10-2**).[18] These tools are used to evaluate the patient for cervical spine injury and to assist in determining whether imaging is necessary.[6,7] Additional screening guidelines are identified in **Box 10-1**; follow facility policies and/or protocols regarding screening for cervical spine injury.[6]

Table 10-12 lists normal extremity movement with associated levels of innervation.

Head

Sudden vision or mental status changes may indicate a possible fat embolism in the cerebral vasculature.[2]

Chest

Assess for a fat embolism within the pulmonary vasculature, which is a complication of long bone fractures. It may be evidenced by acute respiratory difficulty in a patient with multiple injuries and petechiae on the chest.[2]

Pelvis/Perineum

Assess for the presence of priapism. This may be a sign of loss of sympathetic nervous system control and stimulation of the parasympathetic nervous system.

BOX 10-1 American College of Surgeons Guidelines for Screening Patients with Suspected Spine Injury

If the patient exhibits paraplegia or tetraplegia, assume spinal instability.

In patients who are awake, alert, and not under the influence, and who have no neurologic abnormalities, assume the following:

- If there is no presence of neck pain, midline tenderness, or distracting injury, an acute cervical spine fracture or instability is unlikely.
- After the collar is removed and a manual palpation of the neck is performed, if there is no pain, and the patient is able to move the neck without pain, imaging is not necessary.
- If neck pain and midline tenderness are present, imaging is necessary. Multidetector axial CT is recommended where available. The alternative is lateral, AP, and open-mouth odontoid radiographs of the cervical spine and axial CT of any suspicious areas, or the lower cervical spine if not well visualized on radiographs. Views must include the spine down to T1.
  - If images are normal, the cervical collar can be removed. If suspicion for injury remains, replace the collar and consult a spine specialist.

For patients who have an altered level of consciousness or are nonverbal (e.g., children who cannot describe their symptoms), take the following approach:

- Multidetector axial CT is recommended where available.
- The alternative is the same as in the list above, with CT optional in children.
- If the cervical spine is normal, the cervical collar can be removed after evaluation by a physician.
- When in doubt, leave the collar on.

Consult a physician skilled in evaluating and managing patients with spine injuries when spine injury is suspected or determined.

Evaluate patients with neurologic deficits (paraplegia or tetraplegia) rapidly and remove them from the spine board as soon as possible. This is most safely accomplished using the lift and slide or six-person lift technique because logrolling has been shown to cause unacceptable motion in an unstable spine.[24,55]

In patients who require emergency surgery before the completion of a complete spine evaluation:

- Transport the patient carefully, and assume that an unstable spine injury is present.
- Leave the cervical collar on, and strongly consider using a slide sheet or other lateral transfer device, with a team approach, to move the patient to and from the operating table instead of logrolling.[52] The healthcare team should use the safest technique possible based on the staff and handling devices available.
- Remove the patient from the spine board as early as is safely possible.
- Inform the anesthesiologist and surgical team of the status of the spine evaluation.

Vertebral Column Spine Injury

Paraplegia or sensory loss at the level of the chest or abdomen may indicate spinal instability.

For patients who are awake, alert, and not under the influence, and who have no neurologic abnormalities and midline thoracic or lumbar back pain or tenderness, do the following:

- Palpate and inspect the entire spine. If no tenderness is present on palpation and no ecchymosis is noted over the spinous processes, unstable fracture is unlikely, and imaging may not be necessary.

For patients with spine pain or tenderness on palpation or with neurologic deficits, an altered level of consciousness, or suspected intoxication, the following is true:

- AP and lateral radiographs are recommended.
- Thin-cut axial CT is recommended if suspicious areas are seen on radiographs.
- Ensure films are good quality and read by an experienced physician prior to spine clearance.
- Consult a physician skilled in evaluating and managing patients with spine injuries when spine injury is suspected or determined.

AP = anteroposterior; CT = computed tomography.

Data from American College of Surgeons. (2018). Spine and spinal cord trauma. In *Advanced trauma life support: Student course manual* (10th ed., pp. 128–147).

TABLE 10-12 Assessment of Innervation Levels

Movement	Innervation
Extend and flex arms	C5 to C7
Extend and flex legs	L2 to L4
Flexion of foot; extension of toes	L4 to L5
Tighten anus	S3 to S5

Extremities

Inspect for the following:

- Uncontrolled bleeding
- Deformities or tissue abnormalities, which may indicate the presence of fractures or dislocations
- Neurovascular status
- Color, position, and any obvious differences in the injured extremity as compared with the uninjured extremity, such as shortening, rotation, displacement, or loss of function
- Extremity movement and control. Ask the patient to wiggle the toes and fingers and to lift the arms and legs to assess.
- The inability to perform gross extremity movement indicates the possibility of a SCI at or above the level of the extremity.
- Occult peripheral vascular injuries. Assess the ankle brachial index or arterial pressure index to detect.[26]

Palpate for the following:

- The presence of crepitus, step-off deformity, or the development of edema in all extremities
- Skin temperature
- All four extremities, assessing for muscle strength, sensory function, and response to pain and pressure
- Levels of sensory function. Use a pinprick beginning distally and proceeding proximally to aid in localizing the level of injury.[6]
- Pain with passive range of motion of the affected compartment. This can indicate development of or existing compartment syndrome.
- Proprioception. This can be assessed by moving the great toe up, down, or in a neutral position and asking the patient to describe the position.[6]

Interventions

Interventions for musculoskeletal injuries include the following:

- Control of hemorrhage by direct pressure, compression dressings, or tourniquets
- Immobilizing the affected extremity to prevent further injury, bleeding, and pain

Splinting

Splinting is usually performed during or after the secondary survey, dependent on the risk to the patient. Remove clothing and jewelry before splinting and immobilization. Types of splints (**Figure 10-16**) include the following:

- Rigid splints, such as cardboard, plastic, or metal splints. Pad to prevent pressure injury to bony prominences.
- Soft splints or air splints
- Traction splints. Apply for midshaft femur fractures (**Figure 10-17**).
- Custom splints with fiberglass casting materials

Guidelines for splint application include the following[3,64]:

- If the patient has an obvious deformity or bony protrusion, do not attempt to reposition the limb.
- Assess pulse, temperature, color, and pulse quality before and after each attempt to immobilize the limb or move the patient.
    - Note any losses of a previously palpable pulse; changes in temperature, color, or pulse quality; or increased pain.
    - If these findings are present, repositioning of the extremity may be indicated. Remove the splints, and notify the physician.
- When applying a splint or other immobilizing device, include joints above and below the deformity.
    - Avoid movement of the fractured extremity, which can increase bleeding and the risk of fat embolism or result in an inadvertent open fracture.
- Elevate the extremity.
    - If compartment syndrome is suspected, elevate the limb to the level of the heart. Avoid elevating the limb higher than the heart because this can reduce circulation and tissue perfusion.[71]
    - If compartment syndrome is not a risk, elevate the limb above the level of the heart to reduce pain and swelling.
- Assess and treat pain, to include administration of pain medications as prescribed.
- Prepare for procedural sedation according to institutional policy for the reduction of fracture/dislocations.
- Apply ice to reduce swelling and pain for 20 minutes. Do not place ice directly on the skin.
    - If compartment syndrome is suspected, ice is strongly contraindicated.

216 Chapter 10 Spinal and Musculoskeletal Trauma

A Long arm posterior splint
B Sugar tong forearm splint
C Ulnar gutter splint
D Thumb spica splint
E Volar splint
F Posterior ankle splint
G Ankle stirrup splint

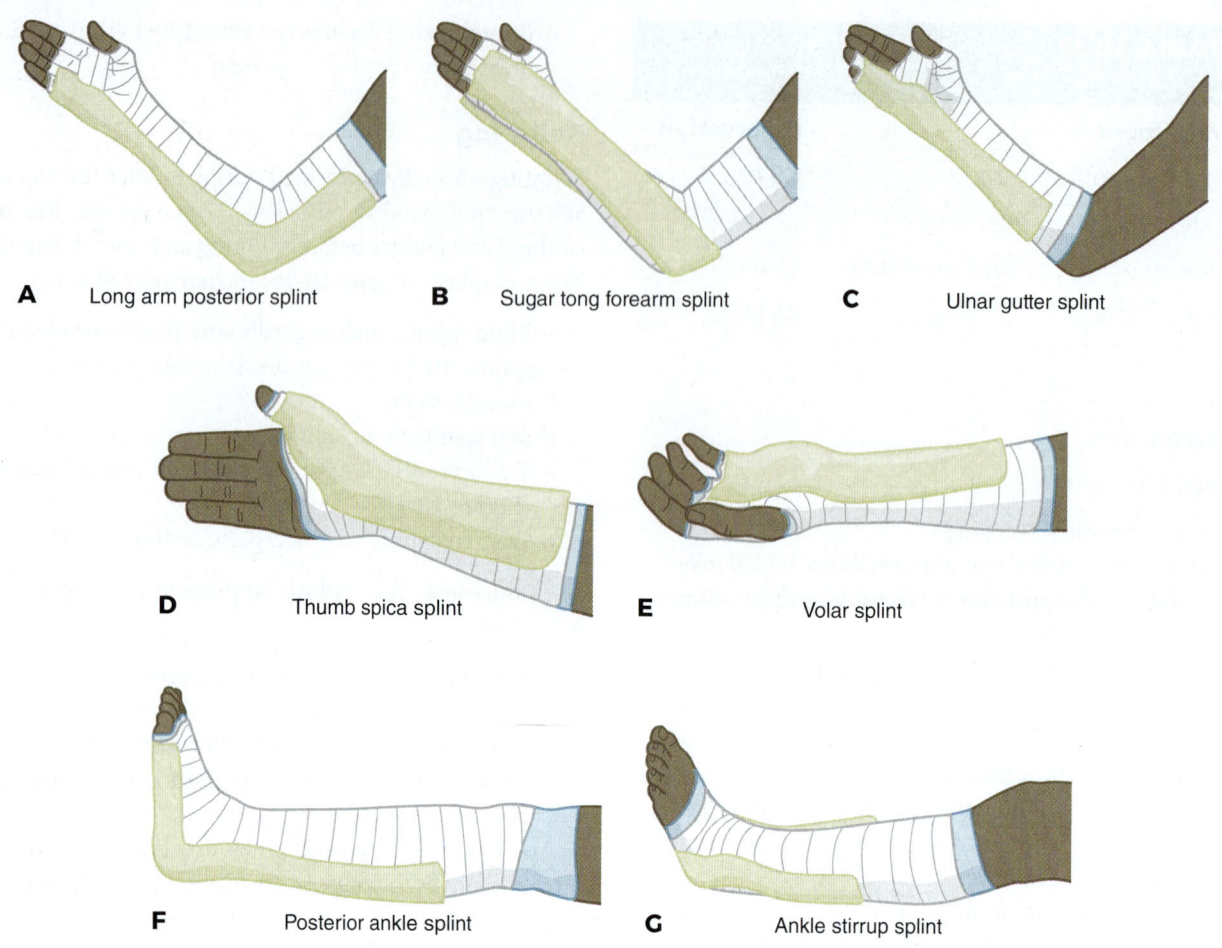

Figure 10-16 *Selected types of splints. The light blue layer is the stockinette, the white layer is the cotton roll, and the beige layer is the splint.* **A.** *Long arm posterior splint.* **B.** *Sugar tong forearm splint.* **C.** *Ulnar gutter splint.* **D.** *Thumb spica splint.* **E.** *Volar splint.* **F.** *Posterior ankle splint.* **G.** *Ankle stirrup splint.*

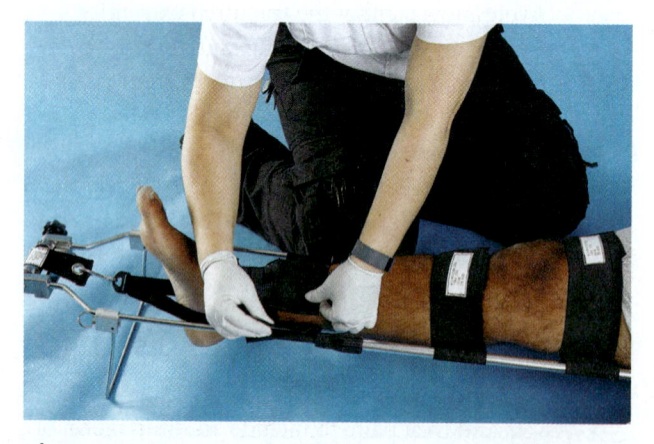

Figure 10-17 *Traction splint for midshaft femur fracture.*
© Jones & Bartlett Learning.

I: Inspect Posterior Surfaces

If a spinal injury is suspected, imaging should be obtained before inspecting the patient's posterior surfaces. However, logrolling may be indicated, as noted earlier, if there is suspicion of penetrating injury causing hemodynamic instability or airway compromise.[45,55] If imaging is deferred or confirms the presence of an unstable spine, extreme caution, with consideration of risks and benefits, is used with any patient movement. The healthcare team uses the safest technique possible based on the available staff and handling devices. Alternate methods to move the patient include air-assisted mattresses and the 6-plus lift and slide.[24,55] If there is a low index of suspicion for a spinal instability, logroll the patient, inspecting the posterior surfaces to assess the vertebral column for deformity, tenderness, open wounds, or impaled objects.

- Palpate the entire vertebral column gently for pain, tenderness, crepitus, or step-off deformities.
- Assess for rectal tone.
    - An alternative to a digital rectal exam (DRE) is to ask the alert patient to squeeze the buttocks together.

- Assess for sacral sparing.
  - When seen in conjunction with focal deficits, the presence of perianal sensation and anal sphincter tone represents an incomplete SCI.[62] Note, however, that perianal sensation and anal sphincter tone may be absent until the resolution of spinal shock.
- Assess for reflexes.
  - In the presence of spinal shock, the patient may present with diminished or absent reflexes. A Babinski or plantar reflex is a pathologic response in anyone age 1 year or older because of dysfunction of upper motor neurons of the corticospinal tract. See Chapter 13, "The Pediatric Trauma Patient," for more information.
  - Deep tendon reflexes are tested with a reflex hammer by tapping sharply on the tendon and observing for a jerk or contraction of the muscle.

Interventions for Selected Injuries

This section covers interventions for open fracture, amputation/penetrating injury, and crush injury and compartment syndrome.

Open Fracture

Interventions for an open fracture include the following[5]:

- Remove gross contaminants.
- Cover open wounds with a moist sterile dressing.
- Administer antibiotics as ordered.
- Administer tetanus according to current Centers for Disease Control and Prevention (CDC) guidelines.

Amputation/Penetrating Injury

Interventions for an amputation/penetrating injury include the following:

- Apply direct pressure on sites with active bleeding, or compress the artery above the bleeding site.
- Elevate the extremity.
- Tourniquets are used when pressure and elevation fail to control bleeding.
  - Pneumatic tourniquets may be required for stabilization of complex injuries.[5]
  - Place tourniquets as close to the amputation site as possible to limit ischemia and nerve compression.
  - Tourniquets may be placed on bare skin or over clothing. Bulky or layered clothing may decrease effectiveness. Do not cover tourniquet with any clothing to ensure that it can be seen by all medical providers.

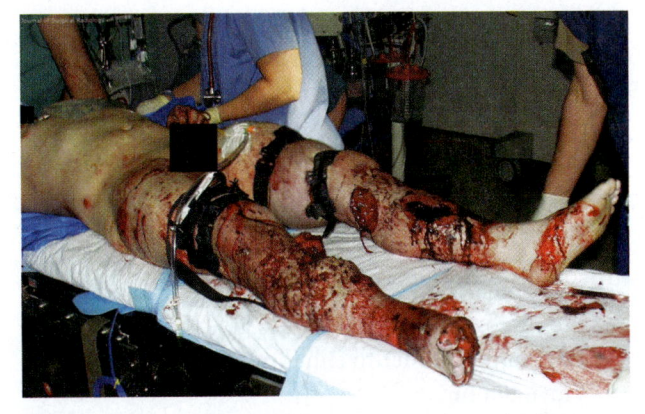

Figure 10-18 *A second tourniquet placed above the first.*
© Surgisphere Corporation. All Rights Reserved. Image used with permission.

  - Clearly mark the time of placement on the device, and document it in the medical record (to track "ischemic time," tourniquets may be left in place for more than 6 hours with only transient nerve dysfunction).[49]
  - If a single tourniquet fails to control bleeding, a second tourniquet may be placed no more than 2 inches above the first (**Figure 10-18**).[22]
  - A tourniquet that is tight enough to control arterial bleeding will be extremely painful to the patient. If a tourniquet is not sufficiently tightened, it may compress veins but not arteries. This will cause congestion of the limb and paradoxical worsening of bleeding.
  - Do not release the tourniquet unless a physician is present and prepared to manage the bleeding, surgically if necessary.
  - Tourniquets are a valuable lifesaving measure for amputations with uncontrolled bleeding and significantly reduce mortality when applied before the development of decompensated shock.
- Remove dirt or debris from the amputated part and the residual limb.
  - Residual limb refers to the part of the body that remains after an amputation. For instance, the part of the thigh that remains following an above-the-knee amputation is the residual limb.[59]
- Keep the amputated part cool by wrapping it in saline-moistened sterile gauze, and then place it in a sealed plastic bag.
  - The bag containing the amputated part is then placed in a second bag containing a mixture of 50% ice and 50% water.
  - Do not allow the amputated part to freeze or be submerged in liquid.
  - Label the bag with appropriate patient identifiers.

- Administer antibiotics as ordered.
- Administer tetanus prophylaxis according to current CDC guidelines.

Crush Injury and Compartment Syndrome

Interventions for crush injury and compartment syndrome include the following:

- Administer an IV isotonic crystalloid solution to increase urinary output to at least 100 mL per hour in order to enhance the excretion of myoglobin.[5]
- Remove casts, splints, or dressings.
- Elevate the limb only to the level of the heart to promote circulation.[71]
- Initiate noninvasive hemodynamic and cardiac monitoring to observe for dysrhythmias.
- Prepare for measuring fascial compartment pressure. This is typically performed by a physician, who inserts a large-caliber needle or catheter into the fascia of the involved muscle and attaches it to a manometer or intercompartmental pressure monitor. A noninvasive method of measuring compartmental pressure is to use near-infrared spectroscopy to measure decreased tissue blood flow.[63] Normal pressure is 0–8 mm Hg (0–1.1 kPa). Elevated readings of 30–40 mm Hg (4–5.3 kPa) are suggestive of ischemia to muscles and nerves; when pressures exceed 30 mm Hg (4 kPa) in any compartment, capillary beds are occluded.
- Anticipate an emergent fasciotomy, if indicated, to decompress the compartment in order to prevent muscle and/or neurovascular damage and loss of the limb. Surgical debridement or amputation may also be necessary.
- Facilitate emergent transfer either to the operating room or to a center with microvascular surgical capabilities for patients with potentially salvageable mangled extremities.

Reevaluation Diagnostic Procedures

Diagnostic procedures include radiographic studies and medications.

Radiographic Studies

Anticipate a CT scan of the cervical, thoracic, and lumbar spine as indicated. If plain radiographic imaging of the cervical spine is used, verify visualization of all cervical vertebrae from the occiput through T1, including lateral, anteroposterior, and open-mouth odontoid views.[6]

Unless contraindicated, magnetic resonance imaging may be used to evaluate ligamentous and cord injuries.[6]

Medications

Hypotension should be treated with a cautious combination of fluid resuscitation and vasopressors. Care should be exercised to avoid overhydration in the SCI patient who is already peripherally vasodilated. Complications of excessive fluid resuscitation can include pulmonary congestion, generalized edema, and abdominal compartment syndrome.

The choice of vasopressor for the hypotensive patient with SCI depends on the level of injury. Possibilities generally include dopamine, epinephrine, norepinephrine, and phenylephrine. Dopamine, epinephrine, and norepinephrine are frequent choices for patients with cervical or high thoracic SCI because of these vasopressors' inotropic, chronotropic, and vasoconstrictive properties. Use of phenylephrine in these patients can worsen existing bradycardia because of its sole vasoconstrictive nature. For patients with a low thoracic SCI with hypotension due primarily to peripheral vasodilation, norepinephrine and phenylephrine work well by providing powerful vasoconstrictive effects.[58]

Administer pain management medications as indicated.

Diagnostics and Interventions for Musculoskeletal Trauma

Additional diagnostic studies for patients with musculoskeletal trauma include the following:

- Anterior-posterior and lateral radiographs of the injured extremity are necessary. Some fractures can be seen only from one angle, which may require an additional oblique view. The images need to include the joints above and below the injury. In children, radiographs of the noninjured extremity may be helpful for comparison.
- CT scans can be used for more definitive evaluation of musculoskeletal trauma and for assessment of damage to surrounding organs. CT scans can also identify organic foreign bodies such as retained splinters.
- Angiography can be performed to identify tears or compressions in the vasculature of the injured extremity.
- Noninvasive near-infrared spectroscopy to measure decreased tissue blood flow can be useful in diagnosing compartment syndrome.

Reevaluation and Post-Resuscitation Care

Reevaluation includes monitoring of neuromuscular status, maintaining homeostasis, and further reevaluation to determine the type and degree of injury. Key points include the following:

- Maintain spinal motion restriction.
- Monitor breathing effectiveness. Patients with disruption of the innervation to the intercostal muscles develop respiratory fatigue and must be monitored closely.
- Monitor changes in sensory and motor function.
- Monitor core temperature to avoid hypothermia.
- Assess the Ps.
- Check urinary output and for the presence of myoglobinuria.
- Maintain control of bleeding (especially after resuscitation with IV fluids or blood products).

Definitive Care or Transport

Prepare the patient for definitive stabilization, operative intervention, hospital admission, or transfer.

If the decision has not already been made, reassess the patient and prepare for interfacility transfer as needed. Careful attention is given to spinal motion restriction during transport as well as serial assessments for changes in condition.[6]

Emerging Trends

As the science of trauma care continues to evolve, interventions to improve patient outcomes are tested, and new standards of care are transitioned into practice. This section on trauma care considerations explores some of the evidence and the potential significance to trauma patient care. In the care of patients with spinal cord and vertebral column injuries, evidence related to cervical spinal clearance, stem cell research, and hypothermia for SCIs is discussed.

Stem Cell Research

Stem cells are unspecialized cells capable of regenerating or proliferating through cell division. They can be induced to become tissue- or organ-specific cells; they are very capable of proliferating. In contrast, nerve cells do not usually repair, duplicate, or replicate.[46] Research is being done on application of stem cells to neurogeneration in spinal cord injuries.[36]

The use of neural stem cells to promote remyelination of nerve cells appears to be promising based on the capability of such cells to promote axonal regeneration through growing axons in the area of ischemia and/or injury.[36,46] Stem cell research in patients with SCI is ongoing.

Hypothermia

Therapeutic hypothermia remains experimental. Research continues to evaluate its efficacy and potential benefit in SCI. The use of hypothermia in the treatment of SCIs has demonstrated possible beneficial effects. Although relatively safe according to research, it is not without potential complications, including systemic hypothermia.[54] Research on hypothermia for its potential to improve neurologic recovery for patients with SCI is ongoing.[54]

Summary

Blunt and penetrating injuries to the vertebral column and skeletal system may result in fractures, subluxations, or dislocations. Knowledge of the MOI—including the type of force applied and the resulting flexion, extension, rotation, or compression—is important during the assessment of the trauma patient.

Although many studies are currently examining the ischemic damage to the spinal cord and regeneration of the myelinated nerve fibers, there is no substitution for the initiation and maintenance of spinal motion restriction.

The Canadian C-Spine Rule and the NEXUS created criteria for clearing patients at low risk for unstable fractures or ligamentous injury to reduce unnecessary imaging. Each institution may have its own policies guiding cervical spine clearance; the criteria in Appendix 10-1 and Appendix 10-2 are provided for reference. Please refer to your institution's policies.

Extremity injuries are usually addressed during the secondary survey. However, some injuries may be life threatening and require immediate intervention for uncontrolled hemorrhage prior to arrival (**Figure 10-19**) or during the primary survey. Consideration is also given to injuries that may result in disability and loss of limb. The secondary survey is carefully conducted to identify all injuries. Early intervention for suspected fractures, including neurovascular assessment before and after any splint application, can help to prevent further injury. Pain is important to consider in musculoskeletal injuries. Splinting and pain medication can be effective in the treatment of pain.

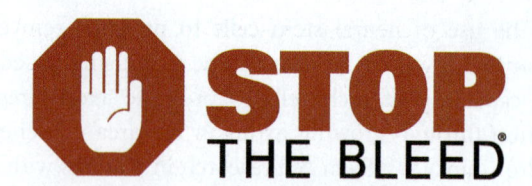

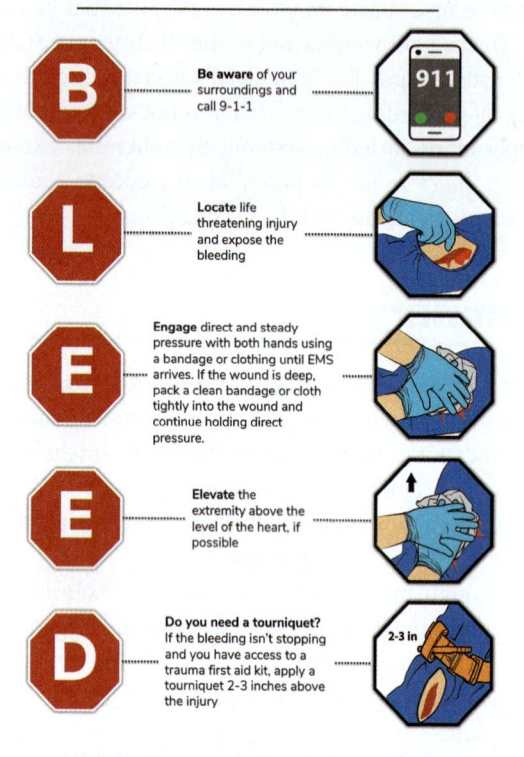

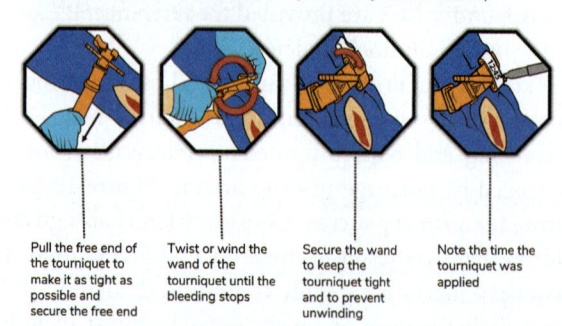

Figure 10-19 *"Stop the Bleed" educational poster.*
© 2021 Emergency Nurses Association.

References

1. Alizadeh, A., Dyck, S. M., & Karimi-Abdolrezaee, S. (2019). Traumatic spinal cord injury: An overview of pathophysiology, models and acute injury mechanisms. *Frontiers in Neurology, 10*, Article 282. https://doi.org/10.3389%2Ffneur.2019.00282

2. Alpert, M., Grigorian, A., Scolaro, J., Learned, J., Dolich, M., Kuza, C. M., Lekawa, M., & Nahmias, J. (2020). Fat embolism syndrome in blunt trauma patients with extremity fractures. *Journal of Orthopaedics 21*, 475–480. https://doi.org/10.1016%2Fj.jor.2020.08.040

3. Althoff, A. D., & Reeves, R. A. (2022, August 8). Splinting. *StatPearls*. StatPearls Publishing. https://www.ncbi.nlm.nih.gov/books/NBK557673/

4. American College of Surgeons. (2018). Geriatric trauma. In *Advanced trauma life support: Student course manual* (10th ed., pp. 214–224).

5. American College of Surgeons. (2018). Musculoskeletal trauma. In *Advanced trauma life support: Student course manual* (10th ed., pp. 148–167).

6. American College of Surgeons. (2018). Spine and spinal cord trauma. In *Advanced trauma life support: Student course manual* (10th ed., pp. 128–147).

7. American College of Surgeons. (2022). *Best practices guidelines: Spine injury*. https://www.facs.org/media/k45gikqv/spine_injury_guidelines.pdf

8. American College of Surgeons. (2022). *Resources for optimal care of the injured patient: 2022 standards*.

9. Anandasivam, N. S., Ondeck, N. T., Bagi, P. S., Galivanche, A. R., Samule, A. M., Bohl, D. D., & Grauer, J. N. (2021). Spinal fractures and/or spinal cord injuries are associated with orthopedic and internal organ injuries in proximity to the spinal injury. *North American Spine Society Journal, 6*, Article 100057. https://doi.org/10.1016/j.xnsj.2021.100057

10. Asif, S., Thaiban, M. A., Alghamdi, A., Alqahtani, M., Suliman, A. A., Alanazi, W., Alharthi, Y., Almatrafi, S., Alshammari, S., Alghamdi, F., & Alsharyah, S. (2021). Management of mangled extremities: Upper vs. lower limb differences. *Journal of Healthcare Sciences*, Article JOHS2021000224. http://doi.org/10.52533/JOHS.2021.1104

11. Assad, W., Alhammoud, A., Younis, M. H., Al Ateeq, A., & Alhaneedi, G. A. (2020). The trend in the management of traumatic hip dislocation in Qatar: A retrospective observational study. *International Journal of Orthopaedics, 7*(6), 1402–1406. http://www.ghrnet.org/index.php/ijo/article/view/3010/3373

12. Bain, K., Parizh, D., Kopatsis, A., & Kilaru, R. (2016). Mangled extremity: To salvage or not to salvage? *BMJ Case Reports*. https://doi.org/10.1136/bcr-2016-218359

13. Ball, C. G. (2015). Penetrating nontorso trauma: The extremities. *Canadian Journal of Surgery, 58*(4), 286–288. http://doi.org/10.1503/cjs.005815

14. Bennett, J., Das, J. M., & Emmady, P. D. (2022, May 11). Spinal cord injuries. *StatPearls*. StatPearls Publishing. https://www.ncbi.nlm.nih.gov/books/NBK560721/

15. Cairns, C., Kang, K., & Santo, L. (2018). *National hospital ambulatory medical care survey: 2018 emergency department summary*

tables. U.S. Department of Health and Human Services, Centers for Disease Control and Prevention, National Center for Health Statistics. https://www.cdc.gov/nchs/data/nhamcs/web_tables/2018-ed-web-tables-508.pdf

16. Clement, C., Stiell, I., Davies, B., O'Connor, A., Brehaut, J., Sheehan, P., Clavet, T., Leclair, C., MacKenzie, T., & Beland, C. (2011). Perceived facilitators and barriers to clinical clearance of the cervical spine by emergency department nurses: A major step towards changing practice in the emergency department. *International Emergency Nursing, 19*(1), 44–52. https://doi.org/10.1016/j.ienj.2009.12.002

17. Criddle, L. M. (Ed.). (2022). Spine and spinal cord injuries. In *TCAR trauma care after resuscitation* (11th ed., pp. 147–161). TCAR Education Programs.

18. Davenport, M. (2017). Cervical spine fracture evaluation workup. *Medscape*. Retrieved August 18, 2017, from http://emedicine.medscape.com/article/824380-overview

19. Dawson-Amoah, K., Raszewski, J., Duplantier, N., & Waddell, B. S. (2018). Dislocation of the hip: A review of types, causes, and treatment. *Ochsner Journal, 18*(3), 242–252. https://doi.org/10.31486/toj.17.0079

20. Denisiuk, M., & Afsari, A. (2022, February 4). Femoral shaft fractures. *StatPearls*. StatPearls Publishing. https://www.ncbi.nlm.nih.gov/books/NBK556057/#:~:text=Femoral%20shaft%20fractures%20(FSF)%20typically,ATLS)%20assessment%20and%20interdisciplinary%20care

21. Ding, W., Hu, S., Wang, P., Kang, H., Peng, R., Dong, Y., & Li, F. (2022). Spinal cord injury: The global incidence, prevalence, and disability from the global burden of disease study 2019. *Spine, 47*(21), 1532–1540. https://doi.org/10.1097/BRS.0000000000004417

22. Donley, E. R., & Loyd, J. W. (2022, July 19). Hemorrhage control. *StatPearls*. StatPearls Publishing. https://www.ncbi.nlm.nih.gov/books/NBK535393/

23. El-Fecky, M. (2021, February 16). Posterior dislocation of the hip. *Radiopaedia*. https://doi.org/10.53347/rID-7265

24. Emergency Nurses Association. (2016). *Avoiding the log roll maneuver: Alternative methods for safe patient handling* [Topic brief]. https://enau.ena.org/Users/LearningActivity/LearningActivityDetail.aspx?LearningActivityID=LJMRSp85WwPew%2bHMK6%2b5YQ%3d%3d

25. Emos, M. C., & Agarwal, S. (2022, August 22). Neuroanatomy, upper motor neuron lesion. *StatPearls*. StatPearls Publishing. https://www.ncbi.nlm.nih.gov/books/NBK537305/#:~:text=Upper%20motor%20neurons%20are%20first,movement%20is%20the%20pyramidal%20tract

26. Feliciano, D. V. (2017). Pitfalls in the management of peripheral vascular injuries. *Trauma Surgery & Acute Care Open, 2*(1), Article e000110. https://doi.org/10.1136/tsaco-2017-000110

27. Fox, A. D. (2014). Spinal shock: Assessment and treatment of spinal cord injuries and neurogenic shock. *Journal of Emergency Medical Services, 39*(11), 64–67. https://www.jems.com/patient-care/assessment-and-treatment-spinal-cord-inj/

28. Gao, T., Huang, F., Xie, Y., Wang, W., Wang, L., Liu-Di, M., Mu, D., Cuy, Y., & Wang, B. (2021). Dynamic changes in the systemic immune response of spinal cord injury model mice. *Neural Regeneration Research, 16*(2), 382–387. https://doi.org/10.4103/1673-5374.290910

29. Godat, L. N., & Doucet, J. J. (2021). Severe crush injury in adults. *UpToDate*. Retrieved October 19, 2022, from https://www.uptodate.com/contents/severe-crush-injury-in-adults/print?sectionName=Crush%20syndrome&search=covid-19&topicRef=7227&anchor=H2157260626&source=see_link

30. Graham, J. K. (2022). Shock, sepsis, and multiple organ dysfunction syndrome. In K. A. McQuillan & M. B. Flynn Makic (Eds.), *Trauma nursing: From resuscitation through rehabilitation* (5th ed., pp. 831–864). Elsevier.

31. Hachem, L. A. (2017). Assessment and management of acute spinal cord injury: From point of injury to rehabilitation. *Journal of Spinal Cord Medicine, 40*(6), 665–675. https://doi.org/10.1080/10790268.2017.1329076

32. Hamilton, R., Kirshblum, S., Sikka, S., Callender, L., Bennett, M., & Prajapati, P. (2018). Sacral examination in spinal cord injury: Is it really needed? *The Journal of Spinal Cord Medicine, 41*(5), 556–561. https://doi.org/10.1080%2F10790268.2017.1410307

33. Harris, B. T., Eichman, E. A., & Burrus, M. T. (2021). Traumatic simultaneous bilateral knee dislocation: A case report. *Cureus, 13*(10), Article e18989. https://doi.org/10.7759/cureus.18989

34. Harrow-Mortelliti, M., Reddy, V., & Jimsheleishvili, G. (2022, January 29). Physiology, spinal cord. *StatPearls*. StatPearls Publishing. https://www.ncbi.nlm.nih.gov/books/NBK544267/

35. Haske, D., Lefering, R., Stock, J. P., & Kreinest, M. (2022). Epidemiology and predictors of traumatic spine injury in severely injured patients: Implications for emergency procedures. *European Journal of Trauma and Emergency Surgery, 48*, 1975–1983. https://doi.org/10.1007/s00068-020-01515-w

36. Huang, L., Fu, C., & Wei, Q. (2021). Stem cell therapy for spinal cord injury. *Cell Transplantation, 30*. https://doi.org/10.1177/0963689721989266

37. Kaji, A. H., & Hockberger, R. S. (2018). Spinal injuries. In R. M. Walls, R. S. Hockberger, & M. Gausche-Hill (Eds.), *Rosen's emergency medicine: Concepts and clinical practice* (9th ed., Vol. 1, pp. 345–371). Elsevier/Saunders.

38. Kaji, A., & Hockberger, R. S. (2022). Spinal column injuries in adults: Definitions, mechanisms, and radiographs. *UpToDate*. Retrieved October 19, 2022, from https://www.uptodate.com/contents/spinal-column-injuries-in-adults-definitions-mechanisms-and-radiographs

39. Lei, F., Ou, D., Huang, X., Pang, M., Chen, X., Yang, B., & Wang, Q. (2019). Surgery versus conservative treatment for type II and II odontoid fractures in a geriatric population. A meta-analysis. *Medicine, 98*(44), Article e10281. https://doi.org/10.1097/MD.0000000000010281

40. Liu, X., Zhang, Y., Wang, Y., & Qian, T. (2021). Inflammatory response to spinal cord injury and its treatment. *World Neurosurgery, 155*, 19–31. https://doi.org/10.1016/j.wneu.2021.07.148

41. Loja, M. N., Sammann, A., DuBose, J., Li, C.-S., Liu, Y., Savage, S., Scalea, T., Holcomb, J. B., Rasmussen, T. E., Knudson, M. M., & AAST PROOVIT Study Group. (2017).

The mangled extremity score and amputation: Time for a revision. *Journal of Trauma and Acute Care Surgery, 82*(3), 518–523. https://doi.org/10.1097/ta.0000000000001339

42. Mayo Clinic. (n.d.). *Chronic exertional compartment syndrome.* http://www.mayoclinic.com/health/medical/IM00124

43. McGee, S. (2012). Examination of the sensory system. In *Evidence-based physical diagnosis* (3rd ed., pp. 567–580). Elsevier.

44. Mondor, E. E. (2022). Trauma. In L. D. Urden, K. M. Stacy, & M. E. Lough (Eds.), *Critical care nursing: Diagnosis and management* (9th ed., pp. 791–830). Elsevier.

45. National Institute for Health and Care Excellence. (2017, November 13). *Fractures (complex): Assessment and management.* https://www.nice.org.uk/guidance/ng37/chapter/Recommendations#hospital-settings

46. National Institutes of Health. (2016). *Stem cell basics.* https://stemcells.nih.gov/info/basics/stc-basics/#stc-II

47. National Spinal Cord Injury Statistical Center. (2019). *Recent trends in causes of spinal cord injury: 2015 SCI data sheet.* https://www.nscisc.uab.edu/Public/Recent%20trends%20in%20causes%20of%20SCI.pdf

48. Nielsen, F. E., Cordtz, J. J., Rasmussen, T. B., & Christiansen, C. F. (2020). The association between rhabdomyolysis, acute kidney injury, renal replacement therapy, and mortality. *Clinical Epidemiology, 12*, 989–995. https://doi.org/10.2147/CLEP.S254516

49. Ode, G., Studnek, J., Seymour, R., Bosse, M. J., & Hsu, J. R. (2015). Emergency tourniquets for civilians. *Journal of Trauma and Acute Care Surgery, 79*(4), 586–591. https://doi.org/10.1097/ta.0000000000000815

50. Okereke, I., & Abdelfatah, E. (2022) Limb salvage versus amputation for the mangled extremity: Factors affecting decision-making and outcomes. *Cureus, 14*(8), Article e28153. https://doi.org/10.7759/cureus.28153

51. Perron, A. D., & Huff, J. S. (2018). Spinal cord disorders. In R. M. Walls, R. S. Hockberger, & M. Gausche-Hill (Eds.), *Rosen's emergency medicine* (9th ed., Vol. 2, pp. 1298–1306). Elsevier.

52. Prasarn, M. L., Horodyski, M., DiPaola, M., DiPaola, C., Del Rossi, G., Conrad, B. P., & Rechtine, G. R. (2015). Controlled laboratory comparison study of motion with football equipment in a destabilized cervical spine: Three spine-board transfer techniques. *Orthopaedic Journal of Sports Medicine, 3*(9), Article 2325967115601853. https://doi.org/10.1177/2325967115601853

53. Ramirez, C., & Menaker, J. (2017). Traumatic amputations. *Trauma Reports.* https://www.reliasmedia.com/articles/140552-traumatic-amputations

54. Ransom, S. C., Brown, N. J., Pennington, Z. A., Lakomkin, N., Mikula, A. L., Bydon, M., & Elder, B. D. (2022). Hypothermia therapy for traumatic spinal cord injury: An updated review. *Journal of Clinical Medicine, 11*(6), Article 1585. https://doi.org/10.3390/jcm11061585

55. Rodrigues, I. F. (2017). To log-roll or not to log-roll–That is the question! A review of the use of the log-roll for patients with pelvic fractures. *International Journal of Orthopaedic and Trauma Nursing, 27*, 36–40. https://doi.org/10.1016/j.ijotn.2017.05.001

56. Russo McCourt, T. (2020). Spinal cord injuries. In K. A. McQuillan & M. B. Flynn Makic (Eds.), *Trauma nursing: From resuscitation through rehabilitation* (5th ed., pp. 454–502). Elsevier.

57. Schmidt, A. H. (2017). Acute compartment syndrome. *Injury, 48*(S1), S22–S25. https://doi.org/10.1016/j.injury.2017.04.024

58. Schuster, J., & Piazza, M. (2016). How should acute spinal cord injury be managed in the ICU? In C. S. Deutschman & P. J. Neligan (Eds.), *Evidence-based practice of critical care* (2nd ed., pp. 583–591). Elsevier.

59. Sears, B. (2020). *Types of lower extremity amputations.* Verywell Health. https://www.verywellhealth.com/types-of-lower-extremity-amputations-2696172

60. Sop, J. L., & Sop, A. (2022, August 8). Open fracture management. *StatPearls.* StatPearls Publishing. https://www.ncbi.nlm.nih.gov/books/NBK448083/

61. Stacy, K. M. (2022). Neurologic anatomy and physiology. In L. D. Urden, K. M. Stacy, & M. E. Lough (Eds.), *Critical care nursing: Diagnosis and management* (9th ed., pp. 534–564). Elsevier.

62. Stahel, P. F., & VanderHeiden, T. (2017). Spinal injuries. In E. E. Moore, D. V. Feliciano, & K. L. Mattox (Eds.), *Trauma* (8th ed., pp. 455–472). McGraw Hill.

63. Starks, I., Frost, A., Wall, P., & Lim, J. (2011). Is a fracture of the transverse process of L5 a predictor of pelvic fracture instability? *Journal of Bone & Joint Surgery, 93*(7), 967–969. https://doi.org/10.1302/0301-620X.93B7.26772

64. Stracciolini, A. (2022). Basic techniques for splinting of musculoskeletal injuries. *UpToDate.* Retrieved October 12, 2022, from https://www.uptodate.com/contents/basic-techniques-for-splinting-of-musculoskeletal-injuries

65. Tepordei, R. T., Stefan, G. T., Cozma, T., Nedelcu, A. H., Ovidiu, A., & Carmen, Z. L. (2014). A comparison of pressure measurement devices used in the acute compartment syndrome of the limbs. *Romanian Journal of Functional and Clinical, Macro- and Microscopical Anatomy and of Anthropology, 13*(3), 369–372. http://revanatomie.ro/en/abstract.php?an_rev=2014&nr_rev=3&nr_art=23

66. Torlincasi, A. M., Lopez, R. A., & Waseem, M. (2022, August 7). Acute compartment syndrome. *StatPearls.* StatPearls Publishing. https://www.ncbi.nlm.nih.gov/books/NBK448124/

67. Tortora, G. J., & Derrickson, B. H. (2021). The autonomic nervous system. In *Principles of anatomy and physiology* (16th ed., pp. 546–568). Wiley.

68. Tortora, G. J., & Derrickson, B. H. (2021). The spinal cord and spinal nerves. In *Principles of anatomy and physiology* (16th ed., pp. 461–492). Wiley.

69. Tortora, G. J., & Derrickson, B. H. (2021). The skeletal system: Bone tissue. In *Principles of anatomy and physiology* (16th ed., pp. 177–201). Wiley.

70. Tortora, G. J., & Derrickson, B. H. (2021). The skeletal system: The axial skeleton. In *Principles of anatomy and physiology* (16th ed., pp. 202–241). Wiley.
71. Walsh, C. (2020). Musculoskeletal injuries. In K. A. McQuillan & M. B. Flynn Makic (Eds.), *Trauma nursing: From resuscitation through rehabilitation* (5th ed., pp. 454–502). Elsevier.
72. Weingart, G., & Kumar, S. (2017). Acute compartment syndrome. *Emergency Medicine, 49*(3), 106–115. https://doi.org/10.12788/emed.2017.0014
73. Whitney, E., & Alastra, A. J. (2022, May 23). Vertebral fracture. *StatPearls*. StatPearls Publishing. https://www.ncbi.nlm.nih.gov/books/NBK547673/
74. Yeung, A. Y., & Garg, R. (2022, January 10). Anatomy, sesamoid bones. *StatPearls*. StatPearls Publishing. https://www.ncbi.nlm.nih.gov/books/NBK578171/
75. Ziu, E., & Mesfin, F. B. (2022, March 3). Spinal shock. *StatPearls*. StatPearls Publishing. https://www.ncbi.nlm.nih.gov/books/NBK448163/

APPENDIX 10-1
Clearing the Cervical Spine

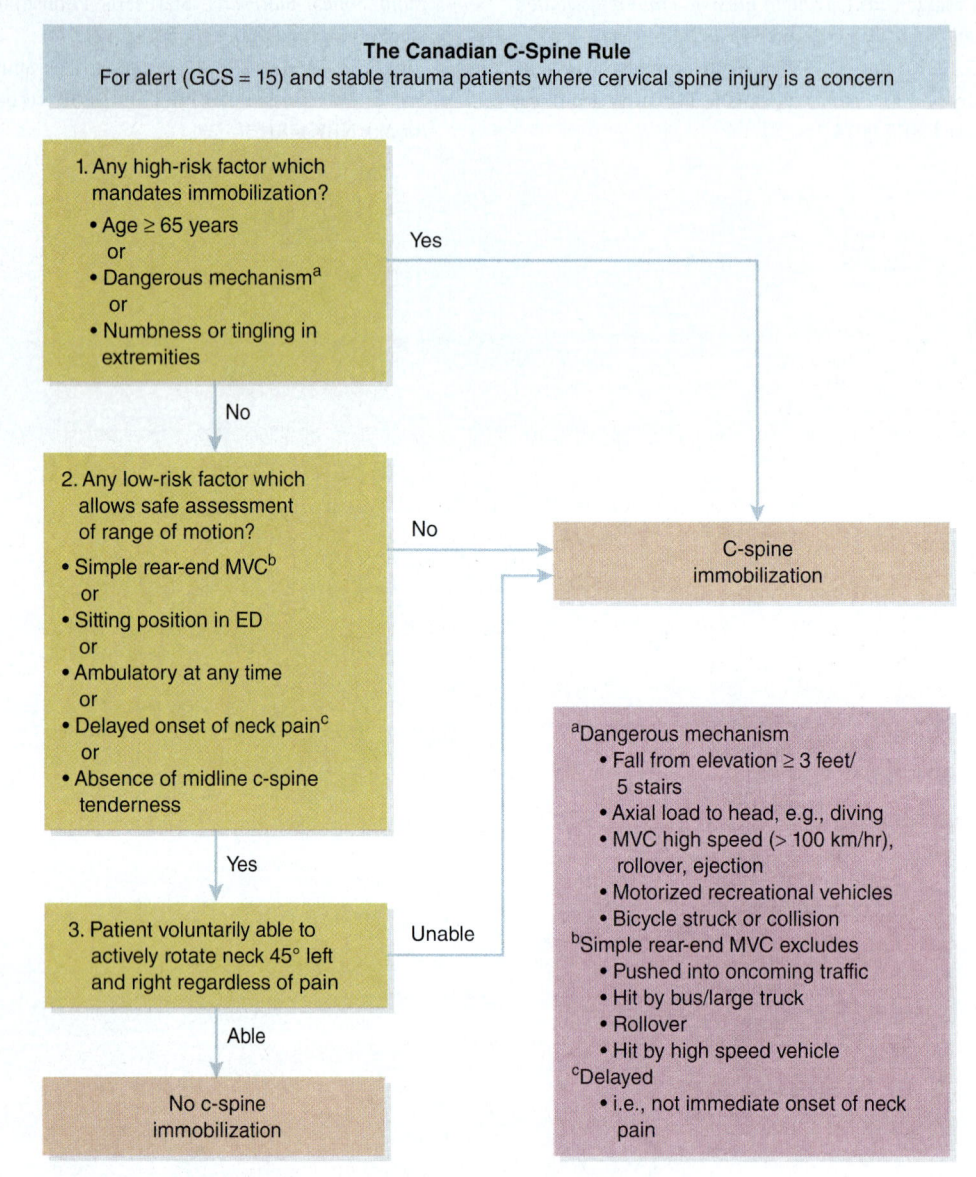

The Canadian C-Spine Rule
For alert (GCS = 15) and stable trauma patients where cervical spine injury is a concern

1. Any high-risk factor which mandates immobilization?
   - Age ≥ 65 years
   or
   - Dangerous mechanism[a]
   or
   - Numbness or tingling in extremities

   → Yes → C-spine immobilization
   → No ↓

2. Any low-risk factor which allows safe assessment of range of motion?
   - Simple rear-end MVC[b]
   or
   - Sitting position in ED
   or
   - Ambulatory at any time
   or
   - Delayed onset of neck pain[c]
   or
   - Absence of midline c-spine tenderness

   → No → C-spine immobilization
   → Yes ↓

3. Patient voluntarily able to actively rotate neck 45° left and right regardless of pain

   → Unable → C-spine immobilization
   → Able ↓

   No c-spine immobilization

[a]Dangerous mechanism
- Fall from elevation ≥ 3 feet/5 stairs
- Axial load to head, e.g., diving
- MVC high speed (> 100 km/hr), rollover, ejection
- Motorized recreational vehicles
- Bicycle struck or collision

[b]Simple rear-end MVC excludes
- Pushed into oncoming traffic
- Hit by bus/large truck
- Rollover
- Hit by high speed vehicle

[c]Delayed
- i.e., not immediate onset of neck pain

ED = emergency department; GCS = Glasgow Coma Scale; MVC = motor vehicle collision.

Reproduced from Clement, C. M., Stiell, I. G., Davies, B., O'Connor, A., Brehaut, J. C., Sheehan, P., Clavet, T., Leclair, C., MacKenzie, T., & Beland, C. (2011). Perceived facilitators and barriers to clinical clearance of the cervical spine by emergency department nurses: A major step towards changing practice in the emergency department. *International Emergency Nursing, 19*(1), 44–52. https://doi.org/10.1016/j.ienj.2009.12.002

APPENDIX 10-2
The NEXUS Criteria for Cervical Spine Clearance

Criteria
No posterior midline cervical spine tenderness is present.
No evidence of intoxication is present.
The patient has a normal level of alertness.
No focal neurologic deficit is present.
The patient does not have a painful distracting injury.

Data from Davenport, M. (2017). Cervical spine fracture evaluation workup. *Medscape*. Retrieved August 18, 2017, from https://emedicine.medscape.com/article/824380-workup

CHAPTER 11

Surface and Burn Trauma

Melanie Stroud, MBA, BSN, RN

OBJECTIVES

Upon completion of this chapter, the learner will be able to:
1. Describe the mechanisms of injury associated with surface and burn trauma.
2. Describe pathophysiologic changes as a basis for assessment for surface and burn injuries.
3. Demonstrate the nursing assessment of the patient with surface and burn injuries.
4. Plan appropriate interventions and evaluate their effectiveness for surface and burn injuries.

Knowledge of normal anatomy and physiology serves as a foundation for understanding anatomic derangements and pathophysiologic processes that may result from trauma. Before reading this chapter, it is strongly suggested that the learner review the following material. Anatomy is not emphasized in the classroom, but it is the basis of physical assessment and skill evaluation, as well as the foundation of questions for testing purposes.

Anatomy and Physiology of the Integumentary System

The integumentary system, or skin, is the largest organ in the body and is composed of the epidermis, dermis, and hypodermis (**Figure 11-1**). The integumentary system serves many vital functions, including the following:

- Protection from environmental hazards, including infection
- Thermoregulation and prevention of excess bodily fluid loss
- Sensory perception
- Vitamin D synthesis, contributing to bone formation and calcium metabolism
- Contributes to innate and adaptive immunity

Epidermis

The epidermis is the outermost layer of skin and the body's first line of defense against environmental threat. It is composed of epithelial cells, is avascular, and receives

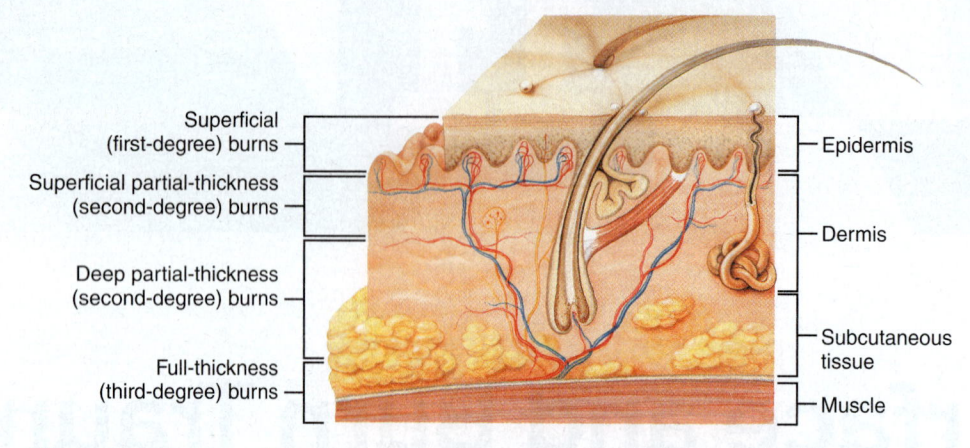

Figure 11-1 *Layers of the skin. The layers of the skin affected depend on the depth of a burn injury.*

nourishment from the dermis and subcutaneous tissue.[28,37] Melanocytes, which are responsible for skin pigmentation, are found within the epidermis. The epidermis is thin in most areas but is thicker on the soles of the feet, the hands, and other areas routinely exposed to pressure and friction.[37] The epidermis of the skin is composed of four layers of cells.[28] It is constantly shedding cells from the outer layer and developing new cells from the basal cell layer. The epidermal layer of the skin regenerates at a rate of complete replacement every month, or faster following an injury. With an intact basal cell layer, regeneration is possible. The epidermis possesses the keratinocytes and other immune cells that are triggered by infection.[30,37]

Dermis

The dermis is located directly beneath the epidermis, has a strong extracellular matrix, and is thicker than the epidermis.[37] The three components of the dermis are *collagen*, a protein that gives skin its mechanical strength; *elastin*, a protein that gives the skin stretch and flexibility; and *ground substance*, which helps to cushion and hydrate the skin.[28,51]

The dermis has two layers. The reticular dermis, the deeper layer, contains nerve endings, hair follicles, sweat and sebaceous glands, fingernails and toenails, and blood vessels. The papillary dermis, the superficial layer, aids in healing and provides nourishment to the epidermis. This layer of skin is highly vascular and plays a role in fluid, electrolyte, and body temperature regulation. The dermis is enriched with leukocytes and serves as a reserve for immune cells in the bloodstream.[30,51]

Unlike the epidermis, the dermis does not continuously regenerate new cells. Instead, repair of damaged dermal cells is dependent on the inflammatory and wound healing processes, especially fibroblasts, which secrete collagen and elastin.[28]

Hypodermis/Adipose Tissue

The subcutaneous tissue, sometimes referred to as the hypodermis or superficial fascia, lies beneath the dermis. This layer is rich in fat and connective tissue and attaches the dermis to the underlying structures. It functions as a heat insulator, nutrition supplier, and mechanical shock absorber. This layer is subdivided into white and subcutaneous white adipose tissue and contains lipid-dependent immune cells. It also provides antimicrobial peptides and factors that defend against infection. Excess fatty tissue, which is not vascular in nature, can delay or complicate wound healing.[30]

Wound Healing

Wound healing is a four-phase process that begins the moment injury occurs.[24,30,32]

Hemostasis Phase

The hemostasis phase is the first phase in the process of wound healing. It occurs immediately following any damage or injury to any tissue or organ. Various cellular responses promote blood clotting and prevent exsanguination, or blood loss, at the site of injury.

- Platelet activation and aggregation are triggered.
- Clotting factors are released, beginning the clotting cascade.
- Vasoconstriction occurs.
- A clot is formed.

Inflammatory Phase

The inflammatory phase begins when the blood vessels dilate and recruit white blood cells, growth factors, antibodies, and enzymes to the site of injury. The inflammation can be characterized by swelling, pain, redness of the tissue, and loss of cellular function. The immune

TABLE 11-1 Pressures Involved in Capillary and Fluid Dynamics

Type of Pressure	Effect
Capillary hydrostatic pressure	Pushes fluid out of the capillary
Tissue (interstitial) hydrostatic pressure	Pushes fluid into the capillary
Capillary (plasma) oncotic pressure	Determined by plasma proteins that are relatively impermeable
	Prevents movement out of the capillary and pulls fluid into the capillary
Tissue (interstitial) oncotic pressure	Dependent on the interstitial protein concentration
	Prevents movement into the capillary and pulls fluid into the interstitial space

Data from Lent-Schochet, D., & Jialal, I. (2022, May 8). Physiology, edema. *StatPearls*. StatPearls Publishing. https://www.ncbi.nlm.nih.gov/books/NBK537065/; Smith, C. C. (2021). Clinical manifestations and evaluation of edema in adults. *UpToDate*. Retrieved September 13, 2022, from https://www.uptodate.com/contents/clinical-manifestations-and-evaluation-of-edema-in-adults/

cells become a defense mechanism, calling attention to the wound healing process and stopping any infection. The following also occur during this phase:

- Vasodilation and capillary permeability increase perfusion to the wound.
- Monocytes and neutrophils infiltrate the area, removing cellular debris and foreign material and fighting infection.
- This process begins within the first 24 hours of injury and can last for weeks to months, depending on severity.

Proliferative or Growth Phase

In this phase, tissue repair and neovascularization occur with the help of keratinocytes and endothelial cells:

- There is proliferation and lateral migration of epithelial cells combined with collagen to resurface the wound bed.
- Activation of keratinocytes assists in closure of the wound and restores the vascular network.
- Growth factors activate endothelial cells.
- Granulation tissues form, and blood flow is restored. The time needed depends on the depth and severity of the wound.
- Tensile strength improves.

Maturation Phase

In the maturation phase, the body attempts to regain normal tissue structure to achieve complete healing:

- This phase can take days to years. Timing is influenced by the severity of injury and nutritional status.
- Tensile strength continues to increase.

- Collagen models scar tissue, reducing the wound's size and visibility.

Capillary and Fluid Dynamics

As noted, the dermis is involved in fluid and electrolyte balance. Four pressures within the interstitial space and vasculature play a role in capillary and fluid dynamics (**Table 11-1**).[35,43] Hydrostatic pressure is the force exerted by fluid pressing against a wall: It is divided into capillary and tissue pressures. Oncotic pressure is created by the presence of nondiffusible molecules such as plasma proteins. It also is classified as capillary or tissue pressure. Tissue edema results from fluid shifts, primarily from the plasma into the extravascular or extracellular space because of changes in endothelial permeability. These shifts cause a depletion in intravascular volume.

In patients with large burns to the skin, these pressures are disrupted. As a consequence, capillary leaking of fluid out of the intravascular space and into the interstitial space occurs and can result in hypovolemia, shock, and death.

Introduction

This chapter addresses both surface trauma and burn injuries, focusing on the effect of these injuries on patient assessment, interventions, and outcomes. Providing care to patients who sustain surface and/or burn injuries is often a labor-intensive process.

Patients who sustain surface or burn trauma require the same resuscitation strategies as any other trauma patient. The primary survey is performed at the same time as any necessary interventions, followed by the secondary survey.

Surface Trauma

Surface trauma is defined as a disruption in the normal anatomic structure and function of the integumentary system. It may be the patient's primary traumatic injury, but more often it occurs concurrently in a patient with multisystem trauma. Traumatic wounds are caused by shearing, tension, or compression.[40] Surface trauma includes the following types of injuries[23,40]:

- Lacerations
- Abrasions
- Avulsions
- Contusions and hematomas
- Puncture wounds
- Missile injuries
- Penetrating injuries
- Frostbite

Surface or soft tissue trauma can involve the skin as well as supporting and underlying structures such as muscles, tendons, ligaments, blood vessels, and nerves. It is essential that the seriousness of these seemingly minor injuries not be minimized because they can result in hemorrhage, loss of limb or function, and death secondary to infection.

Mechanisms of Injury

The following mechanisms of injury (MOIs) are associated with surface injuries[23,40]:

- Falls
- Motor vehicle collisions (MVCs)
- Impact with objects
- Overexertion and strenuous movements
- Cutting or piercing objects
- Crush injures
- Natural and environmental factors
- Foreign bodies
- High-velocity bullet wounds, close-range shotgun injuries, or explosions
- Exposure to chemicals or caustic substances

Knowing the MOI is essential to predicting injury patterns in the trauma patient. Moreover, assessment findings can provide clues to potential underlying tissue and organ damage. See Chapter 3, "Biomechanics and Mechanisms of Injury," for more information.

Pathophysiology as a Basis for Assessment Findings

The wound healing process is complex and requires meticulous and ongoing assessment and monitoring to prevent infection, which remains a leading cause of morbidity and mortality.

Certain wound characteristics predispose some injuries to a greater risk of infection[23,40]:

- Mammalian bites
- Crush injury
- Puncture wounds
- Stellate lacerations
- Wounds with an 8-hour or greater delay in seeking medical treatment

Patients at highest risk for infectious complications include the following groups:

- Older adults
- Infants
- Smokers or others with impaired oxygenation and perfusion
- Patients who are immunocompromised or taking immunosuppressants
- Patients with diabetes or renal failure
- Patients with existing vascular disease

Trauma patients with these comorbidities or risk circumstances often benefit from referral to wound clinics that specialize in optimizing the wound healing process with specialized treatments such as leech therapy, hyperbaric oxygen treatments, negative-pressure wound therapy, and specialty dressings (silver-impregnated products, medical-grade honey, or polyhexamethylene biguanide).[15,28,33,52]

Nursing Care of the Patient with Surface Trauma

When a trauma patient arrives, surface injuries may be a distraction, especially if they are extensive and obvious. They may divert attention away from subtle, but potentially more life-threatening, injuries or situations such as an ineffective airway.

Primary Survey

The primary survey and all life-threatening injuries must be addressed, and the patient stabilized, before addressing surface trauma. Chapter 4, "Initial Assessment," describes the systematic approach to nursing care of the trauma patient. Most surface trauma is addressed in the secondary survey; however, some wounds may require immediate intervention to control hemorrhage.

Secondary Survey

The following assessment parameters are specific to patients with surface injuries.

H: History

Questions to ask during history taking include, but are not limited to, the following:

- When and where did the injury occur? How much time has elapsed since the injury?
- Was the cause of the injury from a clean or dirty source?
- Was the cause of the wound an animal bite, and, if so, is the animal known? Is there a risk of rabies exposure?
- Is there a risk of a retained foreign body? Maintain a high suspicion of a foreign body in all wounds.
- Is there possible tendon involvement, and is there full or partial range of motion?
- Is there possible nerve involvement? Is sensation present at the site? Are there any numbness or tingling sensations? Any laceration of the hand or wrist may involve a tendon or nerve, regardless of how superficial the wound might be.
- Was the injury intentional or unintentional?
- Is the injury work related?
- Does the patient have a history of medical conditions that may affect wound healing (e.g., diabetes, compromised immune system, vascular disease)?
- What medications is the patient taking (e.g., anticoagulants, antihypertensives, steroids)?
- Is the patient's tetanus status up to date?
- If the injury involves the hand or arm, what is the patient's hand dominance?

H: Head-to-Toe Assessment

Inspect for the following:

- The location and type of the wound and any associated injuries
- The effectiveness of hemostasis
- The depth, length, and size of the wound
- The color of the wound and surrounding tissue
- The extent of denuded tissue and visible underlying structures
- Tissue swelling and/or deformity and presence of foreign bodies
- Evidence of any apparent wound contamination or presence of exudate

Palpate for the following (positive findings are suspicious for compartment syndrome):

- Weak or absent distal pulses (late sign)
- Delayed capillary refill
- Firmness on palpation of muscle and soft tissue in the surrounding area
- Distal skin that is cool to the touch
- Pale or cyanotic distal skin
- Decrease in patient sensation

The Ps mnemonic helps the trauma nurse to remember components of the neurovascular assessment, and positive findings are suspicious for compartment syndrome or other neurovascular insult:

- Pain: often out of proportion to the injury and often occurs before changes in pulse quality, skin color, and temperature
- Pallor
- Pulses
- Paresthesia
- Paralysis
- Pressure
- Poikilothermia (inability to regulate temperature; adopts the ambient room temperature)

Compartment syndrome may cause permanent damage with 6 hours, resulting in loss of function and, in cases delayed more than 12 hours, possible amputation.[46] See Chapter 10, "Spinal and Musculoskeletal Trauma," for additional information.

Interventions

The immediate goal when treating surface trauma is to obtain and maintain hemostasis. This is accomplished by applying direct pressure to the site of bleeding. For cases that are not resolved by direct pressure, cauterization and suture ligation of isolated vessels may be necessary. In patients who experience limb injuries for which bleeding cannot be controlled with direct manual pressure, tourniquets have been used successfully. See Chapter 6, "Shock," and Chapter 10, "Spinal and Musculoskeletal Trauma," for more information.

Selected Surface Trauma Injuries

Surface trauma injuries, including types and causes, are discussed in this section.

Abrasion

An abrasion is a partial- or full-thickness wound that denudes the skin, exposing the dermis or subcutaneous skin layer. It does not, however, go deeper than the dermis. This type of injury commonly occurs when the skin is rubbed off by a hard, rough surface, as occurs with falls and bicycle or motorcycle collisions. Abrasions can be mild or severe and can vary in surface area and depth, depending on the mechanism and force involved. Road burn, resulting from a low side crash or laying down a motorcycle, is an example of an abrasion involving a large surface area. If the injured area becomes embedded with gravel and dirt despite vigorous wound cleansing and debridement, it can cause a traumatic tattoo effect on the skin, which is characterized by an irregular black, blue, or gray skin discoloration.[28]

Avulsion

Avulsions are full-thickness wounds caused by a tearing or ripping of skin and soft tissue away from underlying tissues. The wound edges are not well approximated.[28] These injuries often involve the fingers, scalp, and nose, and they can occur as a result of MVCs or working with machinery. A degloving injury is an avulsion in which the skin and tissue is removed, exposing underlying structures, including bone, tendons, and ligaments. Degloving injuries commonly affect the extremities and scalp.[28,41]

Avulsions can occur in bone fractures when soft tissue is torn away from the bone. The extent of these injuries can affect other systems. For example, one prognostic indicator for limb salvage after tibia–fibula fracture is the magnitude of avulsed tissue from the bone shaft.[47] When soft tissue is avulsed, the bone may not receive adequate nutrients through the circulation. Exposed bone and mangle injuries are at highest risk for infection.

Treatment for avulsions depends on the body part and the amount of tissue avulsed. Simple wound care may be adequate in a simple skin avulsion, whereas more extensive avulsions, such as degloving injuries, may require surgical intervention for grafting or amputation.[28]

Contusion and Hematoma

A contusion is a closed wound in which a ruptured blood vessel or capillary bed hemorrhages into the surrounding tissue as a result of blunt trauma (contusion is synonymous with bruise). A hematoma occurs when blood leaks under the skin surface and often forms a palpable mass (blood clot) under the skin.[28,37]

Determining the appropriate treatment requires analysis of the force required to produce the contusion and the potential for trauma to underlying structures, such as compression injury to arteries and nerves, that would cause ischemia.

Laceration

Lacerations are open wounds that result from sharp or blunt forces through the dermis and epidermis, with potential involvement of the underlying structures, such as muscles, tendons, and ligaments. Common causes of lacerations include injuries from tools or machinery. Exploration of deeper lacerations is required to assess the integrity of underlying structures and to evaluate for foreign bodies. Lacerations differ from cuts or incisions, such as those from a knife or broken glass; these have clean, well-approximated edges.[28,39] Lacerations should be assessed to rule out vascular and/or neurologic injuries. Lacerations require debridement and closure. If a laceration is below the fascial level, it might require operative intervention to assess for damage to any underlying structures.[13]

Puncture Wound

Puncture wounds occur when a spearlike object creates an open wound deeper than it is wide. Puncture injuries result from various mechanisms, including the following:

- Superficial wounds, such as stepping on a tack
- Deeper injuries, such as stab wounds
- Injuries from foreign bodies or impalements
- Animal and human bites

Although puncture wounds may appear minor, they carry a potential risk for infection and underlying tissue or organ damage—especially with injuries caused by high pressure, such as a nail or grease gun injury.[28]

When a patient experiences a missile or impalement injury, the foreign body is often more deeply embedded than with other wounds and affects underlying tissue. Large foreign bodies are removed after underlying structures have been assessed. Hemorrhage can result after embedded objects are removed because the item may be providing a means of hemostasis. For example, a piece of glass embedded in the hand may be placing pressure on a branch of a capillary, thus serving to control bleeding. Therefore, premature removal of the glass will result in bleeding. Large, impaled objects are often removed in the operating room by trauma surgeons who can repair damage to deep tissue and vessels. Puncture wounds carry a high infection rate.[28] Risk factors for infection include the following:

- Large or deep wounds
- Contaminated wounds (bite wounds)
- Wounds with osseous involvement
- High-pressure injuries
- Wounds more than 6 hours old
- Human and animal bites

Rabies is a global public health issue and is endemic in some areas of the world.[27] It should be considered when managing animal bite wounds. If the animal is known to the patient or family but not current with immunizations, or if the animal is unknown or wild, rabies prophylaxis and antibiotic therapy may be indicated.[27]

Missile Injuries

Missile injuries include stab wounds, firearm injuries, and other high-pressure puncture wounds.

> **BOX 11-1** Frostbite Interventions
>
> Frostbite interventions include the following:
>
> - Start treatment only after it can be confirmed that the affected area will not be at risk for frostbite again after it is rewarmed because incomplete thawing and refreezing can cause catastrophic injury.[4,22]
> - Initial treatment consists of gently rewarming the affected area over a period of 15–30 minutes in water that is between 40°C and 42°C (104°F to 107.6°F). This is a painful process, and pain medication should be provided.[4] Other considerations include the following:
>   - Ibuprofen will treat pain as well as block prostaglandin production.[4]
>   - Remove wet or constricting clothing and replace with warm blankets.
>   - Give warm fluids by mouth if able to drink.
>   - Reperfusion syndrome can occur with rewarming of large areas, resulting in acidosis, hyperkalemia, and local swelling. Therefore, monitor cardiac status and peripheral perfusion during the rewarming process.[4]
> - Avoid any friction, rubbing, or massaging of the area to preserve tissue integrity.
> - Large, clear blisters that impede movement may be drained, debrided, and bandaged. Large hemorrhagic blisters that impede movement may be drained, but not debrided. Small blisters are maintained intact.
> - Guard against further injury to the area by padding, splinting, and elevating the affected extremity.[4]
> - Prevent or limit the risk of thrombus formation.
>   - The use of thrombolytic medications has been effective in maintaining perfusion and decreasing the need for amputation when administered within 12 hours of thawing an extremity.[4]
>
> Data from American Burn Association. (2018). Cold injuries. In *Advanced burn life support course provider manual: 2018 update* (pp. 86–89); Cochran, A., & Morris, S. E. (2018). Cold-induced injury: Frostbite. In D. N. Herndon (Ed.), *Total burn care* (5th ed., pp. 403–407). Elsevier.

Frostbite

Frostbite occurs when exposure to cold causes tissue to freeze and ice crystals to form.[48] Severe vasoconstriction causes reduced perfusion and injury to the endothelial layer of blood vessels, and a thrombus can form. Frostbite is classified by the American Burn Association as either a mild injury or deep injury, although it is difficult to determine the extent of injury during the initial assessment.[4]

Mild injury includes the following:

- Early rewarming after a brief exposure to the cold.
- Clear blisters to digit tips.
- Bright red or normal skin color.
- Sensation is present.
- Digits are warm.

Deep injury includes the following:

- Delayed warming after prolonged exposure to the cold.
- Hemorrhagic proximal blisters.
- Purple or mottled skin color.
- Sensation is absent.
- Digits are cool.

The severity of frostbite depends on the duration of exposure, temperature, environmental conditions, and the overall health of the exposed person. Less common causes of frostbite include occupational exposures to very cold fluids or direct contact with extremely cold machinery.[4]

Interventions

Healthcare professionals in many parts of the world may never encounter patients with frostbite, while others encounter it regularly, making understanding appropriate interventions necessary to their practice. Frostbite interventions are summarized in **Box 11-1**.

Diagnostics and Interventions for Surface and Burn Trauma

Reevaluation adjuncts for surface and burn trauma include radiographic studies, laboratory studies, and wound care.

Radiographic Studies

Obtain plain films before wound closure to evaluate for foreign bodies and for underlying fractures or joint penetration. Ultrasound may be more useful than radiographs for determining the presence of plastic or wood foreign bodies.

Laboratory Studies

Laboratory studies include the following:

- A complete blood count (CBC) with differential may be obtained to assess for anemia and/or thrombocytopenia from blood loss and for leukocytosis as evidence of possible infection.
- A coagulation profile may be obtained to identify any potential coagulation abnormalities, especially in the setting of deep or large wounds.

All patients with extensive soft tissue trauma should have serial monitoring of/for the following[23]:

- Electrolytes
- Creatine phosphokinase levels
- Hourly urine output (should be recorded)
- Compartment syndrome (close monitoring important)

For infected wounds, wound culture and sensitivity may be useful to guide appropriate antibiotic therapy; this information can be obtained through a swab of viable tissues, tissue biopsy, or needle aspiration. This type of diagnostic study should occur when signs and symptoms of infection are present.[41]

Wound Care

The goals of wound care include the following:

- Promote wound healing
- Prevent complications (infection, limited range of motion)
- Maintain function
- Minimize scar formation

The three basic classifications of closure used for wound healing are primary, secondary, and tertiary:

- Primary wound closure is used for wounds with well-approximated borders and minimal tissue destruction. Simple closure techniques, such as suturing or staples, are used.
- Secondary wound closure is used for infection-prone wounds in which the edges are not easy to approximate. Gauze packing or wound drains may be needed. This method of repair requires formation of granulation tissue from the base of the wound upward.
- Tertiary closure (also known as delayed primary closure) is used for deep wounds that were initially left open and allowed to granulate because of the age of the wound or risk of infection. After this granulation, debridement and sutures are used to bring the wound edges together in order to promote healing.[17,24]

Nursing considerations include the following:

- All wounds may be cleaned with tap water or with normal saline, which is the preferred method of cleansing. This is essential and one of the most effective methods for reducing the risk of wound infections.[28]
- Wound irrigation can reduce the bacterial contamination of the wound and prevent infection. Use a copious amount of irrigation solution. Low-pressure irrigation, such as with a bulb syringe, will help to remove large contaminants, but high-pressure irrigation works best for smaller contaminants and bacteria. Take care not to destroy viable tissue.[26]
- Dirty or deep wounds may require cleansing with an alternative antiseptic solution. If antiseptic solution is used, it is important to avoid substances that may cause increased tissue damage or that are potentially toxic.[28] Follow facility policies and procedures regarding wound cleansing.
- Anesthesia may be required when removing gravel or other foreign materials from the wound or for wound repair.[36] Avoid using lidocaine with epinephrine on the fingers, toes, or any other area where vasoconstriction could cause impaired distal blood circulation.
- Digital blocks using bupivacaine or lidocaine may be used for finger or toe injuries.
- Procedural sedation may be needed for repair of extensive wounds or for repairing wounds in children.
- If necessary, hair removal from around the wound is done with scissors or clippers. Shaving is not recommended because of the potential for infection. Eyebrows should never be clipped or shaved because they may not grow back, or grow back irregularly. Another option for addressing hair when attempting to create a better field of vision is to lubricate the hair and comb away from the wound edges.[17]
- Wounds heal best in a moist, but not wet, environment provided by a proper dressing.[28]
- Prophylactic systemic antibiotics are not routinely used for acute management surface trauma. Topical antimicrobial agents may be used on the wound to reduce the risk of infection.
- Following organizational policies, consider taking photographs of the injury before cleaning or repairing the wounds if the injury was associated with a crime.
- Administer tetanus prophylaxis as indicated. The Centers for Disease Control and Prevention (CDC) provides vaccination resources, including the most recent recommendations for tetanus prophylaxis.[20]

Reevaluation and Post-Resuscitation Care

Reevaluation and ongoing assessment of new wounds include the following issues:

- The ability of the patient to maintain hemostasis of the wound
- The effectiveness of the wound closure modality

Definitive Care or Transport

Consider the need for surgery, admission, or transport to a trauma center as indicated. For patients being discharged, provide education to the patient and family on topics including the following:

- Signs and symptoms of infection, including fever, opening of the wound site, drainage from the wound, redness or red streaks progressing up an extremity, excessive pain or swelling at the site, or numbness or tingling at sites distal to the wounds
- Bathing information with bandage or dressing supplies
- What signs and symptoms to report to their primary care providers
- Instructions regarding suture removal and follow-up
- Infection prevention

Burn Trauma

Burn injuries can have a lifelong impact on patients because of loss of function, scarring, chronic pain, and psychological trauma. Caring for this patient population can be challenging. The patient may have experienced a life-threatening situation necessitating immediate attention, and hypothermia, hypercarbia, and hypoxia may develop. Pain management for these patients can also be difficult. Lengthy recovery, chronic pain, and scarring are common in this patient population.

Epidemiology

Burn injuries are the fourth most common type of trauma worldwide, making it a serious global public health issue.[44] Burns disproportionately affect people in low- to middle-income countries, with burns in such countries accounting for 90% of burns worldwide. In the United States, burns are among the top 10 causes of death for all age groups and the fourth leading cause of death in children. Globally, approximately 11 million burn injuries result in approximately 265,000 fatalities each year. The people most vulnerable to burn injuries are women, children, older adults, and people with disabilities, including those with intellectual disabilities who may not recognize or react appropriately in a dangerous situation.[44,50]

In the United States, 65% of burns occur in the home.[6] The overall survival rate for those with burn injuries is 96% for patients treated at a burn center.[6]

Mechanism of Injury and Biomechanics

Burns are injuries to tissues caused by heat, friction, electricity, radiation, or chemicals.[6] In order of prevalence, the most common mechanisms of burn injury for persons aged 5 years and older are the following:

- Fire/flames
- Scald injuries
- Electrical and chemical

Children younger than 5 years of age are at the highest risk for injury and death from home fires.[4,7] Scalds are the most common MOI in young children, while burns from flames are more common for children between the ages of 5 and 16 years.[50]

Burns can be intentional in cases such as assault, abuse, or self-harm. Pattern burns (such as from a cigarette or identifiable object) or immersion burns (circumferential and sharply demarcated burns to both feet) should raise suspicion of possible maltreatment. See Chapter 17, "Interpersonal Violence," for additional information. Nurses should be mindful that the mechanism and pattern of injury should match the injury history.[4]

Burns are classified by the following categories based on the source of the burn:

- Thermal
- Chemical
- Electrical
- Radiation

Thermal Burns

Thermal burns result from contact with hot objects (contact burns), hot liquids (scalds), or flames. Flame is the predominant cause of burns, particularly for adults who are admitted to burn centers.[2,50]

Scald burns are thermal burns that result from contact with a hot liquid. Young children are commonly injured by pulling a container of hot liquid onto themselves. Injury severity depends on the temperature of the substance and the length of exposure. For instance, the safety standard for the maximum temperature of U.S. residential water heaters is 48.8°C (120°F). According to the American Burn Association,[9] it takes only 3 seconds of skin exposure to liquids at 60°C (140°F) to result in a burn serious enough to require surgical intervention. Hot liquids such as coffee are often served at 79°C (175°F), which can cause immediate severe scald burns when it comes in contact with the skin.[9]

Individuals can sustain burn injuries from hot tar or asphalt. The temperature of these substances can be as high as 230°C (450°F). Very deep burns can occur because of the thickness of the substance combined with the extremely high temperatures. After cooling the tar or asphalt, a petrolatum-based product can be applied to help with emulsification and removal of the tar.[2]

Chemical Burns

Chemical burns result from exposure to acids, alkalis, or organic compounds. There are four mechanisms of injury due to chemicals: inhalation, ingestion, absorption through the mucous membranes or skin, or a combination, such as a scald injury with chemicals in the hot fluid.[3] Acids are organic or inorganic substances that cause coagulation necrosis and protein precipitation.[3] Examples of acids are hydrofluoric acid, carbonic acid, and white phosphorus. Alkalis cause extensive tissue damage by liquification necrosis; thus, they result in deep tissue destruction and necrosis.[3] Examples of alkaline agents are anhydrous ammonia, cement, hydrocarbons, and tar. Organic compounds, such as phenols or petroleum products such as gasoline, tend to dissolve the lipid membrane of the cell wall. Fertilizers and dyes are other examples of organic compounds.

Electrical Burns

Electrical burns are unique in terms of their etiology and severity.

- Electrical burns are caused by direct exposure to an electrical current or a lightning strike. An electrical current can be either direct (DC) or alternating (AC). DC is commonly found in batteries, solar panels, and fuel cells; AC is commonly found in homes and businesses and used in medical devices and electronics. Notably, lightning injuries usually do not traverse the body, but flow around it, potentially creating a shock wave capable of causing fractures and other traumatic injuries.
- The severity of injury is determined by many factors, including the voltage, current (amperage), type of current (AC or DC), path of the current flow, duration of contact, resistance at the point of contact, and individual susceptibility.

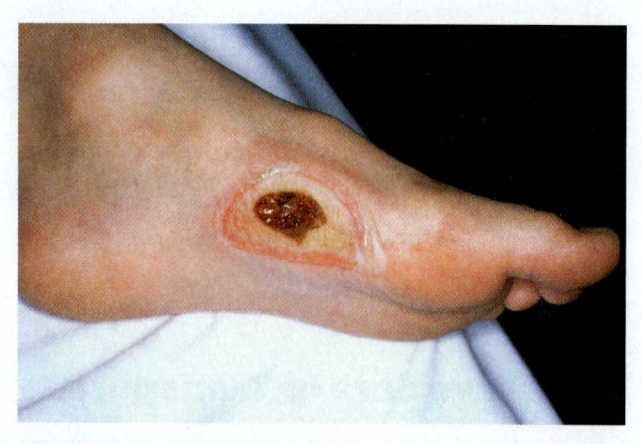

Figure 11-2 Electrical burn.
© Charles Stewart MD, EMDM, MPH.

- Electrical burns frequently are more serious than they appear on the body surface (**Figure 11-2**) and extremities, particularly on fingers or toes.
- Current can travel into blood vessels and nerves, causing local thrombosis and injury to the nerves.
- A small entrance wound, with a clenched fist (contracture), is an indication of a deep soft tissue injury.
- Patients with electrical burns frequently need fasciotomies; these patients should be transferred to a burn center early.

Radiation Burns

Radiation burns result from exposure to thermal radiation, ultraviolet light, or particulate ionizing radiation.[8] Common causes of radiation burns include exposure to the sun (sunburn) and radiation beams used to treat cancer patients. Exposure to radioactive fallout after nuclear explosions or nuclear accidents can also result in beta-radiation burn injuries. See Chapter 19, "Disaster Management," for additional information.

Usual Concurrent Injuries

Patients with selected burn MOIs can be at risk for an inhalation injury, including loss of airway, respiratory failure, and death. Patients who present with thermal burns from fires that occurred in a small or enclosed space are at especially high risk and may experience carbon monoxide or other poisoning. Other concurrent injuries may be identified by considering the MOI and pertinent details from the scene. For example, if the patient jumped from a building during a fire, assess for fractures and organ hemorrhage. If the burn was sustained in an MVC, assess for additional injuries related to the collision. Consider a blunt traumatic injury if the MOI was a blast event. See Chapter 3, "Biomechanics and Mechanism of Injury," for additional information.

Pathophysiology as a Basis for the Assessment Findings of Burn Trauma

The external injury resulting from burn trauma is the destruction of the skin. However, the internal injuries are of equal, if not more, concern in these patients. The pathophysiologic impact of burn injuries primarily depends on the extent and depth of the burn. It is imperative to stop the burning process while proceeding with the primary survey.

Airway Patency

Burns to tissue or exposure to heated gases can cause life-threatening direct injury such as inhalation, but also severe airway edema.[14] A hoarse voice, brassy cough, carbonaceous sputum, burns around the mouth or nares, or stridor may indicate burns to the airway. Signs and symptoms of airway obstruction may be subtle, developing over time and not becoming readily apparent until the patient is in extremis. According to the American Burn Association,[1] indications for early intubation include:

- Significant edema or risk for edema
- Extensive and deep burns to the face
- Burns inside the mouth
- Signs of airway compromise: hoarseness, stridor
- Signs of respiratory compromise: increased work of breathing (accessory muscle use, retractions), poor oxygenation or ventilation
- Difficulty swallowing
- Impairment of protective reflexes with decreased level of consciousness
- Total body surface area (TBSA) burns greater than 40–50%
- Patient transfer for large burns if an airway issue is anticipated, and transfer personnel are not qualified to intubate

Hypoxia, Asphyxia, and Carbon Monoxide Poisoning

Hypoxia can result from an inhalation injury or from carbon monoxide (CO) poisoning. Asphyxia occurs from breathing decreased amounts of oxygen in the inspired air in a closed space where oxygen is being consumed by the fire.[25] Carbon monoxide is a colorless, odorless, and tasteless gas that is released into the air during a fire. Carbon monoxide has a much higher (200–250 times) affinity to the hemoglobin molecule as compared with oxygen.[25] This replaces oxygen in the hemoglobin, creating carboxyhemoglobin (COHb), which reduces blood's oxygen-carrying capacity. Symptoms are related to the percentage of COHb in the blood and vary from tightness over the forehead, headache, confusion, nausea, and vomiting, to more severe symptoms such as syncope, tachycardia, seizures, coma, and death.[25] Measurement of oxygenation and oxygen saturation are best measured with arterial blood gases (ABGs). The pulse oximeter will not differentiate hemoglobin bound to oxygen from hemoglobin bound to CO, making it unreliable.[1]

Carbon monoxide poisoning should be considered for anyone exposed to fire in an enclosed space.[1] Treat the patient with CO poisoning with oxygen until carboxyhemoglobin levels drop to less than 10%. When a patient is placed on 100% oxygen, the half-life of CO is decreased to approximately 1 hour; for this reason, patients presumed to have elevated CO levels should be immediately placed on oxygen therapy.[1] Hyperbaric oxygen for CO poisoning has not been definitely shown to improve neurologic outcomes, and its implementation should not delay transfer to a burn center for definitive treatment.[1,12,31]

> **CLINICAL PEARL**
>
> The pulse oximeter will not differentiate hemoglobin bound to oxygen from hemoglobin bound to CO, making it unreliable.[1,12,25]

Hydrogen cyanide is another product of incomplete combustion of synthetic products such as carpeting, upholstered furniture, plastics, or draperies. When cyanide enters the cells, cells are unable to produce adenosine triphosphate and shift toward anaerobic metabolism. Blood cyanide levels are difficult to measure through routine laboratory studies. Therefore, treatment is prophylactically initiated based on the history of being in an enclosed space, with symptoms of changes in respiratory rate, shortness of breath, headache, confusion, irritation of the eyes and mucous membranes, or lactic acidosis that persists despite fluid resuscitation. The patient should be treated with a hydroxocobalamin cyanide antidote kit.[1,25]

Pulmonary Injury

Pulmonary injury doubles the mortality of patients with burns. The process of pulmonary injury includes the following elements:

- Inhalation of the products of combustion, such as particles of carbon and noxious fumes
- Damage to the mucosal cells of the bronchioles
- Increased permeability of cell membranes, allowing leakage from the cells and causing impaired gas exchange

- Inflammation
- Sloughing of dead cells, which may obstruct the airways
- Mucous hypersecretion, which may obstruct the airways
- Decreased production and/or loss of surfactant, resulting in alveolar collapse
- Spasm of bronchi and bronchioles
- Acute lung injury or acute respiratory distress syndrome
- Secondary complications such as pneumonia

Clinical evidence of a pulmonary injury may not be immediately evident during the resuscitation phase, so it is crucial that the trauma team identify those patients at risk for respiratory compromise and proactively manage and protect the airway.[1,14]

Capillary Leak Syndrome

Edema formation is one of the more challenging management issues of treating burn injuries. The inflammatory response occurs both locally and, in large burns, systemically; this results in a shift of fluid from the intravascular fluid into the interstitial space, sometimes referred to as *third spacing*. In burned tissue, mediators such as histamine, serotonin, prostaglandins, blood products, complement components, and kinins act to increase the vascular permeability of the capillary membrane.[18,44] This increased permeability, referred to as *capillary leak*, allows plasma to pass through the damaged membranes, leaving red blood cells in the intravascular space.[44] In areas of undamaged tissue, permeability may be increased because of the release of the histamines and kinins. Burns greater than 20% TBSA are most commonly vulnerable to this capillary leak.[18]

During capillary leak, large amounts of the fluid infused during resuscitation can seep from the veins into the tissue. This condition can persist for 6–12 hours after the burn injury, until the capillary membranes begin to undergo repair and leakage begins to decrease.[18,32] However, the edema can last much longer. The rate of fluid lost from intravascular spaces depends on the patient's age, burn size and depth, intravascular pressures, and time elapsed since the burn.

The inflammatory response results in the release of numerous substrates, which then lead to further edema and potential cardiac collapse[18,32,44]:

- Release of histamine and prostaglandin leads to vasodilation and increased capillary permeability.
- Thromboxane, a vasoconstrictive substance, causes platelet aggregation and expansion of the zone of coagulation.
- Bradykinin causes increased permeability of the venules, and oxygen-free radicals damage the endothelial cells, which are the basement membrane of new tissue.

Mechanical Obstruction and Circumferential Burns

Circumferential burns to the neck or chest may reduce the ability of the patient to breathe deeply; this is especially prevalent with full-thickness burns because the dry, leathery tissue, known as eschar, is far less compliant than intact healthy skin.[2] An escharotomy may be necessary to relieve the constriction of the chest or extremities.[2]

Loss of Skin Integrity

Loss and destruction of the skin layer results in the loss of vital functions, including thermoregulation and protection against infection. Assessment of the burn surface will reveal a three-dimensional mass of injured tissues (**Figure 11-3**).[32] Burns are divided into three zones[2,32]:

- Zone of coagulation
  - The most severely damaged center of the burn, this area is often necrotic in nature.
  - Debridement of this necrotic tissue is essential for wound healing because it is not capable of regeneration.
  - Skin grafting is a consideration for burns involving the zone of coagulation.
- Zone of stasis
  - This zone surrounds the zone of coagulation.
  - Tissue in this area has been moderately damaged, resulting in decreased tissue perfusion and edema.
  - If wound treatment is timely and appropriate, this tissue may improve to a zone of hyperemia; if not, it may deteriorate to a zone of coagulation.
- Zone of hyperemia
  - This is the outermost area of the burn.

Because of the inflammatory process, blood flow to this area is increased; this results in the best chance for tissue viability, barring infection.

Hypothermia

Patients can become hypothermic, owing to disruption of the normal integumentary function of temperature

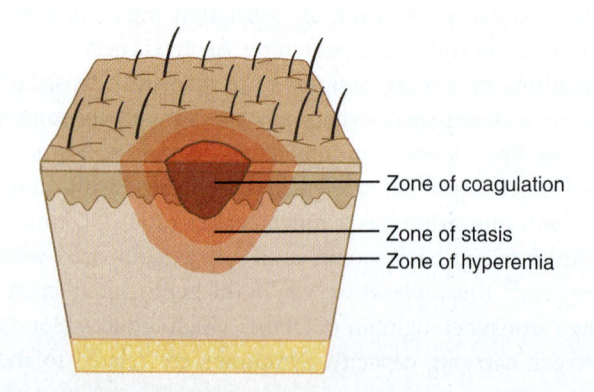

Figure 11-3 *Zones of injury in burns.*

regulation. Hypothermia can help lead to clotting and bleeding disorders such as disseminated intravascular coagulation (DIC). Patients with burns are susceptible to difficulties with thermoregulation. Hypothermia causes vasoconstriction, and a core temperature less than 35°C (95°F) can worsen the burn, in addition to the systemic effects.[5] It is essential to prevent hypothermia by administering warm fluids and blood products, maintaining a warm environment, and using warm blankets.[5]

Nursing Care of the Patient with Burn Trauma

Severe burns can distract from subtle, yet more life-threatening, injuries, resulting in sequela such as an ineffective airway. It is imperative that the trauma team maintain focus on treating life-threatening injuries before treating the burn. Chapter 4, "Initial Assessment," describes the systematic approach to the nursing care of the trauma patient. The following assessment parameters are specific to patients with burn injuries.

Primary Survey and Resuscitation Adjuncts

The primary survey begins with alertness and airway.

A: Alertness and Airway

Assessments and interventions include the following:

- Alertness and the ability to maintain a patent airway.
- If the patient is unable to protect the airway, initiate appropriate interventions to provide a patent airway.
- If fire is the mechanism for a thermal burn, inspect for evidence of extensive and deep facial burns, soot, carbonaceous sputum, singed nasal hairs, erythema or swelling of the oropharynx or nasopharynx, brassy cough, difficulty swallowing, or progressive hoarseness—these signs might indicate an inhalation injury. If they are present, consider prophylactic intubation.
- Consider the need for cervical spine protection based on the MOI.

B: Breathing and Ventilation

Assessments and interventions[1,12,21]:

- Begin administering oxygen at 10–15 L/minute via nonrebreather mask.
- After the primary survey is complete, maintain SpO_2 between 94% and 98% unless there is suspicion of carbon monoxide poisoning.
- Ensure effective ventilation. Observe for adequate chest wall expansion.
- Hyperbaric oxygen may be considered for severe CO poisoning after consultation with a medical toxicologist or poison control center, outside of the resuscitation phase.

C: Circulation and Control of Hemorrhage

Assessment and intervention considerations include the following:

- Avoid obtaining vascular access through burned tissue if possible.
- Follow a fluid resuscitation guideline for calculating the amount of fluid needed to promptly restore intravascular volume and to preserve tissue perfusion in order to minimize tissue ischemia. More definitive calculation of hourly fluid rates is performed during the secondary survey.
- If a pediatric patient has a burn that is obviously > 20% TBSA, and the actual TBSA has not yet been calculated, the following guidelines may be considered until the TBSA has been calculated and the appropriate amount of IV fluid to be administered has been determined[7]:
  - 5 years old and under: 125 mL of LR per hour
  - 6–13 years of age: 250 mL of LR per hour
  - 14 years of age and older: 500 mL of LR per hour
- Under-resuscitation may result in shock and organ failure, especially acute kidney injury.[10]
- Over-resuscitation may result in worsening edema, orbital or abdominal compartment syndrome, pulmonary edema, or cerebral edema.[10]
- Monitor urinary output to assess for effectiveness of volume replacement.
- IV fluids should be warmed.
- IV fluids should be titrated to the patient's physiologic response, according to the patient's urine output.[10,14]

Table 11-2 includes guidelines for fluid resuscitation and target urinary output.[14]

Adult Fluid Replacement Guidelines

Once the TBSA has been determined, fluid replacement guidelines include the following for adults:

- In adults with burn injuries that are more than 20% TBSA, begin fluid resuscitation with lactated Ringer's solution at 2 mL/kg per percentage of TBSA. In adults with electrical burns, begin fluid resuscitation, using 4 mL/kg.
- Half of the fluid is given in the first 8 hours from time of the burn injury, and the remainder is given in the remaining 16 hours.

TABLE 11-2 Resuscitation Fluid Administration Rates and Target Urine Output

Category of Burn	Age and Weight	Adjusted Fluid Rates	Urine Output
Flame or Scald	Adults and older children (≥ 14 years old)	2 mL LR × kg × % TBSA	0.5 mL/kg/hr 30–50 mL/hr
	Children (< 14 years old)	3 mL LR × kg × % TBSA	1 mL/kg/hr
	Infants and young children	3 mL LR × kg × % TBSA Plus a sugar-containing solution at maintenance rate	1 mL/kg/hr
Electrical Injury	All ages	4 mL LR × kg × % TBSA (when possible to calculate) until urine clears	1–1.5 mL/kg/hr until urine clears

LR = lactated Ringer's solution; TBSA = total body surface area.
Reproduced from American College of Surgeons. (2018). Thermal injuries. In *Advanced trauma life support: Student course manual* (10th ed., p. 174).

- In an adult, maintain urinary output at 0.5 mL/kg/hour, or approximately 30–50 mL/hour (always consider the patient's urinary output, comorbidities, and physiologic response before initiating fluid resuscitation). For adults with electrical injuries with evidence of myoglobinuria (dark red or pink-tinged urine), maintain urinary output at 1.0–1.5 mL/kg/hour, or approximately 75–100 mL/hour until the urine is clear.
- Fluid resuscitation rate should be adjusted as needed to maintain adequate urine output.
- Lactated Ringer's solution is the fluid of choice for fluid resuscitation because it approximates intravascular solute contents. Hyperchloremic solutions (e.g., 0.9% sodium chloride) should be avoided.[10,14]

Box 11-2 provides a sample calculation using this formula.

CLINICAL PEARL

Lactated Ringer's Solution

Lactated Ringer's solution is the fluid of choice for fluid resuscitation in burn situations because it approximates the intravascular solute contents. Hyperchloremic solutions (e.g., 0.9% sodium chloride) should be avoided for the burn patient.[10]

Some patients may have greater fluid requirements than the recommended calculations. They include the following groups:

- Infants and children
- Older adults

BOX 11-2 Adult Fluid Replacement Recommendations

Formula: Weight in kg × 2 mL × % TBSA = total amount of fluid to be infused in 24 hours from the time of injury

- Give half of the calculated total during the first 8 hours.
- Give the remaining half over the next 16 hours.

Example: A 100-kg adult patient has sustained a 50% TBSA thermal burn.

- 100 kg × 2 = 200 mL
- 200 mL × 50% TBSA burn = 10,000 mL to be infused over the first 24 hours from the time of the burn.
- 5,000 mL (10,000/2 = 5,000) will be given in the first 8 hours.
- 5,000 mL will be infused over the remaining 16 hours.

TBSA = total body surface area.

- Patients with inhalation injury
- Patients with high-voltage electrical injuries
- Intoxicated patients
- Patients who experience a delayed start of fluid resuscitation

Unlike resuscitation for hemorrhage, burn resuscitation is required to replace ongoing losses from capillary leak syndrome. These higher fluid requirements may arise because of an inability to assess the entirety of burn injury, such as with inhalational and electrical injuries, or they may result from prior dehydration.

Pediatric Fluid Replacement Guidelines

Pediatric fluid replacement guidelines include the following[10,14]:

- For children younger than 14 years, give 3 mL/kg per percentage of TBSA, half during the first 8 hours and the remaining half over the next 16 hours.
- In addition to resuscitation fluid, infants and young children weighing 30 kg or less should be placed on maintenance fluid containing glucose, specifically D5LR. Maintenance therapy is not titrated to urine output.

D: Disability

Patients with burn injuries are usually alert and oriented. If not, consider CO poisoning, preexisting medical conditions, substance use, hypoxia, or concurrent injuries, such as head trauma, that might cause an altered mental status.

E: Exposure and Environmental Control

Maintenance of body temperature is crucial in patients with burns because they have lost their protective skin barrier. Wet dressings should be avoided, and fluid used to clean burns should be warmed.[2]

Exposure

For exposure, do the following:

- Remove all clothing, diapers, and jewelry, especially rings and bracelets that may cause constriction as the extremity swells.
- For superficial burns that are less than 10% TBSA, cool the burned tissue.
  - Apply cool tap water or saline in any practical manner (e.g., wet cloths, lavage) for a brief period (3–5 minutes).
  - Do not apply ice directly to the skin, because it may cause additional tissue damage.
  - Do not immerse the burned area in water.[2]

Environmental Control

To maintain environmental control, do the following:

- Use blankets to keep the patient warm.
- Use caution with cooling interventions because they may contribute to hypothermia.

Reevaluation for Transfer

Consider transfer to a burn center.[11] If transferring the patient to a burn center, coordinate with the receiving burn team to determine the recommended wound care prior to transfer.

The American Burn Association makes the following recommendations with regard to burn care in preparation for transfer to a burn center[2]:

- Avoid delays in transport to a burn center.
- Cover the patient with a clean, dry dressing and keep warm.
- It is not necessary to cleanse extensive wounds before transfer because patients will undergo formal wound evaluation and cleansing at the burn center.
- Do not debride burns or bullae, or break blisters.[3]
- Elevate above the level of the heart any extremity with a burn injury to decrease wound edema.
- Do not apply creams, ointments, or topical antibiotics because they may cause difficulty in assessing the extent of the burn.

F: Full Set of Vital Signs

A reliable blood pressure may be difficult to obtain because of developing edema in the extremities as a result of capillary leak syndrome. Tachycardia is a poor indicator of resuscitation in a burn patient.[3] In adult burn patients who otherwise appear to have received adequate resuscitation, it is common to see a heart rate of 110–120 beats per minute.[10] A persistent heart rate greater than 140 beats per minute should be investigated; it is typically an indication of severe hypovolemia, undertreated pain, agitation, or a combination of all three.[10] Vital signs should be monitored minimally every hour in burns 20% or greater TBSA.[5]

G: Get Monitoring Devices and Give Comfort

Resuscitation adjuncts begin with laboratory studies.

L: Laboratory Studies

Laboratory studies for patients with burns include the following:

- ABGs and oxygenation content of the blood
  - Carboxyhemoglobin levels[34]
    - Healthy nonsmoker: less than 2%
    - Normal smoker: less than 15%
    - Toxic symptoms: 30–50%
    - Life-threatening: more than 50%
- Blood glucose in infants and young children; hypoglycemia may occur because of their reduced glycogen stores.
- Type and screen/crossmatch as indicated for concurrent trauma.
- CBC, especially white blood cells (WBCs), as an indicator of infection.
- Electrolytes, including potassium and magnesium.

- Blood urea nitrogen (BUN) and creatinine as indicators of renal function.
- Creatine kinase as an indicator of rhabdomyolysis.

M: Monitoring

Monitoring includes the following:

- Continuous cardiac monitoring for dysrhythmias for patients—particularly those with electrical burns, underlying cardiac abnormalities, or electrolyte imbalances—is recommended.
- Consider an indwelling urinary catheter to monitor the effectiveness of fluid resuscitation.

N: Nasogastric or Orogastric Tube Insertion

Insert a gastric tube in patients who are intubated, and consider a gastric tube in patients with nausea and vomiting, with burns covering more than 20% TBSA.[5]

O: Oxygenation and Ventilation

Pulse oximetry cannot differentiate oxygen-bound hemoglobin from carboxyhemoglobin, so these readings will not be accurate in the presence of CO saturation.

> **CLINICAL PEARL**
>
> **P: Pain Assessment and Management**
>
> Pain assessment and management include the following considerations:
>
> - Burns can be very painful, and pain management is a priority.
> - Burns cause an increase in metabolism, which can affect medication dosing requirements.
> - Pain medications should be titrated by administering small, frequent intravascular doses. Do not administer pain medications intramuscularly or subcutaneously.

Reevaluation

Consider transfer to a burn center.

Secondary Survey

The following subsections discuss the secondary survey and management of the patient with thermal burns. See the section "Selected Burn Injuries" for a discussion of electrical and chemical burns.

H: History

Example questions specific to patients with thermal burn injuries are as follows:

- If the MOI was a fire, where was the fire located (indoors or outdoors)?
- Did the fire occur in a structure? If so, what type (car, house, commercial structure)?
- How long was the patient in the burning structure? Did the patient have to be removed by firefighters or bystanders from the burning structure?
- At what time did the injury occur?
- Was there exposure to chemicals?
- Were other people injured in the fire?
- Was there a fall, or did the patient jump and have associated injuries?
- Was there a blast?
- Are the circumstances of the burn injury consistent with the burn characteristics? Is there a possibility of abuse?

Obtain an accurate weight of the patient as soon as possible, or obtain the patient's preburn weight. Fluid resuscitation formulas should be based on the preburn weight of the patient. An intentional burn injury should be suspected in children (particularly those very young) and older adults when the history is not consistent with the injuries sustained.[3]

H: Head-to-Toe Assessment

Assess for any concurrent injuries. Determine the depth, extent, and location of the burn wound. All extremities should be examined for pulses, especially in the presence of circumferential burns.

Depth of the Burn

Considerations regarding the depth of the burn include the following[5,18]:

- Temperature of the offending agent.
- Duration of contact with the offending agent.
- Thickness of the epidermis and dermis.
- Blood supply to the area.
- The depth of the burn is reflective of the layers of skin and tissue affected (**Table 11-3**).[2,19]
- Initial assessment is completed to begin fluid resuscitation. Use only partial or full-thickness burns to determine the percent of TBSA for the fluid resuscitation formula.
- Definitive assessment of depth may change over the course of the first 24–48 hours of the wound.

TABLE 11-3 Differentiating Depth of Wounds

Depth	Appearance	Sensation	Healing Time
Superficial	Dry, red, pink Blanches with pressure Soft No skin sloughing or blistering	Painful	5–10 days
Superficial partial thickness	Blisters Moist and weeping with serous exudate Red, pink Blanches with pressure Edematous	Painful to temperature and air	7–21 days
Deep partial thickness	Blisters Wet or waxy dry Red to pale Does not blanch with pressure	Perceptive of pressure only	14–21 days or longer May require grafting
Full thickness	Waxy white to leathery gray to charred and black No blanching with pressure Dry Firm Hair absent or pulls easily from follicle	Perceptive of deep pressure only	Requires surgical grafts
Fourth degree (full thickness)	Extends into fascia and or muscle	Perceptive of deep pressure only or painless	Requires surgical amputation

Data from American Burn Association. (2018). Burn wound management. In *Advanced burn life support course provider manual: 2018 update* (pp. 39–45); Carter, D. W. (2022). Burns. In *The Merck manual for health care professionals*. http://www.merckmanuals.com/professional/injuries_poisoning/burns/burns.html

Extent of the Burn

The modified Lund and Browder chart, the rule of nines, and the rule of palms are some of the evidence-based methodologies to determine the TBSA burned in adult and pediatric patients. Assessing the extent of the burn may include one of the following methods:

- Determine the extent of partial- and full-thickness burn injury using one of the following:
  - The modified Lund and Browder chart is based on age and burned area (**Table 11-4**).
  - The rule of nines (**Figure 11-4**) divides the adult body into areas of 9% or multiples of 9%, except for the perineum, which is 1%.
- The rule of palms (**Figure 11-5**) is used to measure small or scattered burns. A 1% burn is considered the size of the patient's hand, including the fingers.[5]
- The percentage of TBSA is essential to calculating fluid resuscitation.

Location of Burn and Depth of the Burn

Burns identified as high risk include the following[18]:

- Circumferential burns
  - Assess for increasing pressure to the structures located under circumferential burns.
  - Prepare for escharotomy to the chest wall or extremities.

TABLE 11-4 Modified Lund and Browder Chart

	Birth–1	1–4	5–9	10–14	15	Adult
Burned Area			Total Body Surface (%)			
Head	19	17	13	11	9	7
Neck	2	2	2	2	2	2
Anterior trunk	13	13	13	13	13	13
Posterior trunk	13	13	13	13	13	13
Right buttock	2.5	2.5	2.5	2.5	2.5	2.5
Left buttock	2.5	2.5	2.5	2.5	2.5	2.5
Genitalia	1	1	1	1	1	1
Right upper arm	4	4	4	4	4	4
Left upper arm	4	4	4	4	4	4
Right lower arm	3	3	3	3	3	3
Left lower arm	3	3	3	3	3	3
Right hand	2.5	2.5	2.5	2.5	2.5	2.5
Left hand	2.5	2.5	2.5	2.5	2.5	2.5
Right thigh	5.5	6.5	8	8.5	9	9.5
Left thigh	5.5	6.5	8	8.5	9	9.5
Right leg	5	5	5.5	6	6.5	7
Left leg	5	5	5.5	6	6.5	7
Right foot	3.5	3.5	3.5	3.5	3.5	3.5
Left foot	3.5	3.5	3.5	3.5	3.5	3.5

Age (Years) spans columns Birth–1 through Adult.

- Eschar creates restrictive movement and can result in failure to ventilate and/or loss of limb or life.
- Perineal burns are at high risk for contamination or infection.
- Hand or feet burns are at high risk for strictures and require intense rehabilitation.

Interventions

Interventions include the following[18]:

- Assess and manage pain.
- Cover wounds with clean, dry dressings or sheets to minimize exposure to air currents, which can be painful.
- Elevate the head of the bed to 45 degrees unless contraindicated and the extremities above the level of the heart to decrease the development of edema.[2,5]
- If maltreatment is suspected, further investigation and notification of social or child protective services is warranted.
- Administer tetanus prophylaxis as indicated.
- Consider psychological support for the patient and family.

Estimations of TBSA in obese patients is challenging because of the corresponding altered body-mass distribution.[38]

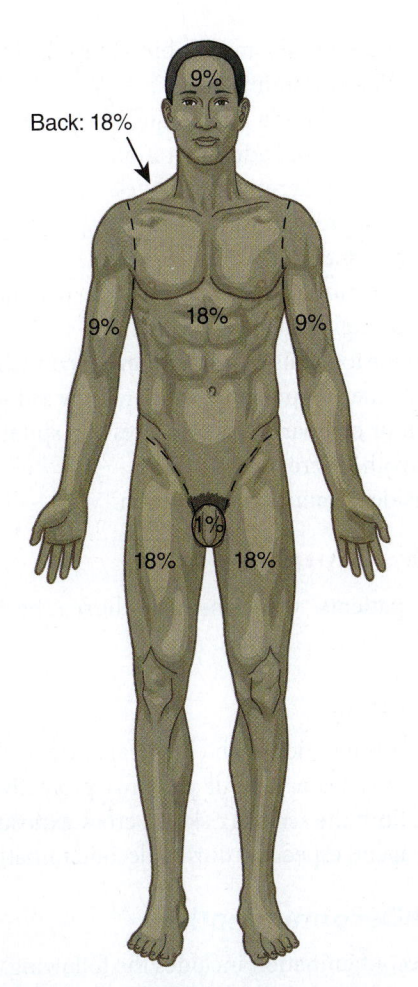

Figure 11-4 *The rule of nines in an adult.*

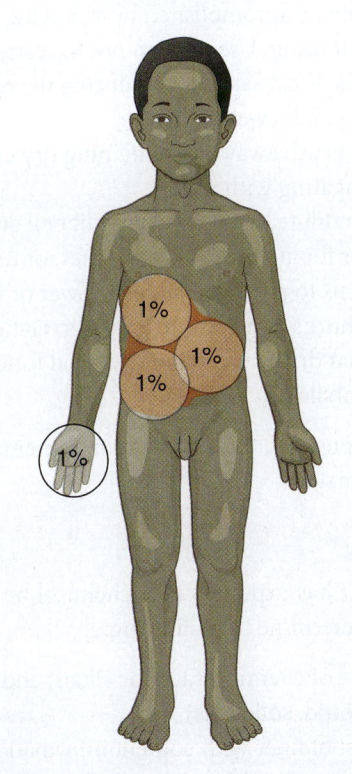

Figure 11-5 *Rule of palms.*

Diagnostics and Interventions for Burns

Reevaluation adjuncts are focused on laboratory studies.

Laboratory Studies

Laboratory studies depend on the burn type and extent of exposure. Ongoing laboratory studies for patients with burns include the following:

- ABGs with carboxyhemoglobin to monitor trends.
- Blood glucose in infants and young children; hypoglycemia may occur because of their reduced glycogen stores.
- CBC, especially WBC, as an indicator of infection in patients with a delayed presentation of a burn injury or when there is a concern for burn wound infection.
- Serum chemistries/electrolytes.
- BUN and creatinine to assess renal function.
- Lactate level urinalysis.

Selected Burn Injuries

Selected burn injuries are discussed in this section.

Electrical Burns

History is particularly important to understanding the effects of electrical burns. This type of burn can be much more serious than it appears. The visible injury may be minor, yet the patient may have sustained deep injury with muscle necrosis and other structural insult. Contractures of an extremity are a sign of severe injury.[3]

H: History

If the patient has experienced an electrical burn, it is important to determine the following:

- The type of current and voltage
  - AC is more dangerous than DC because it causes tetany, which can result in the person tightening their grip on the source of current, thus increasing the exposure.[16]
  - The higher the voltage involved, typically 1,000 volts or more, the greater the size of the internal thermal injury. High-voltage injuries tend to spread out to surrounding structures more than low-voltage injuries do.
- The surface area at point of contact, to help identify areas and extent of burn injury
- The points of contact, to anticipate organs damaged along the path of the current
- Duration of contact with the source, to help determine the possible extent of internal injury
- Any loss of consciousness and any concurrent injuries pertinent to the MOI

H: Head-to-Toe Assessment

It is difficult to assess the damage from electrical burns because much of the injury may be internal. The electrical current enters the body at point of skin contact and travels throughout the body. Thus, it has the potential to damage all types of tissue, including bones, muscles, blood vessels, and nerves—the least resistant to electrical current—before exiting the body.

> **CLINICAL PEARL**
>
> **Electrical Burns**
>
> Do not label the wounds as "exit" or "entrance," but as "contact point" (if known), with a description of the wound.[16]

Assessment findings include the following:

- Wounds or burns to the body
  - Document the assessment of the wounds. Do not label the wounds as "exit" or "entrance," but as "contact point" (if known), with a description of the wound.
- Cardiac dysrhythmias.
  - A frequent cause of death following an electrical injury is cardiac abnormalities. Analyze for abnormal electrocardiogram findings, specifically for ST-segment changes or development of atrial fibrillation, the most common dysrhythmia.[16]
- Rhabdomyolysis with myoglobinuria (see Chapter 21, "Post-Resuscitation Care Considerations," for more information)
  - Urine with myoglobin will appear dark red or brown.
  - Obtain a urinalysis to assess myoglobin levels.
  - Acute kidney injury and renal failure are possible.
  - Obtain BUN and creatinine levels.
  - Determine creatine kinase levels.
  - Consider ABGs with bicarbonate levels for patients with rhabdomyolysis who require alkalization of the urine.
- Fractures
- Seizures

Interventions

Interventions include the following:

- Consider spinal motion restriction based on the MOI.
- Treatment for myoglobinuria includes:
  - Administer an infusion of sodium bicarbonate to alkalize the urine, which promotes the excretion of the myoglobin. Consult a burn center before administering.[3]
  - Prevent oliguria. It is frequently the result of insufficient fluid administration.
  - Normalize serum electrolytes.
  - Decompress any areas with compartment syndrome.
- Monitor cardiac rate and rhythm in patients with low- or high-voltage exposure.
- Monitor for signs and symptoms of compartment syndrome and prepare for fasciotomy as indicated.
- Monitor compartment pressures and splint extremities with severe burns.
- Consider tetanus immunization.

Chemical Burns

Care of patients with chemical burns begins with preparation.

Preparation

The first consideration with chemical burns is the safety of the trauma team. Use of personal protective equipment will limit the serious risk of a cross-exposure to the chemical agent, especially during decontamination.

Patient Decontamination

Patient decontamination includes the following:

- Decontamination of dry chemical exposure can generally be accomplished by removing the patient's clothing. Use caution not to scatter any of the stimulus or causative agent during the removal of clothing and jewelry.
- Lightly brush away any remaining dry chemical before irrigating with water.
  - Then dilute by flushing with liberal amounts of water for at least 20–30 minutes, or until the pH returns to normal, using a shower or hose. Alkaline burns may require longer irrigation.
- Note that dry powder and chemical fumes can also cause inhalation injuries.

See Chapter 19, "Disaster Management," for additional information.

H: History

If the patient has experienced a chemical burn, it is important to determine the following:

- The type of chemical (acid or alkali) and its physical state (liquid, solid, gas)
  - The container with content information can be useful in identifying chemicals.

- The concentration and volume of the chemical
- The route and duration of exposure
- The direct effects of the chemical, such as obvious burning
- Risk for potential systemic effects

Interventions

Interventions include the following:

- Support oxygenation and ventilation, and consider the possibility of inhalation injury.
- Remove the chemical by irrigating the skin until the pH is normal. Generally, the use of neutralizing agents is contraindicated because of the exothermic reactions that often occur. However, it may be appropriate after the patient is stabilized, the initial irrigation has been started, and the substance has been identified.
  - Normal human skin pH is about 5.3.
  - Tap water may be used. Irrigation should be at low pressures to avoid tissue injury.
  - Extensive acid or alkali burns may require several hours of irrigation to achieve neutral pH.
  - Avoid hypothermia by using tepid water.
- Debride any blisters caused by a chemical exposure.
- With tar or asphalt, stop the burning process by using water until the tar or asphalt is cool to the touch, and then use petroleum to assist in removal of the agent.
- Phenols are an acidic form of alcohol and are poorly soluble in water. They are found in most household disinfectants and chemical solvents. For patients with phenol burns, first provide copious irrigation with water, then 50% polyethylene glycol, which increases the solubility of phenols in water. Phenol burns can cause a thick eschar to the affected area if not removed quickly.
  - Consider liver function tests.
- For hydrofluoric acid (used for glass etching, in manufacturing, and as a cleaning agent) burns, irrigate until the skin has returned to a normal pH.
  - Because hydrofluoric acid can cause depletion of calcium, assess calcium levels. Cardiac dysrhythmias and death from hypocalcemia may occur as the fluoride rapidly binds to free calcium in the blood. Closely monitor for cardiac arrhythmias.
  - Topical calcium gel may be applied to the skin to neutralize the fluoride with hydrofluoric acid burns. This is an instance in which a direct neutralizing agent is recommended to treat a chemical exposure.[3,49]

Reevaluation of the Patient with Burn Injury

Provide frequent and ongoing reevaluation of the following:

- The effectiveness of airway and ventilation, including the ongoing ability of the patient to protect the airway and perform adequate ventilation
- The effectiveness of fluid resuscitation, as evidenced by hemodynamic stability and urine output[10]
  - Monitor urine output every hour.
- All associated injuries and the effectiveness of the interventions
- The patient's temperature, so as to prevent hypothermia
- Wound, pulmonary, and systemic signs and symptoms of infections; sepsis is a major risk and can develop any time after the resuscitation phase.[29]
- The patient's pain level and the pain medication's effectiveness

Post-Resuscitation Care

Post-resuscitation care focuses on wound care but can also involve escharotomy.

Wound Care

If the patient will be transferred to or follow up with a burn center, consult with the receiving facility and follow their wound care recommendations. Wound care may include the following measures:

- Initial wound care varies with the type of wound, but it generally includes debridement, topical wound care products, and dressings. This may be done in the emergency department, operating room, or intensive care unit. Wound care and burn debridement should not delay transfer to a burn center.[11]
- Burn debridement and dressing procedures are very painful, so intravenous pain medication should be administered before and during the process. Monitor patients closely after the procedures for respiratory depression.
- Wounds should be cleansed with water, soap, baby shampoo, or chlorhexidine, removing dirt and debris.
- Wound care depends on the location, depth, and extent of the burn.
  - Superficial burns may require topical antibiotics but rarely dressings.
  - Skin grafting may be required for deeper wounds.

- Monitor for hypothermia during wound care. Limit wound care to one extremity or body section at a time.
- Wound healing for larger burns may require weeks or months of inpatient hospital care.
- Reevaluate the effectiveness of interventions.

Escharotomy

An escharotomy is an incision through full-thickness burn eschar down to subcutaneous fat along the length of the circumferential burn. It relieves external constriction that leads to restriction of the chest wall expansion or loss of peripheral perfusion of an extremity. Generally, escharotomies are not needed until several hours into fluid resuscitation and should be done in consultation with a burn center.[2]

Emerging Trends

As the science and evidence of trauma care continue to evolve, tools to improve patient outcomes continue to be trialed and refined. Evidence is tested and replicated, and new standards of care are transitioned into practice. This section on emerging trends explores some of the evidence and the potential significance to trauma patient care. In the care of patients with surface and burn injuries, pain management and computerized protocol-driven resuscitation are two important areas of innovation.

Pain Management

Uncontrolled pain is a challenge when caring for severely burned patients, particularly during wound care procedures. Side effects and reduced efficacy of narcotic pain medications have led care providers to consider alternative means to manage a patient's pain. This includes development of effective pain medication regimens, but also use of nonpharmacologic techniques. Psychological distraction analgesic options—particularly virtual reality pain distraction—are an emerging trend. Researchers and providers are finding that the use of immersive virtual reality pain distraction, used in conjunction with traditional pain medications, can significantly reduce pain in those undergoing wound care. Novel techniques for managing patients' experiences of pain will remain a focus of future advances geared toward improving patient outcomes. The American Burn Association provides a guideline on the management of acute pain for adult patients with burns, including assessment and recommended interventions.[42]

Computerized Protocol-Driven Resuscitation

Optimal burn fluid resuscitation ensures that the least amount of sufficient fluid volume is administered to achieve organ perfusion. A computerized decision-support system (CDSS) uses data obtained from a patient's electronic medical record to assist clinicians in making therapeutic or diagnostic decisions. These algorithms typically take into consideration current infusion rates, hourly urine output, burn size, and time since the burn to calculate a recommended infusion rate or adjustment of the current infusion rate. CDSS-driven burn fluid resuscitation protocols enable nurses to make timely and effective changes to the resuscitation rates without a delay while waiting for provider orders. Additionally, these protocols have demonstrated fewer total volumes delivered, while increasing the percentage of time the urine output goal is achieved.

Summary

The integumentary system is the largest organ in the body. The skin serves many vital functions, such as heat regulation, fluid and electrolyte regulation, and sensory relay. It is also the body's first line of defense against environmental hazards and infection. Surface and burn trauma results in alteration of these normal functions. Trauma resuscitation of patients with skin trauma requires the same resuscitation strategies used for other trauma patients. Once the trauma victim with surface or burn trauma is stabilized, wound care becomes a priority. Infection is a leading cause of morbidity and mortality in these patients. The treatment goal is to promote wound healing, maintain function, prevent complications, minimize disfiguring scars, and optimize the patient's return to activities of daily living.

References

1. American Burn Association. (2018). Airway management and smoke inhalation injury. In *Advanced burn life support course provider manual: 2018 update* (pp. 23–30).
2. American Burn Association. (2018). Burn wound management. In *Advanced burn life support course provider manual: 2018 update* (pp. 39–45).
3. American Burn Association. (2018). Chemical burns. In *Advanced burn life support course provider manual: 2018 update* (pp. 52–58).
4. American Burn Association. (2018). Cold injuries. In *Advanced burn life support course provider manual: 2018 update* (pp. 86–89).
5. American Burn Association. (2018). Initial assessment and management. In *Advanced burn life support course provider manual: 2018 update* (pp. 7–22).
6. American Burn Association. (2018). Introduction. In *Advanced burn life support course provider manual: 2018 update* (pp. 2–6).
7. American Burn Association. (2018). Pediatric burns. In *Advanced burn life support course provider manual: 2018 update* (pp. 59–67).

8. American Burn Association. (2018). Radiation injury. In *Advanced burn life support course provider manual: 2018 update* (pp. 83–85).
9. American Burn Association. (2018). *Scald statistics and data resources.* https://ameriburn.org/wp-content/uploads/2018/12/nbaw2019_statsdataresources_120618-1.pdf
10. American Burn Association. (2018). Shock and fluid resuscitation. In *Advanced burn life support course provider manual: 2018 update* (pp. 31–38).
11. American Burn Association. (2018). Stabilization, transfer, and transport. In *Advanced burn life support course provider manual: 2018 update* (pp. 68–72).
12. American College of Surgeons. (2018). Airway and ventilator management. In *Advanced trauma life support: Student course manual* (10th ed., pp. 23–41).
13. American College of Surgeons. (2018). Musculoskeletal trauma. In *Advanced trauma life support: Student course manual* (10th ed., pp. 148–167).
14. American College of Surgeons. (2018). Thermal injuries. In *Advanced trauma life support: Student course manual* (10th ed., pp. 167–183).
15. Angioi, R., Morrin, A., & White, B. (2021). The rediscovery of honey for skin repair: Recent advances in mechanisms for honey-meditated wound healing and scaffolded application techniques. *Applied Sciences, 11*(11), Article 5192. https://doi.org/10.3390/app11115192
16. Bernal, E., & Arnoldo, B. D. (2018). Electrical injuries. In D. N. Herndon (Ed.), *Total burn care* (5th ed., pp. 396–402). Elsevier.
17. Brancato, J. C. (2021). Minor wound preparation and irrigation. *UpToDate.* Retrieved September 13, 2022, from https://www.uptodate.com/contents/minor-wound-preparation-and-irrigation
18. Cancio, L. C., Bohannon, F. J., & Kramer, G. C. (2018). Burn resuscitation. In D. N. Herndon (Ed.), *Total burn care* (5th ed., pp. 77–86). Elsevier.
19. Carter, D. M. (2022). Burns. In *The Merck manual for health care professionals.* Retrieved September 13, 2022, from http://www.merckmanuals.com/professional/injuries_poisoning/burns/burns.html
20. Centers for Disease Control and Prevention. (n.d.). *Diphtheria, tetanus, and pertussis vaccine recommendations.* https://www.cdc.gov/vaccines/vpd/dtap-tdap-td/hcp/recommendations.html
21. Clardy, P. F., Manaker, S., & Perry, H. (2018). Carbon monoxide poisoning. *UpToDate.* Retrieved September 13, 2022, from https://www.uptodate.com/contents/carbon-monoxide-poisoning
22. Cochran, A., & Morris, S. E. (2018). Cold-induced injury: Frostbite. In D. N. Herndon (Ed.), *Total burn care* (5th ed., pp. 403–407). Elsevier.
23. Demetriades, D., Benjamin, E. R., & Bukur, M. (2021). Soft tissue injuries. In *Color atlas of emergency trauma* (pp. 226–237). Cambridge University Press. https://doi.org/10.1017/9781108776622.011
24. Doughty, D. B., & Sparks, B. (2015). Wound-healing physiology and factors that affect the repair process. In R. A. Bryant & D. P. Nix (Eds.), *Acute and chronic wounds: Current management concepts* (5th ed, pp. 40–62). Mosby Elsevier.
25. Enkhbaatar, P., Sousse, L. E., Cox, R. A., & Herndon, D. N. (2018). The pathophysiology of inhalation injury. In D. N. Herndon (Ed.), *Total burn care* (5th ed., pp. 174–183). Elsevier.
26. Gabriel, A. (2021). Wound irrigation. *Medscape.* Retrieved September 13, 2022, from http://emedicine.medscape.com/article/1895071-overview
27. Ghosh, S., Rana, S., Islam, K., Chowdhury, S., Haider, N., Kafi, M. A., Shah, R. A., Jahan, A. A., Mursalin, H. S., Marma, A. S, Emran Ali, S. M., Hossain, S., Bhowmik, R., Debnath, N. C., Shamsuzzaman, A. K., Ahmed, B. N., Siddiqi, U. R., & Jhora, S. T. (2020). Trends and clinico-epidemiological features of human rabies cases in Bangladesh 2006–2018. *Scientific Reports, 10*(1). https://doi.org/10.1038/s41598-020-59109-w
28. Graham, S. (2020). Wound healing and soft tissue injuries. In K. A. McQuillan & M. B. Flynn Makic (Eds.), *Trauma nursing: From resuscitation through rehabilitation* (5th ed., pp. 229–250). Elsevier.
29. Greenhalgh, D. G. (2019). Management of burns. *New England Journal of Medicine, 380*(24), 2349–2359. https://doi.org/10.1056/NEJMra1807442
30. Gupta, A. (2021). Classification of wounds and the physiology of wound healing. In P. Kumar & V. Kothari (Eds.), *Wound healing research* (pp. 3–53) Springer Nature. https://doi.org/10.1007/978-981-16-2677-7_1
31. Ho, Y. W., Chung, P. Y., Hou, S. K., Chang, M. L., & Kang, Y. N. (2022). Should we use hyperbaric oxygen for carbon monoxide poisoning management? A network meta-analysis of randomized controlled trials. *Healthcare, 10*(7), 1–13. https://doi.org/10.3390/healthcare10071311
32. Jeschke, M. G., van Baar, M. E., Choudhry, M. A., Chung, K. K., Gibran, N. S., & Logsetty, S. (2020). Burn injury. *Nature Reviews: Disease Primers, 6,* Article 11. https://doi.org/10.1038/s41572-020-0145-5
33. Kamath, M. (2020). Role of leech therapy in wound healing—A short review. *Research Journal of Pharmacy and Technology, 13*(10), 5040–5041. https://doi.org/10.5958/0974-360X.2020.00882.3
34. Kinoshita, H., Turkan, H., Vucinic, S., Naqvi, S., Bedair, R., Rezaee, R., & Tsatsakis, A. (2020). Carbon monoxide poisoning. *Toxicology Reports, 7,* 169–173. https://doi.org/10.1016/j.toxrep.2020.01.005
35. Lent-Schochet, D., & Jialal, I. (2022, May 8). Physiology, edema. *StatPearls.* StatPearls Publishing. https://www.ncbi.nlm.nih.gov/books/NBK537065/
36. Lewis, K., & Pay, J. L. (2022). Wound irrigation. *StatPearls.* StatPearls Publishing. https://www.ncbi.nlm.nih.gov/books/NBK538522/?report=classic
37. Lyons, F., & Ousley, L. (2015). Basics of dermatology. In F. Lyons & L. Ousley (Eds.), *Dermatology for the advanced practice nurse* (pp. 15–26). Springer.
38. Moore, R. A., Waheed, A., & Burns, B. (2022). Rule of nines. *StatPearls.* StatPearls Publishing. https://www.ncbi.nlm.nih.gov/books/NBK513287/

39. Newman, R., & Mahdy, H. (2022). Laceration. *StatPearls*. StatPearls Publishing. https://www.ncbi.nlm.nih.gov/books/NBK545166/
40. Park, C. W., Juliano, J. D., & Woodhall, D. (2021). Part 18: Wounds and soft-tissue injuries. In K. Knoop, L. Stack, A. Storrow, & R. Thurman (Eds.), *The atlas of emergency medicine* (5th ed., 18-01–18-04). McGraw Hill.
41. Ramirez, E. G. (2018). Wounds and wound management. In V. Sweet (Ed.), *Emergency nursing core curriculum* (7th ed., pp. 483–496). Saunders Elsevier.
42. Romanowski, K. S., Carson, J., Pape, K., Bernal, E., Sharar, S., Wiechman, S., Carter, D., Liu, Y. M., Nitschke, S., Bhalla, P., Litt, J., Przkora, R., Friedman, B., Popiak, S., Jeng, J. Ryan, C, M., & Joe, V. (2020). American Burn Association guidelines on the management of acute pain in the adult burn patient: A review of the literature, a compilation of expert opinion, and next steps. *Journal of Burn Care & Research, 41*(6), 1129–1151. https://doi.org/10.1093/jbcr/iraa119
43. Smith, C. C. (2021). Clinical manifestations and evaluation of edema in adults. *UpToDate*. Retrieved September 13, 2022, from https://www.uptodate.com/contents/clinical-manifestations-and-evaluation-of-edema-in-adults/
44. Soussi, S., Depret, F., Benyamina, M., & Legrand, M. (2018). Early hemodynamic management of critically ill burn patients. *Anesthesiology, 129*, 583–589. https://doi.org/10.1097/aln.0000000000002314
45. Stewart, B. T. (2022). Epidemiology, risk factors, and prevention of burn injuries. *UpToDate*. Retrieved December 7, 2022, from https://www.uptodate.com/contents/epidemiology-risk-factors-and-prevention-of-burn-injuries?search=epidemiologyof-burn-injuries-globally&source=search_result&selectedTitle=1~150&usage_type=default&display_rank=1
46. Torlincasi, A. M., Lopez, R. A., & Waseem, M. (2022). Acute compartment syndrome. *StatPearls*. StatPearls Publishing. https://www.ncbi.nlm.nih.gov/books/NBK448124/
47. Western Trauma Association. (n.d.). *Management of the mangled extremity*. https://www.westerntrauma.org/western-trauma-association-algorithms/management-of-the-mangled-extremity/introduction/
48. Wheeless, C. R. (2016, November 28). *Frost bite. Wheeless' textbook of orthopaedics*. https://www.wheelessonline.com/muscles-tendons/frost-bite/
49. Williams, F. N., & Lee, J. O. (2018). Chemical burns. In D. N. Herndon (Ed.), *Total burn care* (5th ed., pp. 408–413). Elsevier.
50. Wolf, S. E., Cancio, L. C., & Pruitt, B. A. (2018). Epidemiological, demographic, and outcome characteristics of burn injury. In D. N. Herndon (Ed.), *Total burn care* (5th ed., pp. 14–27). Elsevier.
51. Wysocki, A. B. (2015). Anatomy of skin and soft tissue. In R. A. Bryant & D. P. Nix (Eds.), *Acute and chronic wounds: Current management concepts* (5th ed., pp. 40–81). Mosby Elsevier.
52. Zheng, Y., Wang, D., & Ma, L. Z. (2021). Effect of polyhexamethylene biguanide in combination with undecylenamidopropyl betaine or PsIG on biofilm clearance. *International Journal of Molecular Sciences, 22*(2), 1–12. https://doi.org/10.3390/ijms22020768

CHAPTER 12

The LGBTQ+ Trauma Patient

Steven F. Jacobson, MS, MSN, MBA, RN, CEN, CFRN, CTRN, CPEN, TCRN

OBJECTIVES

Upon completion of this chapter, the learner will be able to:
1. Describe selected terms, definitions, and identities within the LGBTQ+ population.
2. Identify disparities and health risks that affect the LGBTQ+ population.
3. Apply cultural competence and cultural humility to healthcare interactions with the LGBTQ+ population.

Introduction

A recent poll found that 5.6% of Americans surveyed identify as lesbian, gay, bisexual or transgender, which is nearly equivalent to the population of New York State.[38] LGBTQ+ persons remain a vulnerable population with regard to healthcare access and health risks.[52] This chapter introduces lesbian, gay, bisexual, transgender, queer, and other (LGBTQ+) communities, including a brief history, epidemiology, an overview of terms and identities, health disparities, and nursing care considerations. A variety of abbreviations are used throughout the chapter to describe specific communities (e.g., LGB, LGBT, and LGBTQ+) to accurately reflect the cited material and related research. Research on human gender, gender identity, and sexuality is ongoing, and our understanding and terminology will continually evolve.[53]

A Brief History

The American Psychiatric Association (APA) removed homosexuality as a mental disorder from the *Diagnostic and Statistical Manual* in 1973,[19] and in 1990, the World Health Organization declared that homosexuality was no longer considered an illness.[14] These changes signaled the shift in recognition in healthcare that homosexuality is not a condition or diagnosis. This recognition continued as the American Medical Association (AMA), in a policy statement, advocated for physicians to be nonjudgmental regarding sexual orientation and behavior.[2] In spite of this shift in healthcare perspectives by professional medical and nursing organizations, implicit and explicit bias has continued, as with other vulnerable populations.[52]

The declassification of homosexuality as a mental disorder in the 1970s was a starting point for the professional recognition of healthcare needs for this population. However, the emergence of the human immunodeficiency virus (HIV) and acquired immunodeficiency syndrome (AIDS) was associated with the gay community, and the resultant fear and stigmatization further exacerbated the disparity in healthcare. Because some healthcare providers refused to care for patients with AIDS, nurses at San Francisco General Hospital created the first inpatient unit dedicated to caring for patients with AIDS in 1983.[4] Since that time, significant progress has been made regarding funding and research dedicated to HIV/AIDS, and care for sexual and gender minorities is now included.[44]

> **NOTE**
>
> **Want to Learn More History?**
>
> A variety of resources are available that outline important LGBTQ+ leaders and events throughout history. GLSEN has educational material and lesson plans available at https://www.glsen.org/activity/lgbtq-history-timeline-lesson

Epidemiology

Multiple epidemiologic considerations apply to LBGTQ+ communities, including mental health, reproductive health, substance use, risk-taking behaviors, human trafficking, and homelessness.[33,49,52] Evaluation of epidemiologic data in LGBTQ+ populations is challenging because of a lack of questions related to gender and sexual identity in national and statewide health surveys.[33] Despite this limitation, specific healthcare disparities in LGBTQ+ persons have been identified.

Healthcare Disparities and Access to Care

Challenges with healthcare disparities and access to healthcare for the LBGTQ+ community are multifaceted. Some of these challenges have commonalities within the community at large, such as social stigma, marginalization, and explicit or implicit bias, while other disparities are more specific.[44,49] Lesbian women, for example, are less likely than heterosexual women to have mammogram screenings for breast cancer or a Papanicolaou (Pap) test.[52] Studies indicate that limited access to services, decreased quality of care, and worse outcomes are associated with healthcare provider bias.[52] Additionally, LBGTQ adults have higher rates of poverty.[7] Although access to healthcare in the United States has improved since the advent of the Affordable Care Act, barriers continue to exist; for example, most LGBT community health centers are located in major cities and may not be available to people living outside those areas.[44,45]

More than 50% of sexual minorities and 70% of gender minority adults have experienced discrimination and bias from healthcare professionals.[7] Another powerful influence on healthcare disparity is medical mistrust, particularly in specific geographic locations and based on previous experiences with healthcare.[8] Research indicates that up to 23% of transgender people did not see a physician when in need of healthcare because of fear of mistreatment.[37]

Sexual and Reproductive Healthcare

Sexual and reproductive health needs for LGBTQ+ individuals include cancer screenings and treatment, fertility and assistive reproductive technology, pregnancy-related care, sexually transmitted infection (STI) and HIV testing and treatment, and gender-affirming services. It is important that healthcare providers be educated on the unique needs of gender and sexual minorities and provide care that is high quality, equitable, and free from prejudice. High-quality reproductive and sexual healthcare is delivered with consideration of the diversity of the population served while also being tailored to individual needs. While many reproductive health needs within the LGBTQ+ community are the same as, or similar to, those in other communities, there are specific areas of increased risk that must be assessed and treated.[74] Barriers to sexual and reproductive healthcare are exacerbated by provider knowledge deficits regarding the needs of gender-diverse populations.[1]

HIV/AIDS

The HIV that causes AIDS was initially referred to as the gay-related immune deficiency (GRID). The global HIV/AIDS epidemic, which has claimed the lives of 36.3 million people,[76] continues despite remarkable progress in prevention. Studies have demonstrated that the number of individuals with a new diagnosis of HIV in the United States has been reduced by nearly two-thirds since the onset of the epidemic.[10] This marked improvement is related to the advent of highly effective treatments and decreased stigma associated with HIV, as well as decreased prejudice against those with the disease. Additional factors in decreasing HIV infections in gay and bisexual men include pre-exposure prophylaxis (PrEP) (**Table 12-1**),[15,16,34] improved access to testing, and increased condom use.[9] However, new infections are on the rise in Black Americans and transgender individuals.[10,39]

TABLE 12-1 What Are PrEP, PEP, and Treatment as Prevention?

Intervention	Description
Pre-exposure prophylaxis (PrEP)	PrEP is preventive, intended to keep individuals HIV negative by taking antiretroviral medications before HIV exposure. Two medication combinations are currently approved for daily oral use, and in 2021 a long-acting injectable medication was also approved by the Food and Drug Administration. These regimens are considered 99% effective when used correctly. Routine screening and ongoing medical care are necessary.
Post-exposure prophylaxis (PEP)	Following a known or potential exposure to HIV, a 28-day course of antiretroviral medication taken within 72 hours of exposure may decrease the likelihood of infection. Effectiveness is determined by method of exposure and time to treatment. Post-exposure prophylaxis is intended for emergency use only and is not for regular use for repeated exposures.
Treatment as prevention (TasP)	Antiretroviral medication is used to control the virus. An "undetectable" virus level in the blood decreases the likelihood of transmission to others by 96%.
Ending the HIV epidemic	Advances in treatment and public health interventions have significantly reduced the spread and severity of the HIV epidemic. The U.S. Department of Health and Human Services released a federal plan to end the HIV epidemic by 2030 using scientific advances to coordinate resources, expertise, and technology to implement this plan.
Application to the injured patient	Serious, although rare, side effects can occur with some antiretroviral medications. These include kidney problems, lactic acid buildup, and softening of bone structure. These side effects may lead to increased risk for injury and altered response to trauma interventions.

Data from Cohen, M. S. (2019). Successful treatment of HIV eliminates sexual transmission. *The Lancet, 393*(10189), 2366–2367. https://www.thelancet.com/journals/lancet/article/PIIS0140-6736(19)30701-9/fulltext; Cohen, M. S., Chen, Y. Q., McCauley, M., Gamble, T., Hosseinipour, M. C., Kumarasamy, N., Hakim, J. G., Kumwenda, J., Grinsztejn, B., Pilotto, J. H., Godbole, S. V., Mehendale, S., Chariyalertsak, S., Santos, B. R., Mayer, K. H., Hoffman, I. F., Eshleman, S. H., Piwowar-Manning, E., Wang, L., Makhema, J., ... HPTN 052 Study Team. (2011). Prevention of HIV-1 infection with early antiretroviral therapy. *New England Journal of Medicine, 365*(6), 493–505. https://doi.org/10.1056/NEJMoa1105243; HIV.gov. (n.d.). *HIV basics*. U.S. Department of Health and Human Services Minority HIV/AIDS Fund. https://www.hiv.gov/hiv-basics

Reproductive Care

Sexual and reproductive health concerns for the LGBTQ+ population extend beyond HIV and AIDS. As noted earlier, barriers to care, although improving, still exist and include lack of health insurance and access to healthcare.

Sexual minority women are less likely to access reproductive healthcare services than their heterosexual counterparts.[21] These services include counseling and access to contraceptive medications, STI testing and treatment, and cancer screenings, including mammograms and Pap tests.[52] Sexual minority individuals are more likely to seek medical information from peers, the media, and community centers.[63] Sexual minority groups, with the exception of lesbians, are more likely to seek and receive contraceptive counseling.[63] Other sexual minorities are at higher risk of experiencing an unintended pregnancy compared with the nonsexual minority population.[12] Research indicates that healthcare provider knowledge of sexual and reproductive health risks associated with different populations may increase the delivery of appropriate care, such as human papillomavirus vaccines, STI tests, and Pap tests, regardless of sexual orientation.[62]

Evidence indicates that LGBTQ+ populations are among those groups showing the most rapid increases in seeking fertility care.[41] Barriers in fertility care include gender dysphoria, stigmas, psychological distress, cisnormativity, and a lack of specific information related to the LGBTQ+ communities.[41] Also contributing to the challenges associated with fertility and family planning services for LGBTQ+ individuals is a knowledge gap in cultural competence and cultural humility within healthcare.[41]

Mental Health

No global consensus has been reached on the definition of what mental health is, but it is accepted that it is integral to health and a state of mental well-being; mental health is more than the just the absence of mental illness.[27,75] Included in a state of mental well-being, emotional well-being, and physical health are the concepts of autonomy, self-determination, and authenticity.[59] The absence of autonomy support in interpersonal or institutional relations in groups that may be stigmatized can have a negative effect on a person's ability to be authentic to their true selves.[59] Mental health and well-being are foundational to healthy relationships.[51]

Across all age groups, LGBs were 2 to 3 times more likely than heterosexuals to have experienced a mental, behavioral, or emotional disorder that interfered with their life activities.[50] Seventy percent of LGBTQ+ youth ages 13–24 years rated their mental health as "poor."[67] Discrimination, bullying, and isolation are known to negatively affect mental well-being, and LGBTQ adolescents are more likely to be subject to bullying and harassment than their heterosexual counterparts.[6,67]

Adult and school-age transgender and gender nonconforming individuals are exposed to a variety of social stressors that contribute to poor mental health, including discrimination, harassment, bias, and violence.[58,73]

Substance Use Disorders

Substance use and misuse is higher across all age groups in the sexual minority populations than the general population; this includes the use of cannabis, cocaine, methamphetamine, sedatives, hypnotics, hallucinogens, inhalants, and opioids.[40,50] Sexual minority women, compared with heterosexual women, are more likely to engage in heavy alcohol consumption and experience problems related to alcohol use.[40] The minority stress theory may offer some insight into substance use and misuse. However, it does not explain why some individuals develop substance use disorders when most do not.[22] Transgender and nonbinary populations use tobacco, cannabis, and alcohol at higher rates than the general population.[41] Bullying, abuse, trauma, family conflict, and homelessness may be some of the factors that contribute to substance use and misuse when these experiences are internalized, and unhealthy coping mechanisms develop.[22,43]

Substance use, acute stress disorder, and posttraumatic stress disorder are risks for anyone who has suffered a traumatic event; having an awareness of this provides the nurse with an opportunity for early recognition and intervention. See Chapter 18, "Psychosocial Aspects of Trauma Care," for additional information.

Risk-Taking Behaviors

Risk-taking behaviors include unsafe sexual behavior, substance use, binge alcohol drinking, dangerous driving, and illegal activities.[60] Sexual risk-taking behavior is higher in sexual minority youths than in heterosexual youths, with the accompanying higher risk for HIV, other STIs, and pregnancy.[57] Alcohol use is associated with traumatic injury and higher rates of sexual intercourse without a condom.[23] Emerging adulthood is acknowledged as a period of risk-taking in people's lives. An absence of social support and positive influences may negatively impact mental health and increase risk-taking behavior.[47]

Human Trafficking

Human trafficking is categorized as labor and/or sex trafficking and is often referred to as a form of modern slavery.[5] Sex trafficking is defined in part as the "recruitment, harboring, transportation, provision, obtaining, patronizing, or soliciting of a person for the purpose of a commercial sex act (sex trafficking), in which a commercial sex act is induced by force, fraud, or coercion."[68p8] Sex trafficking is a global crisis, and any vulnerable person is at risk across all genders, races, economic status levels, or sexual orientations.[71] Particularly vulnerable groups include undocumented or migrant workers, runaway youths, those with adverse childhood experiences, and LGBTQ+ individuals, all of which can coexist.[5,24,71] Risk factors for trafficking of LGBTQ+ youth may include substance misuse, homelessness, depression, intimate partner violence, absence of financial or emotional support, or a possible history of child sexual abuse.[5,71]

In the care of trauma patients, maintaining a high level of awareness of the possibility of trafficking is essential, particularly for vulnerable groups. It is estimated that during the time an individual is trafficked, 88% will seek medical care. Studies indicate that up to 63% of people who have been trafficked sought care in an emergency department *while being trafficked*.[70] It is unlikely that individuals experiencing trafficking will self-disclose. A trauma-informed approach to care with the understanding of preventing retraumatization is a high priority.[31,70] See Chapter 18, "Psychosocial Aspects of Trauma Care," for additional information on trauma-informed care.

Homelessness

It is estimated that 20–40% of people experiencing homelessness are from the LGBTQ+ populations.[25] Homelessness is a risk factor across all demographics for poor physical and mental health, as well as early death.[26] Persons from the LGBTQ+ communities who are experiencing homelessness are at risk for exploitation, abuse, family rejection, mental and physical issues, and STIs.[46]

Terms, Definitions, and Identities

Understanding the terms and descriptions that LGBTQ+ individuals use to describe themselves will help the nurse provide patients with culturally competent care (**Table 12-2**).[28,29,54,56] However, definitions can vary within LGBTQ+ communities. Each person is unique and may prefer a different identifier, and it is important to defer to their preference for terminology. Continued evolution in terminology is likely.

Gender Identity and Gender Expression

Gender identity usually refers to the person's internal sense of their gender. This can be maleness, femaleness, neither, or both. Gender expression is the external presentation of that person's gender. This presentation can be a person's mannerisms, voice, clothing, or any number of characteristics. Gender does not always equal expression, and expression and identities do not always match genetics.

> **CLINICAL PEARL**
>
> **What Does "Cisgender" Mean?**
>
> When an individual describes or identifies themselves as "cisgender," or sometimes just "cis," it means that they identify with the sex assigned at birth. "Transgender" refers to a person's gender identity differing from the sex assigned at birth or on their birth certificate. In Latin, the word "cis" means "on this side," whereas "trans" means "on the other side."

TABLE 12-2 What Does LGBTQ+ Mean?

Initial or Symbol	Word	Definition
L	Lesbian	A female homosexual. A female who experiences sexual, romantic, or emotional attraction to other females.
G	Gay	Primarily refers to a homosexual person or the trait of being homosexual. Gay is often used to describe homosexual males, but lesbians may also be referred to as gay.
B	Bisexual	A sexual, romantic, or emotional attraction toward more than one gender. Sometimes the term is used to describe an individual attracted to men and women, while others consider it attraction to individuals who are the same and different from one's own gender. Sometimes termed pansexuality.
T	Transgender	An umbrella term for people whose gender identity differs from what is typically associated with the sex they were assigned at birth. It is sometimes abbreviated to trans. It can also be used for an individual who has started or completed the gender reassignment process.[54]
T	Transsexual	Gender identity inconsistent or not culturally associated with the biological sex assigned at birth. Generally considered an antiquated term.
2/T	Two-spirit	A modern umbrella term used by some indigenous North Americans to describe gender-variant individuals within indigenous communities who are seen as having both male and female spirits within them.
Q	Queer	An umbrella term for sexual and gender minorities who are not heterosexual or cisgender.

(continues)

TABLE 12-2 What Does LGBTQ+ Mean? (continued)

Initial or Symbol	Word	Definition
Q	Questioning	The questioning of one's gender, sexual identity, sexual orientation, or all three is a process of exploration by people who may be unsure, still exploring, and concerned about applying a social label to gender or sexuality.
I	Intersex	A variation in sex characteristics, including chromosomes, gonads, or genitals, that does not enable an individual to be distinctly identified as male or female.
A	Asexual (or nonsexual)	Lack of sexual attraction to anyone, or low or absent interest in sexual activity. It may be considered the lack of a sexual orientation, or one of the variations thereof, alongside heterosexuality, homosexuality, and bisexuality.
A	Ally	A person who considers themselves a friend to the LGBTQ+ community.
+	Pansexual (or omnisexual)	Sexual, romantic, or emotional attraction toward people of any sex or gender identity. These individuals may refer to themselves as gender-blind.
+	Agender	Those who identify as having no gender or being without any gender identity. These individuals may also call themselves genderless, gender-free, nongendered, or ungendered.
+	Gender queer	Umbrella term for gender identities that are not exclusively masculine or feminine, which are outside of the gender binary of male or female.
+	Bigender	A gender identity whereby the person moves between feminine and masculine gender identities and behaviors, possibly depending on context. Some express distinct female/feminine and male/masculine personas, while others identify as two genders simultaneously.
+	Gender variant	Behavior or gender expression by an individual that does not match masculine and feminine gender norms. Also referred to as gender nonconformity.
+	Pangender	Describes those who feel they identify as all genders. The term has a great deal of overlap with gender queer. Because of its all-encompassing nature, presentation and pronoun usage varies between individuals who identify as pangender.

Data from GLAAD. (2014). *Media Reference Guide* (11th ed.). https://www.glaad.org/reference#guide; GLSEN. (n.d.). *LGBTQ history*. https://www.glsen.org/lgbtq-history; National Center for Transgender Equality. (2016). *Understanding transgender people: The basics.* https://transequality.org/issues/resources/understanding-transgender-people-the-basics; OK2BEME. (2022). *What does LGBTQ+ Mean?* KW Counselling. https://ok2bme.ca/resources/kids-teens/what-does-lgbtq-mean/

Nursing Care of the LGBTQ+ Patient

Chapter 4, "Initial Assessment," presents the systematic approach to care of the trauma patient. While the primary and secondary survey remain unchanged for the injured LGBTQ+ patient, understanding and support without discrimination, bias, stigma, or shaming is foundational to the practice of nursing.

Reduce Barriers

Healthcare organizations should have policies, procedures, and practices founded in inclusivity for LGBTQ+ patients and their families.[65] Healthcare leaders determine the culture in which care is provided and should set the standard for an organization that promotes respect and prohibits discrimination. Working to eliminate discrimination and the challenges faced by LGBTQ+ populations will contribute to the delivery of equitable, competent, and safe care.[64] Negative bias toward LGBTQ+ persons has the potential to worsen health disparities and negatively impact clinical decision-making.[48] Taking a caring approach with patients in a welcoming and affirming environment may enhance the ability to provide education and interventions.[49]

Transgender Health

Health considerations for transgender persons involve creating safe and effective pathways for these individuals to achieve comfort with their gendered selves. Nursing care of the transgender individual must acknowledge that gender affirmation is a process, not a single step.

Obtaining a "gender narrative" is the process of discussing the individual's history and experiences with their gender awareness, including the process of their gender exploration, acceptance or rejection, and identification. The purpose of obtaining this narrative is collaboration and establishing a plan to approach gender affirmation (**Table 12-3**).[17,69,72] The nurse may care for a patient who

TABLE 12-3 Gender-Affirmation Interventions

System	Intervention(s)
Social dimension	One of the early steps in gender affirmation is the individual's process of self-exploration. This can include reflection, connecting with the community, and, at times, "coming out" as transgender. This is not limited to transgender individuals and applies to many facets of life.
	Additional interventions can include the individual changing their public presentation, tucking, packing, or binding to match their correct gender.
Mental health	Psychotherapy to explore the individual's gender identity, role, and expression.
	Address negative impact of gender dysphoria, enhancing social support, improving body image, and/or promoting resilience.
Voice and communication	Verbal and nonverbal communication are important aspects of human interaction.
	Speech and/or behavioral therapists may be involved in care to facilitate the development of vocal and communication characteristics that align with an individual's gender role expression.
Medical	Hormone therapy is the administration of feminizing or masculinizing hormones.
	Feminizing therapy may also include the administration of anti-androgen medications that reduce or block testosterone.
Surgical	Modification of primary and/or secondary sex characteristics is generally the last, but often most considered, step during the gender-affirmation process.
	Chest surgery can include augmentation or mastectomy.
	The transgender female may undergo penectomy, orchiectomy, vaginoplasty, clitoralplasty, and/or vulvoplasty.
	The transgender male may undergo a hysterectomy, oophorectomy, metoidioplasty, phalloplasty, scrotoplasty, vaginectomy, and/or prosthesis implantation.
	Nongenital surgical interventions may also include surgery on the face or other body systems to create a more masculine or feminine appearance.
Legal	There is no absolute demarcation point for an individual to petition for a change in legal documents. This varies with each individual and can be based on social support, finances, local regulations, and personal desire.

Data from Coleman, E., Radix, A. E., Bouman, W. P., Brown, G. R., de Vries, A., Deutsch, M. B., Ettner, R., Fraser, L., Goodman, M., Green, J., Hancock, A. B., Johnson, T. W., Karasic, D. H., Knudson, G. A., Leibowitz, S. F., Meyer-Bahlburg, H., Monstrey, S. J., Motmans, J., Nahata, L., Nieder, T. O., . . . Arcelus, J. (2022). Standards of care for the health of transgender and gender diverse people, version 8. *International Journal of Transgender Health*, 23(Suppl 1), S1–S259. https://doi.org/10.1080/26895269.2022.2100644; Thompson, J., Hopwood, R. A., deNormand, S., & Cavanaugh, T. (2021). *Medical care of trans and gender diverse adults*. Fenway Health. https://www.lgbtqiahealtheducation.org/wp-content/uploads/2021/07/Medical-Care-of-Trans-and-Gender-Diverse-Adults-Spring-2021.pdf; University of California San Francisco. (2019). *Transition roadmap*. https://transcare.ucsf.edu/transition-roadmap

258 Chapter 12 The LGBTQ+ Trauma Patient

is transitioning; hormone therapy and surgical interventions are on a spectrum and depend on a variety of circumstances. Table 12-4 reviews some physiologic and anatomic changes that the nurse may encounter.[11,17]

When examining a transgender patient, care should be taken to limit the exam only to topics that are relevant to the care of the patient. A gender-affirmative approach would include an inventory of organs that are present, which should be ascertained without assumptions based on perceived gender expression. To obtain information that might be necessary for diagnostics or other aspects of care, a two-step process can be used. First, ask the individual their gender identity, and second, ask what sex they were assigned at birth. The healthcare team should work toward resolving any limitations in the electronic medical record regarding the communication or documentation of this information, particularly regarding any limitations to providing gender-affirming care.

TABLE 12-4 Transgender Physiologic and Anatomic Changes

System	Transgender Man (Female to Male)	Transgender Woman (Male to Female)
Cardiovascular	Testosterone therapy has the potential to increase blood pressure. Hormone therapy may increase the risk of polycythemia.	Estrogen increases the risk of cardiovascular disease in those over 50 with risk factors, as well as the risk for venous thromboembolism.
Neurologic	Hormone therapy affects each person differently and may produce changes in brain size and development. This applies to transgender male and female individuals. Study of the intersection of neuroscience and transgender individuals provides limited data, but studies are ongoing.	
Musculoskeletal	Risk of osteoporosis is increased for up to 3 years after oophorectomy while on long-term hormone therapy. Interruption or insufficient testosterone therapy after oophorectomy may lead to decreased bone density.	Estradiol may decrease muscle mass. Some may experience an increase in bone mineral density.
Integumentary	Testosterone therapy induces acne to a varying degree, as well as male pattern hair loss.	Estradiol may cause softening of the skin and changes in hair distribution.
Gastrointestinal	Abdominal surgery, including hysterectomy, oophorectomy, or use of tissue for phalloplasty may weaken the abdominal wall.	Risk of rectal–vaginal fistula with construction of a neovagina. Hormone therapy may increase the risk of developing gallbladder disease.
Genitourinary	Metoidioplasty is the creation of a phallus from the hormonally enlarged clitoris. The urethra may also be lengthened and redirected during this surgery. Phalloplasty is the surgical construction of a phallus and is used in gender-affirming surgery. Surgical changes to the urethra may vary depending on the individual care plan. Risk of incontinence and development of fistulas is increased.	Construction of a neovagina and redirection of the urethra may result in an increased risk for urinary tract infections, bacterial vaginosis, and the development of fistulas. Spironolactone will increase urine production and may result in dehydration and a decrease in blood pressure.

System	Transgender Man (Female to Male)	Transgender Woman (Male to Female)
Reproductive	Testosterone therapy reduces fertility and, if pregnant, may produce anatomic changes in the developing fetus. Creation of a prosthetic scrotum and testicles may be performed. Some individuals may elect to retain female reproductive organs.	Vaginoplasty will involve redirection of the urethra. Techniques for creating the neovagina include penile inversion, use of a skin graft, and/or use of intestinal tissue. Orchiectomy will result in a significant decrease in testosterone production and irreversible loss of fertility. Hormone therapy will result in the development of breast tissue. Some individuals may elect to have breast augmentation as a part of their gender-affirming treatment.
Endocrine	Possible changes in the body that increase weight gain and increase risk of development of diabetes.	Feminizing hormones may increase the risk of type 2 diabetes.
Psychosocial	Gender-affirming care is associated with decreases in rates of depression, anxiety, suicide, and other negative mental health outcomes in transgender youth. Short-term improvements include improvement of self-image and mental health as they are able to validate their gender identity. Significant decrease in psychological distress. When combined with other affirmative interventions (familial and legal support), there is also a decrease in risk-taking behaviors and adverse health outcomes.[30]	

Multiple gender-affirming interventions are available for transgender people. Not all body systems are affected during interventions, and everyone's path is unique. This list is an overview, but not all encompassing. If there is uncertainty, the best advice is to ask with the desire to learn.

Data from Chan Swe, N., Ahmed, S., Eid, M., Poretsky, L., Gianos, E., & Cusano, N. E. (2022). The effects of gender-affirming hormone therapy on cardiovascular and skeletal health: A literature review. *Metabolism Open, 13,* Article 100173. https://doi.org/10.1016/j.metop.2022.100173; Coleman, E., Radix, A. E., Bouman, W. P., Brown, G. R., de Vries, A., Deutsch, M. B., Ettner, R., Fraser, L., Goodman, M., Green, J., Hancock, A. B., Johnson, T. W., Karasic, D. H., Knudson, G. A., Leibowitz, S. F., Meyer-Bahlburg, H., Monstrey, S. J., Motmans, J., Nahata, L., Nieder, T. O., . . . Arcelus, J. (2022). Standards of care for the health of transgender and gender diverse people, version 8. *International Journal of Transgender Health, 23*(Suppl 1), S1–S259. https://doi.org/10.1080/26895269.2022.2100644

CLINICAL PEARL

Avoid Deadnaming Someone

To deadname someone is to call them by the name they no longer use. For someone who has transitioned or is transitioning, this can be harmful. The process of gender affirmation, including a new name to affirm their correct gender, is important in the process of becoming their true self. Calling someone by a name they no longer use or identify with invalidates their identity.

If legal name verification is required for consent, billing, or other purposes, the nurse can ask the patient to verify the name on their hospital identification band or government identification. Use of this name should be limited to necessary tasks only. Use the individual's updated name and correct pronouns in all other interactions. Some electronic health record systems have features that enable this information to be entered into the patient's record.

Family Presence

Family-centered care and patient involvement in care are essential components of appropriate, safe, and timely healthcare in the trauma setting. This approach is grounded in partnership and collaboration between patients, families, and healthcare providers.[36] It is essential that patients have the support necessary, and the definition of "family" should include the people the patient considers to be family members.[35] See Chapter 18, "Psychosocial Aspects of Trauma Care," for additional information regarding family-centered care.

The Importance of Pronouns

Individuals and organizations can demonstrate inclusivity and communicate safety for gender and sexual minorities through policies and displaying material that is inclusive of LGBTQ+ individuals.[66] It is not, however, enough to have policies and materials; diversity, equity, and inclusivity need to be demonstrated daily in the provision of care. One example of inclusivity is recognizing the importance of an individual's pronouns. Pronouns are useful language tools that enable us to refer to others without using their names. However, it important to know that individuals may not go by the pronoun that we assume applies to them. By using a person's pronouns correctly, nurses send a message of respect and demonstrate the inclusivity of the environment. Asking a simple question, such as, "How should I refer to you?," provides the patient with an opportunity to share not just their name but also their pronouns if they choose to do so. **Table 12-5** provides examples of alternative pronouns to the traditional gendered pronouns for various languages, including use of plural pronouns as singular.[55]

TABLE 12-5 Gender Pronouns, Including Options for Languages without a Gender-Neutral Pronoun

He/She	Him/Her	His/Her	His/Hers	Himself/Herself
They	them	their	theirs	themselves
Zie	zim	zir	zis	zieself
Sie	sie	hir	hirs	hirself
Ey	em	eir	eirs	eirself
Ve	ver	vis	vers	verself
Tey	ter	tem	ters	terself
E	em	eir	eirs	ems

Reproduced from National Institutes of Health Sexual & Gender Minority Research Office, & Office of Gender Diversity, Equity, and Inclusion. (2022, January). *The importance of gender pronouns & their use in workplace communications.* https://dpcpsi.nih.gov/sgmro/gender-pronouns-resource

CLINICAL PEARL

What If I Get It Wrong?

Sometimes we inadvertently misgender someone or use an incorrect pronoun. It's ok! Acknowledge the error, correct it, and move on. Examples include the following:

- When talking with someone who goes by he/him pronouns: "She is experiencing pain, I'm sorry, I mean he is experiencing pain at his surgical site."
- A patient uses they/them pronouns, but other healthcare team members are not aware of this: "The patient I am providing report on in room 15 is named Ronald and uses the pronouns they/them."
- A peer is assuming a set of pronouns you know to be incorrect: "He is resting comfortably right now." Provide a gentle correction using the correct pronoun "She had mentioned earlier that her symptoms had improved today."
- If you aren't certain, politely ask. "What do you like to be called?" is a simple question that communicates respect and acceptance to many generations. You can refer to them by their proper name until you learn their pronouns.

Additional Care Considerations

Cultural competence and cultural humility are integral to all components of trauma care and apply to all individuals regardless of their different backgrounds, beliefs, and identities. It is essential that nurses employ culturally responsive clinical skills to optimize the care provided, as well as communication with the LGBTQ+ community. Pillars of cultural competence include mindfulness, flexibility/adaptability, tolerance, and empathy.[18,61] Cultural humility is a dynamic and lifelong approach to learning and interaction with multiple unique populations. Rather than focusing on achieving knowledge and learning facts associated with various cultures, backgrounds, identities, and beliefs, cultural humility enables understanding of the complexity of identities and reflects a lifelong commitment to self-reflection and redressing power imbalances when working with patients, families, and communities.[32] See Chapter 18, "Psychosocial Aspects of Trauma Care," for additional information."

Diversity, Equity, and Inclusion

The Emergency Nurses Association and other professional organizations have position statements regarding gender inclusivity in healthcare.[3,20] Nurses must ensure that they deliver appropriate, respectful, and inclusive care to all patients, including those who identify as members of the LGBTQ+ population. It is expected that emergency nurses "act with knowledge, compassion, and respect for human dignity and the uniqueness of the individual."[20p1] Diversity alone has the potential to promote stereotypes and emphasize differences instead of commonalities. Diversity, equity, and inclusivity integrate to ensure that all people are accepted and respected for who they are.

> **NOTE**
>
> **Diversity and Inclusion**
>
> "Diversity is being invited to the party: inclusion is being asked to dance."
>
> —Quote attributed to Verna Myers[13]

> **NOTE**
>
> **Nonverbal Communication Matters**
>
> "Body language" is a popular term coined some years ago for the broader concept of nonverbal communication; nonverbal communication includes not only our posture, gestures, facial expressions, and other movement, but also eye contact, intonation, personal distance, and other nonlinguistic aspects of our interactions with others. What we do is just as important as what we say. If the nurse's verbal and nonverbal behaviors contradict one another, the nonverbal communication may override the verbal message. Be aware of your facial expressions, eye movements, intonation, and other nonverbal aspects of your communication with all patients, but particularly with members of minority or LGBTQ+ communities.

Reevaluation and Ongoing Care

The reevaluation process and delivery of ongoing care are the same for the LGBTQ+ individual as they are for all trauma patients. Any hospitalized patient must have the necessary treatment for chronic medical conditions incorporated into their plan of care. An example is a transgender male who is receiving masculinizing hormone therapy as part of their gender-affirmation process. Unless contraindicated, continuation of their care should be provided. Sudden cessation of the ongoing treatment may have deleterious effects. If the medical team is uncertain

> **CLINICAL PEARL**
>
> **Trans Broken Arm Syndrome**
>
> Have you ever broken your arm? Or hand? Or any bone? It is often a painful injury and a very stressful situation. Now consider whether your doctors and nurses focused instead on your gender identity or hormone replacement therapy instead of the fracture right in front of them! This phenomenon is described as "trans broken arm syndrome," and it occurs when a healthcare provider focuses on an individual being transgender or gender nonconforming rather than on the broken arm (or other condition)—or even sees it as somehow related to or causative of the broken arm.
>
> In other words, trans broken arm syndrome occurs when a person's trans status becomes the focus or is blamed for unrelated health problems or injuries. It is a failure to recognize that trans people can have the same healthcare needs as a cisgender person.[42]
>
> Instead of focusing on hormone replacement therapy or what genitalia the person presents with, the healthcare team should, of course, focus on the presenting issue. Ironically, studies have shown that decreased bone density has not been found to be related to long-term testosterone therapy in the trans man; rather, it has been found that the sudden cessation of testosterone therapy could increase the risk of loss of bone density.[17]
>
> The point of discussing trans broken arm syndrome is to emphasize that healthcare providers must put aside their implicit and explicit biases and focus on the patient's actual healthcare needs before they miss something serious, with possibly disastrous consequences.

TABLE 12-6 Internet Resources

Resource	Website
The Trevor Project	www.thetrevorproject.org
GLSEN—Gay, Lesbian & Straight Education Network	www.glsen.org
PFLAG—Parents, Families, and Friends of Lesbians and Gays	www.pflag.org
The Fenway Institute: National LGBTQIA+ Health Education Center	www.fenwayhealth.org/the-fenway-institute/education/
Advancing Effective Communication, Cultural Competence, and Patient- and Family-Centered Care for the Lesbian, Gay, Bisexual, and Transgender (LGBT) Community: A Field Guide by The Joint Commission	www.jointcommission.org/lgbt
WPATH Standards of Care for the Health of Transgender and Gender-Diverse People, Version 8	www.wpath.org/publications/soc
Centers for Disease Control and Prevention (CDC) Lesbian, Gay, Bisexual, and Transgender Health	www.cdc.gov/lgbthealth/index.htm
GLAAD—Gay & Lesbian Alliance Against Defamation	www.glaad.org
National LGBTQIA+ Health Education Center	www.lgbtqiahealtheducation.org
Harvard Implicit Association Test (Project Implicit)	http://implicit.harvard.edu/implicit/
Family Acceptance Project	http://familyproject.sfsu.edu

of the most appropriate plan of care, a medical provider with experience in the care of LGBTQ+ patients should be consulted.

Summary

Empathetic care provided with cultural humility to the LGBTQ+ individual can be enhanced by recognizing differences while finding commonalities. Acceptance of all individuals who seek care enables the nurse to connect with their patients in a way that would otherwise be impossible. Organizations should implement policies and practices of inclusivity for all individuals and integrate the recognition and provision of the unique healthcare needs of the LGBTQ+ population into the expectations for daily practice. **Table 12-6** provides Internet-based resources for helping to do just that.

Simple steps, including using a person's correct pronouns, asking questions when uncertain, and limiting questions to those pertinent to the delivery of care create an environment of dignity and respect. Everyone should be treated as a unique person of incomparable worth, with the right to life and access to healthcare services.

References

1. Agénor, M., Zubizarreta, D., Geffen, S., Ramanayake, N., Giraldo, S., McGuirk, A., Caballero, M., & Bond, K. (2022). "Making a way out of no way:" Understanding the sexual and reproductive health care experiences of transmasculine young adults of color in the United States. *Qualitative Health Research*, 32(1), 121–134. https://doi.org/10.1177/10497323211050051
2. American Medical Association. (2018). *Health care needs of lesbian, gay, bisexual, transgender and queer populations H-160.991.* https://policysearch.ama-assn.org/policyfinder/detail/gender%20identity?uri=%2FAMADoc%2FHOD.xml-0-805.xml
3. ANA Ethics Advisory Board. (2018). ANA position statement: Nursing advocacy for LGBTQ+ populations. *The Online Journal of Issues in Nursing*, 24(1). https://doi.org/10.3912/OJIN.Vol24No01PoSCol02
4. Austin, D. (2014, November). *The unbroken chain: Three decades of HIV/AIDS nursing.* Science of Caring. University of California San Francisco. https://scienceofcaring.ucsf.edu/patient-care/unbroken-chain-three-decades-hivaids-nursing
5. Boswell, K., Temples, H., & Wright, M. (2019). LGBT youth, sex trafficking, and the nurse practitioner's role. *Journal of Pediatric Health Care*, 33(5), 555–560. https://doi.org/10.1016/j.pedhc.2019.02.005

6. Bouris, A., Everett, B., Heath, R., Elsaesser, C., & Neilands, T. (2016). Effects of victimization and violence on suicidal ideation and behaviors among sexual minority and heterosexual adolescents. *LGBT Health, 3*(2), 153–161. https://doi.org/10.1089/lgbt.2015.0037
7. Caceres, B. A., Streed, C. G., Corliss, H. L., Lloyd-Jones, D. M., Matthews, P. A., Mukherjee, M., Poteat, T., Rosendale, N., & Ross, L. M. (2020). Assessing and addressing cardiovascular health in LGBTQ adults: A scientific statement from the American Heart Association. *Circulation, 142*(9), e321–e332. https://doi.org/10.1161/CIR.0000000000000914
8. Cahill, S., Taylor, S. W., Elsesser, S. A., Mena, L., Hickson, D., & Mayer, K. H. (2017). Stigma, medical mistrust, and perceived racism may affect PrEP awareness and uptake in black compared to white gay and bisexual men in Jackson, Mississippi and Boston, Massachusetts. *AIDS Care, 29*(11), 1351–1358. https://doi.org/10.1080/09540121.2017.1300633
9. Centers for Disease Control and Prevention. (n.d.). *Youth risk behavior survey data summary & trends report: 2009–2019.* https://www.cdc.gov/healthyyouth/data/yrbs/pdf/YRBSDataSummaryTrendsReport2019-508.pdf
10. Centers for Disease Control and Prevention. (2021). *HIV surveillance report: Diagnosis of HIV infection in the United States and dependent areas, 2019.* https://www.cdc.gov/hiv/pdf/library/reports/surveillance/cdc-hiv-surveillance-report-2018-updated-vol-32.pdf
11. Chan Swe, N., Ahmed, S., Eid, M., Poretsky, L., Gianos, E., & Cusano, N. E. (2022). The effects of gender-affirming hormone therapy on cardiovascular and skeletal health: A literature review. *Metabolism Open, 13*, Article 100173. https://doi.org/10.1016/j.metop.2022.100173
12. Charlton, B., Everett, B., Light, A., Jones, R., Janiak, E., Gaskins, A., Chavarro, J., Moseson, H., Sarda, V., & Austin, S. (2020). Sexual orientation differences in pregnancy and abortion across the lifecourse. *Women's Health Issues, 30*(2), 65–72. https://doi.org/10.1016/j.whi.2019.10.007
13. Cho, J. H. (2016, May 25). "Diversity is being invited to the party. Inclusion is being asked to dance," Verna Myers tells Cleveland Bar. *cleveland.com*. https://www.cleveland.com/business/2016/05/diversity_is_being_invited_to.html
14. Cochran, S. D., Drescher, J., Kismödi, E., Giami, A., García-Moreno, C., Atalla, E., Marais, A., Vieira, E. M., & Reed, G. M. (2014). Proposed declassification of disease categories related to sexual orientation in the International Statistical Classification of Diseases and Related Health Problems (ICD-11). *Bulletin of the World Health Organization, 92*(9), 672–679. https://doi.org/10.2471/BLT.14.135541
15. Cohen, M. S. (2019). Successful treatment of HIV eliminates sexual transmission. *The Lancet, 393*(10189), 2366–2367. https://www.thelancet.com/journals/lancet/article/PIIS0140-6736(19)30701-9/fulltext
16. Cohen, M. S., Chen, Y. Q., McCauley, M., Gamble, T., Hosseinipour, M. C., Kumarasamy, N., Hakim, J. G., Kumwenda, J., Grinsztejn, B., Pilotto, J. H., Godbole, S. V., Mehendale, S., Chariyalertsak, S., Santos, B. R., Mayer, K. H., Hoffman, I. F., Eshleman, S. H., Piwowar-Manning, E., Wang, L., . . . HPTN 052 Study Team. (2011). Prevention of HIV-1 infection with early antiretroviral therapy. *New England Journal of Medicine, 365*(6), 493–505. https://doi.org/10.1056/NEJMoa1105243
17. Coleman, E., Radix, A. E., Bouman, W. P., Brown, G. R., de Vries, A., Deutsch, M. B., Ettner, R., Fraser, L., Goodman, M., Green, J., Hancock, A. B., Johnson, T. W., Karasic, D. H., Knudson, G. A., Leibowitz, S. F., Meyer-Bahlburg, H., Monstrey, S. J., Motmans, J., Nahata, L., . . . Arcelus, J. (2022). Standards of care for the health of transgender and gender diverse people, Version 8. *International Journal of Transgender Health, 23*(Suppl. 1), S1–S259. https://doi.org/10.1080/26895269.2022.2100644
18. Deardorff, D. K. (2009). *The SAGE handbook of intercultural competence.* SAGE.
19. Drescher, J. (2015). Out of DSM: Depathologizing homosexuality. *Behavioral Sciences, 5*(4), 565–575. https://doi.org/10.3390/bs5040565
20. Emergency Nurses Association. (2018). *Cultural diversity and gender inclusivity in the emergency care setting* [Position statement]. https://enau.ena.org/Users/LearningActivity/LearningActivityDetail.aspx?LearningActivityID=THrAYJXKucnd8WDzgt05Lg%3D%3D&tab=4
21. Everett, B. G., Higgins, J. A., Haider, S., & Carpenter, E. (2019). Do sexual minorities receive appropriate sexual and reproductive health care and counseling? *Journal of Women's Health, 28*(1), 53–62. https://doi.org/10.1089/jwh.2017.6866
22. Felner, J. K., Wisdom, J. P., Williams, T., Katuska, L., Haley, S. J., Jun, H.-J., & Corliss, H. L. (2020). Stress, coping, and context: Examining substance use among LGBTQ young adults with probable substance use disorders. *Psychiatric Services, 71*(2), 112–120. https://doi.org/10.1176/appi.ps.201900029
23. Fenkl, E., Jones, Sandra G., Aronowitz, T., Messmer, P., Olafson, E., Simon, S., & Framil, C. (2020). Risky sex and other personal consequences of alcohol and drug use among sLGBTQ college students. *Journal of the Association of Nurses in AIDS Care, 31*(4), 476–482. https://doi.org/10.1097/JNC.0000000000000161
24. Franchino-Olsen, H. (2019). Vulnerabilities relevant for commercial sexual exploitation of children/domestic minor sex trafficking: A systematic review of risk factors. *Trauma, Violence, & Abuse, 22*(1), 99–111. https://doi.org/10.1177/1524838018821956
25. Fraser, B., Pierse, N., Chisholm, E., & Cook, H. (2019). LGBTQ+ homelessness: A review of the literature. *International Journal of Environmental Research and Public Health, 16*(15), Article 2677. https://doi.org/10.3390%2Fijerph16152677
26. Fusaro, V. A., Levy, H. G., & Shaefer, H. L. (2018). Racial and ethnic disparities in the lifetime prevalence of homelessness in the United States. *Demography, 55*(6), 2119–2128. https://doi.org/10.1007/s13524-018-0717-0
27. Fusar-Poli, P., de Pablo, G. S., De Micheli, A., Nieman, D. H., Correll, C. U., Kessing, L. V., Pfennig, A., Bechdolf, A., Borgwardt, S., Arango, C., & van Amelsvoort, T. (2020). What is good mental health? A scoping review. *European Neuropsychopharmacology, 31*, 33–46. https://doi.org/10.1016/j.euroneuro.2019.12.105

28. GLAAD. (2014). *Media reference guide* (11th ed.). https://www.glaad.org/reference#guide
29. GLSEN. (n.d.). *LGBTQ history*. https://www.glsen.org/lgbtq-history-timeline-lesson
30. Glynn, T. R., Gamarel, K. E., Kahler, C. W., Iwamoto, M., Operario, D., & Nemoto, T. (2016). The role of gender affirmation in psychological well-being among transgender women. *Psychology of Sexual Orientation and Gender Diversity, 3*(3), 336–344. https://doi.org/10.1037/sgd0000171
31. Greenbaum, J., & Albright, K. (2019). *Improving healthcare services for trafficked persons: The complete toolkit*. International Centre for Missing and Exploited Children. https://www.icmec.org/wp-content/uploads/2019/07/Healthcare-Services-for-Trafficked-Persons-6-10-2019.pdf
32. Green-Moton, E., & Minkler, M. (2020). Cultural competence or cultural humility? Moving beyond the debate. *Health Promotion Practice, 21*(1), 142–145. https://doi.org/10.1177/1524839919884912
33. Hafeez, H., Zeshan, M., Tahir, M. A., Jahan, N., & Naveed, S. (2017). Health care disparities among lesbian, gay, bisexual, and transgender youth: A literature review. *Cureus, 9*(4), Article e1184. https://doi.org/10.7759/cureus.1184
34. HIV.gov. (n.d.). *HIV basics*. U.S. Department of Health and Human Services Minority HIV/AIDS Fund. https://www.hiv.gov/hiv-basics
35. Institute for Patient- and Family-Centered Care. (n.d.). *Better together pocket guide for staff*. https://www.ipfcc.org/bestpractices/IPFCC_Better_Together_Staff_Pocket_Print.pdf
36. Institute for Patient- and Family-Centered Care. (n.d.). *Patient and family-centered care*. https://www.ipfcc.org/about/pfcc.html
37. James, S. E., Herman, J. L., Rankin, S., Keisling, M., Mottet, L., & Anafi, M. (2016). *The report of the 2015 U.S. Transgender Survey*. National Center for Transgender Equality. https://www.lgbtagingcenter.org/resources/pdfs/USTS-Full-Report-FINAL.pdf
38. Jones, J. M. (2021, February 24). *LGBT identification rises to 5.6% in latest U.S. estimate*. Gallup.com. https://news.gallup.com/poll/329708/lgbt-identification-rises-latest-estimate.aspx
39. Kaiser Family Foundation. (2020, February 7). *Black Americans and HIV/AIDS: The basics*. https://www.kff.org/hivaids/fact-sheet/black-americans-and-hivaids-the-basics/
40. Kidd, J. D., Paschen-Wolff, M. M., Mericle, A. A., Caceres, B. A., Drabble, L. A., & Hughes, T. L. (2022). A scoping review of alcohol, tobacco, and other drug use treatment interventions for sexual and gender minority population. *Journal of Substance Abuse Treatment, 133*. https://doi.org/10.1016/j.jsat.2021.108539
41. Kirubarajan, A., Patel, P., Leung, S., Park, B., & Sierra, S. (2021). Cultural competence in fertility care for lesbian, gay, bisexual, transgender, and queer people: A systematic review of patient and provider perspectives. *Fertility and Sterility, 115*(5), 1294–1301. https://doi.org/10.1016/j.fertnstert.2020.12.002
42. Knutson, D., Koch, J., Authur, T., Mitchell, T., & Martyr, M. (2016). Trans broken arm: Health care stories from transgender people in rural areas. *Journal of Research on Women and Gender, 7*(1). https://digital.library.txstate.edu/handle/10877/12890
43. Krueger, E., Fish, J., & Upchurch, D. (2020). Sexual orientation disparities in substance use: Investigating social stress mechanisms in a national sample. *American Journal of Preventive Medicine, 58*(1), 59–68. https://doi.org/10.1016/j.amepre.2019.08.034
44. Martos, A. J., Wilson, P. A., & Meyer, I. H. (2017) Lesbian, gay, bisexual, and transgender (LGBT) health services in the United States: Origins, evolution, and contemporary landscape. *PLOS ONE, 12*(7), Article e0180544. https://doi.org/10.1371/journal.Pone.0180544
45. Matsuzaka, S., Romanelli, M., & Hudson, K. (2021). "Render a service worthy of me": A qualitative study of factors influencing access to LGBTQ-specific health services. *SSM – Qualitative Research in Health, 1*, Article 100019. https://doi.org/10.1016/j.ssmqr.2021.100019
46. McCann, E., & Brown, M. (2019). Homelessness among youth who identify as LGBTQ+: A systematic review. *Journal of Clinical Nursing, 18*(11–12). 2061–2072. https://doi.org/10.1111/jocn.14818
47. McDonald, K. (2018). Social support and mental health in LGBTQ adolescents: A review of the literature. *Issues in Metal Health Nursing, 39*(1), 16–29. https://doi.org/10.1080/01612840.2017.1398283
48. McDowell, M., Goldhammer, H., Potter, J., & Keuroghlian, A. (2020). Strategies to mitigate clinician implicit bias against sexual and gender minority patients. *Psychosomatics, 61*(6), 655–661. https://doi.org/10.1016/j.psym.2020.04.021
49. Medina-Martínez, J., Saus-Ortega, C., Sánchez-Lorente, M. M., Sosa-Palanca, E. M., García-Martínez, P., & Mármol-López, M. I. (2021). Health inequities in LGBT people and nursing interventions to reduce them: A systematic review. *International Journal of Environmental Research and Public Health, 18*(22), Article 11801. https://doi.org/10.3390/ijerph182211801
50. Medley, G., Lipari, R., Bose, J., Cribb, D., Kroutil, L., & McHenry, G. (2016, October). Sexual orientation and estimates of adult substance use and mental health: Results from the 2015 National Survey on Drug Use and Health. *NSDUH Data Review*. https://www.samhsa.gov/data/sites/default/files/NSDUH-SexualOrientation-2015/NSDUH-SexualOrientation-2015/NSDUH-SexualOrientation-2015.htm
51. Moagi, M. M., van Der Wath, A. E., Jiyane, P. M., & Rikhotso. (2021). Mental health challenges of lesbian, gay, bisexual and transgender people: An integrated literature review. *Health SA, 26*, Article 1487. https://doi.org/10.4102%2Fhsag.v26i0.1487
52. Morris, M., Cooper, R. L., Ramesh, A., Tabatabai, M., Arcury, T. A., Shinn, M., Im, W., Jaurez, P., & Matthews-Juarez, P. (2019). Training to reduce LGBTQ-related bias among medical, nursing, and dental students and providers: A systematic review. *BMC Medical Education, 19*, Article 325. https://doi.org/10.1186/s12909-019-1727-3
53. Nakamura, N., Dispenza, F., Abreu, R. L., Ollen, E. W., Pantalone, D. W., Canillas, G., Gormley, B., & Vencill, J. A. (2022). The APA Guidelines for Psychological Practice With

Sexual Minority Persons: An executive summary of the 2021 revision. *American Psychologist, 77*(8), 953–962. https://doi.org/10.1037/amp0000939

54. National Center for Transgender Equality. (2016, July 9). *Understanding transgender people: The basics.* https://transequality.org/issues/resources/understanding-transgender-people-the-basics

55. National Institutes of Health, Sexual & Gender Minority Research Office. (2022, January). *The importance of gender pronouns & their use in workplace communications.* https://dpcpsi.nih.gov/sgmro/gender-pronouns-resource

56. OK2BEME.ca. (2022). *What does 2SLGBTQIA+ mean?* KW Counselling. https://ok2bme.ca/resources/kids-teens/what-does-lgbtq-mean/

57. Rasberry, C. N., Lowry, R., Johns, M., Robin, L., Dunville, R., Pampati, S., Dittus, P. J., & Balaji, A. (2018). Sexual risk behavior differences among sexual minority high school students—United States, 2015 and 2017. *Morbidity and Mortality Weekly Report, 67*(36), 1007–1011. https://doi.org/10.15585/mmwr.mm6736a3

58. Reisner, S., Katz-Wise, S., Gordon, A., Corliss, H., & Austin, S. (2016). Social epidemiology of depression and anxiety by gender identity. *Journal of Adolescent Health, 59*(2), 203–208. https://doi.org/10.1016/j.jadohealth.2016.04.006

59. Ryan, W., & Ryan, R. (2019). Toward a social psychology of authenticity: Exploring within-person variation in autonomy, congruence, and genuineness using self-determination theory. *Review of General Psychology, 23*(1), 99–112. https://doi.org/10.1037/gpr0000162

60. Salvatore, C., & Daftary-Kapur, T. (2020). The influence of emerging adulthood on the risky and dangerous behaviors of LGBTQ populations. *Social Sciences, 9*(12), Article 228. https://doi.org/10.3390/socsci9120228

61. Sharifi, N., Adib-Hajbaghery, M., Najafi, M. (2019). Cultural competence in nursing: A concept analysis. *International Journal of Nursing Studies, 99*, Article 103386. https://doi.org/10.1016/j.ijnurstu.2019.103386

62. Solazzo, A. L., Tabaac, A. R., Agénor, M., Austin, S. B., & Charlton, B. M. (2019). Sexual orientation inequalities during provider-patient interactions in provider encouragement of sexual and reproductive health care. *Preventive Medicine, 126*, Article 105787. https://doi.org/10.1016/j.ypmed.2019.105787

63. Tabaac, A. R., Haneuse, S., Johns, M., Tan, A. S. L., Austin, S. B., Potter, J., Lindberg, L., & Charlton, B. M. (2021). Sexual and reproductive health information: Disparities across sexual orientation groups in two cohorts of U.S. women. *Sexuality Research and Social Policy, 18*(3), 612–620. https://doi.org/10.1007/s13178-020-00485-3

64. The Joint Commission. (2011). Introduction. In *Advancing effective communication, cultural competence, and patient- and family centered care for the lesbian, gay, bisexual, and transgender (LGBT) community: A field guide* (pp. 1–6). https://www.jointcommission.org/-/media/tjc/documents/resources/patient-safety-topics/health-equity/lgbtfieldguide_web_linked_verpdf.pdf

65. The Joint Commission. (2011). Leadership. In *Advancing effective communication, cultural competence, and patient- and family centered care for the lesbian, gay, bisexual, and transgender (LGBT) community: A field guide* (pp. 7–10). https://www.jointcommission.org/-/media/tjc/documents/resources/patient-safety-topics/health-equity/lgbtfieldguide_web_linked_verpdf.pdf

66. The Joint Commission. (2011). Provision of care, treatment, and services. In *Advancing effective communication, cultural competence, and patient- and family centered care for the lesbian, gay, bisexual, and transgender (LGBT) community: A field guide* (pp. 11–17). https://www.jointcommission.org/-/media/tjc/documents/resources/patient-safety-topics/health-equity/lgbtfieldguide_web_linked_verpdf.pdf

67. The Trevor Project. (2021). *National survey on LGBTQ youth mental health 2021.* https://www.thetrevorproject.org/survey-2021/

68. The White House. (2021). *The national action plan to combat human trafficking.* https://www.whitehouse.gov/wp-content/uploads/2021/12/National-Action-Plan-to-Combat-Human-Trafficking.pdf

69. Thompson, J., Hopwood, R. A., deNormand, S., & Cavanaugh, T. (2021). *Medical care of trans and gender diverse adults.* Fenway Health. https://www.lgbtqiahealtheducation.org/wp-content/uploads/2021/07/Medical-Care-of-Trans-and-Gender-Diverse-Adults-Spring-2021.pdf

70. Tiller, J., & Reynolds, S. (2020). Human trafficking in the emergency department: Improving our response to a vulnerable population. *Western Journal of Emergency Medicine, 21*(3), 549–554. https://www.ncbi.nlm.nih.gov/pmc/articles/PMC7234705/

71. Toney-Butler, T. J., Ladd, M., & Mittel, O. (2022, July 25). Human trafficking. *StatPearls.* StatPearls Publishing. https://www.ncbi.nlm.nih.gov/books/NBK430910/

72. University of California San Francisco. (2019). *Transition roadmap.* https://transcare.ucsf.edu/transition-roadmap

73. Valentine, S., & Shipherd, J. (2018). A systematic review of social stress and mental health among transgender and gender non-conforming people in the United States. *Clinical Psychology Review, 66*, 24–38. https://doi.org/10.1016/j.cpr.2018.03.003

74. Wingo, E., Ingraham, N., & Roberts, S. (2018). Reproductive health care priorities and barriers to effective care for LGBTQ people assigned female at birth: A qualitative study. *Women's Health Issues, 28*(4), 350–357. https://doi.org/10.1016/j.whi.2018.03.002

75. World Health Organization. (2022, June 17). *Mental health: Strengthening our response.* https://www.who.int/news-room/fact-sheets/detail/mental-health-strengthening-our-response

76. World Health Organization. (2022, July 27). *HIV: Key facts.* https://www.who.int/news-room/fact-sheets/detail/hiv-aids

CHAPTER 13

The Pediatric Trauma Patient

Tibor Bajor, MSN, NP, RN, CPEN

> **OBJECTIVES**
>
> Upon completion of this chapter, the learner will be able to:
> 1. Describe mechanisms of injury associated with the pediatric trauma patient.
> 2. Discuss anatomic, physiologic, and developmental considerations unique to the pediatric patient.
> 3. Plan appropriate interventions and evaluate their effectiveness for pediatric trauma patients.

Introduction

Traumatic injury remains the leading cause of pediatric death worldwide.[1] Evidence suggests significant variation in the quality of trauma care provided and an absence of adherence to evidence-based clinical practice guidelines, highlighting the opportunity for improved standardization of care for the pediatric trauma patient.[50]

The initial treatment algorithm for pediatric trauma follows the same A–J mnemonic used to identify and treat life-threatening injuries in adults. However, the pediatric population has specific challenges; children's growth and development patterns make them a unique population to assess and treat. As they move from infancy through adolescence, children's anatomy and physiology affect injury patterns after trauma.[43] Growth and development influence the child's behavior and risk of traumatic injury. Care of the injured child requires the trauma team to integrate understanding of the child's developmental stage into the care provided. All emergency departments (EDs) must have appropriately sized pediatric equipment readily available for the initial treatment of the injured child.

Epidemiology

Despite significant advances in the prevention, assessment, and management of trauma, it remains the leading cause of morbidity and mortality worldwide in children aged 1–14 years.[1] Globally, injuries result in almost 1 million pediatric deaths each year, and 90% of these injuries are unintentional.[59] Unintentional trauma has a greater impact on morbidity and mortality than any other disease in children. In the United States, more than 7,000 children between the ages of 0 and 19 years died from unintentional injuries in 2019.[22] More than 500,000 pediatric traumatic brain injuries (TBIs) occur each year, resulting in approximately 15,000 hospital admissions for severe TBIs annually.[2]

Mortality due to pediatric trauma is higher in rural areas relative to large metropolitan areas, at 17.6 versus 6.8 deaths, respectively, per 100,000 children.[80] This mortality discrepancy is significant, considering that almost 57% of children in the United States live farther than 30 miles from a pediatric trauma center.[76]

Mechanisms of Injury and Biomechanics

Traumatic events in children often result in multisystem organ injury. In pediatric patients, greater force is distributed throughout the body as a result of trauma because of the child's lesser body mass.[6,43] This force is transmitted through pliable, incompletely calcified bones, limited connective tissues, weaker abdominal walls, organs that are in closer proximity to other organs and structures, and the pediatric patient's smaller physical stature, frequently resulting in multisystem injury.[6,26,43,78] See **Table 13-1** for common mechanisms and associated patterns of injury in the pediatric patient.

Firearm-related deaths across all age groups increased to more than 45,000 between 2019 and 2020.[21] The majority of firearm deaths in children age 0–19 years of age were homicides. However, more than 33% of firearm deaths among children and adolescents (10–19 years of age) were suicide related.[12] Firearm-related injury was the leading cause of death for children 0–19 years of age in 2019 (**Figure 13-1**).[12,29] Fatal drug overdoses and poisonings also increased by 83.6% among children and adolescents during that period, making it the third leading cause of death in that year.[29]

Additional mechanism of injury (MOI) and biomechanical considerations in the pediatric population include the following:

- Approximately 90% of all pediatric trauma is due to blunt injury.[40]
- An abdominal injury is present in 25% of children with major trauma.[68]
- Penetrating injuries are often the result of violence. Because of the compact nature of the organs within the pediatric body, it is likely that a vital structure will be injured.
- MOIs also include drowning, suffocation, burns, and poisonings.[22]
- Sports and recreational injuries in children carry a significant correlation with TBI and musculoskeletal injuries.[56,77]
- Injury from child maltreatment reaches across all age groups and genders. It is important to maintain a high awareness of the potential for maltreatment in all pediatric trauma patients. In cases of suspected child maltreatment, the story of the injury is

TABLE 13-1 Common Mechanisms of Injury and Associated Patterns of Injury in Pediatric Patients

Mechanism of Injury	Common Patterns of Injury
Pedestrian struck by a vehicle	Low speed: Lower extremity fractures
	High speed: Multiple trauma, head and neck injuries, lower extremity fractures
Automobile occupant	Unrestrained: Scalp and facial lacerations, head and neck injuries, and multiple trauma
	Properly restrained: Chest and abdomen injuries, lumbar spinal fractures
Fall from a height	Low: Upper extremity fractures
	Medium: Head and neck injuries, upper and lower extremity fractures
	High: Upper and lower extremity fractures, head and neck injuries, multiple trauma
Fall from a bicycle	Without helmet: Head and neck lacerations, scalp and facial lacerations, upper extremity fractures
	With helmet: Upper extremity fractures
	Striking handlebar: Internal abdominal injuries

Data from American College of Surgeons. (2018). Pediatric trauma. In *Advanced trauma life support: Student course manual* (10th ed., pp. 188–212).

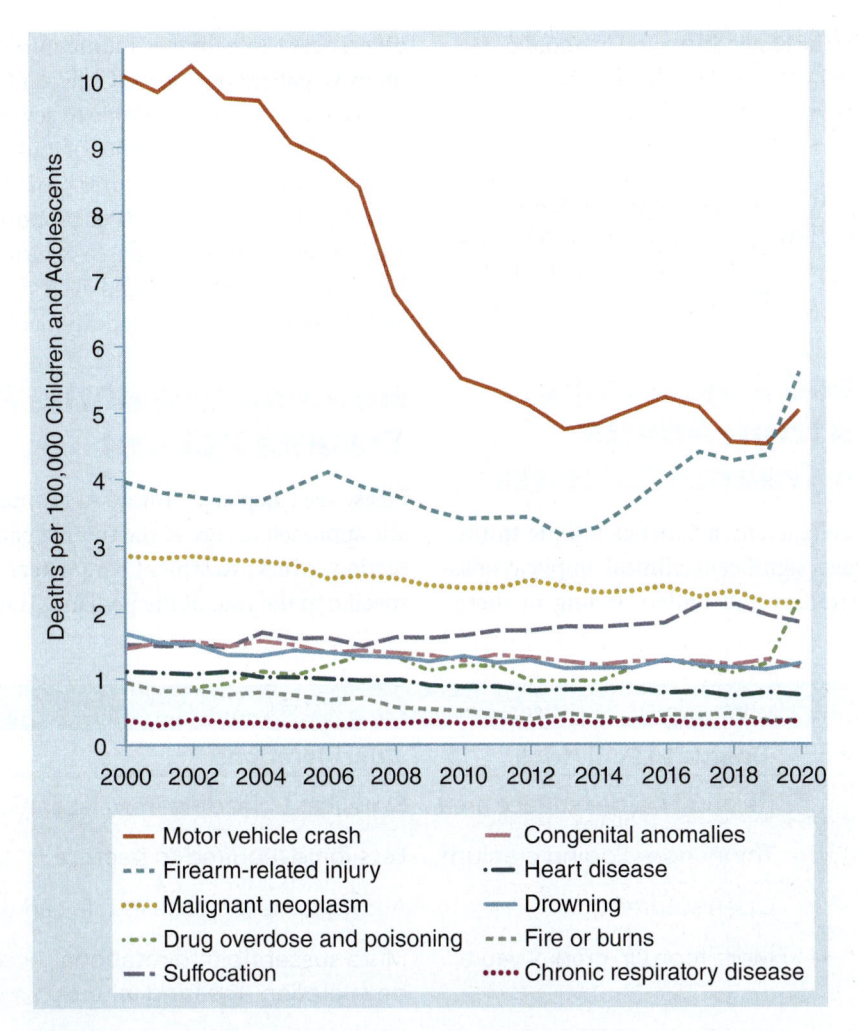

Figure 13-1 Leading causes of death among children and adolescents in the United States, 1999-2020.

From Goldstick, J. E., Cunningham, R. M., & Carter, P. M. (2022). Current causes of death in children and adolescents in the United States. *New England Journal of Medicine, 386*(20), 1955-1956. https://doi.org/10.1056/NEJMc2201761

often unreliable, and the injuries sustained are not congruent with the history provided.[32]

- Children are most often injured, sustain significant trauma, or die when restraints are not used or are not used correctly.[79]

Childhood Growth and Development

Understanding normal childhood growth and development is essential when caring for pediatric trauma patients. This understanding can also assist in anticipating injury and possible indicators of physical maltreatment.[1] Foundational knowledge regarding the pediatric patient's overall body size, greater relative body surface area, and physiologic and immunologic immaturity informs the care provided to the injured child. See **Appendix 13-1** for additional childhood development information.[24] Other injury-related developmental considerations include the following[26,45,70,79]:

- Falls from raised surfaces are a concern because infants are mobile from birth.
- As children learn to crawl, walk, climb, and jump, they become more coordinated.
- Children are easily distracted, have a limited grasp of cause and effect, and lack experience with situations that can cause traumatic injury.
- Children have difficulty judging the speed and distance of oncoming vehicles.
- Young children may have trouble localizing sound and recognizing sounds of danger.
- Children's visual field is lower.
- Toddlers and school-age children are egocentric and believe that if they see the car, the driver sees them.

- Adolescents may be easily distracted by mobile phones.
- Risk-taking behavior is common.

Children with special healthcare needs often develop at different rates, and they may have baseline assessment data that differ from those for commonly accepted parameters. In such cases, the nurse can compare assessment findings with the child's baseline from the caregiver.

Anatomic and Physiologic Differences from Adults in Pediatric Trauma Patients

Anatomic and physiologic characteristics unique to the pediatric patient have significant clinical implications. Maintaining an awareness and understanding of these differences can help the trauma nurse optimize care and improve patient outcomes. Children's relatively small size makes them more susceptible to severe injuries based on the force applied. The absence of muscle mass and incompletely ossified bone structures provide much less protection. In addition, their greater proportional body surface area leaves them vulnerable to environmental toxins and heat loss. See **Table 13-2** and each section in the primary and secondary survey for additional information.[26]

Nursing Care of the Pediatric Trauma Patient

Please see Chapter 4, "Initial Assessment," for the systematic approach to care of the trauma patient. The following section covers assessment parameters and considerations specific to the care of the pediatric trauma patient.

TABLE 13-2 Anatomic and Physiologic Considerations

Anatomic Location	Unique to Pediatrics	Considerations
Head/brain	Relatively larger surface area	Significant bleeding from lacerations
	Thinner developing cranium	Less force required to fracture
	Open sutures	Allows some increase in ICP, can delay diagnosis
	More room in cranial vault	More susceptible to rotational, acceleration/deceleration, shearing injuries
	Large head/weak neck	Prone to hyperflexion/extension injury
Cervical spine	Fulcrum at C2, C3, spinal column flexibility greater than spinal cord	Higher level C-spine injuries and SCIWORA
Airway	Smaller, floppy airway	More prone to obstruction w/ swelling
	Funnel-shaped airway	More prone to pooling secretions/blood
	Cartilage softer	Less prone to fracture
	Short neck	Difficult to assess JVD, tugging
Chest	Thinner, more compliant chest wall	Minimal injury to wall with significant underlying injury
	Heart more anterior and mediastinum mobile	Minimal injury to wall with serious injury to heart/mediastinum
	Lungs susceptible to barotrauma	Must avoid overventilation with B-M
	Smaller airways	Small changes in diameter by secretions or aspiration cause respiratory compromise
	Tidal volume fixed, smaller FRC	Minute ventilation maintained by increasing respiratory rate, rapid desaturation with apnea

Anatomic Location	Unique to Pediatrics	Considerations
Abdomen	Relatively large organs and thin muscle wall	Greater susceptibility to blunt trauma
	Thick visceral capsules	May limit hemoperitoneum, US sensitivity
	Less abdominal fat and elastic ligamentous attachments	Increased vulnerability to acceleration-deceleration, hollow viscus injuries
Skeleton/bones	Incomplete calcification and open epiphyseal plates	Bones more pliable, subject to Salter-Harris fractures
Skin	Greater body surface area	More susceptible to hypothermia
	Thinner skin and less subcutaneous fat	More vulnerable to environmental toxins

ICP = intracranial pressure; SCIWORA = spinal cord injury without radiographic abnormality; JVD = jugular vein distention; B-M = bag mask; FRC = functional residual capacity; US = ultrasound.
Data from Ernst, G. (2020). Pediatric trauma. In J. E. Tintinalli, O. J. Ma, D. M. Yealy, G. D. Meckler, J. S. Stapczynski, D. M. Cline, & S. H. Thomas (Eds.), *Tintinalli's emergency medicine: A comprehensive study guide* (9th ed., 689–697). McGraw Hill.

Pediatric Readiness

The National Pediatric Readiness Project is an ongoing, multiphase initiative dedicated to ensuring that EDs are prepared to care for the unique physiological, emotional, and developmental needs of children experiencing an acute illness or injury.[25,51,52] More than 80% of ill or injured children requiring emergency care are seen and treated in community or general population EDs.[61] The importance of having pediatric-specific competencies and policies, appropriate-sized equipment, and other resources for the care of injured children cannot be overstated.[25,51,52,62]

Preparation

Preparation begins with safety but also includes equipment, nursing, and facilities.

Safe Practice, Safe Care

Because of its complex nature, emergency care of children creates significant potential for medical errors, and children's unique anatomic, physiologic, and developmental characteristics can further compound this potential.[37,64] Performing a systematic, multisystem assessment of the pediatric patient, regardless of the specific MOI, enables easier recognition of multiorgan trauma and rapid intervention in life-threatening injuries.

Patient Equipment

Preparation to care for the injured pediatric patient includes ensuring the availability of necessary pediatric-sized equipment (**Appendix 13-2**). Reference materials, including normal vital sign ranges by age (**Table 13-3**)[8,26,46] and the Glasgow Coma Scale (pediatric) (see **Table 13-4** later in the chapter), should be prominently displayed. Scales should be configured to read in kilograms only. The Emergency Nurses Association, with the support of other professional healthcare associations, has emphasized the importance of children's weight being measured and documented only in kilograms.[37] In addition, length-based resuscitation tapes and guides for appropriately sized equipment and medication dosing should be readily accessible.

Nursing Preparation

Nursing preparation is an integral component of pediatric readiness and may include the following:

- A pediatric care coordinator in nonpediatric specialty EDs.[55]
- Pediatric-specific education and training, including the Emergency Nursing Pediatric Course (ENPC). ENPC provides nurses with an understanding of the unique characteristics of the pediatric population and the preferred management principles.
- Competency evaluation for all clinical staff, to include pediatric skills as well as skills related to the care of the child with special healthcare needs.
- Regular reviews of pediatric trauma cases can assist the trauma team in identifying learning, equipment, and policy needs.
- The use of regular periodic pediatric mock codes may improve the clinical skills of practitioners and improve adherence to the American Heart Association pediatric advanced life support guidelines.[34,53]

TABLE 13-3 Normal Vital Signs for Pediatric Patients

Age	Heart Rate (Beats/Minute)	Respiratory Rate (Breaths/Minute)	Systolic Blood Pressure (mm Hg)
Term neonate, < 1 month	90–190	35–60	67–84
Infant, 1–12 months	90–180	30–55	72–104
Toddler, 1–3 years	80–140	22–40	86–104
Preschooler, 3–5 years	65–120	18–35	89–112
School-age child, 5–12 years	70–120	16–30	90–115
Adolescent, 12–18 years	60–100	12–20	100–130

Data from American Heart Association. (2020). Part 4: Systematic approach to the seriously ill or injured child. *Pediatric advanced life support provider manual*; Ernst, G. (2020). Pediatric trauma. In J. E. Tintinalli, O. J. Ma, D. M. Yealy, G. D. Meckler, J. S. Stapczynski, D. M. Cline, & S. H. Thomas (Eds.), *Tintinalli's emergency medicine: A comprehensive study guide* (9th ed.). McGraw Hill; Lucia, D., & Glenn, J. (2017). Pediatric emergencies. In C. K. Stone & R. L. Humphries (Eds.), *Current diagnosis and treatment: Emergency medicine* (8th ed.). McGraw Hill.

TABLE 13-4 Glasgow Coma Scale

Sign	> 5 years old	2–5 years old	< 2 years old	Score
Eye Opening Examples of nontestable: eye edema, eye dressings	Spontaneous	Spontaneous	Spontaneous	4
	To sound	To sound	To sound	3
	To pressure	To pressure	To pressure	2
	None	None	None	1
	Nontestable	Nontestable	Nontestable	NT
Verbal Response Examples of nontestable: intubation, sedation	Oriented	Oriented	Coos and babbles	5
	Confused	Confused	Irritable/cries	4
	Inappropriate words	Inappropriate words	Cries in response to pressure	3
	Incomprehensible sounds	Incomprehensible sounds	Moans in response to pressure	2
	None	None	None	1
	Nontestable	Nontestable	Nontestable	NT
Motor Response Examples of nontestable: chemical paralysis	Obeys commands	Obeys commands	Moves spontaneously	6
	Localizes (reaches for swab when inserted into nose)	Localizes	Localizes *or* withdraws from pressure	5
	Withdraws from pressure (turns head when swab inserted into nose)	Withdraws from pressure	Withdraws from pressure	4

Sign	> 5 years old	2–5 years old	< 2 years old	Score
	Abnormal flexion with stimulus	Abnormal flexion with stimulus	Abnormal flexion with stimulus	3
	Abnormal extension with stimulus	Abnormal extension with stimulus	Abnormal extension with stimulus	2
	None	None	None	1
	Nontestable	Nontestable	Nontestable	NT
Best Total Score				15

Data from American College of Surgeons. (2018). *Advanced trauma life support: Student course manual* (10th ed., p. 110); Jain, S., & Iverson, L. M. (2021, June 20). Glasgow coma scale. *StatPearls*. StatPearls Publishing. https://www.ncbi.nlm.nih.gov/books/NBK513298/; Institute of Neurological Sciences NHS Greater Glasgow and Clyde. (2015). *Glasgow coma scale: Do it this way*. https://www.glasgowcomascale.org/downloads/GCS-Assessment-Aid-English.pdf?v=3; Wolters Kluwer. (2022). Glasgow coma scale and pediatric Glasgow coma scale. *UpToDate*. Retrieved January 22, 2022, from https://www.uptodate.com/contents/image/print?imageKey=PEDS%2F59662

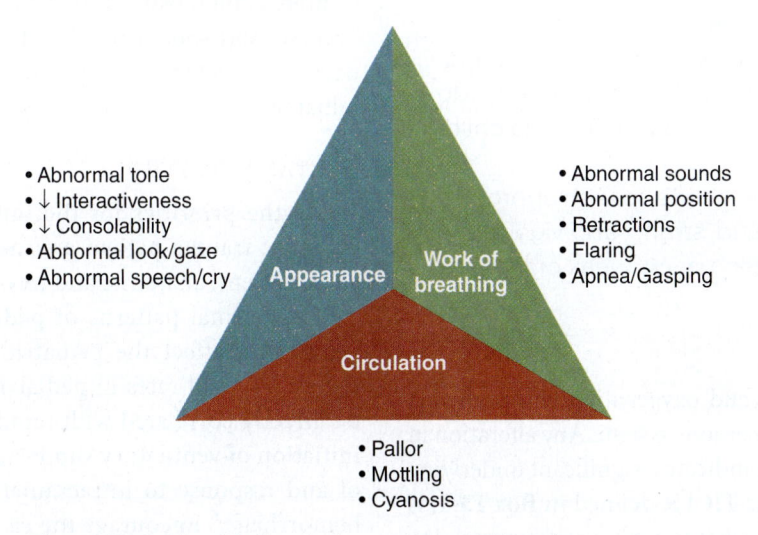

Figure 13-2 *The Pediatric Assessment Triangle.*
From Horeczko, T., Enriquez, B., McGrath, N. E., Gausche-Hill, M., & Lewis, R. J. (2013). The Pediatric Assessment Triangle: Accuracy of its application by nurses in the triage of children. *Journal of Emergency Nursing, 39*(2), 182–189. https://doi.org/10.1016/j.jen.2011.12.020

Facility Preparation

Facility preparation includes the following:

- Patient safety in the ED is a priority for the organization, the hospital, and the ED.[37]
- The care environment, protocols, guidelines, equipment, and other resources are reviewed to ensure a proper pediatric focus and safety.
- Policies and agreements, which incorporate regulatory or governmental mandates, are in place for appropriate transfers to definite care (burn center, pediatric trauma center).

Triage

As the patient arrives, the same across-the-room observation for uncontrolled bleeding is performed, with the appropriate reprioritization if hemorrhage is present. The triage process begins with the Pediatric Assessment Triangle (PAT), which rapidly provides a general impression of the patient's physiologic status and is performed before physical contact is initiated.[27,33,47] The PAT evaluates the following (**Figure 13-2**):

- Appearance
- Work of breathing
- Circulation to the skin

Appearance

The nurse first notes the child's general appearance, which provides essential information regarding the severity of illness or injury. The child's interaction with the caregiver or the environment reveals much about

BOX 13-1 TICLS Mnemonic

The TICLS mnemonic is explained in the following:

- **T**one: Is the muscle tone demonstrated by the child appropriate? Is the child moving their arms and legs, or does the child appear limp or flaccid?
- **I**nteractiveness: Does the child appear to appropriately interact with the environment and/or the caregiver? If age appropriate, does the child play with toys and/or interact with others?
- **C**onsolability: Is the child easily consoled or comforted by the caregiver or a blanket, toy, or pacifier, or is there no consoling the child?
- **L**ook/gaze: If the eyes are open, does the child appear to be alert, or are they staring into space? If the child's eyes are closed, do they open to noise or sound, or is the child just sleeping?
- **S**peech/cry: Is the child's speech appropriate or their cry loud, strong, and vigorous, or is the child's speech or cry weak or listless?

adequacy of ventilation and oxygenation and perfusion to the brain and central nervous system. Any alteration in general appearance may indicate a significant underlying problem. The mnemonic TICLS, defined in **Box 13-1**, is helpful in remembering what to look for when assessing a child's appearance.

Work of Breathing

Assessing the work of breathing provides information on how much effort the child is exerting to ventilate adequately. This reflects the child's oxygenation and ventilation status and includes assessing for the following:

- Abnormal respiratory rate for child's age—too fast or too slow
- Nasal flaring
- Retractions
- Accessory muscle use
- Abnormal upper airway sounds
- Head bobbing
- Position of comfort (tripod, sitting up)

Circulation to the Skin

Circulation to the skin is the third parameter of the PAT and includes looking at the child's skin color in central areas, such as the lips and mucous membranes. The soles of the feet and the palms of the hands may also provide information. Change from the patient's usual color is a strong indicator of poor cardiac output and perfusion. Abnormal circulation to the skin includes the following:

- Color (pallor, mottled, ashen, gray, dusky, or cyanotic)
- Mottling
- Diaphoresis

The PAT can be used to determine whether the child is "sick," "sicker," or "sickest." Even with no abnormalities of the PAT on arrival, the child is still considered "sick." An abnormality of one of the PAT components places the child in the "sicker" category. With abnormalities in two or more components of the PAT, the child is considered "sickest" and should be placed in an area where rapid treatment, including resuscitation, if necessary, can be initiated.

Primary Survey

While the priorities for the initial assessment of the pediatric trauma patient are the same as those for an adult patient, anatomic and physiologic differences, as well as normal patterns of pediatric growth and development, affect the pediatric patient's response to injury. Survival rates in pediatric trauma patients can be directly correlated with rapid airway management, initiation of ventilatory support, and early recognition of and response to intracranial and intra-abdominal hemorrhage.[6] Encourage the caregiver to remain with the child during the initial assessment to help calm the child as well as to provide support and information to the caregivers and family.[78]

A: Airway and Alertness

Assessment of airway and alertness begins with a discussion of pediatric anatomic and physiologic differences and characteristics.

Anatomic and Physiologic Characteristics

Anatomic and physiologic characteristics include the following[6,44,78,79]:

- Infants are preferential nose breathers until 4–6 months of age, and they may more easily develop respiratory distress as a result of nasal congestion.
- Children's relatively smaller airway diameter may cause even minimal amounts of blood, edema, mucus, or foreign objects to partially or completely occlude the airway.

- The tongue size is larger in relation to the oral cavity and may require the use of a tongue depressor, positioning, or airway adjuncts to maintain airway patency.
- A child's trachea and neck are shorter, so an endotracheal tube can be easily dislodged; this may cause a right mainstem bronchus intubation or inadvertent extubation.
- The laryngeal and tracheal cartilage is more pliable, increasing the risk for airway collapse.
- The larynx is cephalad and easily compressed if the neck is hyperextended or flexed.
- The large head results in passive flexion of the cervical spine while in a supine position, which may occlude the airway.
- Lax neck ligaments and incompletely calcified vertebrae place children at a higher risk for spinal cord injury without radiographic abnormalities (SCIWORA).

Assessment

Use the AVPU mnemonic (alert, verbal, pain, unresponsive) to assess the mental status of the pediatric patient. See Chapter 4, "Initial Assessment," for additional information.

- An alert older infant or toddler will recognize their caregiver, be cautious of strangers, and may not respond to commands, which is the expected response.
- It can be difficult to accurately assess the crying child. Observe for signs of an altered mental status, including inconsolability.
- Assess the child's airway for actual or potential obstruction.
- Loose or missing teeth may be normal and not a result of trauma, depending on the age of the child.
  - Assess for bleeding sockets.
  - Anticipate possible aspiration of loose teeth if they become dislodged.
- Assess for cyanosis in the oral mucosa.
  - This is a significant finding and indicative of central cyanosis due to either severe respiratory failure or severe circulatory failure.

Interventions

Interventions include the following:

- Frequent suctioning or placement of a nasal airway (unless contraindicated by facial or head trauma) may be required to keep the pharynx clear of secretions and improve ventilation. It is essential to use the appropriate size and type of suction catheter, and limit duration to less than 30 seconds.
- When inserting an oral airway in the unconscious patient without a gag reflex using the anatomic insertion method, use a tongue blade and insert directly into the oral cavity; slide it over the tongue, using care not to push the tongue back into the airway. The oral airway should curve downward to avoid damage to the soft palate and to limit the potential for subsequent bleeding.
- It is important to use the correct size oral or nasal pharyngeal airway.
  - Oral airway: Measure from the corner of the mouth to the angle of the jaw.
  - Nasopharyngeal: Measure from the bottom of naris to the top of the patient's earlobe.

Spinal Motion Restriction

Alertness and airway include simultaneous cervical spine stabilization:

- Remain in the line of sight when assessing the airway. It is a natural response for the child to turn their head toward a voice.
- Spinal motion restriction (SMR) may frighten and agitate children. Maintain nonthreatening eye contact, and repeatedly reassure the child verbally as SMR interventions are implemented.
- If necessary to accommodate a child's relatively large head, place padding under the patient's shoulders and torso to maintain neutral alignment of the head.
- Assess for appropriate sizing and application of rigid cervical collars to maintain SMR, according to the manufacturer guidelines. Commercial hard and soft collars are available for young children. In the absence of appropriately sized commercial devices, manual stabilization may be necessary.
- For children younger than 1 year, a device that provides spinal immobilization with a rigid cervical collar can be used (**Figure 13-3**).

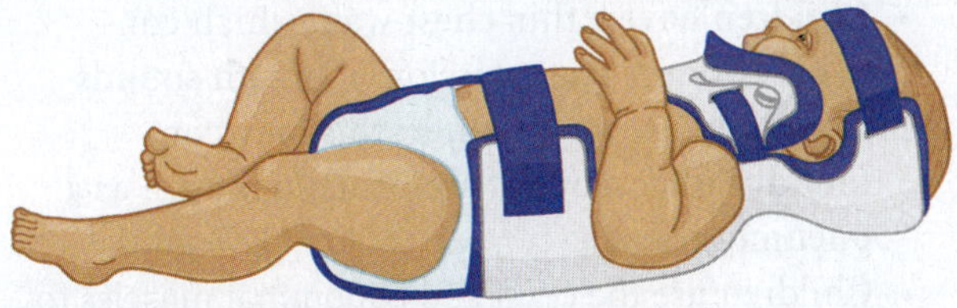

Figure 13-3 *Spinal immobilization with cervical collar.*

- Remove the child from the safety seat while maintaining SMR.
  - One team member stabilizes the infant's head and neck from behind the safety seat, while another lays the safety seat down with the back resting on the stretcher. The infant is removed from the seat and placed onto the stretcher by both team members in a straight motion, with support of the body to maintain spinal alignment.

B: Breathing and Ventilation

The breathing and ventilation assessment follows airway and alertness with SMR.

Anatomic and Physiologic Characteristics

Anatomic and physiologic characteristics include the following[6,44,78,79]:

- The respiratory rate in children is faster than that for adults because of their increased basal metabolic rate (Table 13-3). This contributes to overall insensible fluid losses, which increases the risk for hypovolemia, further exacerbating any blood loss.
- The increased metabolic rate inefficiently uses oxygen. Limited reserves are quickly depleted in times of physiologic stress.
- Respiratory distress may cause an increased respiratory rate and increased work of breathing to maximize ventilation.
  - This requires a large amount of energy, resulting in fatigue and, once physiological reserves are exhausted, decompensation.
- Children have a horizontally oriented rib cage, and weak chest wall and intercostal muscles, resulting in smaller tidal volumes in young children. This decreases children's ability to increase their tidal volume during periods of distress.
- Alveoli have less elastic recoil and lack supportive tissue.
- The diaphragm is more horizontal and is the principal muscle used for inspiration.
- Children have a thin chest wall, which contributes to the transmission of breath sounds from one side to the other; this may confound the presence of abnormalities such as a pneumothorax.
- Children use the chest and abdominal muscles to increase chest expansion. However, these muscles are less developed in children and fatigue quickly.

Assessment

Assessment includes the following:

- Inspect for increased work of breathing:
  - Nasal flaring
  - Retractions
    - Site: Substernal, intercostal, suprasternal, or supraclavicular
    - Severity: Mild, moderate, or severe
  - Head bobbing
  - Expiratory grunting
  - Accessory muscle use (sternocleidomastoid or trapezius)
    - Infants are normally diaphragmatic breathers. In these patients, the diaphragm is the primary muscle of breathing and not an accessory muscle.
- Auscultate for breath sounds. An appropriately sized stethoscope can assist with the accuracy of auscultating the lung fields and lessen the transmission of breath sounds across the chest.
  - Auscultate the following areas[8]:
    - Anterior: Midchest area
    - Lateral: Just under the axilla
    - Posterior: Both sides of the back
- Assess for symmetrical rise and fall of the chest with respirations

Interventions

Interventions include the following:

- For the seriously injured child, a tight-fitting nonrebreather mask with an attached reservoir is recommended.[10]
- If a child requires intubation, the following apply:
  - Cuffed endotracheal tubes (ETTs) are now designed to be high-volume, low-pressure devices that produce a seal at a lower pressure, and the use of cuffed ETTs in young children is increasing. Follow the manufacturer's guidelines regarding air leak and cuff pressure monitoring.
  - If inadequate ventilation is present or ventilation assistance is necessary, begin bag-mask ventilation.
  - Preoxygenate before intubation.[6,44]
  - Attempts at intubation should be no longer than 30 seconds.[44]
  - After intubation, assess for correct placement of the ETT. See Chapter 5, "Airway and Ventilation," for additional information.
  - Secure the ETT at the teeth or gums.
  - A gastric tube decreases gastric distention, facilitates diaphragmatic function and chest expansion, and improves ventilation.[11]

C: Circulation and Control of Hemorrhage

Assessment continues with perfusion and reassessment for hemorrhage, with consideration of pediatric anatomic and physiologic characteristics.

Anatomic and Physiologic Characteristics

Anatomic and physiologic characteristics to consider include the following:

- Normal heart rate varies by age (Table 13-3).
- In children, stroke volume cannot be increased to maintain cardiac output because of smaller contractile mass and shorter myocardial fibers; therefore, tachycardia is the primary mechanism to maintain cardiac output.
- Infants have twice the cardiac output of adults.
- Children have a higher body water composition compared with adults and can easily become dehydrated.
- When compensatory mechanisms are exhausted, decompensation is sudden and rapid.

Tachycardia and delayed capillary refill of more than 3 seconds are signs of poor perfusion in the pediatric trauma patient.[45] Tachycardia is followed by systemic vasoconstriction to increase systemic vascular resistance, resulting in delayed capillary refill, weak distal pulses, and cool, mottled extremities.

Hypovolemic shock as a result of hemorrhage is the most common form of shock in the pediatric trauma patient.[6,78] Hypotension (**Box 13-2**) is a late finding and reflects blood loss of more than one-third of the circulating blood volume, indicating severe compromise to organ perfusion.[6]

Signs of late shock are easy to recognize. The challenge for nurses is to watch closely for early signs of shock in children before they decompensate.

Assessment

Circulatory assessment includes the following:

- Palpate central and peripheral pulses. When cardiopulmonary resuscitation is being provided, the brachial pulse is considered the central pulse in infants under 1 year of age.[7]
- Assess capillary refill; normal is 2 seconds or less.[78] Blanch the forehead, the sole of the foot, or the palm of the hand and observe the time to refill.
- Perform frequent serial assessments with comparison of central and peripheral pulses to determine stability, improvement, or worsening of circulation and perfusion.
- Jugular vein distention can be difficult to assess in infants because of their short necks, particularly when it is accompanied by significant hypovolemia.[9]

Interventions

Goal-directed interventions are determined by the cause and type of shock. Examples of interventions include the following[8,10,14,26,44,78]:

- Rapid vascular access with peripheral intravenous (IV) or intraosseous (IO) access is the priority of care for the patient in shock. It is not necessary to attempt IV access before using the IO route. If peripheral perfusion is compromised and intravascular access is unlikely, IO access may be the best and first choice.[10,78]
- Administer 20 mL/kg bolus of warmed isotonic crystalloid fluid for hypovolemic shock over 5–10 minutes.
  - Use a 10 mL/kg bolus of warmed isotonic crystalloid fluid for neonates, cardiogenic shock, or children at risk of heart failure.
  - Methods of bolus administration vary, depending on available devices such as IV pumps or syringes. One option for administration, depending on the clinical circumstance and organizational protocols, is the pull-push method (**Box 13-3**).
- After each bolus, assess bilateral breath sounds for crackles or other signs of fluid excess.

BOX 13-2 Pediatric Advanced Life Support (PALS) Guidelines for Hypotension

PALS defines hypotension by systolic blood pressure (SBP) as follows:

- Neonate (0 to 28 days old): SPB < 60 mm Hg
- Infants (1–12 months old): SBP < 70 mm Hg
- Children 1–10 years old: SBP < 70 + (2 × age in years) mm Hg
- Children older than 10 years: SBP < 90 mm Hg

These blood pressures defining hypotension commonly overlap with the lower-normal SBP value spectrum.

Data from American Heart Association. (2020). Part 4: Systematic approach to the seriously ill or injured child. In *Pediatric advanced life support provider manual*.

BOX 13-3 Push-Pull Technique for Intravenous Fluid Administration

One technique for efficient delivery of controlled fluid boluses is the push-pull method. Commercially manufactured devices are available for administration of such therapies but are not required. A syringe is attached to a port in the IV tubing. A three-way stopcock or kinking of the IV tubing is used to control the direction of the IV fluid. The fluid is pulled from a bag of IV fluids and then manually pushed to the patient using the syringe. **Figure 13-4** shows an example of the equipment setup.[23,67,74]

A 20 mL syringe works well for very small children and is a precise way to track the volume. One full 20 mL syringe is needed for each kg of weight to administer a 20 mL/kg bolus. For larger children, a larger syringe may be used, but it can cause hand fatigue and is not necessarily faster.

Regardless of syringe size or device, calculate the number of push-pull sequences necessary, and track how many are performed. Using a 60 mL syringe for a 21 kg child, for example, the push-pull process is repeated 7 times to administer 420 mL of fluid for a 20 mL/kg bolus. Using a 20 mL syringe, the push-pull process is repeated 21 times to deliver the same amount. Use care not to contaminate the syringe plunger when using this technique.

Data from Cole, E. E., Harvey, G., Burbanski, S., Foster, G., Thabane, L., & Parker, M. J. (2014). Rapid paediatric fluid resuscitation: A randomized controlled trial comparing the efficiency of two provider-endorsed manual paediatric fluid resuscitation techniques in a simulated setting. *BMJ Open, 4*, Article e0005028. https://doi.org/10.1136/bmjopen-2014-005028; Spangler, H., Piehl, M., Lane, A., & Robertson, G. (2019). Improving aseptic technique during the treatment of pediatric septic shock: A comparison of 2 rapid fluid delivery methods. *Journal of Infusion Nursing, 42*(1), 23–28. https://doi.org/10.1097/NAN.0000000000000307; Toshniwal, G., Ahmed, Z., & Segnstock, D. (2015). Simulated fluid resuscitation for toddlers and young children: Effect of syringe size and hand fatigue. *Paediatric Anaesthesia, 25*(30), 288–293. https://doi.org/10.1111/pan.12573

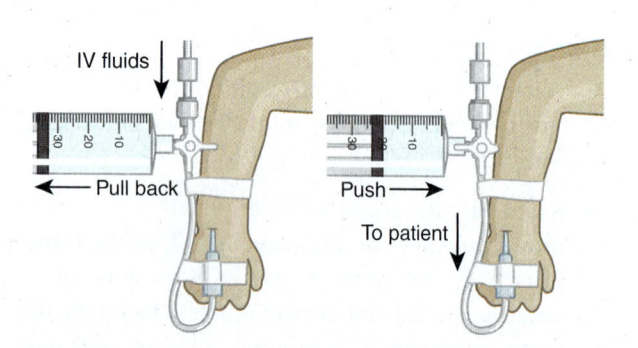

Figure 13-4 Setup for push-pull technique.

- After administering 1–2 isotonic crystalloid fluid bolus, consider early the use of warmed blood balanced products.
- Administer 10 mL/kg of blood for hypovolemic shock due to hemorrhage.
- Epinephrine is administered for anaphylactic shock.
- An antidysrhythmic is used for dysrhythmias associated with a shock state.
- A vasopressor is used for neurogenic shock.
- A pelvic binder may be used for hemorrhage for an unstable pelvis.
- Tranexamic acid may be administered.
- An emergency thoracotomy may be performed; however, this procedure is even less effective in children than in adults.[43]

D: Disability

Disability is the assessment of neurologic status with consideration of pediatric anatomic and physiologic characteristics.

Anatomic and Physiologic Characteristics

Anatomic and physiologic characteristics to consider include[6,15,18,44,78]:

- The brain more than doubles in size by the age of 6 months.[6]
- By 2 years of age, the head has reached 80% of its adult size.[6]
- Because the head is disproportionately large, when infants and children fall, they typically lead with their head, increasing the likelihood of a head injury.
- The posterior fontanel typically closes by 3 months of age and the anterior fontanel by 20 months of age.[44]
- The subarachnoid space is smaller, resulting in a higher likelihood of injury to the brain because of less cushioning.

- Cerebral blood flow progressively increases to twice that of an adult until age 5 years of age, when it begins to decrease. This underscores the susceptibility of children to cerebral hypoxia and hypercarbia.
- Infants have unfused cranial sutures along with open fontanels, enabling expansion of the skull. This can result in more bleeding into the cranial vault before signs of increased intracranial pressure may be noted.
- Early signs of decreased cerebral perfusion include restlessness, crying, fussiness, agitation, and irritability.
- Normal ICP in children is not well established or defined, and it varies with age and time of day. General guidelines for normal ICP in children are as follows[57,69]:
  - 10–15 mm Hg: older children
  - 3–7 mm Hg: younger children
  - 1.5–6 mm Hg: full-term infants
- Intercranial hypertension and cerebral hypoxia occur frequently in children with head trauma, increasing the likelihood of secondary brain injury.

Assessment

Neurological assessment includes the following:

- Consider any pupillary changes or altered level of consciousness to be possible indicators of brain injury, hypoxia, or hypoglycemia, or other abnormalities.
  - Obtain a point-of-care glucose test for any child with an altered mental status.
- Observe behaviors for possible indications of altered mental status—for example, an older infant or toddler who would be expected to exhibit fear or anger toward a stranger. If they do not, this may be an indication of altered mental status.
- Use the Glasgow Coma Scale to evaluate the child's neurologic status (Table 13-4).[6,35,36,81]

Interventions

Interventions include the following:

- Perform a point-of-care glucose test early and often for any child with an altered mental status.
- Assess pupils for shape, consensual size, and reactivity to light.
- Anticipate possible endotracheal intubation for changes in mental status that indicate decreased cerebral blood flow, hypoxia, or fatigue.
- Initiate appropriate interventions to prevent hypoxia, hypotension, or other conditions that may contribute to secondary brain injury.

E: Exposure and Environmental Control

Exposure and environmental control considerations must be assessed in terms of pediatric anatomic and physiologic characteristics.

Anatomic and Physiologic Characteristics

Anatomic and physiologic characteristics include the following:

- Children have a large body-surface-area-to-body-mass ratio, which increases insensible losses through surface evaporation.
- Children are particularly at risk for hypothermia when exposed to cold environments or receiving IV fluids that have not been warmed.[26]
- Children have lesser amounts of body fat than adults, which results in relatively rapid dissipation of body heat when children are exposed to the surrounding environment.
- Hypothermia results in increased oxygen consumption, with resultant hypoxia or acidosis, and contributes to coagulopathy.[26]
- The greater metabolic rate of children relative to adults contributes to increased heat loss.[65]

Assessment

Assessments associated with exposure and environmental control include the following:

- To assess that no life- or limb-threatening abnormalities or hemorrhage have been missed, completely undress the child, including the diaper. This can be done for one area at a time to decrease the risk of hypothermia.
- Observe each exposed area for bleeding, deformities, bruising, rashes, skin discolorations, wounds, and patterned injuries that might be indicative of child maltreatment or other signs of injury or illness.

Interventions

Interventions include the following:

- Implement warming methods, which include, but are not limited to, ambient lights, warming blankets, and warmed intravenous fluids.
- Consider continuous temperature monitoring, such as an indwelling urinary catheter temperature monitor.
- Clothing removal may be upsetting and frightening to the pediatric patient. Provide age-appropriate explanations, and avoid unnecessary exposure (Appendix 13-1).

F: Full Set of Vital Signs and Family Presence

Considerations for vital signs and family presence include the following:

- Use appropriately sized equipment to obtain accurate vital signs.
- Respiratory and heart rates can vary with activity, anxiety, and crying. Attempt to measure vital signs when the pediatric patient is calm, and count both respiration and heart rate for a full minute.
    - Assess the patient while the caregiver holds the child when possible. Obtain the least invasive measurements first. For example, obtain the respiratory rate before obtaining blood pressure.
    - Use toys or bright objects to distract the infant or young child during the assessment.
- When using automated blood pressure devices, ensure the correct sizing of the equipment, and attempt to measure when the child is calm.
    - Adjust the monitor alarm settings to reflect pediatric settings.
    - Assess accuracy of vital sign results if the child is moving or if values are extreme or unexpected.
    - Validate automatic blood pressure readings with a manual blood pressure.
- Promote family-centered care; recognize that the pediatric family may include more than the caregiver, and be supportive.
- Advocate for and encourage family presence at the bedside throughout the ED stay, especially during invasive or frightening procedures and resuscitation. Being present can provide family members with a sense of control and the opportunity to comfort their child. This may reduce fear and anxiety, and improve coping for the child. Additionally, if the child does not survive, having been present may help the family with the grieving process and to understand that everything possible was done.[13,16] Presence of a family member can also facilitate a more accurate assessment by calming and distracting the child.
- A present caregiver can provide accurate information regarding the child's baseline.

See Chapter 18, "Psychosocial Aspects of Trauma Care," for additional information on grieving and trauma-associated stress.

G: Get Monitoring Devices and Give Comfort

The process for getting monitoring devices and giving comfort is the same as that for adults, with the following pediatric-specific considerations.

L: Laboratory Studies

Laboratory study considerations include the following:

- Use pediatric-specific tubes that can accommodate smaller volumes of blood.
- Perform bedside serum glucose testing, and repeat evaluations as needed.
- Children's metabolic demands are greater than those of adults, and glycogen stores in the pediatric liver can be limited. Physiologic stress may rapidly deplete glycogen stores, resulting in hypoglycemia and leading to decreased cardiac contractility, alteration in the level of consciousness, seizures, and acidosis.[8,9]

M: Monitoring

Monitoring considerations include the following:

- Use appropriately sized pediatric equipment.
- Use noninvasive monitors with caution, knowing that movement and crying, poor perfusion, and extreme values can affect the validity of the readings.
- Change monitor alarm settings to reflect normal pediatric parameters for age-based respiratory rate, heart rate, SpO$_2$, and blood pressure.

N: Nasogastric or Orogastric Tube Consideration

Nasogastric or orogastric tube considerations include the following:

- Crying and bag-mask ventilation can cause children to swallow air, leading to gastric distention. Consider decompression with a nasogastric or orogastric tube. Placement of a gastric tube is considered routine care in the intubated patient to minimize aspiration risk.
- A nasogastric tube is contraindicated in the presence of facial fractures or a known or suspected basilar skull fracture.
- Select appropriate sizes of tubes by using a length-based resuscitation tape or other evidence-based resource.

O: Oxygenation

Oxygenation considerations include the following:

- Apply the pulse oximeter probe to a warm extremity for the most accurate results.
    - A warm pack around the hand or foot may help.
    - Other possible locations in the pediatric patient include the side of the hand, the earlobe, or the forehead.
- Consider capnography if indicated.

P: Pain Assessment and Management

Pain assessment and management considerations include the following:

- Pain is consistently poorly assessed and managed in pediatric patients.[31,63]
- Children may have difficulty localizing the source(s) of pain and may not be able to effectively communicate that they are experiencing pain.
- Environmental and emotional factors can potentiate the pain experience in pediatric patients.
- Use an age- and developmentally appropriate pain assessment tool such as the FLACC (face, legs, activity, cry, consolability) scale to assess for pain in *all* injured pediatric patients (**Table 13-5**)[38] (**Figure 13-5**).
- The nurse should advocate for appropriate pain management, including pharmacologic interventions as indicated.
- Nonpharmacologic approaches to pain management can be divided into two categories: physical comfort measures and distracting techniques (**Table 13-6**).[39]
    - Infants find comfort in oral stimulation (pacifiers, breastfeeding, suckling) and physical contact (swaddling/cuddling, rocking). Cold or heat can provide comfort to the older child.
    - Distraction can include interactive toys, bubbles, art, music, and books. Video games and movies are good distractors for the older child.
- Young children are cognitively immature, so they have difficulty managing their fears. Distraction may help with this.
- Assess for signs of traumatic stress. See Chapter 18, "Psychosocial Aspects of Trauma Care," for additional information.

Reevaluation

Assess for the need for pediatric surgical services, intensive care, or specialists (burn center), and prepare for transport if indicated.

The Pediatric Trauma Score is a tool that uses physiologic assessment parameters and can aid in determining the need for transfer to a pediatric trauma center.[6,72]

Secondary Survey, Diagnostics, and Interventions

The secondary survey begins with history taking and the head-to-toe assessment.

TABLE 13-5 Revised FLACC Scale

Variable	0	+1	+2
Face	No expression or smile	Occasional grimace, frown; withdrawn or uninterested. *Appears sad or worried.*	Consistent grimace, quivering chin, clenched jaw, *distressed-looking face, expression of fright or panic*
Legs	Normal position, relaxed, *usual tone and motion to limbs*	Uneasy, restless, tense, *occasional tremors*	Kicking, drawn up, *marked increase in spasticity, constant tremors or jerking*
Activity	Lying quietly, normal position, moves easily, *regular and rhythmic respirations*	Squirming, shifting back and forth, *tense or guarded movements, shallow splinting respirations*	Arched, rigid or jerking *Head banging, breath holding, gasping or severe splinting*
Cry	None	Moans or whimpers, occasional complaint, *occasional verbal outburst or grunt*	Crying steadily, screams or sobs, frequent complaints, *repeated outbursts, constant grunting*
Consolability	Content and relaxed	Reassured by occasional touching/hugging or being talked to, distractible	Difficult to console or comfort, *pushing away, resisting care or comfort measures*

Note. The areas where the revised scale differs from the original FLACC scale appear in italics.

Modified from Kjeldgaard Pendersen, L., Rahbek, O., Nikolajsen, L., & Møller-Madsen, B. (2015). The revised FLACC score: Reliability and validation for pain assessment in children with cerebral palsy. *Scandinavian Journal of Pain, 9*, 57–61. https://doi.org/10.1016/j.sjpain.2015.06.007

Wong-Baker FACES® Pain Rating Scale

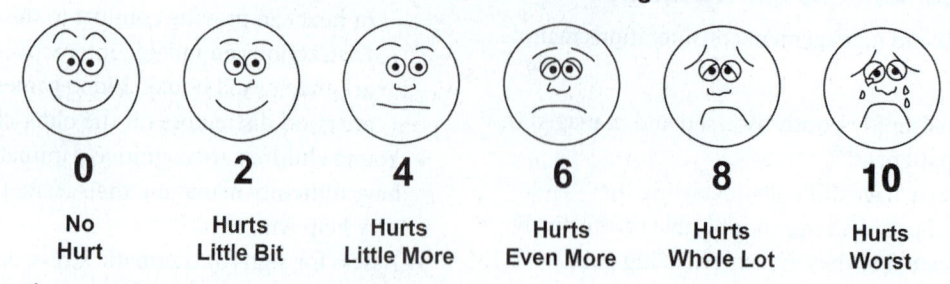

0	2	4	6	8	10
No Hurt	Hurts Little Bit	Hurts Little More	Hurts Even More	Hurts Whole Lot	Hurts Worst

Figure 13-5 *Faces Pain Scale–Revised.*
© 1983 Wong-Baker FACES Foundation. www.WongBakerFACES.org. Used with permission. Originally published in *Whaley & Wong's nursing care of infants and children.* © Elsevier Inc.

TABLE 13-6 Nonpharmacologic Approaches to Pain Management in Children

Physical Comfort (Infants and Young Children)	Distraction Techniques (All Ages)
Rocking	Blowing bubbles
Cuddling/swaddling	Conversation/asking questions
Pacifiers	Sound, music, art
Touch: stroking, rubbing, patting	Books, interactive games, puppets
	Imagery, controlled deep breathing
	Video games

Data from Krauss, B., Calligaris, L., Green, S., & Barbi, E. (2016). Current concepts in management of pain in children in the emergency department. *The Lancet, 387*(10013), 83–92. https://doi.org/10.1016/S0140-6736(14)61686-X

History

History includes one or both of the following:

- Obtain additional history from prehospital providers. Inquire about any pain medication that may have been given.
- Obtain history from caregivers or family. SAMPLE is a mnemonic that can be used to obtain history.
  - **S**igns and symptoms associated with the illness or injury
  - **A**llergic to medications, foods, substances, or the environment
  - **M**edications, including those routinely administered and/or given for this illness/injury. Ask about the last dose administered, over-the-counter medications, and supplements.
  - **P**ast medical and/or surgical history, including immunizations
  - **L**ast meal/output (void and bowel movement) and menstrual period
  - **E**vents leading up to the current illness or injury

Head-to-Toe

Older infants, toddlers, and preschool-age children may respond better to a least-invasive-to-most-invasive approach to the assessment, rather than a head-to-toe progression. Engage a child life specialist if available.

- Head
  - Palpate the infant for full or bulging fontanels or sunken fontanels.
- Chest
  - The pediatric patient's ribs are more cartilaginous, so fractures are not common. When present, rib fractures indicate significant force transmitted across the chest, accompanied by the high possibility of damage to underlying structures.
  - A mobile mediastinum allows a greater degree of shift to the right or left in the presence of pneumothorax, hemothorax, and/or tension pneumothorax.
- Abdomen
  - Anatomic and physiologic characteristics
    - The abdominal muscles are thin and less developed, so abdominal organs are not well protected.
    - The liver is more anterior and less protected by the ribs.
    - The kidneys are more mobile and less protected by fat.
    - The sigmoid colon and ascending colon are more mobile within the peritoneum and at greater risk for deceleration injuries.
    - The duodenum has an increased vascular supply. Injury can lead to increased blood loss or hematoma formation.[60]

- Assessment
  - Inspect the abdomen for distention. Determine whether distension may be gastric dilation from swallowing air while crying or from bag-mask–assisted ventilations.
  - Crying interferes with the assessment for guarding, tenderness, and rigidity. Provide distraction, involve the caregiver, or take the time for the patient to become calm before assessing.
- Pelvis and genitalia
  - The urinary bladder is significantly less protected in the pediatric patient than the adult because of its position above the pelvic ring, less adipose tissue, and underdeveloped muscles. Pelvic fractures are also present in approximately 57% of children with bladder rupture. However, bladder injuries in the presence of a pelvic fracture range from 0.5% to 18.6%.[66]
  - Assessing for rectal tone in the pediatric patient can be upsetting and can contribute to a reduction in the patient's cooperation, potentially limiting ongoing systemic assessments.
    - Assess by observing for an anal wink with rectal temperature unless contraindicated.
    - Perform this last, and include the caregiver to comfort and hold the patient at the end of the assessment.
- Extremities
  - Pediatric patients have pliable, incompletely calcified bones that may mask significant underlying trauma.
  - Greenstick and buckle/torus fractures of the bones occur frequently in children because of the pliability and cartilaginous nature of young bones.
  - Because of the ossification process in children, comparison views for extremity radiographs will assist in identifying injury.

Diagnostics and Interventions

Diagnostics and interventions center primarily on radiographic and sonographic studies. Although uncommon, diagnostic peritoneal lavage may be considered by the trauma team.[6]

Radiographic Studies

Trauma centers are limiting the use of unnecessary computed tomography (CT) scans during evaluation of the injured child. Evidence demonstrates that radiation from CT scanners correlates with an increased risk of cancer, especially when the exposure occurs in childhood.[6,49] Although CT scanning is indicated at times, the American College of Surgeons recommends that scanning occur only when absolutely necessary and with the lowest amount of radiation possible, and when the results of the scan will impact patient management.[6] Alternatives might include ultrasonography, magnetic resonance imaging (MRI), or radiographs.[49]

Focused Assessment with Sonography for Trauma (FAST)

The FAST exam has limited sensitivity in pediatric patients for identifying peritoneal bleeding, but it can be useful for the hypotensive patient who is too unstable to undergo CT. Practice in this area is evolving rapidly as physicians use the FAST exam as an extension of the physical exam.[6] Management of the patient is not determined by the FAST exam, but the presence or absence of hemodynamic stability.[6]

Diagnostic Peritoneal Lavage

Diagnostic peritoneal lavage (DPL) is no longer considered the preferred diagnostic method to rule out intra-abdominal bleeding in children. However, DPL may still be used in some cases, such as when an injured child cannot be transported to CT, and FAST is not available.[6] Accuracy and expertise with FAST have lessened the need for the more invasive DPL.

Selected Injuries

This section presents selected injuries and associated considerations.

Head Injury

Head injury considerations include the following:

- Suspect severe brain injury in a pediatric trauma patient with bulging fontanels. Rapid consultation with a neurosurgeon is indicated.[6]
- Children under 3 years of age are at risk for worse outcomes for a brain injury compared with children older than 3 years.[6]
- Hypotension and hypoxia contribute to a poor outcome following a head injury.[6]
  - Hypotension due to hemorrhage in a child with a serious brain injury is the highest risk factor and can have catastrophic consequences.[6]
- Persistent vomiting posttrauma can be an indication of increased ICP.
- Significant bleeding can occur after scalp lacerations because of the head's extensive vascularity.
- Considerations for disposition following a TBI include medical or surgical intervention, observation, and discharge. The Pediatric Emergency Care Applied Research Network (PECARN) criteria

284 Chapter 13 The Pediatric Trauma Patient

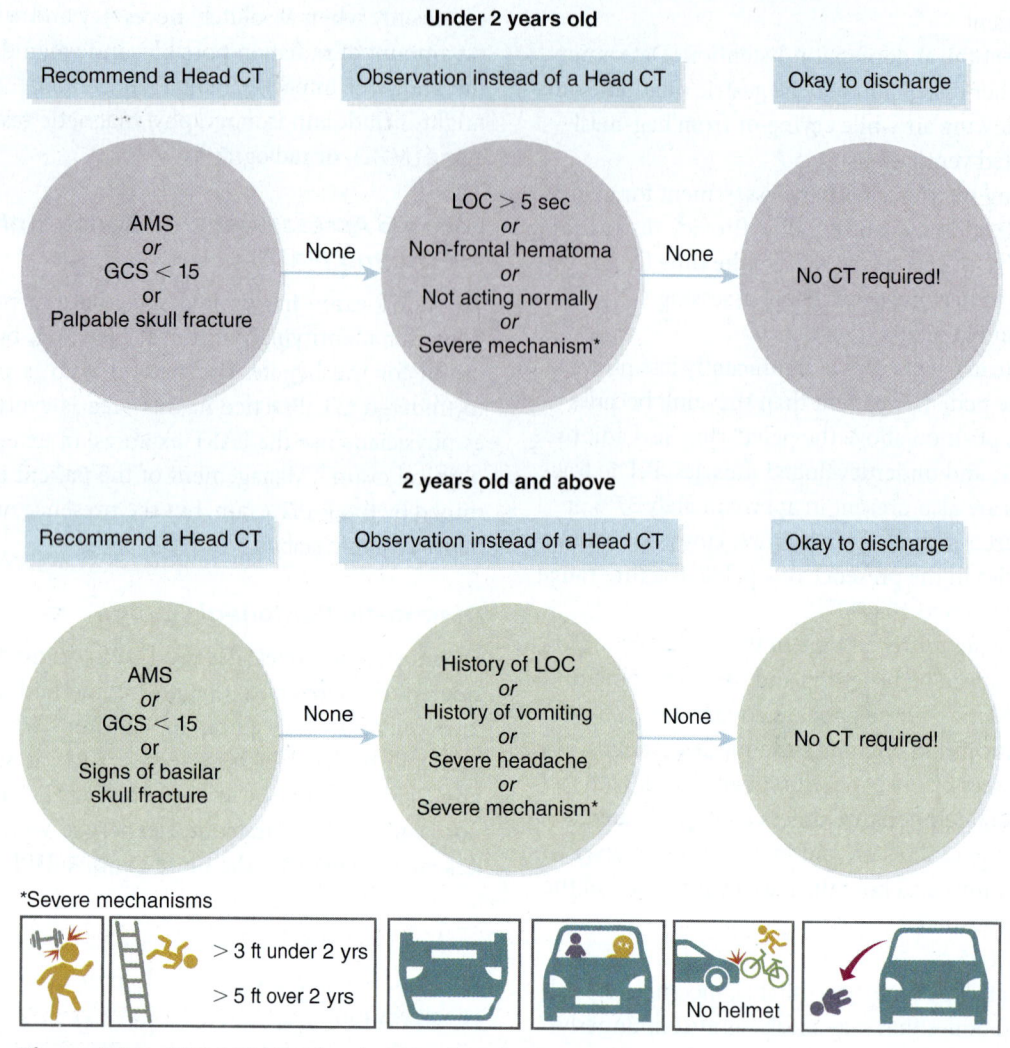

Under 2 years old

Recommend a Head CT: AMS or GCS < 15 or Palpable skull fracture → None →

Observation instead of a Head CT: LOC > 5 sec or Non-frontal hematoma or Not acting normally or Severe mechanism* → None →

Okay to discharge: No CT required!

2 years old and above

Recommend a Head CT: AMS or GCS < 15 or Signs of basilar skull fracture → None →

Observation instead of a Head CT: History of LOC or History of vomiting or Severe headache or Severe mechanism* → None →

Okay to discharge: No CT required!

*Severe mechanisms: > 3 ft under 2 yrs; > 5 ft over 2 yrs; No helmet

Figure 13-6 PECARN Pediatric Head CT Rule.
AMS = altered mental status; GCS = Glasgow Coma Scale; LOC = loss of consciousness.

(**Figure 13-6**) can assist in identifying patients who require observation only, thus limiting children's exposure to ionizing radiation.

Cervical Spine Injury

Cervical spine injury considerations include the following:

- Although not common, children are at risk for cervical spine injury because of their disproportionately large head, weak musculature and lax ligaments supporting the spine and spinal cord, flat facet joints, and open growth plates with unossified vertebrae.[6,42]
- If any signs or symptoms of spinal cord injury are present despite negative radiographic evidence, assume that an unstable spinal injury exists, and maintain SMRs.
- Appropriate early removal of cervical collars promotes comfort, decreases anxiety and fear, decreases risk for skin breakdown and pressure injury, and may lower the risk of aspiration in pediatric patients.[71]
- Dislocations and subluxations of the vertebrae with injury to ligaments are more common in children younger than 8 years.[42]

Adult screening tools such as the National Emergency X-Radiography Utilization Study (NEXUS) criteria may be helpful for older children and adolescents but have limitations for younger children.[41] Young pediatric patients rarely meet the criteria, and those younger than 9 years may require alternative diagnostic approaches such as radiographs or CT.[6] Risk factors for cervical spine injury in pediatric patients include the following[41]:

- High-risk motor vehicle crash
- Diving
- Altered mental status
- Neck pain
- Focal neurologic deficits

- Torticollis
- Significant injury to the torso
- Predisposing condition that can be related to cervical spine injury

Maintain SMR if symptoms are present, even in the face of negative radiographs or CT imaging. SCIWORA can be diagnosed with MRI.

Abdominal Injury

Blunt abdominal trauma is the third most common cause of trauma-related death in children.[26,78] It is also the most common area of missed injury that results in death.[26,78] Injury to the abdomen includes the following considerations:

- Pediatric patients are more susceptible to abdominal injury than adults. Bruising, pain, abrasions, lacerations, or Chance fractures may indicate the need for additional diagnostics.[6,78]
- The liver and spleen are the most commonly injured abdominal organs in children and can result in severe hemorrhage.[78]

Management is based on the patient's hemodynamic stability and the need for continued blood replacement therapy. Liver and spleen injuries may be managed nonoperatively in the hemodynamically stable pediatric patient.[26] Preservation of the spleen is a high priority because of the organ's immunologic functions. If surgery is necessary, the focus is on repair, not removal.[28]

Musculoskeletal Injury

Injuries involving the growth plates may result in growth abnormalities and have lifelong implications, such as length discrepancies in arms or legs, scoliosis, kyphosis, or gait disturbances. For the child with a growth plate injury, anticipate referral to an orthopedic specialist for follow-up.

Maltreatment

Child maltreatment is associated with significant morbidity and mortality. It is considered an adverse childhood event (ACE) and, as such, not only can cause lifelong physical issues but also carries significant mental health consequences. See Chapter 18, "Psychosocial Aspects of Trauma Care," for additional information. Approximately 80% of deaths related to child abuse occur in children under 5 years of age, and 40% occur in children younger than 1 year.[1] Abusive head injury results in greater incidence of diffuse axonal injury and subdural bleeding compared with unintentional head injury.[1] Head trauma is the most common and most lethal MOI in child maltreatment.[1,78]

Screening for maltreatment in the ED is an important aspect of trauma care. Each facility should have clearly defined policies and procedures for the screening, forensic processes (including history and documentation expectations), treatment, and reporting of suspected child abuse to the appropriate agencies and law enforcement. In many countries, nurses must report suspected child abuse (mandated reporters) to the appropriate agency, such as child protective services. Other considerations include the following[6,17,78]:

- Injuries inconsistent with developmental stage (Appendix 13-1)
- Injuries inconsistent with history and/or MOI
- History of repeated injuries with visits to the same or different EDs
- Prolonged time between injury and seeking of medical care
- Bruising suspicious for abuse:
  - Present in nonmobile infants
  - Patterned (looped cord or bite mark)
  - In protected areas[58]
    - TEN-4: Bruising to torso, ears, or neck in children under 4 years of age
    - FACES P: Bruising to the frenulum, angle of the jaw/ear, cheek, eyelid, subconjunctiva, and patterned injuries
- Injuries in various stages of healing
- Rib fractures in children younger than 18 months—70% are caused by abuse
- Fractures of long bones in children under the age of 3 years

The absence of bruising does not rule out abuse; children can experience serious injury without bruising, such as head trauma and abdominal trauma.[17] See Chapter 17, "Interpersonal Violence," for additional information.

Burns

The majority of burns in children up to 5 years of age are scald burns that occur in the home.[5] Scald burns can be accidental; however, scalding is also a common form of child abuse.[5] Thermal burns from flame are more common in older children and adolescents.[5] See Chapter 11, "Surface and Burn Trauma," for additional information, including resuscitation, fluid resuscitation, and calculation of total body surface area percentage.

Other considerations in the pediatric patient include the following:

- Stop the burning process. Remove all clothing, including the diaper.
- Keep patients covered to prevent heat loss.
- Advocate for appropriate management of pain using pharmacologic and nonpharmacologic interventions. Burns should be covered to decrease pain from air current movement.

- Anticipate the possibility of airway compromise. Edema is a significant risk factor in children.[5]
- Young children may require early intubation because of their inherently smaller airway.[5]
- Rapidly consider placement of an IO if intravenous vascular access is unlikely or unsuccessful.
- Anticipate transfer to a burn center for children with full-thickness burns; inhalation injury; electrical burns; and burns to the face, genitalia, hands, or feet.[5]

Psychosocial Considerations

Psychosocial considerations when caring for the injured child include the following:

- Traumatic injuries are frightening and painful.
- Use an appropriate evidence-based pain scale to assess pain. If a child is unresponsive, assume that pain is present based on injuries sustained and MOI.
- ACEs can have lifelong impact on health and well-being.
- The traumatic event that resulted in the child being brought to the ED, as well as the ED experience itself, can become an ACE. See Chapter 18, "Psychosocial Aspects of Trauma Care," for additional information.
- Understanding emotional, cognitive, and physical development is essential when caring for an injured child (Appendix 13-1).
- If available, involve a child life specialist in the care of the injured child.
- Both the child and the caregivers need to perceive that they are in a safe place with skilled staff.
- Communication is vital for both the child and the caregivers. Recognize the importance of both verbal and nonverbal communication.
- Communicate with the child at eye level, using language appropriate to their developmental stage (Appendix 13-1).
- Be honest. Do not tell a child something will not hurt when it will.
- When possible, allow the child to hold onto a favorite toy or item that comforts them, such as a blanket.
- Encourage the family to ask questions and to be actively involved in the child's care.

Disaster Management

Pediatric considerations in disaster management include the following:

- Pediatric disaster preparedness includes, but is not limited to, pediatric-sized equipment, resources for staff, and education that includes weight-based medication principles, anatomic and physiologic differences in children, normal vital sign parameters, family reunification processes, and mental health resources.
- Children separated from families during a disaster are very vulnerable and at risk for significant sequelae, including mental trauma, abuse, and exploitation.[3]
- Children may not understand how to flee from danger.[4]
- Children may actually move toward danger, not recognizing the threat.[4]
- Children's proximity to the ground and increased respiratory rate may make them more vulnerable to some chemical and biological agents.
- Thinner skin in children leads to increased systemic absorption of biological and chemical agents.
- Children will likely require additional assistance during the decontamination process.
- Use warm water when decontaminating; prevent hypothermia.
- To assist with reunification, document any personal effects, including backpacks, bags, jewelry, or any other identifying objects.
- On the child's skin, use a permanent marker to record any important identifying characteristics.

Reevaluation and Post-Resuscitation Care

Reevaluation and post-resuscitation care include the following considerations:

- Ongoing assessment and evaluation of interventions include frequent, serial reevaluation of the primary survey, monitoring for changes in vital signs, and continued reevaluation and management of pain and identified injuries. These actions, along with monitoring urine output, will help to guide therapy.
- Continue to monitor and treat serum glucose levels for hypoglycemia, especially in infants and young children, whose glycogen stores may become rapidly depleted.

Patient Safety

Safety of the injured pediatric patient in the emergency setting can consume many resources, but it is essential to prevent further injury. Infants and younger children need constant supervision in the absence of a caregiver, and they require cribs or isolettes to help prevent falls from a stretcher. Other risks for falls include older children who may attempt to remove themselves from SMR devices or try to ambulate unassisted while under the effects of opioids and/or with compromised balance from an injury.

The assistance of social services may be necessary to ensure family reunification if the patient arrives without a primary caregiver. A child life therapist and child life techniques can be helpful for promoting normalcy and calmness during difficult procedures.

Safety also includes ensuring that the patient's weight is obtained and documented in kilograms to avoid medication errors. When it is not possible to obtain an actual weight, a length-based resuscitation tape can be used. This is a temporary measure until an actual weight in kilograms can be obtained.

Definitive Care or Transport

Care and transport considerations include the following:

- Consider the need for transfer to a pediatric trauma or burn center early in the care and management of the injured child for better outcomes. See Chapter 20, "Transition of Care for the Trauma Patient," for additional information.
- The patient's status, injuries, and needs for definitive care are considered when determining the team members needed for the transport team. Pediatric patients have better outcomes and fewer unplanned events when transported by a specialized pediatric team.[19]
- Provide follow-up and clear discharge instructions, such as information on gradual and incremental return to play for all patients diagnosed with TBI, including those with concussions. Returning to play while symptoms persist places the patient at risk for secondary brain injury, which is more likely to be fatal in the pediatric patient.[48]
- Have information readily available for referral to the closest pediatric trauma center for transfer or consult.

Emerging Trends

Emerging trends in the area of pediatric trauma care include reduction in the use of unnecessary radiation, changes in motor vehicle design to reduce traumatic injuries in children, and pediatric resuscitative endovascular balloon occlusion of the aorta (REBOA).

Reduction of the Use of Unnecessary Radiation

As noted earlier, ionizing radiation exposure in children may increase their lifetime risk of developing some types of malignancies. Trauma teams can use PECARN guidelines and other evidence-based algorithms to safely reduce CT scans among hemodynamically stable patients. Some children may undergo MRI, plain film, or ultrasound imaging instead of CT scans. Studies show that nonpediatric trauma centers are more likely to overradiate pediatric trauma patients.[49,54] Research is ongoing into the use of advanced imaging, including contrast-enhanced ultrasound, ultrafast MRI, and improvements in CTs, in an effort to limit radiation exposure.[30,49,75]

Motor Vehicle Design to Reduce Traumatic Injuries in Children

Efforts to reduce motor vehicle crashes through better car design or roadway engineering improvements will decrease the incidence of injured children. These efforts are ongoing. In addition, enforcement of stronger laws addressing child car seats and drunk drivers, as well as graduated driving laws for teenagers, will continue to reduce pediatric injuries.

Pediatric Resuscitative Endovascular Balloon Occlusion of the Aorta

REBOA is used in some trauma centers as an intervention for hemorrhagic shock due to noncompressible hemorrhage in the chest, abdomen, and pelvis in the adult population.[6,73] Recent evidence indicates that REBOA may also be an intervention for use in severely injured children when immediate control of hemorrhage may not otherwise be possible.[73] Although promising, further research is needed, given the myriad of anatomic and physiologic differences between children and adults, including the effect of REBOA on the child who has a TBI.[20,73]

Summary

Pediatric trauma care requires familiarity with the unique responses of the injured pediatric patient. The systematic approach of the primary survey is the same for adults and children, but the clinical manifestations of complications and interventions may vary based on the patient's age, size, and development. Knowledge of normal growth and development assists the trauma nurse in approaching the pediatric patient and providing appropriate care. Trauma-informed care is vital in the pediatric population. Identification of the primary caregivers and integration of their perspectives and input into care can promote optimal pediatric trauma care. **Table 13-7** identifies internet resources related to the care of pediatric patients.

TABLE 13-7 Internet Resources

Internet Resource	Web Address
Emergency Nurses Association	www.ena.org
Society of Trauma Nurses	www.traumanurses.org
American Academy of Pediatrics	www.aap.org
American College of Emergency Physicians	www.acep.org
American College of Surgeons	www.facs.org/trauma
Pediatric Trauma Society	www.pediatrictraumasociety.org
Emergency Medical Services for Children Innovation & Improvement Center	https://emscimprovement.center
Centers for Disease Control and Prevention	www.cdc.gov/injury
Injury Free Coalition for Kids	www.injuryfree.org
Safe Kids Worldwide	www.safekids.org
SageDiagram (free TBSA calculator)	www.sagediagram.com
Image Gently Campaign	www.imagegently.org
Pediatric Emergency Care Applied Research Network (PECARN)	www.pecarn.org
American Association of Neurological Surgeons	www.aans.org

Note. This is not a comprehensive list.

References

1. Acker, S. N., & Kulungowski, A. M. (2019). Error traps and culture of safety in pediatric trauma. *Seminars in Pediatric Surgery, 28*(3), 183–188. https://doi.org/10.1053/j.sempedsurg.2019.04.022
2. Allen, K. A. (2016). Pathophysiology and treatment of severe traumatic brain injuries in children. *Journal of Neuroscience Nursing, 48*(1), 15–27. https://doi.org/10.1097/JNN.0000000000000176
3. American Academy of Pediatrics. (2018). *Family reunification following disasters: A planning tool for health care facilities.* https://downloads.aap.org/AAP/PDF/AAP%20Reunification%20Toolkit.pdf
4. American Academy of Pediatrics. (2019). How children are different. In *Pediatric disaster preparedness and response topical collection.* https://downloads.aap.org/AAP/PDF/Topical-Collection-Chapter-1.pdf?_ga=2.47117728.66921406.1667602181-2072806600.1667081229
5. American Burn Association. (2018). Pediatric burns. In *Advanced burn life support course provider manual: 2018 update* (pp. 59–67).
6. American College of Surgeons. (2018). Pediatric trauma. In *Advanced trauma life support: Student course manual* (10th ed., pp. 188–212).
7. American Heart Association. (2020). Part 2: Review of BLS and AED for infants and children. In *Pediatric advanced life support manual* (pp. 13–26).
8. American Heart Association. (2020). Part 4: Systematic approach to the seriously ill or injured child. In *Pediatric advanced life support manual* (pp. 37–70).
9. American Heart Association. (2020). Part 9: Recognizing shock. In *Pediatric advanced life support manual* (pp. 165–188).
10. American Heart Association. (2020). Part 10: Managing shock. In *Pediatric advanced life support manual* (pp. 189–228).
11. American Heart Association. (2020). Part 13: Post-cardiac arrest care. In *Pediatric advanced life support manual* (pp. 261–278).
12. Andrews, A. L., Killings, X., Oddo, E. R., Gastineau, K. A., & Hink, A. B. (2022). Pediatric firearm injury mortality epidemiology. *Pediatrics, 149*(3), Article e2021052739. https://doi.org/10.1542/peds.2021-052739
13. Auerbach, M., Butler, L., Myers, S. R., Donoghue, A., & Kassam-Adams, N. (2021). Implementing family presence during pediatric resuscitations in the emergency department: Family-centered care and trauma-informed care best practices comment. *Journal of Emergency Nursing, 47*(5), 689–692. https://doi.org/10.1016/j.jen.2021.07.003
14. Balamuth, F., Fitzgerald, J. C., & Weiss, S. L. (2021). Shock. In K. N. Shaw & R. G. Bachur (Eds.), *Fleisher & Ludwig's textbook of pediatric medicine* (8th ed., pp. 72–86). Wolters Kluwer.
15. Banta-Wright, S. A. (2020). Developmental management of infants. In *Burns' pediatric primary care* (7th ed., pp. 92–108). Elsevier.

16. Bradley, C. (2021). Family presence and support during resuscitation. *Critical Care Nursing Clinics of North America*, 33(3), 333–342. https://doi.org/10.1016/j.cnc.2021.05.008
17. Brown, C. L., Yilanli, M., & Rabbit, A. L. (2022). Child physical abuse and neglect. *StatPearls*. StatPearls Publishing. https://www.ncbi.nlm.nih.gov/books/NBK470337/
18. Butterfield, R. J., & Huether, S. E. (2019). Alterations of neurologic function in children. In K. L. McCance & S. E. Huether (Eds.), *Pathophysiology* (8th ed., pp. 619–643). Elsevier.
19. Calhoun, A., Keller, M., Shi, J., Brancato, C., Donovan, K., Kraus, D., & Leonard, J. (2016). Do pediatric teams affect outcomes of injured children requiring inter-hospital transport? *Prehospital Emergency Care*, 21(2), 192–200. https://doi.org/10.1080/10903127.2016.1218983
20. Campagna, G. A., Cunningham, M. E., Hernandez, J. A., Chau, A., Vogel, A. M., & Naik-Mathuria, B. J. (2020). The utility and promise of resuscitative endovascular balloon occlusion of the aorta (REBOA) in the pediatric population: An evidence-based review. *Journal of Pediatric Surgery*, 55, 2128–2133.
21. Centers for Disease Control and Prevention. (n.d.). *Fast facts: Firearm violence prevention.* https://www.cdc.gov/violenceprevention/firearms/fastfact.html
22. Centers for Disease Control and Prevention. (n.d.). *Injuries among children and teens.* https://www.cdc.gov/injury/features/child-injury/index.html
23. Cole, E. E., Harvey, G., Burbanski, S., Foster, G., Thabane, L., & Parker, M. J. (2014). Rapid paediatric fluid resuscitation: A randomized controlled trial comparing the efficiency of two provider-endorsed manual paediatric fluid resuscitation techniques in a simulated setting. *BMJ Open*, 4, Article e0005028. https://doi.org/10.1136/bmjopen-2014-005028
24. Conway, A. (2012). From the start. In *Emergency Nursing Pediatric Course provider manual* (4th ed., pp. 25–49). Emergency Nurses Association.
25. Emergency Medical Services for Children Innovation & Improvement Center. (n.d.). *National Pediatric Readiness Project.* https://emscimprovement.center/domains/pediatric-readiness-project/
26. Ernst, G. (2020). Pediatric trauma. In J. E. Tintinalli, O. J. Ma, D. M. Yealy, G. D. Meckler, J. S. Stapczynsk, D. M. Cline, & S. H. Thomas (Eds.), *Tintinalli's emergency medicine: A comprehensive study guide* (9th ed., pp. 789–797). McGraw Hill.
27. Fernandez, A., Ares, M. I., Martinez-Indart, L., Mintegi, S., & Benito, J. (2017). The validity of the Pediatric Assessment Triangle as the first step in the triage process in a pediatric emergency department. *Pediatric Emergency Care*, 33(4), 234–238. https://doi.org/10.1097/pec.0000000000000717
28. Gillory, L., & Naik-Mathuria, B. (2017). Pediatric abdominal trauma. In D. E. Wesson & B. Naik-Mathuria (Eds.), *Pediatric trauma: Pathophysiology, diagnosis, and treatment* (2nd ed., pp. 215–238). CRC Press.
29. Goldstick, J. E., Cunningham, R. M., & Carter, P. M. (2022). Current causes of death in children and adolescents in the United States. *New England Journal of Medicine*, 386(20), 1955–1956. https://doi.org/10.1056/NEJMc2201761
30. Gräfe, D., Roth, C., Weisser, M., Krause, M., Frahm, J., Voit, D., & Hirsch, F. W. (2020). Outpacing movement—Ultrafast volume coverage in neuropediatric magnetic resonance imaging. *Pediatric Radiology*, 50(12), 1751–1756. https://doi.org/10.1007/s00247-020-04771-5
31. Hartshorn, S., Durnin, S., Lyttle, M. D., & Barrett, M. (2022). Pain management in children and young adults with minor injury in emergency departments in the UK and Ireland: A PERUKI service evaluation. *BMJ Paediatrics Open*, 6, e001273. https://doi.org/10.1136/bmjpo-2021-001273
32. Hoedeman, F., Puiman, P. J., Smits, A. W., Dekker, M. I., Diderich-Lolkes de Beer, H., Laribi, S., Lauwaert, D., Oostenbrink, R., Parri, N., Garcia-Castrillo Riesgo, L., & Moll, H. A. (2021). Recognition of child maltreatment in emergency departments in Europe: Should we do better? *PLOS ONE*. https://doi.org/10.1371/journal.pone.0246361
33. Horeczko, T., Enriquez, B., McGrath, N. E., Gausche-Hill, M., & Lewis, R. J. (2013). The Pediatric Assessment Triangle: Accuracy of its application by nurses in the triage of children. *Journal of Emergency Nursing*, 39(2), 182–189. https://doi.org/10.1016/j.jen.2011.12.020
34. Hutchinson, J., Waggoner, B., Gephart, B., Case, L. A., Pearcy, A., & Zehner, S. (2020). The implementation of pediatric quarterly mock codes and its impact on resuscitation skills compliance. *Journal of Pediatric Nursing*, 55, 266–269. https://doi.org/10.1016/j.pedn.2020.09.005
35. Institute of Neurological Sciences NHS Greater Glasgow and Clyde. (2015). *Glasgow Coma Scale: Do it this way.* https://www.glasgowcomascale.org/downloads/GCS-Assessment-Aid-English.pdf?v=3
36. Jain, S., & Iverson, L. M. (2021, June 20). Glasgow Coma Scale. *StatPearls.* StatPearls Publishing. https://www.ncbi.nlm.nih.gov/books/NBK513298/
37. Joseph, M. M., Mahajan, P., Snow, S. K., Ku, B. C., Saidinejad, M., American Academy of Pediatrics Committee on Pediatric Emergency Medicines, American College of Emergency Physicians Pediatric Emergency Medicine Committee, & Emergency Nurses Association Pediatric Committee. (2022). Optimizing pediatric patient safety in the emergency care setting. *Pediatrics*, 150(5). https://doi.org/10.1542/peds.2022-059673
38. Kjeldgaard Pendersen, L., Rahbek, O., Nikolajsen, L., & Møller-Madsen, B. (2015). The revised FLACC score: Reliability and validation for pain assessment in children with cerebral palsy. *Scandinavian Journal of Pain*, 9, 57–61. https://doi.org/10.1016/j.sjpain.2015.06.007
39. Krauss, B., Calligaris, L., Green, S., & Barbi, E. (2016). Current concepts in management of pain in children in the emergency department. *The Lancet*, 387, 83–92. https://doi.org/10.1016/S0140-6736(14)61686-X
40. Lee, L. K., & Farrell, C. (2022). Trauma management: Approach to the unstable child. *UpToDate.* Retrieved November 14, 2020, from https://www.uptodate.com/contents/trauma-management-approach-to-the-unstable-child
41. Leonard, J. C. (2020). Cervical spine injury in infants and children. In J. E. Tintinalli, O. J. Ma, D. M. Yearly, G. D.

Meckler, J. S. Stapczynski, D. M. Cline, & S. H. Thomas (Eds.), *Tintinalli's emergency medicine: A comprehensive study guide* (9th ed., pp. 706–709). McGraw Hill.

42. Leonard, J. C. (2022). Evaluation and acute management of cervical spine injuries in children and adolescents. *UpToDate.* Retrieved November 11, 2022, from https://www.uptodate.com/contents/evaluation-and-acute-management-of-cervical-spine-injuries-in-children-and-adolescents

43. Letton, R. W., & Johnson, J. J. (2017). The ABCs of pediatric trauma. In D. E. Wesson & B. Naik-Mathuria (Eds.), *Pediatric trauma: Pathophysiology, diagnosis, and treatment* (2nd ed., pp. 51–60). CRC Press.

44. Lewis, C. A. (2022). The pediatric patient. In L. D. Urden, K. M. Stacy, & M. E. Lough (Eds.), *Critical care nursing: Diagnosis and management* (9th ed., pp. 974–996). Elsevier.

45. Logee, K. (2020). Pediatric emergencies. In V. Sweet & A. Foley (Eds.), *Sheehy's emergency nursing* (7th ed., pp. 556–575). Elsevier.

46. Lucia, D., & Glenn, J. (2017). Pediatric emergencies. In C. K. Stone & R. L. Humphries (Eds.), *Current diagnosis and treatment: Emergency medicine* (8th ed., pp. 964–1016). McGraw Hill.

47. Ma, X., Liu, Y., Du, M., Ojo, O., Huang, L., Feng, X., Gao, Q., & Wang, X. (2021). The accuracy of the Pediatric Assessment Triangle in assessing triage of critically ill patients in emergency pediatric department. *International Emergency Nursing, 58,* Article 101041. https://doi.org/10.1016/j.ienj.2021.101041

48. Mahajan, P. (2019). Minor head trauma. In M. Tenenbein, C. G. Macias, G. Q. Sharieff, L. G. Yamamoto, & R. Schafermeyer (Eds.), *Strange and Schafermeyer's pediatric emergency medicine* (5th ed., pp. 31–36). McGraw Hill.

49. Marin, J. R., Rodean, J., Hall, M., Alpern, E. R., Aronson, P. L., Chaudhari, P. P., Cohen, E., Freedman, S. B., Morse, R. B., Peltz, A., Samuels-Kalow, M., Shah, S. S., Simon, H. K., & Neuman, M. I. (2020). Trends in use of advanced imaging in pediatric emergency departments, 2009–2018. *JAMA Pediatrics, 174*(9), Article e202209. https://doi.org/10.1001/jamapediatrics.2020.2209

50. Moore, L., Freire, G., Ben Abdeljelil, A., Berube, M., Tardif, P. A., Gnanvi, E., Stelfox, H. T., Beaudin, M., Carsen, S., Stang, A., Beno, S., Weiss, M., Labrosse, M., Zemek, R., Gagnon, I. J., Beaulieu, E., Berthelot, S., Klassen, T., Turgeon, A. F., . . . Yanchar, N. (2022). Clinical practice guideline recommendations for pediatric injury care: Protocol for a systematic review. *BMJ Open, 12*(4), Article e060054. https://doi.org/10.1136/bmjopen-2021-060054

51. Newgard, C. D., Lin, A., Goldhaber-Fiebert, J. D., Marin, J. R., Smith, M., Cook, J. N. B., Mohr, N. M., Zonfrillo, M. R., Puapong, D., Papa, L., Cloutier, R. L., Burd, R. S., & Pediatric Readiness Study Group. (2022). Association of emergency department pediatric readiness with mortality to 1 year among injured children treated at trauma centers. *JAMA Surgery,* Article e217419. https://doi.org/10.1001/jamasurg.2021.7419

52. Newgard, C. D., Lin, A., Olson, L. M., Cook, J. N. B., Gausche-Hill, M., Kuppermann, N., Goldhaber-Fiebert, J. D., Malveau, S., Smith, M., Dai, M., Nathens, A. B., Glass, N. E., Jenkins, P. C., McConnell, K. J., Remick, K. E., Hewes, H., Mann, N. C., & Pediatric Readiness Study Group. (2021). Evaluation of emergency department pediatric readiness and outcomes among U.S. trauma centers. *JAMA Pediatrics, 175*(9), 947–956. https://doi.org/10.1001/jamapediatrics.2021.1319

53. Odia, O., Meadows, M. E., & Oluwole, I. (2018). Assessing the usefulness of a mock code curriculum. *Pediatrics, 142*(1 Meeting Abstract), Article 590. https://publications.aap.org/pediatrics/article/142/1_MeetingAbstract/590/2909/Assessing-the-Usefulness-of-a-Mock-Code-Curriculum?autologincheck=redirected

54. Ohana, O., Soffer, S., Zimlichman, E., & Klang, E. (2018). Overuse of CT and MRI in paediatric emergency departments. *British Journal of Radiology, 91*(1085). https://doi.org/10.1259%2Fbjr.20170434

55. Owusu-Ansah, S., Moore, B., Shah, M. I., Gross, T., Brown, K., Gausche-Hill, M., Remick, K., Adelgais, K., Rappaport, L., Snow, S., Wright-Johnson, C., Leonard, J. C., Lyng, J., Fallat, M., Committee on Pediatric Emergency Medicine, Section on Emergency Medicine, & EMS Subcommittee, Section on Surgery. (2020). Pediatric readiness in emergency medical services systems. *Pediatrics, 145*(1), Article e20193308. https://doi.org/10.1542/peds.2019-3308

56. Patel, D. R., Yamasaki, A., & Brown, K. (2017). Epidemiology of sports-related musculoskeletal injuries in young athletes in United States. *Translational Pediatrics, 6*(3), 160–166. https://doi.org/10.21037%2Ftp.2017.04.08

57. Pedersen, S. H., Lilja-Cyron, A., Astrand, R., & Juhler, M. (2019). Monitoring and measurement of intracranial pressure in pediatric head trauma. *Frontiers in Neurology, 10,* Article 1376. https://doi.org/10.3389%2Ffneur.2019.01376

58. Pierce, M. C., Kaczor, K., Lorenz, D. J., Bertocci, G., Fingarson, A. K., Makoroff, K., Berger, R. P., Bennett, B., Magana, J., Staley, S., Ramaiah, V., Fortin, K., Currie, M., Herman, B. E., Herr, S., Hymel, K. P., Jenny, C., Sheehan, K., Zuckerbraun, N., . . . Leventhal, J. M. (2021). Validation of a clinical decision rule to predict abuse in young children based on bruising characteristics. *JAMA Network Open, 4*(4), Article e215832. https://doi.org/10.1001/jamanetworkopen.2021.5832

59. Pinkham, L., Botelho, F., Khan, M., Guadagno, E., & Poenaru, D. (2022). Teaching trauma in resource-limited settings: A scoping review of pediatric trauma courses. *World Journal of Surgery, 46*(5), 1209–1219. https://doi.org/10.1007/s00268-021-06419-3

60. Povilavičius, J. (2020). Surgical management of blunt duodenal injuries in children. *International Journal of Pediatric Surgery, 1*(2). Article 1007. http://www.medtextpublications.com/open-access/surgical-management-of-blunt-duodenal-injuries-in-children-540.pdf

61. Remick, K., & Cramer, A. (2020). Hear our voice: Every child, every day—Pediatric emergency care services in the United States. *Clinical Pediatric Emergency Medicine, 21*(2), Article 100781. https://doi.org/10.1016/j.cpem.2020.100781

62. Remick, K., Gaines, B., Ely, M., Richards, R., Fendya, D., & Edgerton, E. A. (2019). Pediatric emergency department readiness among U.S. trauma hospitals. *Journal of Trauma and Acute Care Surgery, 86*(5), 803–809. https://doi.org/10.1097/TA.0000000000002172

63. Rugg, C., Woyke, S., Ausserer, J., Voelckel, W., Paal, P., & Strohle, M. (2021). Analgesia in pediatric trauma patients in physician-staffed Austrian helicopter rescue: A 12-year registry analysis. *Scandinavian Journal of Trauma, Resuscitation and Emergency Medicine, 29*, Article 161. https://doi.org/10.1186/s13049-021-00978-z

64. Selbst, S. M., & Krill, K. (2020). Medical errors in the pediatric emergency department: Don't make these mistakes! *Contemporary Pediatrics, 37*(12), 24–26. https://www.contemporarypediatrics.com/view/medical-errors-in-the-pediatric-emergency-department-don-t-make-these-mistakes

65. Singer, D. (2021). Pediatric hypothermia: An ambiguous issue. *International Journal of Environmental Research and Public Health, 18*(21), Article 11484. https://doi.org/10.3390%2Fijerph182111484

66. Singer, G., Arbeutz, C., Tscgauner, S., Castellani, C., & Till, H. (2021). Trauma in pediatric urology. *Seminars in Pediatric Surgery, 30*(4), Article 151085. https://doi.org/10.1016/j.sempedsurg.2021.151085

67. Spangler, H., Piehl, M., Lane, A., & Robertson, G. (2019). Improving aseptic technique during the treatment of pediatric septic shock: A comparison of 2 rapid fluid delivery methods. *Journal of Infusion Nursing, 42*(1), 23–28. https://doi.org/10.1097/NAN.0000000000000307

68. Spijkerman, R., Bulthuis, L. C., Hesselink, L., Nijdam, T. M., Leenen, L. P., & de Bruin, I. G. (2021). Management of pediatric blunt abdominal trauma in a Dutch level one trauma center. *European Journal of Trauma and Emergency Surgery, 47*(5), 1543–1551. https://doi.org/10.1007/s00068-020-01313-4

69. Srinivasan, V. (2017). *Pediatrics increased intracranial pressure.* Cancer Therapy Advisor. https://www.cancertherapyadvisor.com/home/decision-support-in-medicine/pediatrics/increased-intracranial-pressure/#:~:text=Normal%20ICP%20values%20are%20less,require%20treatment%20in%20most%20instances

70. Stavrinos, D., Pope, C. N., Shen, J., & Schwebel, D. C. (2018). Distracted walking, bicycling, and driving: Systematic review and meta-analysis of mobile technology and youth crash risk. *Child Development, 89*(1), 118–128. https://doi.org/10.1111/cdev.12827

71. Talbot, L. J., & Kenney, B. D. (2017). Clearance of the cervical spine in children. In D. E. Wesson & B. Nauj-Mathuria (Eds.), *Pediatric trauma pathophysiology, diagnosis, and treatment* (2nd ed., pp. 63–73). CRC Press.

72. Tepas, J. J., III, Mollitt, D. L., Talbert, J. L., & Bryant, M. (1987). The Pediatric Trauma Score as a predictor of injury severity in the injured child. *Journal of Pediatric Surgery, 22*(1), 14–18. https://doi.org/10.1016/S0022-3468(87)80006-4

73. Theodorou, C. M., Trappey, A. F., Beyer, C. A., Yamashiro, K. J., Hirose, S., Galante, J. M., Beres, A. L., & Stephenson, J. T. (2021). Quantifying the need for pediatric REBOA: A gap analysis. *Journal of Pediatric Surgery, 56*(8), 1395–1400. https://doi.org/10.1016/j.jpedsurg.2020.09.011

74. Toshniwal, G., Ahmed, Z., & Segnstock, D. (2015). Simulated fluid resuscitation for toddlers and young children: Effect of syringe size and hand fatigue. *Paediatric Anaesthesia, 25*(3), 288–293. https://doi.org/10.1111/pan.12573

75. Trinci, M., Piccolo, C. L., Ferrari, R., Galluzzo, M., Ianniello, S., & Miele, V. (2019). Contrast-enhanced ultrasound (CEUS) in pediatric blunt abdominal trauma. *Journal of Ultrasound, 22*(1), 27–40. https://doi.org/10.1007/s40477-018-0346-x

76. United States Government Accountability Office. (2017). *Pediatric trauma centers: Availability, outcomes, and federal support related to pediatric trauma care.* https://www.gao.gov/assets/690/683914.pdf

77. Waltzman, D., Womack, L. S., Thomas, K. E., & Sarmiento, K. (2020). Trends in emergency department visits for contact sports-related traumatic brain injuries among children—United States, 2001–2018. *Morbidity and Mortality Weekly Report, 69*(27), 870–874. http://doi.org/10.15585/mmwr.mm6927a4

78. Wathen, B., & Recicar, J. (2020). Trauma in the pediatric patient. In K. A. McQuillan & M. B. Flynn Makic (Eds.), *Trauma nursing: From resuscitation through rehabilitation* (5th ed., pp. 677–703). Elsevier.

79. Waunch, A., & Zaky, K. (2020). Pediatric trauma. In V. Sweet & A. Foley (Eds.), *Sheehy's emergency nursing: Principles and practice* (7th ed., pp. 517–536). Elsevier.

80. West, B. A., Rudd, R. A., Sauber-Schatz, E. K., & Ballesteros, M. F. (2021). Unintentional injury deaths in children and youth, 2010–2019. *Journal of Safety Research, 78*, 322–330. https://doi.org/10.1016/j.jsr.2021.07.001

81. Wolters Kluwer. (2021). Glasgow Coma Scale and Pediatric Glasgow Coma Scale. *UpToDate.* Retrieved January 22, 2022, from https://www.uptodate.com/contents/image/print?imageKey=PEDS%2F59662

APPENDIX 13-1
Childhood Development

Physical and Motor Development	Intellectual or Psychosocial Development	Language Development	Pain	Death
Infant Development (Ages 1 Month–1 Year)				
Growth: Period of most rapid growth; infant weight gain, approximately 28.3 g/day; weight doubles by the age of 6 months and triples by the age of 1 year	Trust versus mistrust (Erikson): When physical needs are consistently met, infants learn to trust self and environment; common fears (after the age of 6 months) include separation and strangers	Sensorimotor period: Infants learn by the use of their senses and activities	Infants do experience pain; the degree of pain perceived is unknown	Infants do not understand the meaning of death; the developing sense of separation serves as a basis for a beginning understanding of the meaning of death
Toddler Development (Ages 1-2 Years)				
Growth: Rate significantly slows down, accompanied by a tremendous decrease in appetite; general appearance is potbellied, exaggerated lumbar curve, wide-based gait, and increased mobility	Autonomy versus shame and doubt (Erikson): Increasing independence and self-care activities; expanding the world with which the toddler interacts; need to experience the joy of exploring and exerting some control over body functions and activity while maintaining support of an "anchor" (primary caregiver); common fears include separation, loss of control, altered rituals, and pain	Sensorimotor period: Cognition and language not yet sophisticated enough for children to learn through thought processes and communication	No formal concept of pain related to immature thought process and poorly developed body image; react as intensely to painless procedures as to those that hurt, especially when restrained; intrusive procedures, such as taking a temperature, are distressing; react to pain with physical resistance, aggression, negativism, and regression; rare for toddlers to fake pain; verbal responses concerning pain are unreliable	Understanding of death still limited; belief that loss of significant others is temporary; reinforced by developing sense of object permanence (objects continue to exist even if they cannot be seen); repeated experiences of separations and reunions; magical thinking; belief in TV shows (cartoon characters)

APPENDIX 13-1 Childhood Development

Preschool Development (Ages 3–5 Years)

Growth: Weight gain of 2 kg/year; height gain of 6–8 cm per year; usually are half of adult height by the age of 2 years; general appearance of "baby fat" and protuberant abdomen disappear	Initiative versus guilt (Erikson): Greater autonomy and independence; still intense need for caregivers when under stress; initiate activities, rather than just imitating others; age of discovery, curiosity, and development of social behavior; sense of self as individual; common fears include mutilation, loss of control, death, dark, and ghosts	Preoperational (Piaget): Time of trial-and-error learning; egocentric (experiences from own perspective); understand explanations only in terms of real events or what their senses tell them; no logical or abstract thought; coincidence confused with causation; magical thinking continues; difficulty distinguishing between reality and fantasy; may see illness or injury as punishment for "bad" thoughts or behavior; imaginary friends; fascination with superheroes and monsters	Pain perceived as punishment for bad thoughts or behavior; difficulty understanding that painful procedures help them get well; cannot differentiate between "good" pain (resulting from treatment) and "bad" pain (resulting from injury or illness); react to painful procedures with aggression and verbal reprimands ("I hate you" and "You're mean")	Incomplete understanding of death fosters anxiety because of fear of death; death is seen as an altered state of consciousness in which a person cannot perform normal activities, such as eating or walking; perceive immobility, sleep, and other alterations in consciousness as deathlike states; associate words and phrases ("put to sleep") with death; death is seen as reversible (reinforced by TV and cartoons); unable to perceive inevitability of death as the result of their limited time concept; view death as punishment

School-Age Children (Ages 6–10 Years)

Growth: Relatively latent period	Industry versus inferiority (Erikson): Age of accomplishment, increasing competence, and mastery of new skills; successes contribute to positive self-esteem and a sense of control; need parental support in times of stress (may be unwilling or unable to ask); common fears include separation from friends, loss of control, and physical disability	Concrete operations (Piaget): Beginning of logical thought; deductive reasoning develops; improved concept of time; awareness of possible long-term consequences of illness; more sophisticated understanding of causality; still interpret phrases and idioms at face value	Reaction to pain affected by past experiences, parental response, and the meaning attached to it; better able to localize and describe pain accurately; pain can be exaggerated because of heightened fears of bodily injury, pain, and death	Concept of death more logically based; understand death as the irreversible cessation of life; view death as a tragedy that happens to others, not themselves; when death is an actual threat, may feel responsible for death and experience guilt

(continues)

Adolescent Development (Ages 11–18 Years)

Physical and Motor Development	Intellectual or Psychosocial Development	Language Development	Pain	Death
Growth: For females, growth spurt begins at the age of 9.5 years; for males, growth spurt begins at the age of 10.5 years; at puberty, secondary sex characteristics begin to develop between the ages of 8 and 13 years for females and between the ages of 10 and 14 years for males	Identity versus role confusion (Erikson): Transition from childhood to adulthood; quest for independence often leads to family dissension; major concerns: establishing identity and developing mature sexual orientation; risk-taking behaviors include feeling that nothing bad can happen to them; common fears include changes in appearance or functioning, dependency, and loss of control	Concrete to formal operations (Piaget): Memory fully developed; concept of time well understood; adolescents can project to the future and imagine potential consequences of actions and illnesses; some adolescents do not achieve formal operations	Can locate and quantify pain accurately and thoroughly; often hyperresponsive to pain; react to fear of changes in appearance or function; in general, highly controlled in responding to pain and painful procedures	Understanding of death similar to that of adults; intellectually believe that death can happen to them but avoid realistic thoughts of death; many adolescents defy the possibility of death through reckless behavior, substance abuse, or daring sports activities

Reproduced from Conway, A. (2012). From the start. In *Emergency nursing pediatric course provider manual* (4th ed., pp. 25–49). Emergency Nurses Association.

APPENDIX 13-2
Pediatric Readiness in the Emergency Department

Pediatric Readiness in the Emergency Department

This checklist is based on the American Academy of Pediatrics (AAP), American College of Emergency Physicians (ACEP), and Emergency Nurses Association (ENA) 2018 joint policy statement "Pediatric Readiness in the Emergency Department," which can be found online at:
https://pediatrics.aappublications.org/content/pediatrics/142/5/e20182459.full.pdf.

Use this tool to check if your hospital emergency department (ED) has the most critical components listed in the joint policy statement.

Administration and Coordination of the ED for the Care of Children

☐ Physician Coordinator for Pediatric Emergency Care (PECC)*
- Board certified/eligible in EM or PEM (preferred but not required for resource limited hospitals)
- The Physician PECC is not board certified in EM or PEM but meets the qualifications for credentialing by the hospital as an emergency clinician specialist with special training and experience in the evaluation and management of the critically ill child.

☐ Nurse Coordinator for Pediatric Emergency Care (PECC)*
- CPEN/CEN (*preferred*)
- Other credentials (e.g., CPN, CCRN)

* An Advanced Practice Provider may serve in either of these roles. Please see the guidelines/toolkit for further definition of the role(s).

Physicians, Advanced Practice Providers (APPs), Nurses, and Other ED Healthcare Providers

☐ Healthcare providers who staff the ED have periodic pediatric-specific competency evaluations for children of all ages. Areas of pediatric competencies include any/all of the following:
- Assessment and treatment (e.g., triage)
- Medication administration
- Device/equipment safety
- Critical procedures
- Resuscitation
- Trauma resuscitation and stabilization
- Disaster drills that include children
- Patient- and family-centered care
- Team training and effective communication

Guidelines for QI/PI in the ED

☐ The QI/PI plan includes pediatric-specific indicators
- Data are collected and analyzed
- System changes are implemented based on performance
- System performance is monitored over time

Please see the guidelines/toolkit for additional details.

ED Policies, Procedures, and Protocols

Policies, procedures, and protocols for the emergency care of children. *These policies may be integrated into overall ED policies as long as pediatric-specific issues are addressed.*

☐ Illness and injury triage
☐ Pediatric patient assessment and reassessment
☐ Identification and notification of the responsible provider of abnormal pediatric vital signs
☐ Immunization assessment and management of the under-immunized patient
☐ Sedation and analgesia, for procedures including medical imaging
☐ Consent, including when parent or legal guardian is not immediately available
☐ Social and behavioral health issues
☐ Physical or chemical restraint of patients
☐ Child maltreatment reporting and assessment
☐ Death of the child in the ED
☐ Do not resuscitate (DNR) orders
☐ Children with special health care needs
☐ Family and guardian presence during all aspects of emergency care, including resuscitation
☐ Patient, family, guardian, and caregiver education
☐ Discharge planning and instruction
☐ Bereavement counseling
☐ Communication with the patient's medical home or primary care provider as needed.
☐ Telehealth and telecommunications

All-Hazard Disaster Preparedness

The written all-hazard disaster-preparedness plan addresses pediatric-specific needs within the core domains including:

☐ Medications, vaccines, equipment, supplies and trained providers for children in disasters
☐ Pediatric surge capacity for injured and non-injured children
☐ Decontamination, isolation, and quarantine of families and children of all ages
☐ Minimization of parent-child separation
☐ Tracking and reunification for children and families
☐ Access to specific behavioral health therapies and social services for children
☐ Disaster drills include a pediatric mass casualty incident at least every two years
☐ Care of children with special health care needs

Evidence-Based Guidelines

☐ Evidence-based clinical pathways, order sets or decision support available to providers in real time

Inter-facility Transfers

☐ Written pediatric inter-facility transfer agreements

☐ Written pediatric inter-facility transfer guidelines. These may include:
- Criteria for transfers (e.g., specialty services)
- Criteria for selection of appropriate transport service
- Process for initiation of transfer
- Plan for transfer of patient information
- Integration of family-centered care
- Integration of telehealth/telecommunications

Guidelines for Improving Pediatric Patient Safety

Pediatric patient and medication safety needs are addressed in the following ways:

☐ Children are weighed in kilograms only
☐ Weights are recorded in kilograms only
☐ For children who require emergency stabilization, a standard method for estimating weight in kilograms is used (e.g., a length-based system)
☐ Infants and children have a full set of vital signs recorded
- A full set of vital signs includes temperature, heart rate, respiratory rate, pulse oximetry, blood pressure, pain, and mental status when indicated in the medical record

☐ CO^2 monitoring for children of all ages
☐ Process for safe medication delivery that includes:
- Prescribing
- Administration
- Disposal

☐ Pre-calculated drug dosing and formulation guides
☐ 24/7 access to interpreter services in the ED
☐ Timely tracking and reporting of patient safety events

Guidelines for ED Support Services

☐ Medical imaging capabilities and protocols address age- or weight-appropriate dose reductions for children

☐ All efforts made to transfer completed images when a patient is transferred from one facility to another

☐ Collaboration with radiology, laboratory and other ED support services to ensure the needs of children in the community are met

Please see the guidelines/toolkit for additional details

Guidelines for Medication, Equipment and Supplies

Pediatric equipment, supplies, and medications are appropriate for children of all ages and sizes (see list below), and are easily accessible, clearly labeled, and logically organized.

☐ ED staff is educated on the location of all items
☐ Daily method in place to verify the proper location and function of pediatric equipment and supplies
☐ Medication chart, length-based tape, medical software, or other systems is readily available to ensure proper sizing of resuscitation equipment and proper dosing of medications
☐ Standardized chart or tool used to estimate weight in kilograms if resuscitation precludes the use of a weight scale (e.g., length-based tape)

Medications

☐ Analgesics (oral, intranasal, and parenteral)
☐ Anesthetics (eutectic mixture of local anesthetics; lidocaine 2.5% and prilocaine 2.5%; lidocaine, epinephrine, and tetracaine; and LMX 4 [4% lidocaine])
☐ Anticonvulsants (benzodiazepines, levetiracetam, valproate, carbamazepine, fosphenytoin, and phenobarbital)
☐ Antidotes (common antidotes should be accessible to the ED, e.g., naloxone)
☐ Antipyretics (acetaminophen and ibuprofen)
☐ Antiemetics (ondansetron and prochlorperazine)
☐ Antihypertensives (labetalol, nicardipine, and sodium nitroprusside)
☐ Antimicrobials (parenteral and oral)
☐ Antipsychotics (olanzapine and haloperidol)
☐ Benzodiazepines (midazolam and lorazepam)
☐ Bronchodilators
☐ Calcium chloride and/or calcium gluconate
☐ Corticosteroids (dexamethasone, methylprednisolone, and hydrocortisone)
☐ Cardiac medications (adenosine, amiodarone, atropine, procainamide, and lidocaine)
☐ Hypoglycemic interventions (dextrose, oral glucose)
☐ Diphenhydramine
☐ Epinephrine (1mg/mL [1M] and 0.1 mg/mL [IV] solutions)
☐ Furosemide
☐ Glucagon
☐ Insulin
☐ Magnesium sulfate
☐ Intracranial hypertension medications (mannitol, 3% hypertonic saline)
☐ Neuromuscular blockers (rocuronium and succinylcholine)
☐ Sucrose solutions for pain control in infants
☐ Sedation medications (midazolam, etomidate and ketamine)
☐ Sodium bicarbonate (4.2%)
☐ Vasopressor agents (dopamine, epinephrine and norepinephrine)
☐ Vaccines (tetanus)

APPENDIX 13-2 Pediatric Readiness in the Emergency Department

Equipment/Supplies: General Equipment

- ☐ Patient warming device (infant warmer)
- ☐ IV blood and/or fluid warmer
- ☐ Restraint device
- ☐ Weight scale, in kilograms only (no opportunity to weigh or report in pounds), for infants and children
- ☐ Tool or chart that relies on weight (kilograms) used to assist physicians and nurses in determining equipment size and correct drug dosing (by weight and total volume)
- ☐ Pain scale assessment tools that are appropriate for age
- ☐ Rigid boards for use in CPR
- ☐ Pediatric-specific AED pads

Equipment/Supplies: Vascular Access

Arm boards
- ☐ infant
- ☐ child

☐ Atomizer for intranasal administration of medication

Catheter-over-the-needle device
- ☐ 22 gauge
- ☐ 24 gauge

Intraosseous needles or device
- ☐ pediatric
- ☐ IV administration sets with calibrated chambers and extension tubing and/or infusion devices with the ability to regulate the rate and volume of infusate (including low volumes)

IV solutions
- ☐ Normal saline
- ☐ Dextrose 5% in 0.45% normal saline
- ☐ Lactated Ringer's solution
- ☐ Dextrose 10% in water

Equipment/Supplies: Fracture-Management Devices

Extremity splints (including femur splints)
- ☐ pediatric

Cervical Collar
- ☐ infant
- ☐ child

Equipment/Supplies: Monitoring Equipment

Blood pressure cuffs
- ☐ neonatal
- ☐ infant
- ☐ child

- ☐ Doppler ultrasonography devices
- ☐ ECG monitor and/or defibrillator with pediatric and adult capabilities, including pediatric-sized pads and/or paddles
- ☐ Pulse oximeter with pediatric and adult probes
- ☐ Continuous end-tidal CO2 monitoring

Equipment/Supplies: Respiratory

Endotracheal Tubes
- ☐ uncuffed 2.5 mm
- ☐ uncuffed 3.0 mm
- ☐ cuffed or uncuffed 3.5 mm
- ☐ cuffed or uncuffed 4.0 mm
- ☐ cuffed or uncuffed 4.5 mm
- ☐ cuffed or uncuffed 5.0 mm
- ☐ cuffed or uncuffed 5.5 mm
- ☐ cuffed 6.0 mm

Feeding Tubes
- ☐ 5F
- ☐ 8F

Laryngoscope Blades
- ☐ straight: 0
- ☐ straight: 1
- ☐ straight: 2
- ☐ curved: 2

Magill Forceps
- ☐ pediatric

Nasopharyngeal Airways
- ☐ infant
- ☐ child

Oropharyngeal Airways
- ☐ size 0
- ☐ size 1
- ☐ size 2
- ☐ size 3

Stylets for endotracheal tubes
- ☐ pediatric
- ☐ infant

Suction Catheters
- ☐ infant (6-8F)
- ☐ child (10-12F)

Rigid Suction Device
- ☐ pediatric

Bag-mask device, self-inflating
- ☐ infant (250 ml)
- ☐ child (450-500 ml)

Non-rebreather masks
- ☐ infant
- ☐ child

Clear Oxygen masks
- ☐ infant
- ☐ child

Masks to fit bag-mask device adaptor
- ☐ neonatal
- ☐ infant
- ☐ child

Nasal cannula
- ☐ infant
- ☐ child

Gastric tubes
- ☐ infant (8F)
- ☐ child (10F)

Equipment/Supplies: Specialized Pediatric Trays or Kits

Difficult airway supplies and/or kit

Contents to be based on pediatric patients served at the hospital and may include some or all of the following:
- ☐ supraglottic airways of all sizes
- ☐ needle cricothyrotomy supplies
- ☐ surgical cricothyrotomy kit
- ☐ video laryngoscopy

Newborn delivery kit (including equipment for initial resuscitation of a newborn infant)
- ☐ umbilical clamp
- ☐ scissors
- ☐ bulb syringe
- ☐ towel

Urinary catheterization kits and urinary (indwelling) catheters
- ☐ infant
- ☐ child

Additional Recommendations for High-Volume EDs (>10,000 Pediatric Patient Visits per Year)	
☐ Alprostadil (prostaglandin E1) <u>Central venous catheters</u> ☐ 4.0F ☐ 5.0F ☐ 6.0F ☐ 7.0F <u>Chest tubes</u> ☐ infant (8–12F catheter) ☐ child (14–22F catheter) ☐ adult (24–40F catheter) OR pigtail catheter kit (8.5–14F catheter) ☐ Hypothermia thermometer ☐ Inotropic agents (e.g., digoxin and milrinone) <u>Laryngoscope blade</u> ☐ size 00 <u>Lumbar puncture tray, spinal needles</u> ☐ infant ☐ child	<u>Noninvasive ventilation</u> ☐ continuous positive airway pressure OR high-flow nasal cannula <u>Self-inflating bag-mask device</u> ☐ pediatric ☐ Tube thoracostomy tray <u>Tracheostomy tubes</u> ☐ size 0 ☐ size 1 ☐ size 2 ☐ size 3 ☐ size 4 ☐ size 5 ☐ size 6 <u>Umbilical vein catheters</u> ☐ 3.5F ☐ 5.0F ☐ Video laryngoscopy

Revised: April 5, 2021

Produced by the AAP, ACEP, ENA and the EMSC Innovation and Improvement Center

American Academy of Pediatrics — DEDICATED TO THE HEALTH OF ALL CHILDREN

American College of Emergency Physicians — ADVANCING EMERGENCY CARE

ENA — EMERGENCY NURSES ASSOCIATION

EIIC — Emergency Medical Services for Children Innovation and Improvement Center

Courtesy of AACP, ACEP, ENA, & EMSC Innovation and Improvement Center. (2021). Pediatric readiness in the emergency department. https://media.emscimprovement.center/documents/NPRP_Checklist_Final_Apr2021_LEqqleE.pdf

CHAPTER 14

The Obese Trauma Patient

Nycole D. Oliver, DNP, APRN, RN, FNP-C, ACNP-AG, CEN, FAEN

OBJECTIVES

Upon completion of this chapter, the learner will be able to:
1. Describe mechanisms of injury associated with the obese trauma patient.
2. Describe pathophysiologic changes as a basis for assessment of the obese trauma patient.
3. Demonstrate the nursing assessment of the obese trauma patient.
4. Plan appropriate interventions for the obese trauma patient.
5. Evaluate the effectiveness of nursing interventions for the obese trauma patient.

Introduction

Obesity is a condition increasing in prevalence and has been shown to increase morbidity and mortality in trauma patients.[24] The terms "obese" and "bariatric" are often used interchangeably, although "bariatric" has a more specific definition: It comes from the ancient Greek word *baros*, meaning "weight,"[14] and describes the field of medicine that offers research on, prevention of, and treatment for obesity. *Bariatric* is defined as "having to do with the causes, prevention, and treatment of obesity." However, more specific definitions are necessary to identify and classify patients and discuss trauma care for this unique patient population.

The World Health Organization (WHO) uses body mass index (BMI) to define the degree to which a person is considered overweight.[59] BMI is calculated by dividing a person's weight in kilograms by the individual's height in meters squared. The WHO has developed the following classifications for obesity[59]:

- Underweight: BMI less than 18.5 kg/m^2
- Normal weight: BMI between 18.5 kg/m^2 and 24.9 kg/m^2
- Overweight (pre-obese): BMI between 25 kg/m^2 and 29.9 kg/m^2
- Obese: BMI of 30 kg/m^2 or greater

Obesity is frequently subdivided into categories:

- Class 1: BMI of 30 to < 35
- Class 2: BMI of 35 to < 40
- Class 3: BMI of 40 or higher (sometimes categorized as "severe" obesity)[10]

When a patient reaches a BMI of 40 kg/m² or greater, the individual is considered morbidly obese. In children and teens, age- and gender-specific tables are used that take into account developmental changes to determine BMI and degree of obesity.[27] An obese patient's health is often significantly impacted by diseases such as hypertension, hyperlipidemia, obstructive sleep apnea, diabetes mellitus, chronic kidney disease, and others; as BMI increases, the prevalence of these disorders also tends to increase.[1,45,49] This chapter covers special considerations in the care of the trauma patient with obesity, including epidemiology, pathophysiology, and mechanisms of injury, as well as nursing care considerations in this special population.

Epidemiology

The rates of obesity are increasing around the world, tripling in prevalence between 1975 and 2016.[59] In 2016, more than 650 million adults and 39 million children were classified as obese.[59] **Figure 14-1** shows the increase over time in levels of obesity among selected countries in North America, Europe, and Asia.[45] Australia shows similar growth in obesity rates: in 2017–2018, around 2 in 3 (67%) Australians aged 18 and older, and 1 in 4 (25%) children and adolescents aged 5–17 years, were overweight or obese.[3,44]

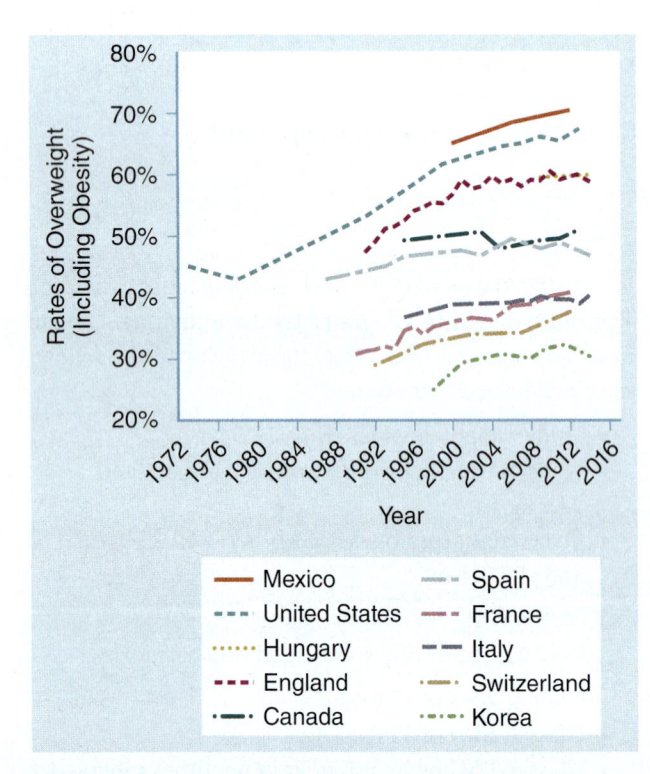

Figure 14-1 *World obesity.*

Reproduced from Organisation for Economic and Co-operative Development. (2017). *Obesity update 2017*. https://www.oecd.org/els/health-systems/Obesity-Update-2017.pdf

In keeping with this trend, increasing numbers of obese trauma patients are presenting to the emergency department for care. Both physicians and nurses report challenges in the assessment and care of this group, including difficulties with measuring vital signs, diagnostic testing, venipuncture, intravenous (IV) cannulation, patient positioning and mobilization, urinary catheterization, airway management, resuscitative measures, and other general procedures.[45,49] Difficulty finding appropriately sized equipment is common.[49] Healthcare provider education regarding this population can assist the trauma nurse to be better prepared to care for these patients.

Mechanisms of Injury and Biomechanics

Research related to patterns and severity of injury in obese patients shows mixed data over the past few decades. BMI has been identified as an independent risk factor for mortality and other adverse outcomes following blunt trauma, such as infectious complications, acute respiratory distress syndrome, hematologic complications, and decubitus ulcers.[17,24] Bariatric patients who experience orthopedic trauma have higher rates of complications and hospitalization compared with individuals of normal weight.[24] Further evidence shows that bariatric patients have a greater risk of pulmonary complications and multiorgan failure with increased mortality after severe blunt trauma, which is attributable not to obesity alone but also to comorbidities such as diabetes.[24,48] Several factors are associated with higher mortality rates for patients with obesity, including greater incidence of specific injuries, improper fit of safety equipment or inability to use it at all, not following safety practices, and comorbidities.[24,34]

Notably, studies have found increased mortality for bariatric patients involved in frontal motor vehicle collisions (MVCs).[24] Specific injuries more common in obese patients include spinal, upper torso, and upper and lower extremity fractures.[24] Obese patients may initially sustain fewer injuries, but their injuries tend to be more severe. These patients have longer hospital and intensive care unit lengths of stay, with lower survival rates compared with those of patients who are of a normal weight.[16,24] Morbidly obese drivers in severe MVCs have an increased mortality rate; one study demonstrated a 52% greater risk of mortality compared with drivers of a normal weight and an 84% increase in mortality in motorists with morbid obesity who did not use protective equipment.[16,34]

These poor outcomes among morbidly obese drivers and passengers may be related to decreased use of seat belts. In one of the largest studies to date, normal-weight drivers were 67% more likely to wear seat belts than morbidly obese drivers.[12] If obese persons do wear a seat belt, they are at an increased risk to wear it inappropriately, suggesting that seat belts may not be designed with the obese/morbidly obese in mind.[12]

Among individuals of all weights, those who wear seat belts experience fewer injuries than those who do not.[18]

Risk for, and response to, injury are influenced by comorbid conditions and factors associated with obesity, such as sleep apnea, obesity hypoventilation syndrome, decreased endurance and reserve, diabetes, and gastroesophageal reflux disease. For example, drivers with untreated sleep apnea are often drowsy while driving, translating into a 243% higher risk for vehicular collisions as compared with drivers without sleep apnea.[12,25,46] These obesity-related comorbidities result in considerable challenges to management of the patient during trauma, including increased rates of infection and thrombosis, inadequate wound healing, and problems with intubation and ventilation.[46]

Pathophysiologic Differences in the Trauma Patient with Obesity

Patients with a BMI greater than 30 kg/m² can have functional and physiologic differences relative to normal-weight patients that may contribute to poorer outcomes and delayed functional recovery after a traumatic injury.[45] Increased BMI has also been associated with hypertension, renal insufficiency, diabetes, and cardiovascular disease, which are factors known to complicate trauma care and increase risk of poor outcomes. These factors are further explained throughout the chapter.[12,45,46]

Airway changes in obese patients can include a larger neck circumference, increased chin and neck tissue, and extra parapharyngeal tissue, which can limit the ability to open the patient's mouth, decrease neck mobility, and increase upper airway resistance.[45] Increased adipose tissue in the thoracic cage can decrease chest wall compliance.[45]

Figure 14-2 shows the difference between the airway of a bariatric patient and a normal-weight patient.[30] The airway of a patient of normal weight is often maintained best in a supine position; for the obese patient, this may not be the case. In the supine position, the chest and diaphragm can become obstructed because of excess abdominal mass, hindering effective ventilation.[45] These differences can lead to airway management and intubation difficulties; such challenges have also been attributed to increased neck circumference with decreased mobility, shorter neck, and increased accumulation of fat in the oral cavity and cheeks of bariatric patients.[45,48]

Obesity can have a significant effect on the respiratory system.[45,49] In a patient with excessive weight, expiratory reserve volume is reduced, which in turn reduces the functional residual capacity. Closure of the smaller airways leads to collapsed alveoli and a chronic state of

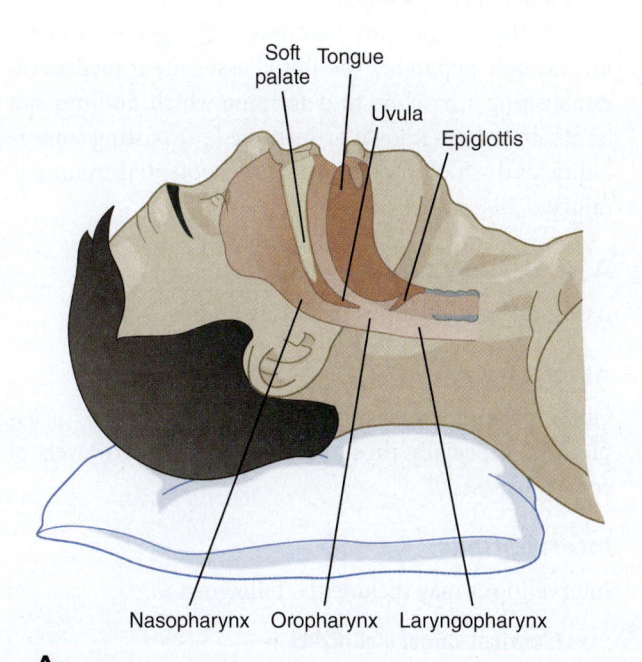

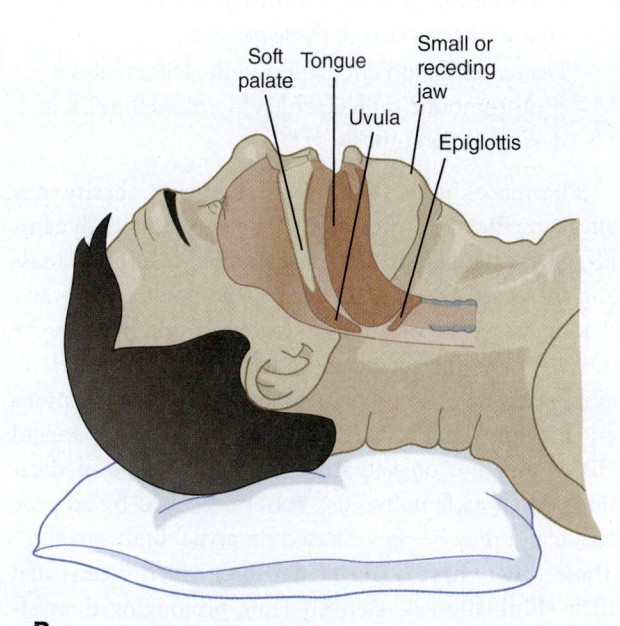

Figure 14-2 A. *Airway of a normal-body-weight patient.* **B.** *Airway of an obese patient.*

microatelectasis in the bases of the lungs, resulting in ineffective gas exchange.[45,48,49] Dyspnea at rest, a higher respiratory rate, lower tidal volumes, and increased minute ventilation have also been identified in obese individuals.[45] It is vital to anticipate difficulty with bag-mask ventilations caused by pathophysiological changes of the obese patient.[48]

Obese patients have increased abdominal and visceral adipose tissue, which is associated with a multitude of comorbid conditions, including the following[12,37,46,49]:

- Respiratory compromise and obesity hypoventilation syndrome.
- Hypertension and cardiovascular disease.
- Gastroesophageal reflux disease.
- Depression.
- Diabetes mellitus and hyperglycemia.
- Idiopathic intracranial hypertension (formerly called pseudotumor cerebri).
- Renal insufficiency.
- Deep vein thrombosis and pulmonary embolism.
- Delayed venous return resulting from increased intra-abdominal pressure creates a high risk for deep vein thrombosis and pulmonary embolus in the bariatric patient.
- Compromise from injury and/or decreased mobility due to lower extremity injury further increases the risk.
- The main pathophysiological background of the elevated thrombotic risk in the obese patient is represented by inflammation; C-reactive protein, a sensitive marker of inflammation, may represent the common pathway for the risk of arterial and venous thrombosis in these patients.
- Decreased blood circulation in the legs creates a prothrombotic milieu, which increases the risk of deep vein thrombosis.[12,31,39]

Pharmacokinetic factors associated with obesity may affect medication metabolism and pharmacodynamics. Obese patients have both increased lean body mass and increased fat mass. Muscle tissue holds more water than fat tissue; medications that are hydrophilic (dissolve in water) are distributed more to lean tissue and less to adipose tissue.[13,45,49] In general, hydrophilic medications (such as morphine) are dosed based on ideal body weight (IBW) and not on actual weight.[45] Lipophilic medications (such as fentanyl) are better absorbed by adipose tissue and may be dosed based on actual body weight.[45] These agents have a longer half-life, which means that their elimination is relatively slow, prolonging their effects. Renal function is also a factor in medication clearance, especially in patients with comorbidities of diabetes or hypertension.[12,45,49] Consider consultation with a clinical pharmacist to review appropriate drug dosing in bariatric patients.

In many patients, obesity causes alterations in joint cartilage and bone metabolism. A BMI greater than 30 kg/m^2 is linked to an increase in musculoskeletal injuries, leading to early development of osteoarthritic disorders.[37] **Table 14-1** outlines both physiologic changes seen in obesity and signs and symptoms related to such changes.

Nursing Care of the Obese Trauma Patient

Nursing care of the bariatric trauma patient begins with proper preparation and is followed by the primary survey.

Preparation

It is important to be prepared with equipment in a variety of appropriate sizes, such as stretchers, blood pressure cuffs, and cervical spine collars, before the trauma patient's arrival. Education regarding the special considerations of caring for obese patients can also serve as a foundation for the trauma team to provide competent, safe, and sensitive trauma care.

Primary Survey and Resuscitative Measures

Obese patients with lower BMI levels may be able to adequately compensate with little noticeable difference in their assessment parameters. As the BMI level increases, expect physiologic and functional changes to become increasingly apparent. The initial assessment focuses on establishing a baseline to determine which findings can be attributed to a known or suspected preexisting comorbidity, and which may be related to potential traumatic injury.

A: Alertness and Airway

Assess and consider needed interventions.

Assessment

Obese patients are at high risk for gastric reflux or aspiration, especially those patients with altered levels of consciousness.[12,46]

Interventions

Interventions may include the following:

- Cervical spinal stabilization
  - Blanket or towel rolls, wedges, and tape can be used to assist stabilization.[36] Commercially

TABLE 14-1 Pathophysiologic Changes Related to Obesity and Morbid Obesity

System	Alterations	Related Disorder	Signs and Symptoms Affecting Trauma Patients
Ventilatory	Narrowed airway, larger tongue, relaxed pharyngeal muscle Respiratory insufficiency due to chest-wall weight, decreased chest-wall compliance, and increased airway resistance[12,16,17,24,25,36,37,45,46,48,49]	Increased adipose tissue and/or larger neck circumference Increased work of breathing	Oxygen saturation likely lower in supine position Abnormal airway sounds, such as snoring in supine position Dyspnea with very mild exertion, positional dyspnea Hypoxia, hypercapnia, hypoxemia Daytime drowsiness common in undiagnosed sleep apnea; may contribute to MVCs
Cardiovascular	Ventricular remodeling[8,12,15,16,17,23,24,31,32,37,45,48,52] › Left ventricle hypertrophy and decreased compliance › Increased cardiac output › Diastolic dysfunction	Hypertension Increased left ventricular load	Muffled heart sounds
	Accelerated rate of coronary atherosclerosis Increased IAP thought to contribute to development of hypertension as well as lower extremity circulatory disorder Venous insufficiency Elevated blood viscosity due to increased leptin	Right- and left- sided heart failure Pulmonary hypertension Varicose veins Venous stasis Pulmonary embolism	Compensatory tachycardia ECG changes: › PR, QRS, and QT intervals prolonged › ST depression, or flattening of T waves › Low QRS voltage › Arrhythmias › Higher incidence of atrial fibrillation › Premature ventricular contractions common Edema in the lower extremities
	Increased circulatory volume	Obesity	Lymphedema and hypertension
Endocrine	Elevated insulin levels and resistance to endogenous insulin, cholesterol production	Metabolic syndrome Type 2 diabetes Dyslipidemia Polycystic ovarian syndrome	Elevated blood glucose levels

(continues)

TABLE 14-1 Pathophysiologic Changes Related to Obesity and Morbid Obesity (continued)

System	Alterations	Related Disorder	Signs and Symptoms Affecting Trauma Patients
Musculoskeletal	Weight-bearing joint deterioration due to excess weight[43,55] Compression of spinal vertebrae due to weight load	Osteoarthritis Low back pain	Degenerative symptoms: › Joint pain, particularly in the lower hips, knees, and ankles › Limited range of motion of extremities › Limited flexibility › Increased incidence of joint replacement Back pain, neurologic symptoms
	Increase in uric acid Gait and balance changes related to weight distribution with increased BMI	Gout	Pain, swelling, and redness of affected area Decreased mobility
Gastrointestinal	Increased IAP, inability to lower esophageal sphincter to withstand this pressure[1,12,42,49]	Gastroesophageal reflux	Reports of reflux from awake patient or potential aspiration symptoms in altered consciousness
	Increased liver size due to fatty deposits	Nonalcoholic fatty liver disease	Elevated liver function studies, often asymptomatic
	Abdominal muscle-wall weakness, increased IAP	Hernias	Pain, bulging on palpation of abdomen
Genitourinary	Insulin resistance and IAP causation[1,39,49]	Renal dysfunction	Elevated BUN and creatinine levels
	Increased urinary bladder pressure related to IAP	Urinary stress incontinence	Urinary urgency, leakage Rhabdomyolysis
Neurologic	Increased intracranial pressure due to IAH[12,24,47]	Idiopathic intracranial hypertension (pseudotumor cerebri)	Headaches, visual disturbances
Skin	Venous stasis in lower extremities[1,24,28]	Cellulitis	Early breakdown of skin in moist areas and areas of pressure points, including occiput
	Excess skin accumulation	Intertrigo under skin folds	
Psychological	Psychological disturbances[37,49]	Depression Low self-esteem Social isolation	

MVCs = motor vehicle collisions; IAP = intra-abdominal pressure; ECG = electrocardiogram; BUN = blood urea nitrogen; BMI = body mass index; IAH = intra-abdominal hypertension.

available stabilization devices may not fit the obese patient with a shorter, thicker neck.
- Anticipate the need for additional personnel when transferring, repositioning, or turning the patient.
• Airway
  - Use a two-handed bilateral jaw-thrust maneuver with airway adjuncts for optimal airway control.[45,55]
  - Anticipate the need for early intubation if airway compromise is a risk.
  - Anticipate difficulties with intubation.[48]
  - The reverse Trendelenburg position will benefit the patient in terms of both airway maintenance and work of breathing.[16,24,49]
• Place the patient in a position with the head elevated during intubation, with the external auditory canal parallel with the sternal notch to enable better visualization of pharyngeal landmarks.[24,45] This position is known as the *ramped* position (**Figure 14-3**).[1,7,9,16,45] Blankets can be used to elevate the head and torso into this position.
• Awake intubation using fiber-optic technology may be preferable because it preserves pharyngeal and laryngeal muscle tone.[16,36] Fiber-optic visualization also provides a superior view of the glottis in many patients.[53]
• Selection of the provider with the most experience in difficult airway management is recommended.[16,45]

Drug-Assisted Intubation

Drug-assisted intubation medication dosage for patients remains controversial.

• Evidence at this time supports using lean body weight (LBW) when determining the dose for induction agents, IBW for rocuronium and other nondepolarizing agents, and total body weight (TBW) for succinylcholine.[45,60] **Table 14-2** provides information that can be used to rapidly estimate medication dosages in emergent situations.[9]
• Monitor the patient closely for desaturation. Increased oxygen consumption leads to rapid desaturation in the obese patient; a patient with a higher BMI may desaturate in as little time as 1 minute.[24]
• Placing the patient in reverse Trendelenburg position to 25 degrees prolongs the safe apnea time, as does preoxygenation with a bag-mask device.[16,24,49]

If intubation is unsuccessful, a supraglottic device such as the laryngeal mask airway or multilumen airway is acceptable for use in the bariatric patient.[7,16,60] Other useful devices include an endotracheal tube introducer.

TABLE 14-2 Information for Rapidly Estimating Medication Dosages to Facilitate Intubation

Height (in.)	Height (cm)	IBW[a] (kg)	Approximate LBW in Class III Obesity[b] (kg)
Female			
60	152	46	52
65	165	57	60
70	178	68	70
75	191	80	80
Male			
60	152	50	63
65	165	62	73
70	178	76	85
75	191	89	97
80	203	103	112

IBW = ideal body weight; LBW = lean body weight; BMI = body mass index; TBW = total body weight.

[a] IBW male = 50 kg + (2.3 kg × height in inches over 5 feet); IBW female = 45.5 kg + (2.3 kg × height in inches over 5 feet). Full metric formula: IBW male = × (height in meters)^2; IBW female = 22 × (height in meters − 10 cm)^2.

[b] Approximate LBW in class III obesity (BMI 40–45 kg/m^2) for dosing emergency medications; LBW estimate (kg) = (9,270 × TBW)/(A + B × BMI), where A and B are 6,680 and 216, respectively, for males and 8,780 and 244, respectively, for females.

Data from Brown, C. A. (2021). Emergency airway management in the morbidly obese patient. *UpToDate*. Retrieved May 1, 2022, from https://www.uptodate.com/contents/emergency-airway-management-in-the-morbidly-obese-patient

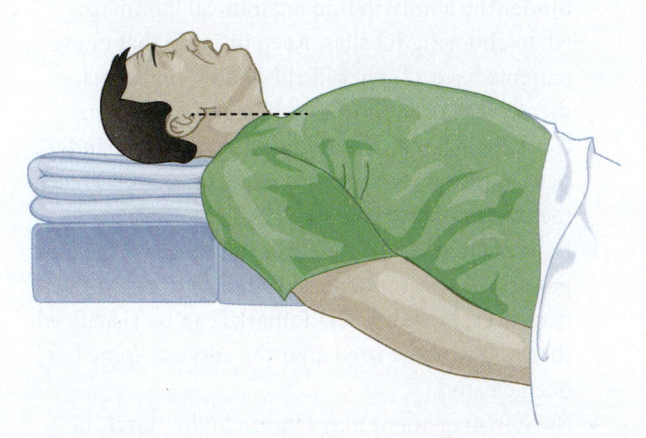

Figure 14-3 *Patient in ramped position for better visualization with intubation.*

Obtaining tracheal access may be necessary in patients when intubation fails. In such a case, surgical cricothyrotomy is the technique of choice.[43] Use of an endotracheal tube is recommended because the standard cricothyrotomy tube may be too short.[53] Tracheostomy is less desirable in this patient population because of increased complications and procedure difficulty.[53]

B: Breathing and Ventilation

Assess the patient and consider needed interventions.

Assessment

Assess as follows:

- Inspect for the following:
  - Increased work of breathing, especially when in a supine position. Weakened respiratory muscles may quickly lead to fatigue and respiratory failure.
  - Monitor level of consciousness: Lethargy, mental status changes, and restlessness may indicate hypoxia.
  - The obese patient has less chest wall mobility; assessing for equal chest rise and fall as well as symmetry may be challenging.[23]
  - Subcutaneous emphysema over the chest wall is significant; auscultation of breath sounds and percussion may not be as useful in detecting chest injuries because of the effects of subcutaneous tissue in muffling accurate sound transmission from the lungs.[41]
- Auscultate for the following:
  - Breath sounds can be muffled through additional soft tissue.[41]
  - Displace skin folds over the lung area to auscultate lung sounds.

Interventions

Interventions include the following:

- As soon as the cervical spine is cleared, unless otherwise contraindicated, place the patient in an upright position to improve access and chest excursion.
  - Placing the patient in a lateral left position or elevating the head of the bed in reverse Trendelenburg position at 25 degrees may help the patient with adequate ventilation.[16,24,49]
- Anticipate potential use of bilevel positive airway pressure (BiPAP).
  - This can be a useful intervention prior to intubation to provide adequate ventilation, especially in patients with a history of sleep apnea.[60]
  - BiPAP can be useful in patients with flail chest injury or any other blunt chest trauma.[11]
- Prior to application, ensure that the patient has an intact swallow function, gag reflex, and cough mechanism.[5]
- Use two- to three-person bag-mask ventilation with oropharyngeal or nasopharyngeal airways in place, unless contraindicated, if manual ventilation is required.[7]

C: Circulation and Control of Hemorrhage

Assess and consider needed interventions.

Assessment

Heart sounds may be muffled in the obese patient, and pulses may be difficult to palpate through adipose tissue. Positioning the patient on the left side (unless contraindicated) and listening over the left lateral chest wall may improve auscultation.[23]

Interventions

Interventions include the following:

- Volume resuscitation should be based on IBW. Monitor the volume of fluid resuscitation closely to avoid overload—some obese patients with cardiac comorbidities may not tolerate aggressive fluid administration.[35]
- Conversely, obese patients have a larger circulating fluid volume; this may make fluid resuscitation difficult, possibly resulting in patients receiving insufficient fluid resuscitation during trauma.[23]
- Use guided ultrasound for catheter placement if there is difficulty obtaining IV access.[1,16,45,49]
- Consider the use of intraosseous (IO) access devices. Move directly to the use of an intraosseous device if there is difficulty in obtaining IV access. Consider that extra adipose tissue over IO sites may hinder the ability to find anatomical landmarks when choosing IO sites. Keep in mind that obese patients have a higher likelihood of joint replacement, which can limit the choice of access sites. Consider a larger size IO needle if needed. Underpenetration is a common complication of IO placement with obese patients.[48]
- External jugular cannulation attempts may be impaired because of increased adipose tissue in the neck area; however, if landmarks can be visualized, these sites can be used after the cervical spine has been cleared.
- Burn management may require higher levels of fluid replacement, and patients with burn injuries will be at high risk of infection.[12]

Resuscitative Measures

Accuracy of vital signs can be a problematic issue with an obese patient.

F: Full Set of Vital Signs

Obtaining an accurate blood pressure reading in an obese patient can be a challenge. The following recommendations include those resulting from research using automated blood pressure devices:

- Use an appropriately sized cuff.
- A cuff that is too small can produce a false high pressure reading.[2]
- The forearm can be used for blood pressure measurement; however, results may be higher than pressures taken in the upper arm.[2]
- Obtaining the correct cuff size for the forearm is essential, and the circumference of the forearm should be measured midway between the elbow and wrist; remember to keep placement of the cuff consistent for accurate trending of blood pressures.
- Center the cuff between the elbow and the wrist, with the arm supported at the level of the heart. Accurate blood pressure may be difficult to obtain with obese patients. Arterial line readings may be necessary to determine responsiveness to fluid resuscitation measures.[2,48]

Conduct palpation of anatomic landmarks before performing an electrocardiogram (ECG). Placement of ECG leads in obese patients may be difficult, but these leads should be placed under the breast-area tissue when possible.[26] If the patient goes to the operating room, the anesthesia provider may remove all chest leads for surgical preparation and instead place them on the shoulders and left leg. Greater chest circumference will cause lead placement that is wider than on a standard-sized person; however, the landmarks of the midclavicular and midaxillary lines are the same for all patients.

G: Get Monitoring Devices and Give Comfort

Address the L, M, N, O, and P elements:

- L: Laboratory studies
  - Additional laboratory studies related to comorbid conditions as indicated
  - Arterial blood gases to evaluate ventilation status
  - Liver function studies and renal studies to compare baseline values and rule out significant pathology
- M: Monitoring devices
  - Difficulty finding appropriately sized equipment is common.[49]
  - Make sure that equipment, such as stretchers, blood pressure cuffs, and cervical spine collars, is available in a variety of appropriate sizes.
  - Utilize appropriately sized monitoring equipment.
- N: Nasogastric or orogastric tube consideration
  - If a patient's history includes recent bariatric surgery, blind placement of a nasogastric or orogastric tube is contraindicated because it may disrupt the suture lines of the new stomach or perforate the smaller stomach.
  - Tubes may be safely placed using fluoroscopy if indicated.[50]
- O: Oxygenation and ventilation
  - Continuously monitor oxygenation status and capnography.
  - Higher concentrations of supplemental oxygen may be necessary to achieve adequate oxygenation.
  - Conversely, obese patients have higher rates of chronic obstructive pulmonary disorder, so the risk of hyperoxia may also include the loss of ventilatory drive. Monitor and maintain SpO_2 between 92% and 96%.[6]
- P: Pain assessment and management
  - Pain medication dosing is based on IBW or normal weight parameters and not on actual weight.[19]
  - Lipophilic medications are taken up by adipose tissue and released slowly back into the bloodstream. Medications that are lipophilic—including benzodiazepines, propofol, and fentanyl—should be titrated according to effects and the patient's response monitored closely.[19,45,49]

Emergency Resuscitation

Although obesity can make resuscitation efforts more challenging, no modifications to basic or advanced life support procedures are recommended by the American Heart Association's Advanced Cardiovascular Life Support Guidelines.[38] Defibrillation is best accomplished using a biphasic defibrillator, which delivers energy from one contact point or pad to the other and then reverses direction back to the source. There is no current evidence that supports the need for higher energy levels, larger pads, or any change in the algorithm for defibrillation with obese patients.[38] In the case of cardiopulmonary resuscitation, providers of small to medium build may not be able to produce enough pressure on the chest of an obese person to perform effective compressions. Physical exhaustion may set in earlier.[48]

Secondary Survey

The secondary survey includes the history and head-to-toe assessment. The secondary (and tertiary) surveys can be very challenging for obese patients. Barriers to obtaining a thorough and complete secondary survey include difficulty in finding anatomical landmarks, overhanging pannus, excessive skin with skin folds, and difficulty the patient may have with moving extremities or changing positions.[48]

H: History

The trauma nurse should consider several questions when obtaining the history of an obese patient.

- What is the patient's current weight and height?
  - Weight may be used for adequate medication dosing. Studies have shown that physicians and nurses are able to estimate a patient's weight within 10% of the actual weight less than 70% of the time and that parent or patient estimates are most accurate.[56]
  - Use of a bed or stretcher with weight measurement capability is ideal for the obese patient who may lack mobility. Check this equipment for upper weight limits before use.
- What medical problems does the patient have?
  - Known medical history and potential undiagnosed conditions are both important factors.
  - Be alert for signs of comorbidities that have yet to be identified.
    - Ask about increased thirst, urination, dry mouth, headaches, or fatigue, because these may indicate the presence of metabolic syndrome or elevated glucose levels.
    - Symptoms such as snoring, daytime drowsiness and fatigue, difficulty concentrating, memory problems, irritability and depression, frequent night awakening, observed apnea, or a choking sensation during sleep can indicate undetected sleep apnea.[12,50]
- Does the patient have a history of bariatric surgery?
  - A patient who has undergone surgery may be in one of several stages of weight loss, may have achieved limited success, or may have rebounded with weight gain occurring at some point after the original surgery.
  - Determine the type of procedure, any complications (such as leak, bleeding, bowel obstruction), and when it was performed.[33,58]
  - Patients who have not been compliant with dietary and vitamin recommendations may have deficiencies in their protein or vitamin levels. Patients who have undergone gastric bypass, for example, are more likely to have iron and vitamin B_{12} deficiencies and may have baseline anemia that affects laboratory studies.
- Which medications is the patient taking?
  - Obese patients may be taking medications to treat several comorbid conditions. It is important to determine the patient's use of the following medications:
    - Antidiabetic medications, including last dose
    - Diuretics[20]
    - Antihypertensives
    - Antilipidemics
    - Anticoagulants and salicylates
    - Antianginals, including calcium-channel blockers, beta-adrenergic blockers, and nitrates
    - Antacids and histamine antagonists
    - Antidepressants
    - Bronchodilators and corticosteroids
    - Appetite suppressants—may cause tachycardia, increased blood pressure, paresthesia, dyspepsia, and abdominal pain, which can be confused with trauma-related injury symptoms[29]
    - Chronic pain medications, including nonsteroidal anti-inflammatory medications
  - Because of altered absorption following bariatric surgery, many patients may be taking vitamin supplements.
  - Ask about over-the-counter medications, alternative and herbal remedies, and the use of energy supplements or drinks.

H: Head-to-Toe Assessment

Peripheral pulses may need to be assessed using Doppler ultrasound. The presence of lymphedema related to the patient's obesity can make it very difficult to palpate distal pulses.[48] Bowel sounds of the obese patient may be difficult to hear. The excess adipose tissue of the abdomen may mask a pregnant abdomen; pregnancy tests on all obese females of childbearing age who have not had a hysterectomy or tubal ligation should be performed.[23]

Reevaluation Measures

Of particular importance is thromboembolism prevention.

Thromboembolism Prevention

The obese patient is at higher risk for thrombus formation and for serious complications from thromboembolism. Standard prevention measures include sequential compression devices, prophylactic anticoagulant therapy, and early mobilization.[31]

Patients who are discharged with reduced mobility after fractures may need anticoagulation medication as well as discharge instructions related to signs and symptoms of thromboembolism. Fracture stabilization choices may be altered because of the need for custom-fit splints that allow for the anticipated swelling.[21] Patients with a BMI greater than 40 kg/m^2 will need specialty beds to help prevent complications of immobility.

Radiographs

Depending on a facility's availability of equipment, it may be difficult to obtain quality radiographic images. Load capacity and the ability to accommodate the dimensions of the obese patient are just some of the barriers. The increased mass of the patient reduces the contrast of images.[48] It may be helpful for the trauma nurse to assist in positioning the head of the bed at 10–15 degrees (unless contraindicated) to obtain chest radiographs.[23]

Computed Tomography and Magnetic Resonance Imaging

Be aware of weight limits and size restrictions of the computed tomography (CT) scanning equipment; gantry aperture diameter may not be large enough to accommodate the obese patient. When CT scanners and magnetic resonance imaging (MRI) machines are of adequate size, the patient may have difficulty raising their arms above their head for testing.[48] Prepare alternative options in advance. Artifacts and poor quality of imaging related to the increased mass of the patient may make accuracy of diagnostic interpretation difficult when obtaining CT and MRI.[48]

Ultrasound/FAST Exam

The use of ultrasound to obtain urgent diagnostic information may be the only possible option, especially in rural or small community hospitals with no other alternatives. This can be challenging because morbid obesity is often a contraindication to using ultrasound. Considerations to help overcome this barrier include having an experienced provider use the ultrasound. Placing the patient in a modified lateral position may help to displace some of the excess body mass, particularly when attempting to scan through the flank during the focused assessment with sonography for trauma (FAST) exam. Some visceral and pericardial fat can often be misinterpreted for fluid or clotted blood.[48]

Staff and Patient Safety

Staff safety during procedures is a consideration when caring for obese patients. The weight of an extremity in a patient with a BMI greater than 40 kg/m^2 may exceed the safe lifting load for a single caregiver, and lifting devices should be used in all aspects of care to help prevent staff and patient injury. Consideration should be given to preplanning and training in the use of techniques and devices to assist in transfer, positioning, and nursing care procedures.

Lateral transfer devices should be used to help prevent skin shearing and staff injury. Such devices include slider boards and friction-reduction devices, as well as air-assisted lateral transfer aids. Friction-reduction sheets and air transfer cushions need to be placed on the stretcher before patient use. With the lateral air transfer device, air flows through the inflated mattress to provide a thin cushion of air to move the patient laterally, reducing the work of transfer.[4]

Providing a safe environment for the obese patient involves the following key components:

- Knowing the weight capacity of conventional equipment (stretchers, wheelchairs, toilets) and the capacity and size of openings of CT and MRI tables and openings
- Being familiar with safe use of the bariatric equipment available in the department
- Demonstrating confidence in the ability to safely care for obese patients and ensure the safety of other caregivers

Patient Dignity

Obese patients often experience discrimination and bias in healthcare settings.[51,54] Physicians, nurses, and other staff members may have negative beliefs and opinions about causes of obesity and characteristics of obese patients, which can translate into care that lacks sensitivity or that even may be openly prejudicial. The challenges of providing care to obese patients can also lead the trauma nurse to exhibit frustration, an emotion that the obese patient may perceive as a negative reaction directed at them.

To provide sensitive care for obese patients, follow these guidelines:

- *Protect patient privacy.* Provide adequately sized gowns and draping, and obtain the patient's weight in a discreet manner.
- *Demonstrate tact regarding weight issues.* References to "large size," "big boy," "obesity," or "excess fat" are often offensive to patients with obesity. Terms such as "weight problem" or "excess weight" are often less emotionally charged.[51,54]
- *Be sensitive to the obese patient's past encounters with healthcare providers.* Many have suffered embarrassment from the use of improperly sized equipment, insensitive comments, and even openly discriminatory behavior. Be aware of nonverbal communication.

A heightened sensitivity to these issues is needed in the care of the obese patient to overcome self-protective barriers and develop a trusting relationship that will facilitate care.[51,54]

Reevaluation and Post-Resuscitation Care

Continued assessment of the airway and ventilation is the highest priority in obese trauma patients, to include monitoring for the following conditions:

- Signs of impending airway or respiratory compromise
- Signs of gastric reflux, which can lead to pulmonary aspiration, particularly in a supine patient
- Signs and symptoms of pulmonary embolism, given that both obesity and trauma are independent risk factors for this complication[1,24,31]

Because of the numerous challenges in evaluation and treatment of obese patients, prolonged immobilization can occur.[14] Ongoing reevaluation includes monitoring for the following complications:

- Pressure-induced rhabdomyolysis from muscle breakdown (see Chapter 10, "Spinal and Musculoskeletal Trauma")
- Acute compartment syndrome in compromised extremities (see Chapter 10)
- Skin breakdown, particularly on the occiput area of the head and between skin folds, along with areas of bony prominence[57]
- If using BiPAP, monitor for the following[40]:
  - Skin breakdown across the bridge of the nose due to mask pressure
  - Gastric insufflation and potential regurgitation and aspiration

Definitive Care or Transport

Bariatric centers of excellence are located throughout the United States. Consider whether the patient needs to be cared for at a trauma center and/or bariatric center of excellence. Ensure that transport services are aware of the patient's size and have the appropriate equipment and staff to transport the patient safely.

Emerging Trends

Obese trauma patients require special handling to prevent injuries to both the patient and staff. Assistive devices such as bariatric hospital beds, overhead/ceiling lifts, stand-up lifts, and sliding boards can greatly increase safety when caring for these patients.[22] Consulting with a bariatric nurse coordinator (if available) when planning care/protocols specifically for obese trauma patients will significantly improve safe patient handling for both obese patients and healthcare workers.

Summary

Trauma nurses are encountering increasing numbers of trauma patients who are overweight or obese. This patient population is a vulnerable group because of the presence of functional and physiologic changes, and these patients are at high risk for airway and breathing complications. Standard assessments and interventions may need to be modified, and equipment must be available for use in a variety of sizes. Trauma care goals are aimed at diagnosis and management of injury, despite challenges presented by body habitus and limited diagnostic capabilities, while preserving the dignity of the patient.

References

1. Anderson, M. R., & Shashaty, M. G. S. (2021). Impact of obesity in critical illness. *CHEST, 160*(6), 2135–2145. https://doi.org/10.1016/j.chest.2021.08.001
2. Arnold, A., & McNaughton, A. (2018). Accuracy of non-invasive blood pressure measurements in obese patients. *British Journal of Nursing, 27*(1), 35–40. https://doi.org/10.12968/bjon.2018.27.1.35
3. Australian Institute of Health and Welfare. (2021, June 29). *Inequalities in overweight and obesity and the social determinants of health*. https://www.aihw.gov.au/reports/overweight-obesity/inequalities-overweight-social-determinants-health/summary
4. Barlow, R. D. (2018). No time to rest. *Healthcare Purchasing News, 42*(2), 40–42. https://www.hpnonline.com/sourcing-logistics/article/13000959/no-time-to-rest
5. Batabyal, R. A., & O'Connell, K. (2018). Improving management of severe asthma: BiPAP and beyond. *Clinical Pediatric Emergency Medicine, 19*(1), 69–75. httsp://doi.org/10.1016/j.cpem.2018.02.007
6. Beasley, R., Chien, J., Douglas, J., Eastlake, L., Farah, C., King, G., Moore, R., Pilcher, J., Richards, M., Smith, S., & Walters, H. (2017). Target oxygen saturation range: 92–96% versus 94–98%. *Respirology, 22*(1), 200–202. https://doi.org/10.1111/resp.12879
7. Belle-Franklin, A., & Thompson, S. R. (2018). Out-of-hospital resuscitation of obese patients: Myths, challenges and the evidence. *Whitireia Nursing & Health Journal, 25*, 82–90. https://search.informit.org/doi/10.3316/informit.280990911390242
8. Brashers, V. L. (2019). Alterations of cardiovascular function. In S. H. K. McCance & S. E. Huether (Eds.), *Pathophysiology* (8th ed., pp. 1059–1114). Elsevier.

9. Brown, C. A. (2021). Emergency airway management in the morbidly obese patient. *UpToDate*. Retrieved May 1, 2021, from https://www.uptodate.com/contents/emergency-airway-management-in-the-morbidly-obese-patient

10. Centers for Disease Control and Prevention. (n.d.). *Overweight and obesity: Defining adult overweight and obesity*. https://www.cdc.gov/obesity/basics/adult-defining.html

11. Chawla, R., Dixit, S. B., Zirpe, K. G., Chaudhry, D., Khilnani, G. C., Mehta, Y., Khatib, K. I., Jagiasi, B. G., Chanchalani, G., Mishra, R. C., Samavedam, S., Govil, D., Gupta, S., Prayag, S., Ramasubban, S., Dobariya, J., Marwah, V., Sehgal, I., Jog, S. A., & Kulkarni, A. P. (2020). ISCCM guidelines for the use of non-invasive ventilation in acute respiratory failure in adult ICUs. *Indian Journal of Critical Care Medicine, 24*(Suppl. 1), S61–S81. https://doi.org/10.5005/jp-journals-10071-G23186

12. Chen, J. L., Urman, R. D., & Moon, T. S. (2020). The trauma patient with obesity: Anesthetic challenges. *International Anesthesiology Clinics, 58*(3), 58–65. https://doi.org/10.1097/aia.0000000000000279

13. Climent, E., Benaiges, D., & Pedro-Botet, J. (2021). Hydrophilic or lipophilic statins? *Frontiers in Cardiovascular Medicine, 8*, Article 687585. https://doi.org/10.3389/fcvm.2021.687585

14. Davis, C. P. (Ed.). (2021, March 29). Medical definition of bariatrics. *MedicineNet*. Retrieved December 6, 2021, from https://www.medicinenet.com/bariatrics/definition.htm

15. Davis, L. L., & Nolan, M. Z. (2021). The influence of obesity on care of adults with cardiovascular disease. *The Nursing Clinics of North America, 56*(4), 511–525. https://doi.org/10.1016/j.cnur.2021.07.002

16. Di Giacinto, I., Guarnera, M., Esposito, C., Falcetta, S., Cortese, G., Pascarella, G., Sorbello, M., & Cataldo, R. (2021). Emergencies in obese patients: A narrative review. *Journal of Anesthesia, Analgesia and Critical Care, 1*(1), Article 13. https://doi.org/10.1186/s44158-021-00019-2

17. Drury, B., Kocharians, C., Dong, F., Tran, L., Beroukhim, S., Hajjafar, R., Vara, R., Wong, D., Woodward, B., & Neeki, M. M. (2021). Impact of obesity on mortality in adult trauma patients. *Cureus, 13*(2), Article e13352. https://doi.org/10.7759/cureus.13352

18. Elkbuli, A., Dowd, B., Spano, P. J., II, Hai, S., Boneva, D., & McKenney, M. (2019). The association between seatbelt use and trauma outcomes: Does body mass index matter? *American Journal of Emergency Medicine, 37*(9), 1716–1719. https://doi.org/10.1016/j.ajem.2018.12.023

19. Erstad, B. L., & Barletta, J. F. (2020). Drug dosing in the critically ill obese patient—A focus on sedation, analgesia, and delirium. *Critical Care, 24*, 1–8. https://doi.org/10.1186/s13054-020-03040-z

20. Evans, P. L., Prior, J. A., Belcher, J., Mallen, C. D., Hay, C. A., & Roddy, E. (2018). Obesity, hypertension and diuretic use as risk factors for incident gout: A systematic review and meta-analysis of cohort studies. *Arthritis Research & Therapy, 20*(1), Article 136. https://doi.org/10.1186/s13075-018-1612-1

21. Frye, S. K., & Geigle, P. R. (2021). A comparison of prefabricated and custom made resting hand splints for individuals with cervical spinal cord injury: A randomized controlled trial. *Clinical Rehabilitation, 35*(6), 861–869. https://doi.org/10.1177/0269215520983486

22. Gallagher, S., Alexandrowiz, M., Fritz, R., Kumpar, D., Miller, M., McNaughton, C., & Nowicki, T. (2020). Bariatric space, technology, and design: A round table. *Workplace Health & Safety, 68*(7), 313–319. https://doi.org/10.1177/2165079920911549

23. Gamaly, M. (2020). Trauma in the bariatric patient. In K. A. McQuillan & M. B. Flynn Makic (Eds.), *Trauma nursing: From resuscitation through rehabilitation* (5th ed., pp. 719–737). Elsevier.

24. Gray, S., & Dieudonne, B. (2018). Optimizing care for trauma patients with obesity. *Cureus, 10*(7), Article e3021. https://doi.org/10.7759/cureus.3021

25. Gurubhagavatula, I., Sullivan, S., Meoli, A., Patil, S., Olson, R., Berneking, M., & Watson, N. F. (2017). Management of obstructive sleep apnea in commercial motor vehicle operators: Recommendations of the AASM Sleep and Transportation Safety Awareness Task Force. *Journal of Clinical Sleep Medicine, 13*(5), 745–758. https://doi.org/10.5664/jcsm.6598

26. Hadjiantoni, A. S. (2020). *Is the correct anatomical placement of the electrocardiogram (ECG) electrodes essential to diagnosis in the clinical setting: A systematic review* [Unpublished manuscript]. https://doi.org/10.21203/rs.3.rs-74147/v1

27. Hales, C. M., Carroll, M. D., Fryar, C. D., & Ogden, C. L. (2017, October). *Prevalence of obesity among adults and youth: United States, 2015–2016* (NCHS Data Brief No. 288). National Center for Health Statistics. https://www.cdc.gov/nchs/data/databriefs/db288.pdf

28. Hirt, P. A., Castillo, D. E., Yosipovitch, G., & Keri, J. E. (2019). Skin changes in the obese patient. *Journal of the American Academy of Dermatology, 81*(5), 1037–1057. https://doi.org/10.1016/j.jaad.2018.12.070

29. Hocking, S., Dear, A., & Cowley, M. A. (2017). Current and emerging pharmacotherapies for obesity in Australia. *Obesity Research & Clinical Practice, 11*(5), 501–521. https://doi.org/10.1016/j.orcp.2017.07.002

30. Hostetler, M. A. (2008). Use of noninvasive positive-pressure ventilation in the emergency department. *Emergency Medical Clinics of North America, 26*, 929–939. https://doi.org/10.1016/j.emc.2008.07.008

31. Hotoleanu, C. (2020). Association between obesity and venous thromboembolism. *Medicine and Pharmacy Reports, 93*(2), 162–168. https://doi.org/10.15386/mpr-1372

32. Inanir, M., Sincer, I., Erdal, E., Gunes, Y., Cosgun, M., & Mansiroglu, A. K. (2019). Evaluation of electrocardiographic ventricular repolarization parameters in extreme obesity. *Journal of Electrocardiology, 53*, 36–39. https://doi.org/10.1016/j.jelectrocard.2018.12.003

33. Jafri, A., Lo Menzo, E., Szomstein, S., & Rosenthal, R. J. (2020). Management of complications of bariatric operations. In M. Patti, M. Di Corpo, & F. Schlottmann (Eds.), *Foregut surgery* (pp. 273–282). Springer. https://doi.org/10.1007/978-3-030-27592-1_29

34. Joseph, B., Hadeed, S., Haider, A. A., Ditillo, M., Joseph, A., Pandit, V., Kulvatunyou, N., Tang, A., Latifi, R., & Rhee, P. (2017). Obesity and trauma mortality: Sizing up the risks in

motor vehicle crashes. *Obesity Research and Clinical Practice, 11*(1), 72–78. https://doi.org/10.1016/j.orcp.2016.03.003

35. Kaseer, H. S., Patel, R., Tucker, C., Elie, M.-C., Staley, B. J., Tran, N., & Lemon, S. (2021). Comparison of fluid resuscitation weight-based dosing strategies in obese patients with severe sepsis. *American Journal of Emergency Medicine, 49,* 268–272. https://doi.org/10.1016/j.ajem.2021.06.036

36. Katsevman, G. A., Daffner, S. D., Brandmeir, N. J., Emery, S. E., France, J. C., & Sedney, C. L. (2020). Complexities of spine surgery in obese patient populations: A narrative review. *Spine Journal, 20*(4), 501–511. https://doi.org/10.1016/j.spinee.2019.12.011

37. Kinder, F., Giannoudis, P. V., Boddice, T., & Howard, A. (2020). The effect of an abnormal BMI on orthopaedic trauma patients: A systematic review and meta-analysis. *Journal of Clinical Medicine, 9*(5), Article 1302. https://doi.org/10.3390/jcm9051302

38. Kleinman, M. E., Goldberger, Z. D., Rea, T., Swor, R. A., Bobrow, B. J., Brennan, E. E., Terry, M., Hemphill, R., Gazmuri, R. J., Hazinski, M. F., & Travers, A. H. (2018). 2017 American Heart Association focused update on adult basic life support and cardiopulmonary resuscitation quality: An update to the American Heart Association Guidelines for Cardiopulmonary Resuscitation and Emergency Cardiovascular Care. *Circulation, 137*(1), e7–e13. https://doi.org/10.1161/CIR.0000000000000539

39. Lai, H. H., Helmuth, M. E., Smith, A. R., Wiseman, J. B., Gillespie, B. W., & Kirkali, Z. (2019). Relationship between central obesity, general obesity, overactive bladder syndrome and urinary incontinence among male and female patients seeking care for their lower urinary tract symptoms. *Urology, 123,* 34–43. https://doi.org/10.1016/j.urology.2018.09.012

40. Mahran, M. M., Said El-Kalla, R., Abd El khalek Sallam, A., Ahmed El Heniedy, M., & Mohey El-deen EL-Gendy, H. (2021). Noninvasive bi-level positive airway pressure ventilation in blunt chest trauma. *Journal of Advances in Medicine and Medical Research, 33*(22), 8–15. https://doi.org/10.9734/JAMMR/2021/v33i2231154

41. Marshall, J. (2020). Nursing considerations for anaesthesia of the obese patient. *Veterinary Nursing Journal, 35*(7), 202–204. https://doi.org/10.1080/17415349.2020.1795027

42. Maspero, M., Bertoglio, C. L., Morini, L., Alampi, B., Mazzola, M., Girardi, V., Zironda, A., Barone, G., Magistro, C., & Ferrari, G. (2021). Laparoscopic ventral hernia repair in patients with obesity: Should we be scared of body mass index? *Surgical Endoscopy, 36,* 2032–2041. https://doi.org/10.1007/s00464-021-08489-9

43. Mazza, F., Venturino, M., Turello, D., Gorla, A., Degiovanni, C., Locatelli, A., & Melloni, G. (2021). Cricothyroidotomy in the emergency setting: Indications, techniques and outcomes. *Signa Vitae, 17*(3), 31–41. https://doi.org/10.22514/sv.2021.063

44. Organisation for Economic Co-operation and Development. (2017). *Obesity update 2017.* https://www.oecd.org/els/health-systems/Obesity-Update-2017.pdf

45. Parker, B. K., Manning, S., & Winters, M. E. (2019). The crashing obese patient. *Western Journal of Emergency Medicine, 20*(2), 323–330. https://doi.org/10.5811/westjem.2018.12.41085

46. Pucher, P. H., Tanno, L., Hewage, K., & Bagnall, N. M. (2017). Demand for specialized training for the obese trauma patient: National ATLS expert group survey results. *Injury, 48*(5), 1058–1062. https://doi.org/10.1016/j.injury.2017.02.027

47. Razeghi Jahromi, S., Ghorbani, Z., Martelletti, P., Lampl, C., Togha, M., & School of Advanced Studies of the European Headache Federation. (2019). Association of diet and headache. *The Journal of Headache and Pain, 20*(1), Article 106. https://doi.org/10.1186/s10194-019-1057-1

48. Richardson, S., & Harris, S. (2018, November). Managing the bariatric patient in the ED setting. *Emergency Nurse New Zealand,* 9–15. https://www.nzno.org.nz/Portals/0/Files/Documents/Groups/Emergency%20Nurses/Journals/ENN46_CENNZ%20Journal_Nov%202018_.pdf

49. Schetz, M., De Jong, A., Deane, A. M., Druml, W., Hemelaar, P., Pelosi, P., Pickkers, P., Reintam-Blaser, A., Roberts, J., Sakr, Y., & Jaber, S. (2019). Obesity in the critically ill: A narrative review. *Intensive Care Medicine, 45*(6), 757–769. https://doi.org/10.1007/s00134-019-05594-1

50. Sechser, N. R., Overhue, H. L., & Van Guilder, G. P. (2021). An oral myofunctional exercise prescription for obstructive sleep apnea. *ACSM's Health & Fitness Journal, 25*(3), 35–43. https://doi.org/10.1249/FIT.0000000000000670

51. Smigelski-Theiss, R., Gampong, M., & Kuraski, J. (2017). Weight bias and psychosocial implications for acute care of patients with obesity. *AACN Advanced Critical Care, 28*(3), 254–262. https://doi.org/10.4037/aacnacc2017446

52. Subramaniam, R., Pushparaj, H., & Aravindan, A. (2021). Preoperative evaluation of the morbidly obese patient. In A. C. Sinha (Ed.), *Oxford textbook of anaesthesia for the obese patient* (pp. 167–180). https://doi.org/10.1093/med/9780198757146.003.0017

53. Sultana, A., Wadhwa, A., & Berkow, L. C. (2020). Alternate airway strategies for the patient with morbid obesity. *International Anesthesiology Clinics, 58*(3), 1–8. https://doi.org/10.1097/aia.0000000000000277

54. Wakefield, K., & Feo, R. (2017). Confronting obesity, stigma and weight bias in healthcare with a person centred care approach: A case study. *Australian Nursing & Midwifery Journal, 25*(1), 28–31. https://search.informit.org/doi/10.3316/INFORMIT.909958228125391

55. Wan, L., Shao, L. J., Liu, Y., Wang, H. X., Xue, F. S., & Tian, M. (2019). A feasibility study of jaw thrust as an indicator assessing adequate depth of anesthesia for insertion of supraglottic airway device in morbidly obese patients. *Chinese Medical Journal, 132*(18), 2185–2191. https://doi.org/10.1097/CM9.0000000000000403

56. Wells, M., Goldstein, L. N., & Bentley, A. (2017). The accuracy of emergency weight estimation systems in children—A systematic review and meta-analysis. *International Journal of Emergency Medicine, 10,* Article 29. https://doi.org/10.1186/s12245-017-0156-5

57. Williamson, K. (2020). Nursing people with bariatric care needs: More questions than answers. *Wounds UK, 16*(1), 64–71. https://www.wounds-uk.com/download/wuk_article/8403
58. Windish, R., & Wong, J. (2019). Review article: Postoperative bariatric patients in the emergency department: Review of surgical complications for the emergency physician. *Emergency Medicine Australasia, 31*(3), 309–313. https://doi.org/10.1111/1742-6723.13252
59. World Health Organization. (2021). *Obesity and overweight* [Fact sheet]. https://www.who.int/news-room/fact-sheets/detail/obesity-and-overweight
60. Wynn-Hebden, A., & Bouch, D. C. (2020). Anaesthesia for the obese patient. *BJA Education, 20*(11), 388–395. https://doi.org/10.1016/j.bjae.2020.07.003

CHAPTER 15

The Older Trauma Patient

Milagros Tabije-Ebuen, DNP, MSN-NE, RN, CEN, PCCN, CCRN

OBJECTIVES

Upon completion of this chapter, the learner will be able to:
1. Describe mechanisms of injury associated with the older adult trauma patient.
2. Describe age-related anatomic and physiologic changes as a basis for assessment of the older adult trauma patient.
3. Demonstrate the nursing assessment of the older adult trauma patient.
4. Plan appropriate interventions for the older adult trauma patient.
5. Evaluate the effectiveness of nursing interventions for the older adult trauma patient.

Introduction

Every country in the world is experiencing growth in the number and proportion of older people.[65] Globally, the number of people over 60 years of age is expected to nearly double between 2020 and 2050, from 1.4 to 2.1 billion.[65] As the age of populations increases, so does the need for increased knowledge of the unique vulnerabilities of the older adult. The predictable decline at a cellular level associated with aging directly impacts physiologic reserves and the ability to respond to injury. Appropriate prioritization and early management of the injured older adult can improve outcomes while minimizing morbidity and mortality. Physiologic and anatomic changes associated with aging, preexisting conditions, polypharmacy, and unique psychosocial considerations mandate a multidisciplinary approach to the care of the injured older adult.[2]

Epidemiology

Advances in the management of chronic diseases, along with an emphasis on preventive medicine, have contributed to people living longer, often with more active lifestyles.[33,44] Increased physical activity in the older adult significantly increases the likelihood of injury.[33] Up to 33% of fatal injuries occur in the older adult as a result of mechanisms such as falls and motor vehicle crashes.[47] Falls are the leading cause of injury-related morbidity and mortality, accounting for nearly 60% of nonfatal

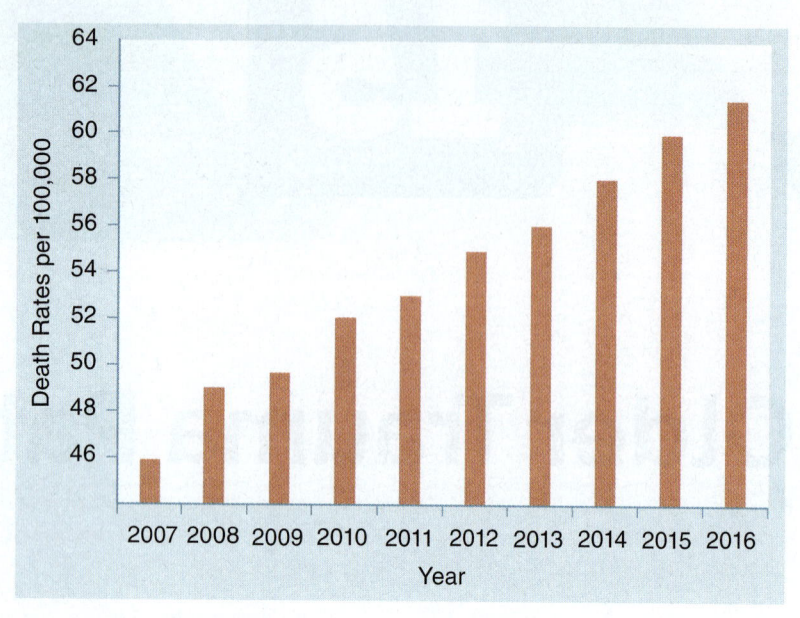

Figure 15-1 U.S. fall death rates increased 30% from 2007 to 2016 for older adults.

injury-related emergency department (ED) visits in the United States in 2020.[10] Globally, more than 600,00 deaths every year are attributed to falls,[8] and fall-related deaths in the United States have increased 30% (**Figure 15-1**).[12] Injuries most associated with falls in the older adult include intracranial hemorrhage, fractures, and thoracic or abdominal injuries.[44]

Physiologic changes that increase trauma-related mortality may begin as early as 50 years of age, highlighting the importance of understanding the impact of age on injury outcomes.[9,18,44]

Decreased physiologic reserve, accompanied by impaired compensatory mechanisms, comorbidities, and polypharmacy, is among the factors that increase the severity of injuries, incidence of complications, and mortality rate in this population, *even with minor trauma*.[33,66] Additionally, injured older adults in the United States are undertriaged, defined as transport to a nontrauma center, by up to 50%.[58]

In addition to these factors, it is important to understand common mechanisms of injury in this population.

Mechanisms of Injury in the Older Adult

Consideration of mechanism of injury can direct the trauma team to potential injuries (**Table 15-1**).[16]

Falls, motor vehicle collisions (MVCs), including pedestrian-related collisions, burns, and penetrating injures are common causes of fatal and nonfatal injury in adults 65 years and older.[1,18]

Falls

In the older adult population, falls are the leading cause of injury-related death, hospital admissions for trauma, and loss of independence in the United States and globally.[11] As noted previously, the rate of death due to falls has risen sharply in recent years, with an approximate 30% increase in the past decade[12] (Figure 15-1). An older adult falls every second, and every year 36 million falls lead to 8 million injuries, 3 million ED visits, 950,000 hospitalizations, and 32,000 deaths.[12] Falls account for 25% of all hospital admissions and 40% of all nursing home admissions. Of those admitted, 40% do not return to independent living, and 25% die within a year[33,38]: In a 2016 study, females older than 65 years of age had the highest rate of fall-related injuries.[62]

Falls in older adults are primarily low-energy trauma (LET) events that occur from a standing height or lower. They are often caused by conditions such as wet surfaces, poor lighting, inadequate footwear, and cluttered pathways, along with weakness, gait, and balance impairments, and use of psychoactive medications.[38,61] Falls can also occur as a result of the following factors[38,61]:

- Syncope due to dysrhythmias, venous pooling, orthostatic hypotension, hypoxia, anemia, or hypoglycemia
- Alcohol and medications (antihypertensives, antidepressants, diuretics, and hypoglycemia agents)
- Changes in postural stability, balance, motor strength, and coordination

TABLE 15-1 Incidents by Mechanism of Injury

Mechanism	Number	Percent	Deaths	Case Fatality Rate
Fall	380,800	44.18	16,623	4.37
Motor vehicle traffic	223,866	25.97	10,343	4.62
Struck by, against	55,662	6.46	755	1.36
Transport, other	39,269	4.56	903	2.30
Cut/pierce	35,565	4.13	776	2.18
Firearm	36,325	4.21	5,557	15.30
Pedal cyclist, other	14,730	1.71	207	1.41
Other specified and classifiable	13,682	1.59	522	3.82
Hot object/substance	8,401	0.97	36	0.43
Fire/flame	7,877	0.91	467	5.93
Unspecified	7,834	0.91	433	5.53
Machinery	8,101	0.94	99	1.22
Natural/environmental, bites and stings	5,868	0.68	62	1.06
Other specified, not elsewhere classifiable	4,059	0.47	74	1.82
Overexertion	2,613	0.30	12	0.46
Pedestrian, other	2,845	0.33	177	6.22
Natural/environmental, other	2,387	0.28	38	1.59
Suffocation	885	0.10	240	27.12
Poisoning	413	0.05	8	1.94
Drowning/submersion	375	0.04	72	19.20
Adverse effects, medical care	224	0.03	11	4.91
Adverse effects, drugs	102	0.01	7	6.86
Not known/not recorded	10,005	1.16	403	4.03
Total	861,888	100	37,825	4.39

Reproduced from Chang, M. C. (Ed.). (2016). *The National Trauma Data Bank 2016: Annual report*. American College of Surgeons. https://www.facs.org/~/media/files/quality%20programs/trauma/ntdb/ntdb%20annual%20report%202016.ashx. The content reproduced from the NTDB remains the full and exclusive copyrighted property of the American College of Surgeons. The American College of Surgeons is not responsible for any claims arising from works based on the original data, text, tables, or figures.

- Slower reaction times
- Poor visual acuity and visual attention
- Reduction of proprioceptive and vibratory sensation
- Hearing impairment
- Increased sway
- Poor positional control
- Environmental hazards

Most falls occur at home (60%), with an additional 30% occurring in the community, and 10% in nursing homes or other institutions.[35] Often, falls occur while the older adult patient is engaged in everyday activities, such as walking on stairs, going to the bathroom, or working in the kitchen. Many older patients fail to inform their healthcare providers about fall incidents, which therefore go unnoticed and are untreated.[61] Older adults are

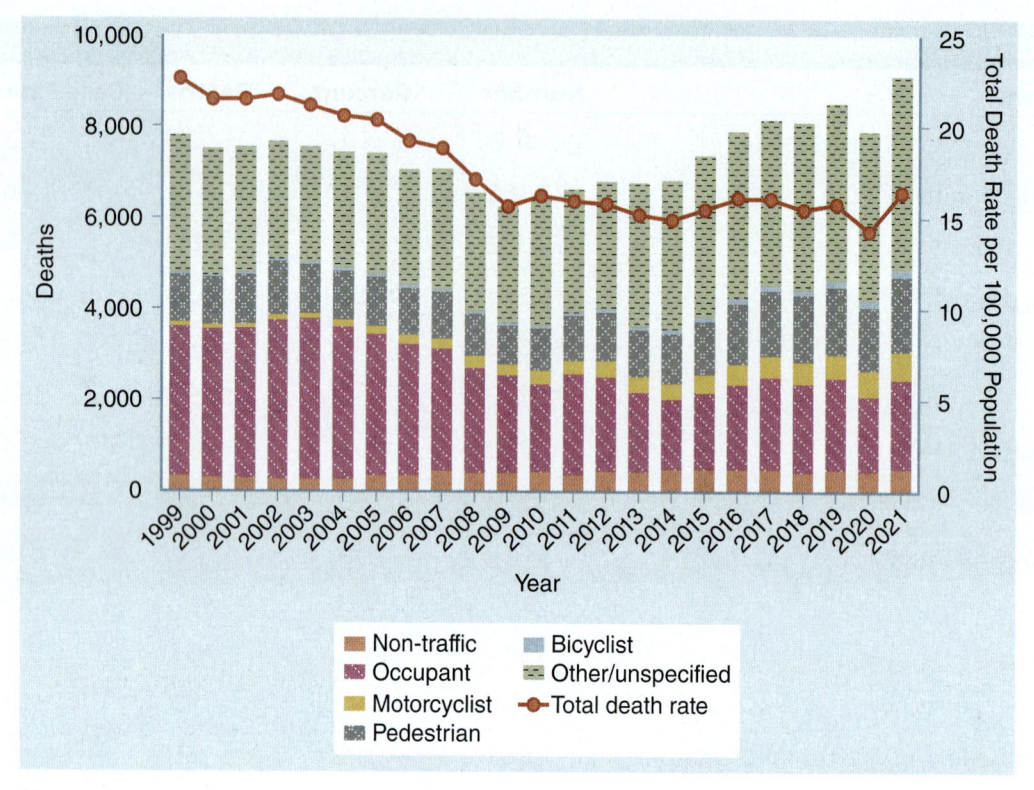

Figure 15-2 *Fatalities in motor vehicle crashes of those aged 65 and older by person type, 1999–2020.*

often undertriaged after experiencing a LET fall from a standing height. Mortality and disability can be affected by the undertriage of older patients. Falls (or LET) and high-energy trauma (such as MVCs) are categorized and often triaged differently, but the mortality and morbidity rates are similar for both. Patients with LET should be triaged at a higher level of urgency until they are assessed, and all the predisposing factors (medications, medical history) are considered.[7]

The most common injuries resulting from falls in the older adult include the following[16,21]:

- Lacerations and contusions
- Traumatic brain injury
- Fractures, especially of the hip

After a fall, many older adults cannot get up without assistance, which can result in further complications. When a person falls and lies motionless for many hours, the weight of the body results in compression of muscle tissue, placing the patient at risk for rhabdomyolysis (see Chapter 10, "Spinal and Musculoskeletal Trauma," for more information). Rhabdomyolysis can lead to many serious complications, including the following[64]:

- Acute kidney injury
- Hyperkalemia and other electrolyte imbalances
- Fluid shifting, hypovolemic shock
- Fat embolism and acute respiratory distress syndrome
- Coagulopathies (disseminated intravascular coagulopathy and fibrinolysis)
- Sepsis and multiple organ dysfunction syndrome

Motor Vehicle Collisions

In 2020, more than 48 million licensed drivers were aged 65 and over in the United States.[14] The number of older drivers over the past decade has increased by 60%.[11] Overall, the number of motor vehicle deaths combined (MVCs, pedestrian collisions, bicycling) has increased 20% over the last decade (**Figure 15-2**).[42]

In 2020, approximately 200,000 older adults were treated in EDs for crash injuries, and approximately 7,500 died in traffic crashes.[14] Age-related physiologic changes can affect the ability to drive. These include changes in vision, hearing, perception, muscle flexibility, and reflexes.[24] A single drink can affect the driving ability of older drivers; they may become "intoxicated" below the federal legal blood alcohol concentration level of 0.08%.[52]

The percentage of alcohol-impaired drivers involved in fatal crashes has increased in older populations and decreased in drivers under 55 years of age (**Table 15-2**).[60]

TABLE 15-2 Alcohol-Impaired Drivers Involved in Fatal Crashes, by Age Group, Sex, and Vehicle Type, 2011 and 2020

Drivers Involved in Fatal Crashes by Age Group	2011 Total Drivers	2011 BAC: .08+ g/dL Number	2011 BAC: .08+ g/dL % of Total	2020 Total Drivers	2020 BAC: .08+ g/dL Number	2020 BAC: .08+ g/dL % of Total	Change in % with BAC = .08+ g/dL 2011 and 2020
15–20	4,362	852	20%	4,561	790	17%	−3%
21–24	4,488	1,448	32%	4,884	1,288	26%	−6%
25–34	8,549	2,538	30%	11,933	3,100	26%	−4%
35–44	7,084	1,694	24%	8,896	2,004	23%	−1%
45–54	7,513	1,564	21%	7,731	1,506	19%	−2%
55–64	5,572	763	14%	7,294	1,157	16%	+2%
65–74	2,960	231	8%	4,116	496	12%	+4%
75+	2,528	125	5%	2,810	199	7%	+2%
Total	43,840	9,287	21%	53,890	11,022	20%	−1%

Modified from U.S. Department of Transportation National Highway Traffic Safety Administration. (2022). *Traffic safety facts: 2020 data.* https://crashstats.nhtsa.dot.gov/Api/Public/ViewPublication/813294

MVCs involving older adult drivers are less likely to be related to speed. Instead, the physiologic changes just noted affect the older adult's ability to drive safely in the following situations[19,24]:

- At intersections (due to limited peripheral vision)
- Merging into traffic when another vehicle is traveling faster (due to reduced reaction time)
- When another car is in the older driver's blind spot (due to limited peripheral vision and kyphosis)
- When it is dark (due to loss of visual acuity)

Older patients have injury patterns that differ from those seen in younger adults and are susceptible to serious injury from minor trauma. Twenty-five percent of injured older adults will sustain chest trauma, including rib fractures and flail chest, which can exacerbate underlying cardiopulmonary disease.[18,40] **Table 15-3** describes physiologic changes in older adults that may increase their risk of injury. Additional considerations include the following[34,36,50,54]:

- Rib fractures are common as a result of bone demineralization, with geriatric patients having double the morbidity and mortality of younger adults.
- Complications from these injuries may lead to acute respiratory problems due to hypoventilation, such as respiratory failure/hypoxia, pneumonia, and pleural effusion. There is a relationship between the number of ribs fractured and mortality.
- Lower cervical injuries are common because of degenerative changes and relative immobility of the lower cervical spine. Injury incidence is increased at the craniocervical junction, particularly at C2 and the odontoid.
- Minor head injury can result in significant intracranial injury; older adults have three times the incidence of long-term functional disability as younger adults.
- Older patients presenting with lateral pelvic fractures are more likely to hemorrhage.

Pedestrian-Related Collisions

While the overall probability of a vehicle colliding with a pedestrian has decreased in recent years, pedestrian fatalities have increased, especially in the geriatric population.[4] Greater severity of injury and worse outcomes for adults 50 years of age and older are associated with low-velocity pedestrian collisions.[4] Older adults are at high risk for pedestrian-related collisions and have higher rates of morbidity and mortality.[4] Strategies to prevent pedestrian deaths should include consideration of the needs of the older population.[44] See Chapter 3, "Biomechanics and Mechanisms of Injury," for more information.

Most pedestrians involved in collisions receive injuries not only from contact with the vehicle but also from subsequent contact with the ground. The older population has been found to sustain more tibial, pelvic, chest,

TABLE 15-3 Anatomic and Physiologic Changes in the Older Adult

System	Changes with Aging
Airway	› Atrophy of oral mucosa may lead to loose or poorly fitting dentures (full or partial) that may obstruct the airway. › Relaxed musculature of the oropharynx may result in aspiration. › Decreased gag and cough reflexes predispose the older adult to aspiration, infection, and bronchospasm. › Temporomandibular and cervical arthritis make intubation more difficult.
Cervical spine	Older adults are predisposed to cervical injury and/or discomfort from the rigid spine board because of the following: › Osteoporosis › Changes in bone density › Ankylosing spondylitis › Osteopenia › Development of spinal stenosis › Frequent injury of the odontoid process › Increasing rigidity of the C4 to C6 levels; lever action causes fractures above and below these points › Rigidity from neurologic disorders (Parkinson disease) or from spinal surgery › Kyphosis, which limits cervical range of motion, inhibiting the ability to see oncoming traffic or crossing signals
Breathing	› Older adults experience a loss of strength in the muscles of respiration and diminished endurance, leading to easier fatigue. › Costal cartilage calcification decreases inspiratory and expiratory force and chest expansion/elasticity; increases the respiratory rate; and reduces tidal volume. › Respiratory fatigue occurs more easily, resulting in hypoxia. › Older adults have decreased ability to compensate for hypoxia. › Older adults have a higher rate of complications, even following minor thoracic injuries, including pulmonary edema, atelectasis, and pneumonia. › Decreased cough strength due to anatomic changes of the thorax (anterior curvature or kyphosis; decrease in thoracic cavity size; and rib space narrowing, which decreases the length of the intercostal muscles). › Small airways lose recoil, resulting in potential airway collapse, air trapping, and uneven distribution of ventilation. › Pain, injury, and extended supine positioning can reduce arterial oxygen saturation and cardiac output.

Circulation	› Limited ability to increase heart rate and cardiac output in response to physiologic stress
	› Variations in adrenergic responses due to changes to the parasympathetic and sympathetic systems:
	  • Heart rate > 90 beats/min may indicate significant physiologic stress.
	  • Orthostatic hypotension may result from loss of sensitivity of baroreceptors.

System	Changes with Aging
	› Hypoperfusion is poorly tolerated because of declining cardiac reserve.
	› Left ventricular thickening and decrease in pacemaker cells in the sinoatrial and atrioventricular nodes decrease filling capacity and delay filling time.
	› Muscle mass reduction and atrial stiffening result in decreased contractility.
	› Reduction in total body water increases risk for dehydration.
	› Anemia is caused by nutritional deficiencies, chronic inflammatory disease, and chronic renal disease.
Neurologic	› Brain tissue atrophy results in the following conditions: • Stretching of the parasagittal bridging veins, predisposing them to tearing with injury • Additional space in the cranial vault, resulting in substantial bleeding before the onset of symptoms • Higher incidence of chronic subdural hematomas › Other potential factors include the following: • Increased likelihood of anticoagulant/antiplatelet medication use • Alcohol abuse, which adds to brain atrophy and causes liver damage that can increase bleeding tendencies • Antipsychotic and dopamine antagonist drugs and medications for glaucoma, which may affect neurologic examination
	› Nerve cells transmit signals more slowly, reducing reflexes and sensation; this leads to problems with movement, safety, and pain perception and control.
	› Accumulation of the protein beta-amyloid, which may signal developing cognitive impairment over time.
	› Increased risk of sleep disorders, delirium, and pain perception.
Skin and tissue	› Diminished autonomic response and thinner skin limit thermoregulation (impaired heat conservation, production, and dissipation).
	› Increased risk of skin breakdown results from: • Skin aging from lifestyle, diet, heredity, sun exposure, and other habits (smoking) • Breakdown of elastin • Obesity • Loss and loosening of subcutaneous fat, thinning of the skin • Decrease in vascular supply to the skin • Decreased ability to sweat • Immobility
Renal	› Some renal changes may be due to cardiovascular changes.
	› A decreased number of nephrons, loss of renal mass, and loss of functional glomeruli limit the ability to concentrate urine.
	› Decrease in the glomeruli filtration rate impairs electrolytes and water balance.
	› Diminished sense of thirst, leading to dehydration.

(continues)

TABLE 15-3 Anatomic and Physiologic Changes in the Older Adult (continued)

System	Changes with Aging
Musculoskeletal	Fat and fibrous tissue replace lean body mass, so only 15% of the total body mass is muscle by age 75, producing the following effects: › Diminished force of contractile muscle › Increased weakness and fatigue › Poor exercise tolerance › Slower, limited movement › Slower and shorter gait, unsteadiness
Endocrine	› Thyroid function (T_3 and T_4) decreases, slowing metabolism. › Parathyroid levels rise, increasing the risk of osteoporosis. › Metabolic syndrome (decreased sensitivity to insulin) increases, blunting the effects of insulin. › Aldosterone production drops, predisposing older adults to orthostatic hypotension and dehydration.

Data from Jubert, P., Lonjon, G., Garreau de Loubresse, C., & Bone and Joint Trauma Study Group. (2013). Complications of upper cervical spine trauma in elderly subjects. A systematic review of the literature. *Orthopaedics & Traumatology: Surgery & Research, 99,* S301–S312. https://doi.org/10.1016/j.otsr.2013.07.007; Lee, S. Y., Shih, S. C., Leu, Y. S., Chang, Y. H., Lin, H. C., & Ku, H. C. (2017). Implications of age-related changes in anatomy for geriatric-focused difficult airways. *International Journal of Gerontology, 11,* 130–133. https://doi.org/10.1016/j.ijge.2016.11.003; Sadro, C. T., Sandstrom, C. K., Verma, N., & Gunn, M. L. (2015). Geriatric trauma: A radiologist's guide to imaging trauma patients aged 65 years and older. *RadioGraphics, 35*(4), 1263–1285. https://doi.org/10.1148/rg.2015140130; Smith, C. M., & Cotter, V. T. (2016). Age-related changes in health. In M. Boltz, E. Capezuti, T. Fulmer, & D. Zwicker (Eds.), *Evidence-based geriatric nursing protocols for best practice* (5th ed., pp. 23–42). Springer.

spinal, and brain trauma after pedestrian MVCs compared with children.[4] Age-related changes also can contribute to these pedestrian-related collisions,[54] including the following factors:

- Kyphosis, which can decrease cervical range of motion, limiting the older adult's ability to see oncoming traffic or crossing signals
- Inability to walk quickly because of potential decreases in agility, gait, balance, and coordination
- Reduced reaction time, with slowing of processing powers
- Decreased hearing
- Loss of visual acuity and peripheral vision as a result of vestibular apparatus changes

Age-Related Anatomic and Physiologic Changes

Two categories of factors impact the older patient's response to illness and injury: Nonmodifiable changes occur as a result of the natural aging process (refer to Table 15-3), while other changes are due to modifiable factors, such as lifestyle.

Nonmodifiable Factors

Nonmodifiable factors that occur through aging can affect how the older adult responds to stress, illness, temperature, medications, trauma, and blood loss. Each patient is unique in their response to aging, illness, and injury.

Modifiable Factors

Modifiable factors that influence the older adult's ability to respond to illness and injury include the following:

- Lifestyle
  - Use/misuse of alcohol or tobacco
  - Use of illicit drugs
  - Misuse of prescription medication and/or polypharmacy
  - Weight (obesity)
- Socioeconomic characteristics
  - Live alone
- Diet
  - Healthy diet
  - Unhealthy diet
- Failure to eat because of illness or depression, loss of appetite, or financial restrictions

- Physical activity
    - Active
    - Inactive

Nursing Care of the Geriatric Trauma Patient

The following assessment parameters are specific to the older adult trauma patient. An important concept to remember is that older adults may display atypical presentations of disease, infection, and trauma. Refer to Chapter 4, "Initial Assessment," for the systematic approach to the nursing care of the trauma patient.

Preparation and Triage

Prehospital and ED triage of the older adult can be challenging. The mechanism of injury and vital signs can be misleading triage tools in older adult trauma patients because of their susceptibility to significant injuries from even relatively minor mechanisms or trauma.[18,33,50,66] This leads to a lower threshold for field triage of older trauma patients directly to a designated/verified trauma center.[58]

Primary Survey and Resuscitation Adjuncts

Primary survey and resuscitation adjuncts begin with the patient's alertness and airway.

A: Alertness and Airway with Cervical Spine Stabilization

Aging changes body structure, so the older adult may be prone to structural and functional changes surrounding the airway. In opening and clearing the airway of the older adult patient, also assess for the following[1,36,40,44]:

- Decreased gag reflex and diminished cough reflex
- Presence of full or partial dentures or the attrition of teeth
- Thin, smooth, and dry oral mucosa with a loss of elasticity
- Musculoskeletal degenerative changes such as osteoarthritis
- Increased body mass index—"double chin"
- Possible neurologic sequelae due to strokes, such as a loss of or decrease in the function of the glossopharyngeal or hypoglossal nerves, resulting in diminished control in swallowing and tongue movement

Interventions

Interventions include the following:

- Because loss of muscle mass, osteoporosis, osteoarthritis, and kyphosis can contribute to discomfort and skin breakdown in the older patient, consider padding bony areas and facilitate removal from the spine board as quickly as possible.
- The routine use of the "neutral position" adopted for cervical spine stabilization may not be appropriate in the older patient because it may inappropriately hyperextend the cervical spine. Using the "chin–brow horizontal" angle may be more appropriate.[46] The chin–brow horizontal angle is the angle of a line running from the brow to the chin when the patient is horizontal on a flat surface.
- The mucosa is thinner in older adults, and the older patient may be on anticoagulant therapy. Use caution when inserting an oral or nasal airway and when suctioning. Either of these procedures can result in swelling, bleeding, or hemorrhage.[36]

B: Breathing and Ventilation

Breathing and ventilation considerations include the following:

- Assess and monitor the work of breathing; older adults may have a lack of physiologic reserves.
- Consider early ventilatory support, especially with multiple rib fractures.
- Consider leaving dentures in place if they fit well and the patient requires bag-mask ventilation; intact dentures may help ensure a tighter-fitting mask.

Interventions

Interventions include the following:

- If spontaneous breathing is present, deliver supplemental oxygen using the most appropriate method the patient will tolerate.
- All seriously injured individuals should have oxygen delivered at the highest concentration in a manner that is appropriate for their medical condition and history.
- Consider using a nonrebreather at a flow rate sufficient to keep the reservoir inflated during inspiration, usually 12–15 L.
- Use care during intubation because arthritis and osteoporosis have the following effects:
    - Limited visualization of the vocal cords from decreased mobility with the jaw thrust
    - Increased possibility of cervical spine injury during instrumentation[36]

C: Circulation and Control of Hemorrhage

Maintenance of homeostasis in an older adult trauma patient can be difficult. Owing to their limited cardiac reserves, older adults may deteriorate quickly without exhibiting the usual expected changes in vital signs, urinary output, and physiologic responses.[44]

The older adult's heart and baroreceptors have a limited response to the body's normal release of catecholamines (adrenaline and norepinephrine), which are needed to increase heart rate and cardiac output.[54] The administration of medications such as beta blockers and cardiac glycosides can further limit this response. Regardless of the history of the older adult patient, a heart rate of greater than 90 beats per minute may indicate significant physiologic stress and increases the risk of mortality.[43] Additionally, a systolic blood pressure of less than 110 mm Hg is considered hypotension in adults older than 65 years of age because of changes to systemic vascular resistance accompanied by the possibility of preexisting hypertension.[1]

Interventions

Interventions include the following:

- Consider smaller fluid boluses, with reassessment for signs of fluid overload (increased work of breathing or crackles on auscultation of lung sounds) after every bolus.
- Consider early administration of packed red blood cells to maintain adequate tissue perfusion and oxygenation while correcting any coagulopathy.[39,63]
- If indicated, initiate hemorrhage control measures such as pressure dressings, a tourniquet, and vitamin K for control of internal and external bleeding if the patient takes any anticoagulant medications.[63]
- Trend endpoints of resuscitation as well as lactate and/or base deficit levels.
- Consider the use of thromboelastography, rotational thromboelastometry (TEG, ROTEM) in monitoring coagulation in patients with trauma-induced coagulopathy.[7,39,63]

Cardiac dysfunction may be the cause or the result of trauma in the older adult. Any complaint of chest pain warrants further investigation for either a pathophysiologic or a traumatic cause. When assessing the older adult patient, ask questions such as the following:

- Did the pain begin before the injury, possibly precipitating the injury?
- Did the pain begin directly after the trauma, possibly indicating tissue damage?
- Was there shortness of breath or any other symptoms before the chest pain?

D: Disability (Neurologic Status)

Head trauma can result in both acute and chronic subdural hematoma. Cerebral atrophy causes tension on the parasagittal bridging veins, making them more susceptible to rupture and increasing the risk for subdural hematoma even with minor trauma to the head. There is also an increased incidence of intracerebral hematomas among the older adult population, which may be caused by anticoagulant use.

Severe head injury with hypotension is associated with high mortality.[55] (See Chapter 7, "Head Trauma.") Cerebral atrophy causes increased space within the skull and allows bleeding to accumulate before the patient exhibits signs and symptoms of increased intracranial pressure. Consider the following factors:

- Maintain a high index of suspicion for bleeding to the brain.
- Consider the need for computed tomography of the brain early in the resuscitation.
- Continuously monitor the patient for signs of increased intracranial pressure.

Altered mental status in the older adult patient may have several possible causes aside from the traumatic injury. Changes in neurologic status require a full investigation to rule out the following conditions:

- Hypoglycemia
- Hypoxia
- Hyperthermia or hypothermia
- Anxiety, disorientation, agitation, and confusion
- Dementia or mental health issue

Delirium Interventions

Interventions include the following:

- If a head injury is suspected in the older adult, the trauma management is the same, and early computed tomography is recommended.
- Close monitoring and frequent reorientation are needed for the confused patient.

E: Exposure and Environmental Control

Older adults are at increased risk for hypothermia and resulting complications. As the adult ages, normal body temperature becomes more difficult to regulate (refer to Table 15-2). Factors contributing to the risk of compromised thermoregulation include the following:

- Loss of subcutaneous fat and thinning of the skin
- Decreased ability to sweat
- Neurologic changes
- Chronic cardiac or thyroid conditions
- Poor nutrition
- Psychotropic medications

The risk is increased when the older adult is exposed to temperature extremes at the site of the trauma or in the ED. Such a patient may present with either hypothermia or hyperthermia. When obtaining a history from the patient, family, or prehospital providers, identifying the location where the trauma occurred is important. For instance, determine whether there was prolonged extraction from a vehicle with exposure to high or low temperatures.

Hyperthermia should be considered, especially following a fall where exposure and environmental temperature are factors. Signs and symptoms of hyperthermia include the following[15]:

- Headache
- Vertigo
- Syncope
- Dehydration
- Rapid respirations
- Confusion
- Agitation
- Delirium
- Hallucinations
- Convulsions

Interventions

Because maintenance of normothermia is so important in the older adult trauma patient, regulate the ambient temperature in the trauma room as needed, apply warm blankets, and administer warmed intravenous fluid. When using mechanical warming devices, such as forced-air blankets or fluid warmers, monitor the temperature closely to avoid thermal burns to fragile skin.

Resuscitation Adjuncts

Resuscitation adjuncts include vital signs, laboratory studies, monitoring, and pain assessment and management.

F: Full Set of Vital Signs

In addition to comorbidities and medication history, baseline changes in respiration and pulse may be present in the older adult's vital signs.

G: Get Monitoring Devices and Give Comfort

Get the following resuscitation adjuncts.

L: Laboratory Studies

It is important to perform glucose (point-of-care testing), arterial blood gas (base excess), lactate, prothrombin time, partial thromboplastin time, and coagulation studies, along with the use of thromboelastography.[5,7,63] Use of anticoagulants and antiplatelet medications is common among older adults. Alcohol use and changes in the liver can affect clotting. An increased international normalized ratio has been associated with increased mortality in the older adult trauma patient.[7,28] Both an elevated lactate level (greater than 2) and an abnormal base deficit (less than −6) have been associated with major injury and mortality in trauma patients.[5,37]

M: Monitoring

An electrocardiogram may be indicated, particularly if the patient has a history of cardiac disease or chest trauma, or has since developed signs and symptoms of myocardial ischemia surrounding the traumatic event.

N: Nasogastric or Orogastric Tube

Consider the need for placement of a nasogastric or orogastric tube to evacuate stomach contents and relieve gastric distention. If the patient has been intubated, place a gastric tube to decrease gastric distention and increase diaphragmatic excursion. Consider additional interventions listed in Chapter 4.

O: Oxygenation and Ventilation

Pulse oximetry measures oxygenation, not ventilation. Consider weaning oxygen based on oximetry to avoid hyperoxia. Use end-tidal carbon dioxide monitoring for intubated or sedated patients to measure ventilation. Consider additional interventions listed in Chapter 4.

P: Pain Assessment and Management

The older adult trauma patient who is anxious, is confused, or has dementia may not be able to accurately report pain, so it is important for trauma nurses to assess behavioral cues, subtle signs of discomfort, and common pain responses to injuries. Older adults are frequently undermedicated because of the failure to appropriately assess them for pain, fear of overmedicating them, and lack of knowledge of pain medications.[28,57]

When using opioids for pain relief, consider the following:

- Obtain an accurate body weight before starting opioid administration, and calculate doses accordingly.
- Use of smaller doses is indicated. Remember to "start low, go slow."
- Monitor the patient closely for decreased respirations and blood pressure.
- Monitor any alteration in level of consciousness and any reports of dizziness.

Because some age-related compromise to the respiratory system is likely to exist in older adults, failure to aggressively manage pain from rib contusions and fractures may result in increased respiratory complications and disability.[1,44] According to the American College of Surgeons, "mortality risk increases for each additional rib fractured."[1(p221)]

Controlling pain in patients with fractured ribs is essential for preventing secondary complications (i.e., atelectasis, pneumonia, and even progression to chronic pain). Alternatives to opioid use in pain management include continuous intercostal nerve blocks for rib fractures using long-acting anesthetics. These nerve blocks can be placed safely in a patient who is anticoagulated.

Reevaluation

Reevaluation includes the following:

- Consider early transfer to a trauma center.
- If signs of internal hemorrhage are present, consider a focused assessment with sonography for trauma ultrasound and/or chest and/or pelvis radiograph.

Secondary Survey and Reevaluation

The secondary survey and additional diagnostics and interventions start with history.

H: History

For the older adult patient, a pertinent medical history is crucial. In addition to the findings in the primary survey, it is important that the trauma nurse ask pertinent questions about a patient's comorbidities and all current and recently discontinued medications. Include questions about multiple prescribers, compliance, or obstacles to taking prescribed medications. Discuss patient preferences for care and specific health outcome goals, including determining if the patient has completed an advance care directive.[31]

Comorbidities

As a result of advances in medicine, more adults are living longer with chronic diseases and comorbidities, sometimes necessitating the use of multiple medications. These comorbidities, as well as medication effects, affect the number and severity of complications, and the mortality and morbidity experienced by older patients.

Older adults may present with preexisting conditions, so it is important for the trauma nurse to consider their impact on patient assessment and interventions. Comorbidities may result in a cascade of effects, where one system impacts another, resulting in increased morbidity and mortality.[17,18]

Comorbid factors to be assessed in the older trauma patient who has experienced a fall include the following[17,18,44]:

- Acute problems
  - Cardiac disease, such as myocardial infarction or arrhythmia
  - Stroke
  - Postural hypotension
  - Hypovolemia
- Chronic problems
  - Neurologic disease, such as dementia or parkinsonism
  - Neuropathy
  - Balance problems that can occur post stroke or brain injury
  - Medication such as analgesics, antihistamines, anticoagulants, sleeping aids, or antidepressants

In addition to the aging process, comorbidities can decrease the physiologic reserves in the older adult trauma patient.[17,18,44] The body loses its ability to function above its basic level in times of stress. This may be the result of the sympathetic response being circumvented by cardiac disease, pacemakers, or medications. The inability to increase heart rate to compensate for decreased volume can conceal that a patient is hemorrhaging, so it is essential that the trauma nurse consider the complete presentation and history to obtain a true representation of the patient's condition.

Loss of physiologic reserve is a primary factor resulting in the following outcomes[17,18,44,54]:

- Increased complications
- Decreased independence
- Increased morbidity or mortality following a traumatic event

Medications

It is important to obtain a current list of medications, herbal supplements, recreational drugs, and over-the-counter medications that the patient is using and to consider their potential contributing and complicating effects[20]:

- Antihypertensives
  - Beta blockers: prevent the increase in heart rate that is an expected compensatory response in patients with hypovolemia, shock states, pain, or stress
- Antiplatelet medications: aspirin, adenosine diphosphate receptor (ADP)/P2Y inhibitors (e.g., clopidogrel, ticagrelor), or anticoagulants (e.g., warfarin, heparin, enoxaparin, apixaban, dabigatran, rivaroxaban)
  - These medications are the most frequently prescribed in the older adult[5,37,39] and increase the

possibility of intracranial, internal, or retroperitoneal bleeding.
- Diabetes medications: biguanides, dipeptidyl peptidase-4 (DPP-4) inhibitors, insulin, or glucagon-like peptides
    - If a patient is taking any diabetes medications, a change in the level of consciousness or mentation may be due to abnormal blood sugar levels.
- Medications that depress the central nervous system, such as opioids, benzodiazepines, anticholinergics, alcohol, and recreational drugs, may affect balance and judgment.
    - Check the patient for any medication patches.
    - Ask whether the patient has received any pain medications in the past or is currently on any pain medications.
        - If so, what was prescribed and how much, and how did the patient respond or react?
        - Did the medication cause excessive sedation?
        - What, if any, adverse effects did the patient experience?
    - Inquire about and observe for behaviors of misuse of a prescription and over-the-counter medication. Be sure to obtain an alcohol level and toxicology screen.
- Nitroglycerin
    - May increase injury risk due to decreased blood pressure.

H: Head-to-Toe Assessment
See Chapter 4 for comprehensive assessment information.

Urinary Catheter Considerations
Older adults are vulnerable to infections, and insertion of a urinary catheter increases the risk of a catheter-acquired urinary tract infection.[44] This type of infection is common and can result in more severe complications (i.e., sepsis, prostatitis and epididymitis in males, pyelonephritis, endocarditis, and increased length of stay) in the older adult population. If a urinary catheter is clinically indicated, it should be discontinued as soon as possible.[44] Consider alternative methods of output measurement before inserting a urinary catheter.[23]

I: Inspect Posterior Surfaces
To help prevent pressure sores and decrease the discomfort associated with being immobilized on a spine board, expedite removing the board. If not done earlier, this can be done when inspecting the posterior if there are no contraindications to logrolling. If logrolling the patient is contraindicated because of potential unstable spine, pelvis, or other injuries, alternate methods to move the patient include air-assisted mattresses and the 6-plus lift-and-slide.[22,48] In the older adult, even 30–45 minutes of lying on a spine board can cause skin breakdown.[25,26] Physiologic changes due to osteoporosis, osteoarthritis, and kyphosis increase the discomfort of the rigid spine board in older adults, and the loss of subcutaneous fat and thinning of the skin with aging means that they have less padding. The skin's blood vessels are more fragile, resulting in easier bruising, bleeding under the skin, and skin tears in the older adult. Once off the board, frequent turning may help to prevent the formation of pressure sores.

Reevaluation and Post-Resuscitation Care

The older adult has limited physiologic reserves; frequent reassessments are important to quickly identify any changes in vital signs, pain, injuries, and the effectiveness of any interventions implemented that may indicate a deterioration in their condition. Reassessment of the primary survey is also of the upmost importance in this population.

Definitive Care or Transport

Two important topics related to definitive care or transport of the older adult trauma patient are the relationship between length of stay and adverse events and the risk of rib fractures.

Length of Stay and Adverse Events
Increased length of stay in the ED has been associated with worse outcomes and increased mortality across all trauma patient populations, but in the older adult trauma patient, ED boarding is more likely to result in an adverse event.[18,30,41] Older adults tend to take more medications and have more comorbidities, and these factors increase the risk of an adverse event.

Rib Fractures
Blunt chest trauma from falls, MVCs, and assault are common sources of rib fractures in older adults, whose morbidity and mortality increase with each additional rib fractured.[1] In the older adult, first rib fractures, bilateral rib fractures, pneumothorax, or hemothorax are associated with increased morbidity, while bilateral pneumothoraces and more than five rib fractures are associated with increased mortality.[44] The number of rib fractures also increases the likelihood of pneumonia, hypoventilation, pneumothorax, and respiratory failure.[17]

Older adults with rib fractures may be discharged from the ED with mild oral analgesia and an incentive spirometer. Many of these individuals develop pulmonary complications because of tenderness around the injured area and pain during movement, coughing, and/or breathing. These complications can be seen within 48–72 hours post injury because of inadequate respiratory effort; they lead to increased work of breathing, atelectasis, and an inability to clear secretions.[6] Given this risk, it is imperative that analgesia for rib fracture be started early, not just for pain management and patient comfort, but also as an attempt to prevent the complications that may follow over the subsequent days. Pain management may consist of the following:

- Simple analgesia: nonsteroidal anti-inflammatory drug, either oral or transdermal
- Lidocaine transdermal patches (also can be purchased as over-the-counter products)
- An opioid alone or in conjunction with the nonsteroidal anti-inflammatory drug
- Regional anesthetic (thoracic epidural)
- Continuous intercostal nerve block with the use of a pump, which has been found to decrease hospital length of stay (**Figure 15-3**)[6]
- Operative fixation for multiple rib fractures[17]

Elder Maltreatment

Maltreatment of older adults is defined by the Centers for Disease Control and Prevention as "an intentional act or failure to act that causes or creates a risk of harm to an older adult."[13] This includes neglect and physical, sexual, emotional, psychological, or financial abuse; older adults often experience more than one type of abuse.[13,49] It is estimated that 1 out of 10 older adults living at home and who are 60 years of age and older have experienced abuse or neglect.[13,29] The ED is in a unique position to identify and intervene for victims of elder abuse; however, maltreatment of older adults often goes undetected.[49]

Suspected maltreatment is reported according to the protocol established by the individual facility and jurisdiction. In the United States, healthcare workers are

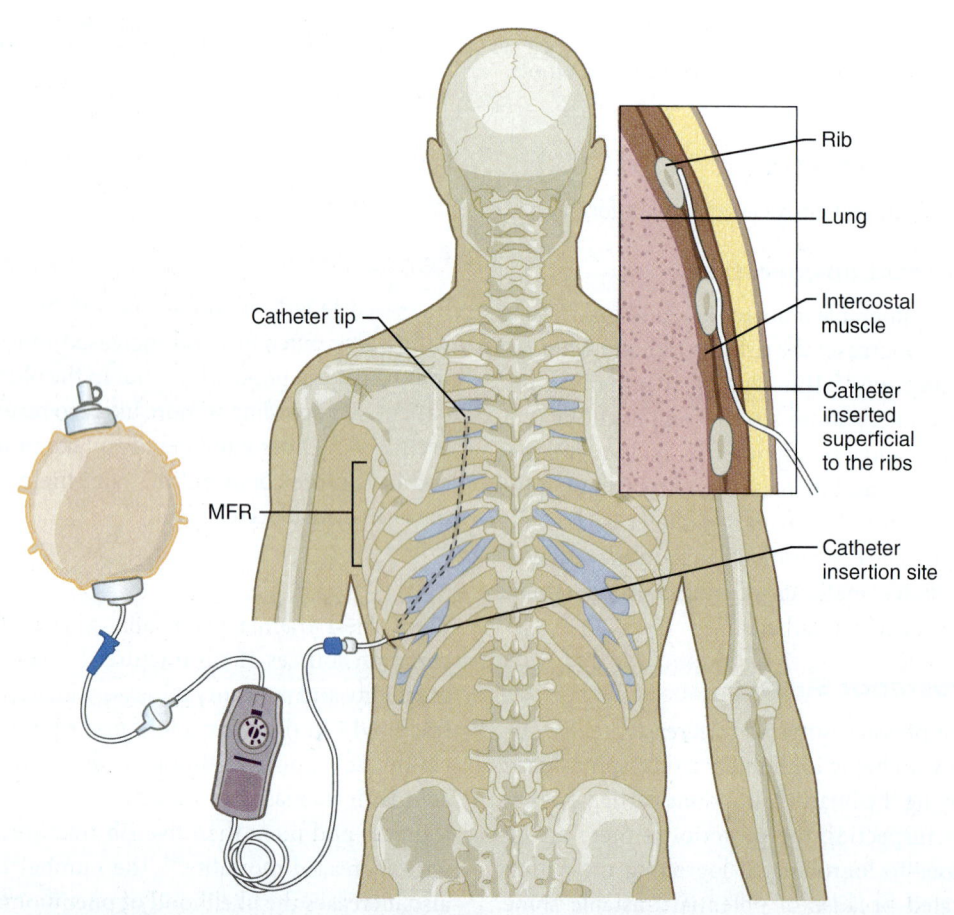

Figure 15-3 *Continuous intercostal nerve block system.*

mandated reporters of suspected abuse. When assessing older adults, completely undress the patient and assess for any of the following signs of physical abuse or neglect[49]:

- Bruising in unusual locations
- Burns
- Multiple fractures
- Markings or scars to the wrist or ankle areas
- Bald patches or hematomas to the scalp
- Subconjunctival bleeding
- Soft tissue injuries in the mouth
- Genital or rectal injury
- Dehydration
- Malnutrition
- Pressure injuries/decubitus
- Poor hygiene and/or dirty clothing

Other possible indicators of maltreatment include the following:

- Injury inconsistent with history
- Unexplained injuries
- Frequent ED visits
- Care sought from multiple physicians or EDs
- Delay in seeking care (injury or illness)
- Caregiver describes patient as "accident prone"

Victim risk factors for maltreatment include[56]:

- Chronic illness
- Physical disability
- Functional impairment
- Mental health impairments
- Substance misuse
- Dependency on others (physical, financial, emotional)
- Ineffective coping mechanisms
- Self-neglect
- Previous abuse by a person(s) other than the current perpetrator
- Serious problems with relationships, including with the perpetrator

See Chapter 17, "Interpersonal Violence," for more information regarding maltreatment of the older adult.

Emerging Trends

The increasing population of older adults poses significant challenges for the available healthcare resources.

Promotion of geriatric-focused emergency medicine services and EDs is a challenge for ED providers. A few of these challenges facing dedicated geriatric EDs relate to ED staffing, training, and education; availability of validated screening tools; and sustained support from the hospital administration.[51] Older patients do not come in just with a chief complaint, but often have comorbidities that may need to be addressed. In addition, functional limitations in this population may be a challenge upon presentation to the ED. Social issues can be very challenging but must be addressed upon discharge. These factors, if not taken into account, may send the patient into a trajectory that leads back to the ED in the form of readmission.

As we address some of these challenges, we will describe what a geriatric ED should look like. Following are five essentials that need to be thought through when designing a "geriatric-friendly" ED[45]:

1. Design the right physical setting.
    a. Include special furniture, equipment, and visual elements:
        i. Nonskid and nonglare floors
        ii. Pressure-reducing mattresses
        iii. Quieter areas
        iv. Low beds
        v. Extra glasses to be able to read forms
2. Build an interdisciplinary team to address some of the complex issues with which these patients present.
3. Hone the screening and triage processes.
    a. Screen for dementia, delirium, and geriatric syndromes. Recognizing delirium among older adult ED patients is challenging, however.
    b. Screening instruments include the following:
        i. The modified Confusion Assessment Method for the Emergency Department (mCAM-ED) tool to assess delirium in the ED. It can be used to assess patients with and without dementia and applies a minimal screening and assessment burden on the patient.[27]
        ii. Patient vulnerability assessment tool.
        iii. Stop and watch tool (used in assisted living but can easily be used at triage).[32]
        iv. **SPICES** (**S**kin integrity, **P**roblems eating, **I**ncontinence, **C**onfusion, **E**vidence of falls, **S**leep disturbance)—a screening tool for frailty risks.[3]
4. Provide a robust geriatric training/educational program for all providers.
5. Be vigilant about metrics. Monitor hospital admission rates, readmission rates, transfers, patient outcomes, and patient experience.

Other Trends

The use of telehealth can improve transitions of care from a facility to home. Telehealth can offer immediate virtual rounding that takes place while a home health nurse or therapist is visiting with a patient. These collaborative "virtual visits" can improve teamwork between agencies and primary care physicians while improving the patient experience and decreasing readmission rates.

Interpersonal violence advocates are bringing visibility to maltreatment experienced by older adults. June 15 has been designated as the international World Elder Abuse Day. This day brings awareness to some of the obstacles and challenges that elder abuse patients face.[59] The National Clearinghouse on Abuse in Later Life (NCALL) has a course that deals with some of the challenges that elder abused individuals face when seeking shelter[53]:

- Misalignment between the older survivors' needs and traditional safety planning
- True peer advocacy for older adults who find that they are the only survivors of their age group in the program
- Accessibility and restrictive policies

Summary

Age-related changes can complicate the assessment of the older adult trauma patient. Presence of comorbidities and the individual response to illness and injury make each patient unique. Failure to recognize the impact of those age-related changes, acknowledge the patient's medications and history, and understand the older adult's response to physical and emotional stress can result in poorer outcomes. For an older adult with multiple injuries, early consideration of transfer to a trauma center may reduce mortality and morbidity.

References

1. American College of Surgeons. (2018). Geriatric trauma. In *Advanced trauma life support* (10th ed., pp. 214–224).
2. American College of Surgeons. (2022). *Resources for optimal care of the injured patient: 2022 standards*. https://www.facs.org/~/media/files/quality%20programs/trauma/ntdb/ntdb%20annual%20report%202016.ashx
3. Aronow, H. U., Borenstein, J., Haus, F., Braunstein, G. D., & Bolton, L. B. (2014). Validating SPICES as a screening tool for frailty risks among hospitalized older adults. *Nursing Research and Practice*, Article 846759. http://doi.org/10.1155/2014/846759
4. Baltazar, G. A., Bassett, P., Pate, A. J., & Chendrasekhar, A. (2017). Older patients have increased risk of poor outcomes after low-velocity pedestrian–motor vehicle collisions. *Pragmatic and Observational Research, 8*, 43–47. https://doi.org/10.2147%2FPOR.S127710
5. Bar-Or, D., Salottolo, K. M., Orlando, A., Mains, C. W., Bourg P., & Offner, P. J. (2013). Association between a geriatric trauma resuscitation protocol using venous lactate measurements and early trauma surgeon involvement and mortality risk. *Journal of the American Geriatrics Society, 61*, 1358–1364. https://doi.org/10.1111/jgs.12365
6. Britt, T., Sturm, R., Ricardi, R., & Labond, V. (2015). Comparative evaluation of continuous intercostal nerve block or epidural analgesia on the rate of respiratory complications, intensive care unit, and hospital stay following traumatic rib fractures: A retrospective review. *Local and Regional Anesthesia, 8*, 79–84. https://doi.org/10.2147/LRA.S80498
7. Calland, J. F., Ingraham, A. M., Martin, N., Marshall, G. T., Schulman, C. L., Stapleton, T., & Barraco, R. D. (2012). Evaluation and management of geriatric trauma: An Eastern Association for the Surgery of Trauma practice management guideline. *Journal of Trauma Acute and Care Surgery, 73*, S345–S350. https://doi.org/10.1097/TA.0b013e318270191f
8. Carter, B., Short, R., Bouamra, O., Parry, F., Shipway, D., Thompson, J., Baxter, M., Lecky, F., & Braude, P. (2022). A national study of 23 major trauma centres to investigate the effect of frailty on clinical outcomes in older people admitted with serious injury in England (IFiTR1): A multicenter observational study. *The Lancet: Healthy Longevity, 3*, e540–e548. https://doi.org/10.1016/S2666-7568(22)00122-2
9. Caterino, J. M., Valasek, T., & Werman, H. A. (2010). Identification of an age cutoff for increased mortality in patients with elderly trauma. *The American Journal of Emergency Medicine, 28*(2), 151–178. https://doi.org/10.1016/j.ajem.2008.10.027
10. Centers for Disease Control and Prevention (n.d.). *10 leading causes of nonfatal emergency department visits, United States, 2020*. https://wisqars.cdc.gov/nonfatal-leading
11. Centers for Disease Control and Prevention. (n.d.). *Common injuries as we age*. https://www.cdc.gov/stillgoingstrong/about/common-injuries-as-we-age.html
12. Centers for Disease Control and Prevention. (n.d.). *Facts about falls*. https://www.cdc.gov/homeandrecreationalsafety/falls/adultfalls.html
13. Centers for Disease Control and Prevention (n.d.). *Fast facts: Preventing elder abuse*. https://www.cdc.gov/violenceprevention/elderabuse/fastfact.html
14. Centers for Disease Control and Prevention. (n.d.). *Older adult drivers*. https://www.cdc.gov/transportationsafety/older_adult_drivers/index.html
15. Centers for Disease Control and Prevention. (n.d.). *Warning signs and symptoms of heat-related illness*. https://www.cdc.gov/disasters/extremeheat/warning.html#text
16. Chang, M. C. (Ed.). (2016). *The National Trauma Data Bank 2016 annual report*. American College of Surgeons. https://www.facs.org/~/media/files/quality%20programs/trauma/ntdb/ntdb%20annual%20report%202016.ashx
17. Clare, D., & Zink, K. (2021). Geriatric trauma. *Emergency Medicine Clinics of North America, 39*(2), 257–271. https://doi.org/10.1016/j.emc.2021.01.002
18. Colwell, C. (2021). Geriatric trauma: Initial evaluation and management. *UpToDate*. Retrieved August 29, 2022, from

https://www.uptodate.com/contents/geriatric-trauma-initial-evaluation-and-management?search=Geriatric%20trauma:%20Initial%20evaluation%20and%20management&source=search_result&selectedTitle=1~150&usage_type=default&display_rank=1

19. Crandall, M., Streams, J., Duncan, T., Mallet, A., Greene, W., Violano, P., Christmas, A. B., Barraco, R., & Eastern Association for the Surgery of Trauma Injury Control and Violence Prevention Committee. (2015). Motor vehicle collision-related injuries in the elderly: An Eastern Association for the Surgery of Trauma evidence-based review of risk factors and prevention. *Journal of Trauma and Acute Care Surgery, 79*, 152–158. https://doi.org/10.1097/TA.0000000000000677

20. Dalton, T., Rushing, M. R., Escott, M. E. A., & Monroe, B. J. (2015). Complexities of geriatric patients. *Journal of Emergency Medical Services, 40*(11). https://www.jems.com/patient-care/complexities-of-geriatric-trauma-patients/

21. Deprey, S. M., Biedrzycki, L., & Klenz, K. (2017). Identifying characteristics and outcomes that are associated with fall-related fatalities: Multi-year retrospective summary of fall deaths in older adults from 2005–2012. *Injury Epidemiology, 4*(21). https://doi.org/10.1186%2Fs40621-017-0117-8

22. Emergency Nurses Association. (2016). *Avoiding the log roll maneuver: Alternative methods for safe patient handling* [Topic brief]. https://enau.ena.org/Users/LearningActivity/LearningActivityDetail.aspx?LearningActivityID=LJMRSp85WwPew%2bHMK6%2b5YQ%3d%3d

23. Galen, B. T. (2015). Underpad weight to estimate urine output in adult patients with urinary incontinence. *Journal of Geriatric Cardiology, 12*(2), 189–190. http://www.jgc301.com/en/article/doi/10.11909/j.issn.1671-5411.2015.02.016

24. Gurwell, M. (2018, January 7). The role of exercise in older driver safety. *The Legal Examiner*. http://www.legalexaminer.com/automobile-accidents/the-role-of-exercise-in-older-driver-safety-2/

25. Ham, W., Schoonhoven, L., Schuurmans, M. J., & Leenen, L. (2014). Pressure ulcers from spinal immobilization in trauma patients: A systematic review. *Journal of Trauma and Acute Care Surgery, 76*(4), 1131–1141. https://doi.org/10.1097/TA.0000000000000153

26. Ham, W., Schoonhoven, L., Schuurmans, M. J., & Leenen, L. (2017). Pressure ulcers in trauma patients with suspected spine injury: A prospective cohort study with emphasis on device-related pressure ulcers. *International Wound Journal, 14*(1), 104–111. https://doi.org/10.1111/iwj.12568

27. Hasemann, W., Grossmann, F. F., Stadler, R., Bingisser, R., Breil, D., Hafner, M., Kressig, R. W., & Nickel, C. H. (2018). Screening and detection of delirium in older ED patients: Performance of the modified Confusion Assessment Method for the Emergency Department (mCAM-ED): A two-step tool. *Internal and Emergency Medicine, 13*, 915–922. https://doi.org/10.1007/s11739-017-1781-y

28. Hogas, A. L., Grall, M., & Hoon, S. L (2016). Pain management. In M. Boltz, E. Capezuti, T. Fulmer, & D. Zwicker (Eds.), *Evidence-based geriatric nursing protocols for best practice* (5th ed., pp. 263–282). Springer.

29. Hoover, R. M., & Pollson, M. (2014). Detecting elder abuse and neglect: Assessment and intervention. *American Family Physician, 89*(6), 453–460. https://www.aafp.org/afp/2014/0315/p453.html

30. Hymel, G., Leskovan, J. J., Thomas, Z., Greenbaum, J., & Ledrick, D. (2020). Emergency department boarding of non-trauma patients adversely affects trauma patient length of stay. *Cureus, 12*(9), Article e10354. https://doi.org/10.7759/cureus.10354

31. Institute for Healthcare Improvement. (2022). *Age-friendly health systems: Guide to recognition for geriatric emergency department accredited sites*. https://forms.ihi.org/hubfs/Guide%20to%20Recognition%20for%20GEDA%20Sites_FINAL.pdf

32. Interact Assisted Living. (2014). *Stop and watch: Early warning tool*. Pathway Health. https://pathway-interact.com/download/stop-and-watch-early-warning-tool-3/

33. Joseph, B., & Scalea, T. (2020). The consequences of aging on the response to injury and critical illness. *Shock, 54*(2), 144–153. https://doi.org/10.1097/SHK.0000000000001491

34. Jubert, P., Lonjon, G., Garreau de Loubresse, C., & Bone and Joint Trauma Study Group. (2013). Complications of upper cervical spine trauma in elderly subjects: A systematic review of the literature. *Orthopaedics & Traumatology: Surgery & Research, 99*(Suppl. 6), S301–S312. https://doi.org/10.1016/j.otsr.2013.07.007

35. Lee, A., Lee, K. W., & Khang, P. (2013). Preventing falls in the geriatric population. *Permanente Journal, 17*(4), 37–39. https://doi.org/10.7812%2FTPP%2F12-119

36. Lee, S. Y., Shih, S. C., Leu, Y. S., Chang, Y. H., Lin, H. C., & Ku, H. C. (2017). Implications of age-related changes in anatomy for geriatric-focused difficult airways. *International Journal of Gerontology, 11*(3), 130–133. https://doi.org/10.1016/j.ijge.2016.11.003

37. Levine, M., & Alkhawan, L. (2016, August 21). Geriatric trauma and medical illness: Pearls and pitfalls. *emDOCs*. http://www.emdocs.net/geriatric-trauma-medical-illness-pearls-pitfalls/

38. Lukaszyk, C., Harvey, L., Sherrington, C., Keay, L., Tiedemann, A., Coombes, J., Clemson, L., & Iver, R. (2016). Risk factors, incidence, consequences and prevention strategies for falls and fall-injury within older indigenous populations: A systematic review. *Australian and New Zealand Journal of Public Health, 40*(6), 564–568. https://doi.org/10.1111/1753-6405.12585

39. Mador, B., Nascimento, B., Hollands, S., & Rizoli, S. (2017). Blood transfusion and coagulopathy in geriatric trauma patients. *Scandinavian Journal of Trauma Resuscitation and Emergency Medicine, 25*, Article 33. https://doi.org/10.1186/s13049-017-0374-0

40. Mondor, E. E. (2022). Trauma. In L. D. Urden, K. M. Stacy, & M. E. Lough (Eds.), *Critical care nursing: Diagnosis and management* (9th ed., pp. 791–830). Elsevier.

41. Morley, C., Unwin, M., Peterson, G. M., Stankovich, J., & Kinsman, L. (2018). Emergency department crowding: A systematic review of causes, consequences and solutions. *PLoS One, 13*(8). Article e0203316. https://doi.org/10.1371/journal.pone.0203316

42. National Safety Council. (2022). *Road users: Older drivers*. https://injuryfacts.nsc.org/motor-vehicle/road-users/older-drivers/
43. Navaratnarajah, A., & Jackson, S. H. D. (2017). The physiology of ageing. *Medicine, 45*(1), 6–9. https://doi.org/10.1016/j.mpmed.2016.10.008
44. Plummer, E. (2020). Trauma in the elderly. In K. A. McQuillan & M. B. Flynn Makic (Eds.), *Trauma nursing: From resuscitation through rehabilitation* (5th ed., pp. 705–718). Elsevier.
45. Ponte, M. (2016, May 17). *5 essentials of a geriatric emergency department*. HealthLeaders. https://www.healthleadersmedia.com/clinical-care/5-essentials-geriatric-emergency-department?page=0%2C5
46. Rao, P. J., Pha, K., Mobbs, R. J., Wilson, D., & Ball, J. (2016). Cervical spine immobilization in the elderly population. *Journal of Spine Surgery, 2*(1), 41–46. https://www.ncbi.nlm.nih.gov/pmc/articles/PMC5039838/pdf/jss-02-01-041.pdf
47. Rivera Drew, J. A., & Xu, D. (2020). Trends in fatal and nonfatal injuries among older Americans. *American Journal of Preventive Medicine, 59*(1), 3–11. https://doi.org/10.1016/j.amepre.2020.01.008
48. Rodrigues, I. F. (2017). To log-roll or not to log-roll—That is the question! A review of the use of the log-roll for patients with pelvic fractures. *International Journal of Orthopaedic and Trauma Nursing, 27*, 36–40. https://doi.org/10.1016/j.ijotn.2017.05.001
49. Rosen, T., Stern, M. E., Elman, A., & Mulcare, M. R. (2018). Identifying and initiating intervention for elder abuse and neglect in the emergency department. *Clinics in Geriatric Medicine, 34*(3), 435–451. https://doi.org/10.1016/j.cger.2018.04.007
50. Sadro, C. T., Sandstrom, C. K., Verma, N., & Gunn, M. L. (2015). Geriatric trauma: A radiologist's guide to imaging trauma patients aged 65 years and older. *RadioGraphics, 35*(4), 1263–1285. https://doi.org/10.1148/rg.2015140130
51. Schumacher, J. G., Hirshon, J., Hogan, T., Magidson, P., & Chrisman, M. (2017). Trends in geriatric emergency medicine for older adult patients. *Innovation in Aging, 1*(Suppl. 1), 111. https://doi.org/10.1093/geroni/igx004.461
52. Sklar, A. L., Boissoneault, J., Fillmore, M. T., & Nixon, S. J. (2014). Interaction between age and moderate alcohol effects on simulated driving performance. *Psychopharmacology, 231*(3), 557–566. https://doi.org/10.1007/s00213-013-3269-4
53. Slye, S., & Brandl, B. (2017, June 14). *Recognizing the emergency housing & shelter needs of older survivors on World Elder Abuse Awareness Day*. National Network to End Domestic Violence. https://nnedv.org/latest_update/housing-shelter-world-elder-abuse/
54. Smith, C. M., & Cotter, V. T. (2016). Age-related changes in health. In M. Boltz, E. Capezuti, T. Fulmer, & D. Zwicker (Eds.), *Evidence-based geriatric nursing protocols for best practice* (5th ed., pp. 23–42). Springer.
55. Spaite, D. W., Hu, C., Bobrow, B. J., Chikani, V., Sherrill, D., Barnhart, B., Gaither, J. B., Denninghoff, K. R., Viscusi, C., Mullins, T., & Adelson, P. D. (2017). Mortality and prehospital blood pressure in patients with major traumatic brain injury: Implications for the hypotension threshold. *JAMA Surgery, 152*(4), 360–368. https://doi.org/10.1001/jamasurg.2016.4686
56. Storey, J. E. (2020). Risk factors for elder abuse and neglect: A review of the literature. *Aggression and Violent Behavior, 50*, Article 101339. https://doi.org/10.1016/j.avb.2019.101339
57. Tabije-Ebuen, M. (2018). Evaluation of knowledge and attitudes by healthcare providers regarding pain in the ED and ICU. *International Journal of Anesthesia and Relaxation, 2*(3), 19–32. https://www.biocoreopen.org/ijar/Evaluation-of-Knowledge-and-Attitudes-by-HealthCare-Providers-Regarding-Pain-in-the-ED-and-ICU.php
58. Uribe-Leitz, T., Jarman, M. P., Sturgeons, D. J., Harlow, A. F., Lipsitz, S. R., Cooper, Z., Salim, A., Newgard, C. D., & Haider, A. H. (2020). National study of triage and access to trauma centers for older adult. *Annals of Emergency Medicine, 75*(2), 125–135. https://doi.org/10.1016/j.annemergmed.2019.06.018
59. USC Center for Elder Justice. (n.d.). *World Elder Abuse Awareness Day*. University of Southern California. https://eldermistreatment.usc.edu/weaad-home/
60. U.S. Department of Transportation National Highway Traffic Safety Administration. (2022). *Traffic safety facts: 2020 data*. https://crashstats.nhtsa.dot.gov/Api/Public/ViewPublication/813294
61. Vaishya, R., & Vaish, A. (2020). Falls in older adults are serious. *Indian Journal of Orthopaedics, 54*, 69–74. https://doi.org/10.1007/s43465-019-00037-x
62. Verma, S. K., Willetts, J. L., Corns, H. L., Marucci-Wellman, H. R., Lombardi, D. A., & Courtney, T. K. (2016). Falls and fall-related injuries among community-dwelling adults in the United States. *PLoS One, 11*(3), Article e0150939. https://doi.org/10.1371/journal.pone.0150939
63. Wise, R., Faurie, M., Malbrain, M., & Hodgson, E. (2017). Strategies for intravenous fluid resuscitation in trauma patients. *World Journal of Surgery, 41*, 1170–1183. https://doi.org/10.1007/s00268-016-3865-7
64. Wongrakpanich, S., Kallis, C., Prasad, P., Rangaswami, J., & Rosenzweig, A. (2018). The study of rhabdomyolysis in the elderly: An epidemiological study and single center experience. *Aging and Disease, 9*(1), 1–7. https://doi.org/10.14336%2FAD.2017.0304
65. World Health Organization. (2021). *Fact sheet: Aging and health*. https://www.who.int/news-room/fact-sheets/detail/ageing-and-health
66. Ziegenhain, F., Scherer, J., Kalbas, Y., Neuhas, V., Lefering, R., Teuben, M., Sprengel, K., Pape, H. C., Jensen, K. O., & Trauma Register DGU. (2021). Age-dependent patient and trauma characteristics and hospital resource requirements—Can improvement be made? An analysis from the German Trauma Registry. *Medicina, 57*(4), Article 330. https://doi.org/10.3390%2Fmedicina57040330

CHAPTER 16

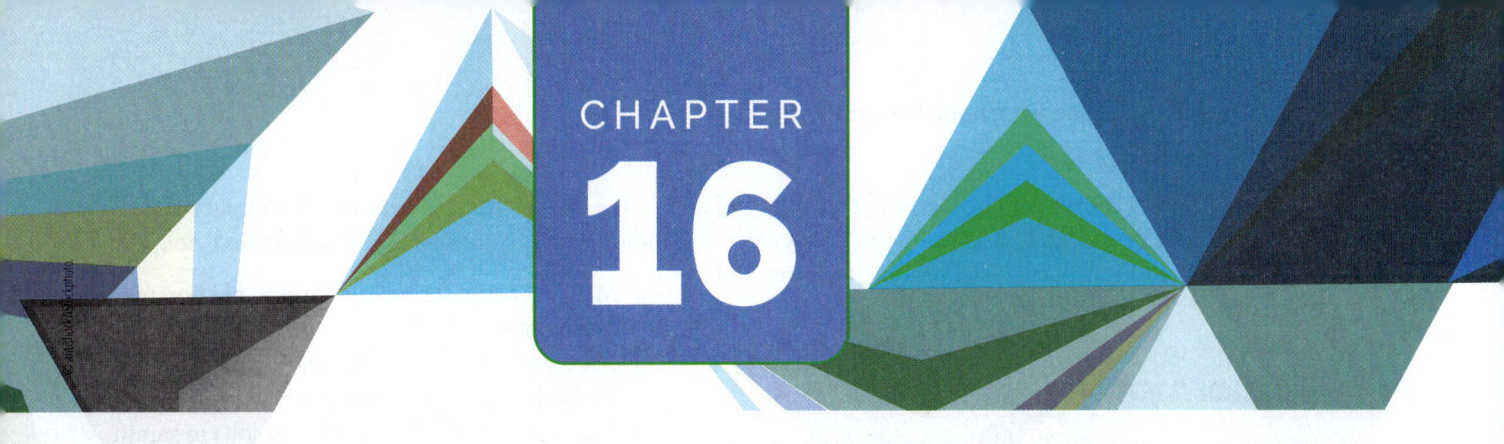

The Pregnant Trauma Patient

Judy Stevenson, DNP, APRN-CNS, ACCNS-AG, RN-BC, CCRN, CEN, CSRN, CPEN, TCRN, NH DP-BC

OBJECTIVES

Upon completion of this chapter, the learner will be able to:
1. Describe mechanisms of injury associated with the pregnant trauma patient and fetus.
2. Describe physiologic and developmental changes as a basis for assessment of the pregnant trauma patient and fetus.
3. Identify potential complications for the pregnant trauma patient.
4. Demonstrate the nursing assessment of the pregnant trauma patient and fetus.
5. Plan appropriate interventions for the pregnant trauma patient and fetus.
6. Evaluate the effectiveness of nursing interventions for the pregnant trauma patient and fetus.

Introduction

Trauma is a leading cause of death for women of reproductive age and the leading cause of nonobstetric death in pregnant women across the globe.[8,20,33] Every woman of reproductive age should be considered pregnant until proved otherwise by a definitive pregnancy test or pelvic ultrasound.[8,18,21,29] Although there are unique considerations and issues for an injured woman during pregnancy, trauma resuscitation priorities for the injured pregnant and nonpregnant trauma patient remain the same.[8,38] Despite this recognition, studies have shown that healthcare providers erroneously deviate from standard trauma principles when caring for a pregnant trauma patient.[30] During the resuscitative phase of treatment, pregnancy should not limit or restrict any diagnostic or pharmacologic treatment.[6,29] Assessment of the pregnant trauma patient is complicated by maternal anatomic and physiologic adaptations designed to nourish the second patient, the fetus. Optimal resuscitation of the mother affords the best fetal outcome.[8,34,37] A multidisciplinary approach is necessary to optimize outcomes for both the mother and her fetus. It is important to access obstetric consultation early in the resuscitation process as the trauma team simultaneously manages two patients: the mother and the fetus. The Emergency Nurses Association and the Association of Women's Health, Obstetric and Neonatal Nurses, in a joint consensus statement, provide guidance for the emergency care of patients during pregnancy and the postpartum period, including recognition that emergency nurses require specialized education, training, and competencies in the care of this special population.[31]

Epidemiology

Trauma is not only the leading cause of death among women of childbearing age but also the leading non-obstetric cause of maternal death and disability during pregnancy.[13,19,20,24,33,34,38] It is estimated that 8% of all pregnancies are complicated by trauma,[3,30] with 50% of nonobstetric maternal mortalities due to trauma.[11]

Other important epidemiologic factors include the following:

- There is no single predictor of fetal outcomes, although some studies report maternal injury severity score, abdominal injury, presence of shock, gestational age, and coagulopathy as factors that can contribute.[34] Major trauma is associated with a 40–50% risk of fetal death.[24] Among maternal injuries resulting in fetal death, pelvic fracture is the most common.[24]
- Maternal hemorrhage and disseminated intravascular coagulation (DIC) can contribute to maternal death.[17,28]
- Pregnancy alters the pattern of injury, and the gravid patient is more prone to abdominal trauma as gestation progresses.[18]
- Hemorrhage is the leading cause of maternal death due to trauma.
- The most common cause of fetal death is maternal death.[8,24]
- Evidence suggests that premature delivery, low birth weight, and fetal demise are posttraumatic issues, even when the mother experiences minor injuries.[29,34,40] Minor trauma accounts for as many as 50% of fetal deaths related to trauma, emphasizing the importance of close monitoring.[36,38]
- Injured pregnant women are more likely to be hospitalized even when experiencing less severe injury.[33]
- The physiologic response of the mother is to maintain her own survival, even if this adversely impacts the fetus.[6]

Mechanisms of Injury and Biomechanics

Blunt trauma is responsible for the majority of maternal injuries and occurs 10 times more often in this population than penetrating trauma.[15,29]

The most common mechanisms of injury (MOIs) are motor vehicle collisions (MVCs), falls, and violence.[38,40]

- MVCs account for more than 50% of all traumas during pregnancy.[40]
- MVCs and penetrating trauma are responsible for the highest proportion of maternal deaths.[29]
- Penetrating abdominal trauma results in significantly higher fetal mortality compared with blunt trauma: 75% and 10%, respectively.[18]
- Approximately 1 in 4 pregnant women will fall, and most of these incidences will occur after 32 weeks' gestation; less than 10% cause serious injury to mother or fetus.[18,20]

The incidence of intentional injury from interpersonal violence rises during pregnancy, ultimately occurring in as many as 20% of all pregnancies.[38] Knowing the exact number of women experiencing interpersonal violence during pregnancy is difficult to ascertain because not all patients seek care from a healthcare provider or facility. Those who do present for care may have seemingly minor injuries such as lacerations, bruises, and welts.[18] However, homicide is "a common cause of trauma-associated death among pregnant and postpartum women today."[18(p639)] It is essential to screen all women; 10% of women killed were assaulted in the month before.[18] See Chapter 17, "Interpersonal Violence," for additional information. Additional research findings on violence during pregnancy include the following:

- Pregnant women are twice as likely to experience violent trauma as nonpregnant women.[15]
- Intimate partner violence may be more common during pregnancy than conditions women are routinely screened for, such as gestational diabetes or preeclampsia.[2,4]
- A leading cause of death during pregnancy and the postpartum period is homicide.[44]
- Gunshot wounds, stabbings, and strangulation are the most common mechanisms of injury associated with maternal death to due violence.[38]
- As the pregnancy progresses, the growing uterus is more likely to sustain injury by direct impact or penetrating trauma.[38]

The severity of violence may escalate during pregnancy or the postpartum period.[41] The potential for direct injury to the fetus increases with each trimester.[3]

- Blunt maternal abdominal trauma or pelvic fractures may cause fetal skull fractures and intracranial hemorrhage. Clavicle and long-bone injuries may also occur in utero. Abdominal trauma can

also be severe enough to cause placental rupture or abruption.
- Gunshot wounds to the maternal abdomen and uterus are frequently associated with fetal injury and death.

MOIs such as falls or MVCs might also be caused by pregnancy-related pathology (e.g., seizure from pregnancy-induced hypertension).[6]

The incorrect use of a seatbelt during pregnancy can contribute to injury. Not using a restraint presents a higher risk of premature delivery and fetal death.[8,35]

- Lap belt use alone, without the shoulder restraint, enables forward flexion and uterine compression, which can result in uterine rupture or abruptio placentae.
- A lap belt worn too high over the gravid uterus may produce uterine rupture from direct uterine force on impact. Lap and shoulder restraints together provide a reduction in the likelihood of fetal injury.[35]
- The lap seatbelt should be placed below the dome of the uterus to decrease risk of uterine injury.[35] The shoulder harness should be positioned across the clavicle and then between the breasts.[24]
- Airbag deployment does not appear to increase pregnancy-specific risks,[8] although airbag deployment predicts severity of the mechanism of trauma.

Anatomic and Physiologic Changes During Pregnancy as a Basis for Assessment Findings

Pregnancy causes major physiological changes and can alter anatomical relationship to nearly every organ system.[8,18,20] Anatomic and physiologic changes in pregnancy can confound the typical assessment findings associated with trauma. Understanding these changes is critical to the accurate assessment and evaluation of the pregnant trauma patient.

Cardiovascular Changes

Cardiovascular changes during pregnancy include the following:

- Pregnancy results in a hypervolemic, hyperdynamic state. Total blood volume increases, improving maternal tolerance to hemorrhage. The pregnant patient can lose as much as 30–40% (1,200–1,500 mL) of her circulating volume before a significant drop in blood pressure occurs.[18] Sudden and profound changes in vital signs can occur. Early signs of maternal hemorrhage may be reflected by signs of fetal distress.[8,18]
- Resting heart rate increases 10–20 beats/minute to help meet the increased metabolic demands of mother and fetus and results in increased cardiac output.[8,16] Cardiac output increases 20% by the eighth week of gestation and increases by 40% by weeks 20–28 of gestation.[18]
- Although patients with heart rates greater than 100 beats/minute should be assessed for shock and other possible causes of tachycardia,[6] it is of the utmost importance to recognize that shock due to hemorrhage may be present without tachycardia or hypotension.[16]
- Increased hormonal levels (estrogen, progesterone) cause vasodilation, resulting in a decrease in systemic vascular resistance and pulmonary vascular resistance.[8,18] Peripheral resistance decreases, causing a small decrease in systolic blood pressure and a more marked decrease in diastolic blood pressure. The pregnant patient in shock may appear warm and dry because of this vasodilation.
- Supine hypotension syndrome (aortocaval compression) may occur after 20 weeks' gestation as the aorta and inferior vena cava are compressed by the uterus and its contents when the patient is supine. Venous return decreases, and cardiac output falls by up to 30–40%.[16,29,37,38] The patient may report acute nausea and dizziness and appear pale and diaphoretic or hypotensive.[18]
- As the uterus becomes increasingly gravid, pushing the diaphragm upward, the heart muscle shifts slightly. This can result in electrocardiogram changes, which can be normal in pregnancy; these include atrial and ventricular ectopy, A waves and inverted T waves, ST segment depression, and left axis shift of QRS.[18]
- Increased blood flow to the uterus and placenta, and engorged pelvic vessels increase the risk of hemorrhage with maternal pelvic fractures.[24]
- Catecholamine-mediated vasoconstriction of uterine vessels in response to hemorrhage shunts blood to the mother and away from the fetus. Fetal hypoperfusion, evidenced by fetal tachycardia (greater than 160 beats/minute) or bradycardia (less than 120 beats/minute) and changes in fetal movement, can occur before signs of maternal shock become apparent.[8,18]

Respiratory Changes

Respiratory changes include the following:

- Hormonal changes result in ventilatory changes. Capillary engorgement of the upper respiratory

passages increases the risk of nasopharyngeal bleeding and upper airway obstruction.[18]
- Minute ventilation—the amount of air inhaled and exhaled in 1 minute—increases as respiratory rate increases and tidal volume decreases.[6,24]
- Oxygen consumption increases, and functional reserve capacity decreases as the gravid uterus compresses the bases of the lungs; this places the mother and fetus at increased risk for hypoxia.[37,43]
- As the gravid uterus presses on the diaphragm, functional residual capacity decreases. In turn, the pregnant patient breathes at a faster rate, decreasing the partial pressure of carbon dioxide (PCO_2) levels; this results in a state of respiratory alkalosis.[6,18]
- The diaphragm is pushed upward by the expanding uterus.[24]

Hematologic Changes

Hematologic changes include the following:

- By week 30 of pregnancy, the amount of circulating plasma has increased to 30–50% above its original volume, resulting in a dilutional or physiologic anemia and a proportional decrease in hematocrit.[6,8,18] Normal hemoglobin by term is 10–14 g/dL.[24]
- An increase in fibrinogen levels and clotting factors results in a hypercoagulable state that increases the risk for thromboembolism and DIC.[29,38]
- Pregnancy is a hypercoagulable state, which leads to increased risk of clot formation.[6,18]

Neurologic Changes

Eclampsia is a complication of late pregnancy that can result in neurologic changes, including seizures.[8] The enlarged uterus can cause compression of pelvic nerves or vascular stasis, leading to sensory changes in the lower extremities.

Gastrointestinal Changes

Gastrointestinal changes include the following:

- The abdominal organs are displaced laterally and cephalad by the enlarging uterus, so they lie in the upper abdomen.[8]
- The abdominal wall muscles are stretched and lax and may mask typical findings of guarding and rigidity.[8] Abdominal palpation is less reliable.
- Bowel sounds are less audible.
- The prolonged emptying time of the gastrointestinal tract increases the risk of aspiration.[6,29]
- An increase in gastric secretions makes the gravid patient more prone to gastric reflux, passive regurgitation, and aspiration. Gastric emptying is delayed.[18,29]

Renal and Genitourinary Changes

Renal changes include the following:

- Urinary stasis increases the risk for urinary tract infection.
- Urinary frequency increases because of the increase of renal blood flow and the resulting increased glomerular filtration rate.[8] The mother feels additional pressure as the uterus compresses the bladder.
- Serum creatinine and urea nitrogen decrease to approximately one-half of normal prepregnancy levels. During pregnancy, glycosuria is common.[8]
- As pregnancy progresses, the urinary bladder, which is attached to the wall of the uterus, elevates out of the pelvis, becoming an abdominal organ; its vulnerability to injury is thus increased.[8,18]

Reproductive Changes

Reproductive changes include the following:

- The production of amniotic fluid acts as a cushion to protect the fetus through the absorption of energy.
- Fetal heart rate normal range is 120–160 beats/minute.[8]
- The uterus remains an intrapelvic organ until approximately 12 weeks of gestation. By 20 weeks, the uterus is at the umbilicus, and between 34–36 weeks, it reaches the costal margin.[8]
- The uterus receives 20% of the patient's cardiac output during the third trimester. The cardiac output can be greatly influenced by the mother's position.[8] The pelvic vessels are engorged and can contribute to massive retroperitoneal bleeding following a pelvic injury from blunt trauma.[8]

Musculoskeletal Changes

Musculoskeletal changes include the following:

- Softening and relaxation of the sacral ligaments and pubic symphysis make the pelvis more flexible.
- The widening pelvis and heavy abdomen result in an unsteady gait and a change in the center of gravity, predisposing the patient to falls.[12]
- Musculoskeletal changes during pregnancy contribute to a propensity for orthopedic injuries.[40]

Selected Injuries and Emergencies

The selected injuries and emergencies of the pregnant patient and fetus discussed here include preterm labor, abruptio placentae, uterine rupture, and maternal cardiopulmonary arrest/fetal delivery.

Abdominal and Pelvic Injuries

The bowel is somewhat protected in blunt abdominal trauma because uterine placement pushes it into the upper abdomen. In penetrating trauma to the upper abdomen during late gestation, complex intestinal injury can occur. Clinical signs of peritoneal irritation are less evident in pregnant women, so abdominal exams may provide less information.[8,34] Additionally, the uterine walls become thinner, and the uterus and its contents (placenta and fetus) are more vulnerable to injury.[24] Amniotic fluid embolism is a rare but catastrophic and often fatal event that may present as cardiopulmonary collapse, an anaphylaxis-type reaction, and/or right or left heart failure.[18] In the third trimester, the fetal head is often positioned into the pelvis. Pelvic fractures can result in fetal skull fracture or serious intracranial injury to the fetus.[8] Fetal mortality is 35% in the presence of a maternal pelvic fracture.[24] The risk of hemorrhage following a pelvic fracture is increased because of dilated pelvic vasculature.[24] The risk of bladder injury is also increased because it rises out of the pelvis during pregnancy.[6]

Preterm Labor

Preterm labor is the most common obstetric complication in the pregnant trauma patient, occurring in as many as 25% of patients.[24] Contractions are experienced by up to 40% of women who are alert but may go undetected in unconscious or intubated patients.[24] Common causes of preterm labor include placental abruption, hypoxia, and hypovolemia.[24] Assessment findings for preterm labor include the following:

- More than six uterine contractions per hour
- Abdominal or low back pain, pressure, or cramping
- Vaginal bloody show or bleeding
- Passage of mucous plug
- Rupture of amniotic membranes
- Cervical dilation and/or effacement

Interventions for preterm labor include ongoing monitoring of fetal heart rate and uterine contractions, admission or transfer to a tertiary care unit, and neonatology consultation.[3,43] Tocolytic agents such as magnesium sulfate or terbutaline may be effective in halting preterm labor in the hemodynamically stable patient; however, caution should be used because contractions may be a result of less obvious maternal instability.[18] Tocolytic agents are contraindicated in the presence of placental abruption.[3] With preterm labor or high risk of preterm labor at 24 or more weeks' gestation, the administration of betamethasone for fetal lung maturation is considered, even with minor trauma.[38,43] If rupture of membranes occurs, the nurse will need to document the date and time of rupture. Note the amount, color, odor, and presence of meconium in the amniotic fluid. Communicate these findings in any handoff report on the patient.[18]

Abruptio Placentae

Abruptio placentae, or placental abruption, is the premature separation of a portion of the placenta from the uterine wall. This disrupts maternal–fetal circulation, interrupting oxygen supply to the fetus.[18] In the later stages of pregnancy, the placenta loses elasticity, which may contribute to abruptio placentae.[3] Acceleration/deceleration forces can shear the relatively inelastic placenta from the elastic uterus, resulting in abruption.[40] Abruptio placentae most commonly occurs in the second or third trimester and is the second most common cause of fetal death in the pregnant patient.[18] The effects on the fetus depend on the amount of functional placenta that remains attached to the uterine wall. Even minor injuries can result in abruptio placentae.[8] Any blunt abdominal trauma places the pregnant patient at risk for an abruption. Maternal mortality is low unless bleeding goes undetected[18]; however, 32% of fetal deaths were caused by placental abruption in a review of fetal demise associated with pelvic fractures.[24] Placental abruption may also cause premature labor.

Placental abruption may occur in as many as 50% of patients with major injuries.[24] Assessment findings for abruptio placentae include the following[8,18,23]:

- Dark red vaginal bleeding (the amount is variable and may be absent because of concealed hemorrhage). Bleeding occurs in up to 70% of cases.
- Abdominal or back pain (sudden onset, sharp, constant)
- Fetal distress (alteration in fetal heart rate and rhythm)
- Uterine irritability and rigidity with tetanic contractions (boardlike uterus)
- Preterm labor; frequent contractions
- Maternal shock presentation disproportionate to the amount of visible vaginal bleeding
- Rising fundal height
- DIC developing as late as 48 hours after the initial trauma

The classic triad of vaginal bleeding, abdominal pain, and uterine irritability associated with abruptio placentae may not be present in the trauma patient.[24] Trauma patients may have concealed abruption and may not exhibit vaginal bleeding or painful contractions. The edges of the placenta may enclose the bleeding internally.[24] A high degree of suspicion is warranted when the fetal heart rate is less than 110 beats/minute or greater than 160 beats/minute. Placental abruption is a clinical diagnosis.[22] A computed tomography (CT) scan should be considered in the evaluation of high-risk maternal trauma to evaluate for maternal and fetal injuries.[22] A CT may be more beneficial than an ultrasound because 40% of abruption hemorrhages are retroperitoneal.[45]

Interventions for placental abruption include close monitoring of maternal vital signs for a progressing shock condition, aggressive management of hypovolemic shock, ongoing monitoring of the fetal heart rate and uterine contractions, and admission or transfer to a tertiary care unit with appropriate consultations of obstetrics and neonatology providers. Sonography may be a possibility but is not considered a reliable test for placental abruption and should not delay treatment or transfer.[10] Serial coagulation studies will assist with recognizing DIC. In extreme cases, an emergent transfer to the operating room for cesarean section may improve maternal survival with a nonviable fetus or may improve maternal and fetal survival even if premature delivery becomes necessary.

Uterine Rupture

Actual tearing or laceration of the uterus is rare[42] but may occur in patients with extreme compression injury or with a history of prior cesarean sections. Uterine rupture is associated most commonly with blunt trauma to the abdomen and with pelvic fractures and injuries to the bladder.[18] It carries a high maternal and fetal mortality.[24,38]

Assessment findings for uterine rupture include the following[3,6,45]:

- Sudden onset of sharp abdominal or suprapubic pain
- Abdominal tenderness, guarding, rigidity, or rebound tenderness
- Asymmetry of the uterus
- Palpation of fetal parts
- Maternal shock
- Slowing or absent fetal heart tones
- Vaginal bleeding (may or may not be present)
- Radiograph may show extension of fetal extremities or abnormal fetal positioning

With uterine rupture, fetal survival is rare.[24,45] Aggressive shock management and emergent laparotomy with hemorrhage control are needed to improve the chance of maternal and fetal survival.[18,45] DIC is a complication of abruptio placentae and uterine rupture.[18,28]

Maternal Cardiopulmonary Arrest

Causes of maternal cardiac arrest for the pregnant trauma patient most often include hemorrhage or hypoxia, but they can result from any trauma-related causes. It is both a medical and surgical emergency. Decision-making depends on the possible cause of the cardiac arrest and its estimated duration.[1] It is important to consider a perimortem cesarean section or resuscitative hysterotomy in any moribund patient at 20 weeks' uterine size or later, though the clinical decision to perform such a procedure is complex.[37] When the return of spontaneous maternal circulation does not rapidly occur, delivery of the fetus may improve the effectiveness of resuscitative efforts when the uterus is no longer gravid and potentially causing aortocaval compression.[35,37] Priorities for pregnant women in cardiac arrest should include high-quality cardiopulmonary resuscitation, relief of aortocaval compression with lateral uterine displacement,[9] and identification of the cause of cardiac arrest with the appropriate interventions.[37] Estimation of gestational age and assessment of fetal heart activity can be obtained rapidly while cardiopulmonary resuscitation (CPR) is being performed.

To optimize the fetal outcome, the American Heart Association recommends that a cesarean section be performed within 5 minutes of maternal arrest and that the fetus be rapidly delivered with unsuccessful maternal resuscitative attempts.[9] It is unlikely that chest compressions alone will adequately perfuse the fetus.[1] It is essential that a team capable of neonatal resuscitation be present.[9,38] Begin basic life support and advanced life support according to American Heart Association guidelines, and continue them throughout the procedure.[37] Remember the following points when performing CPR on a pregnant patient:

- Manually displace the uterus to the left and upward during chest compressions to minimize aortocaval compression for any pregnant patient with gestational age greater than 20 weeks or if the fundal height is at or above the level of the umbilicus. According to the American Heart Association,[9(p148)] follow these steps:
  - Stand to the left side of the patient, level with the top of the uterus.
  - Reach across the midline with both hands and pull the gravid uterus leftward and upward toward your abdomen (**Figure 16-1A**).

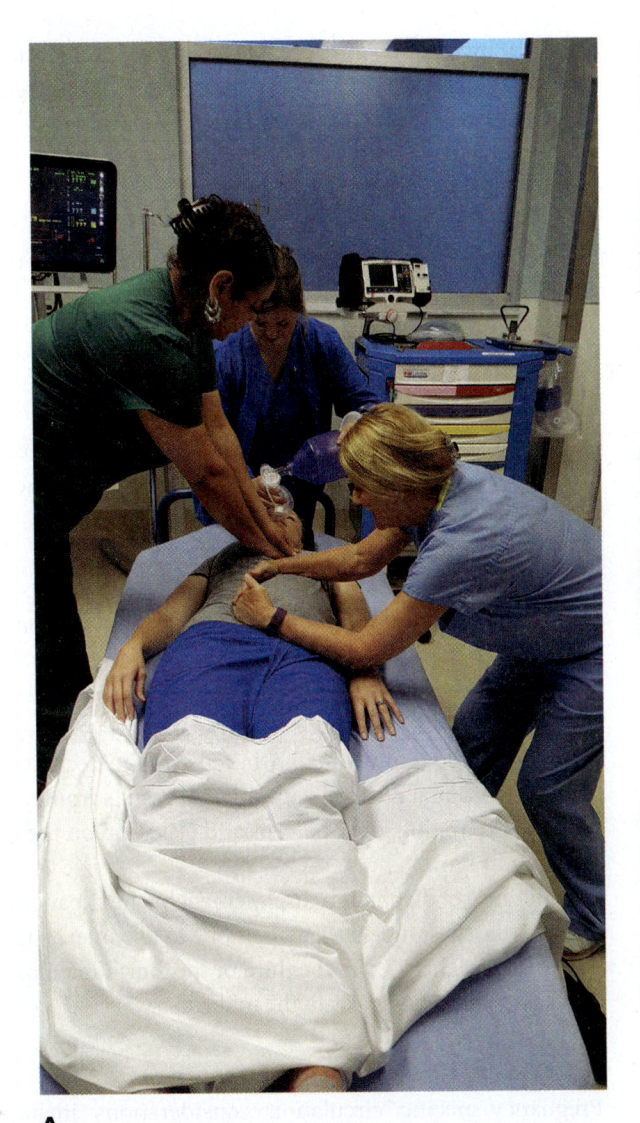

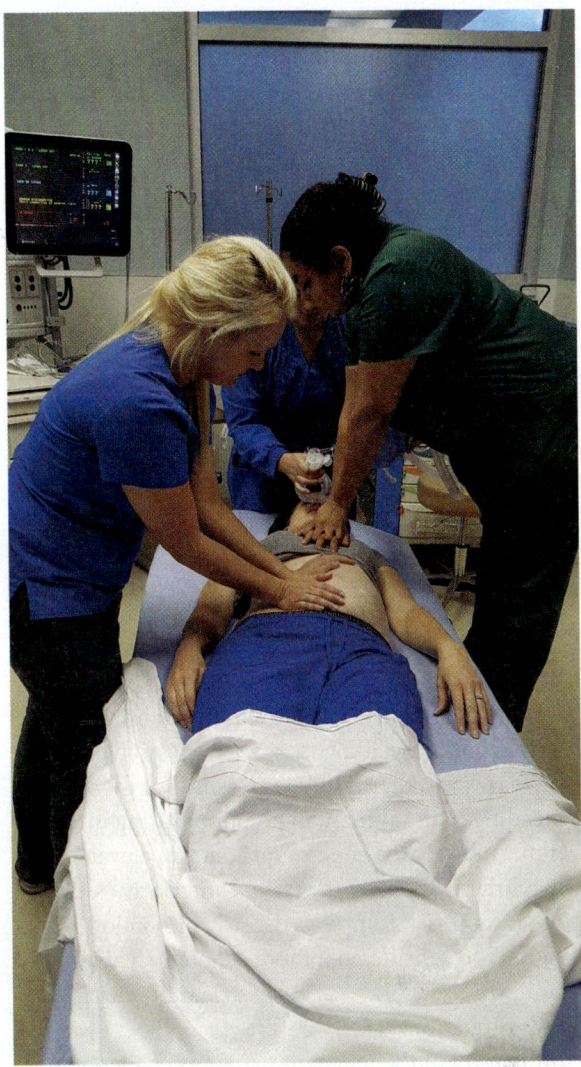

Figure 16-1 A. *Displacing the uterus off the vena cava by pulling to the left.* **B.** *Displacing the uterus off the vena cava by pushing to the left, CPR in progress.*
Courtesy of Terri Repasky.

- If you cannot stand on the left side of the patient, push the uterus to the patient's left and upward (**Figure 16-1B**).
- Defibrillate according to ACLS guidelines as you would a nonpregnant patient; do not delay defibrillation. No significant shock is transferred to the fetus. Remove fetal monitors before shock.[9,18]
- After maternal resuscitation, an undelivered fetus remains susceptible to the effects of hypothermia, acidosis, hypoxia, and hypotension, all of which may occur during this period.[37]

A perimortem cesarean section must be organized, and simulation drills have been recommended to increase emergency preparedness.[18,25]

Nursing Care of the Pregnant Trauma Patient

Trauma in pregnancy can elicit a sense of anxiety even with an experienced trauma team. The systematic approach is the same as for any other injured patient, while recognizing nonetheless that two patients require care. It is essential to initially focus on the mother by beginning with the triage and prioritization process and proceeding to the primary survey. Fetal survival is enhanced by providing optimal care to the mother.[34]

Triage and Prioritization

A valid and reliable triage method is used to prioritize patients in the emergency care setting. The Maternal

Fetal Triage Index, which was developed by the Association of Women's Health, Obstetric and Neonatal Nurses, is a valid and reliable five-level triage tool that may assist in the triage of obstetric trauma patients.[7]

Pregnancy introduces complexity with the addition of a second patient. An additional team designated for decision-making regarding pregnancy and delivery should be consulted before arrival if possible.[30]

Primary Survey

See Chapter 4, "Initial Assessment," for the systematic approach to care of the trauma patient. The following assessment parameters are specific to pregnant trauma patients.

A: Airway

Pregnancy-specific airway concerns include the following:

- Hormonal changes (estrogen-mediated fluid retention) of pregnancy can contribute to upper airway edema.[16,18,27] Edema can obscure visualization of the glottis by laryngoscopy.[27] Airway edema increases vascularity and increases the risk of bleeding with minor manipulation during intubation.[3,27] Increased abdominal contents elevate the diaphragm and shift the larynx anteriorly.[6]
- Aspiration risk is increased. Early intubation should be considered if there is potential airway compromise.[6,11,18,45] An orogastric tube should follow intubation.[45]
- Intubation of the pregnant patient is challenging.[27] Anesthesia literature shows significantly higher rates of failed intubation.[11,27]
- During intubation, consider a smaller endotracheal tube because of airway edema.[11,27] After two attempts at intubation without success, a failed intubation should be considered, and a difficult airway algorithm should be implemented.[27]
- Mallampati scores increase as pregnancy progresses.[27] Standard bedside tests for airway assessment (neck circumference, thyromental distance, and Mallampati score) may fail to predict a difficult airway.[27,45]
- Optimizing patient positioning through the use of "ramping," or "head up," should be considered when possible.[11]
- Cricoid pressure has been recommended in the pregnant patient despite the lack of evidence to support the technique in this setting.[16,45]
- Because of the altered respiratory physiology, adequate preoxygenation should be done before intubation.[45]
- Succinylcholine during rapid sequence intubation should be given at a lower dose because of reduced concentrations of pseudocholinesterase during pregnancy.[24]

B: Breathing

Pregnancy-specific breathing considerations include the following:

- Maternal oxygen saturation should be greater than or equal to 96% to ensure adequate fetal oxygenation.[18]
- Fetal hypoxia has known detrimental effects; therefore, considerations include earlier advanced airway management for the trauma patient.[37]
- The desaturation rate during periods of apnea is faster because of the increase in oxygen consumption, tidal volume, and minute ventilation.[6,16] Continuing the administration of oxygen using a nasal cannula during intubation may increase the time to desaturation during the period of apnea.[27] Hypoxia occurs more quickly because of the decrease in functional residual capacity that results from the expanding gravid uterus and elevation on the diaphragm.[16]
- Because of diaphragm displacement by the expanding uterus, chest tube placement is one to two intercostal spaces higher[3,19,24] in the third or the fourth intercostal space and anterior to the midaxillary line.[45]

C: Circulation

Pregnancy-specific circulation considerations include the following:

- Maintain a high index of suspicion for blood loss even without vital sign changes or other signs of hypovolemia.[8]
- Position the patient on the side to prevent supine hypotension from aortocaval compression if she is greater than 20 weeks' gestation. A 15-degree tilt of the long board to the left or lateral displacement of the uterus can release pressure on the inferior vena cava.[6,18,38] The left lateral position is preferred, but tilting to either side may be beneficial if the patient has injuries that interfere with left lateral positioning. Displacing the uterus off the aorta and vena cava increases cardiac output.[8,18]
- Femoral venous access should be avoided when possible because of potential uterine compression of the vena cava.[24]
- Severe bleeding can occur without the physical signs of hypovolemia usually seen (tachycardia and hypotension).[16] During hypovolemia, blood flow is

shunted from the placenta and uterine circulation to perfuse the mother's organs, causing severe fetal compromise.[16] Uterine blood flow is directly dependent on maternal mean arterial pressure.[11]

- Permissive hypotension is not recommended during pregnancy.[24] Any episode of hypotension should be immediately investigated.[24]
- Up to 35% of blood volume can be lost in the absence of hemodynamic instability in the pregnant patient.[11,16] Volume replacement should be commenced early, and vascular access should be secured above the level of the diaphragm.[11,16] **Table 16-1** provides a classification of blood loss states.
  - Consider blood administration early to avoid further increase in physiological anemia of pregnancy.
  - Whole blood is considered a potentially good alternative to blood component therapy.[3]
  - Administer O-negative blood products to avoid alloimmunization in Rh-negative mothers. When available, typed and cross-matched blood should be administered.[3,8,45]
- The use of vasopressors in pregnant women should be limited to patients with intractable hypotension or who are unresponsive to fluid resuscitation because of adverse effects on uteroplacental perfusion.[3,8,20]
- Tranexamic acid is recommended in pregnancy per local trauma guidelines.[11,24]
- A maternal focused assessment with sonography for trauma (FAST) exam should be done to evaluate maternal injuries. This is a priority because maternal shock and death are the leading causes of fetal death in trauma patients.[30] Maternal resuscitation is essential to survival of the fetus.[30]
- A fetal FAST exam should be performed as an adjunct to the primary survey immediately following the maternal exam.[30] This should be done by an obstetrician to provide information, such as gestational age, placental location, fetal presentation, and viability, that is essential for management decisions.[19,30]
- Evaluation of the fetus is a part of the circulation assessment.
- Monitor fetal heart rate and uterine contractions in all pregnancies greater than 20 weeks' gestation.
- Initiate continuous fetal monitoring (cardiotocography) early in the resuscitation of the mother for pregnancies at 20 weeks' gestation or more.[8,29]

TABLE 16-1 Blood Loss Classes

Class	Blood Loss	Pulse	Blood Pressure	Other
Class 1	< 1,200 mL Up to 15% blood volume	< 100 beats/minute	May increase	
Class 2 Mild	1,200–1,500 mL Up to 30% blood volume	> 100 beats/minute	Narrow pulse pressure, orthostatic hypotension Mean arterial pressure decreases 10–15%	Cold, pale
Class 3 Moderate	1,500–2,000 mL 30–35% blood volume	> 120 beats/minute	Hypotension Mean arterial pressure decreases 25–30%	Oliguria Tissue hypoxia
Class 4 Severe	> 2,000 mL > 40% blood volume	> 140 beats/minute	Mean arterial pressure < 50 mm Hg	Mental change Anuria Tissue hypoxia Disseminated intravascular coagulation

Modified from Huls, C., & Detlefs, C. (2018). Trauma in pregnancy. *Seminars in Perinatology, 42*, 13–20. https://doi.org/10.1053/j.semperi.2017.11.004

- An abnormal fetal heart rate response to uterine contractions may be the result of maternal hypovolemia or fetal hypoxia from an underlying pathology, such as placental separation or uterine rupture.
  - Cardiotocography monitors both the fetal heart rate and uterine contractions.
- An open thoracotomy with open-chest cardiac massage for women in cardiac arrest may be considered when the cardiac arrest has a possibly reversible cause.[1]

D: Disability

Pregnancy-specific disability considerations include the following:

- Any altered level of consciousness or seizure should be evaluated for possible eclampsia, in addition to a potential maternal head injury.[3,6]
- Appropriate sizing and application of cervical collars may not be possible because of pregnancy-related neck edema, increased adipose tissue, and increased breast size. In these situations, manual in-line stabilization must be performed.[20]

In a pregnant patient, D can also stand for "displacement" of the uterus if this has not already been done.[45]

Secondary Survey

The secondary survey begins with history before moving to the head-to-toe assessment.

H: History

Ask these questions when taking the patient's history:

- What was the MOI?
- For events related to MVCs:
  - Was the patient wearing a safety restraint device?
  - How was the restraint positioned?
- For events related to falls:
  - What was the height of the fall?
  - What was the surface on which the patient landed?
  - Which body part impacted the surface?
- Obstetric questions
  - When was the last normal menstrual period? Consider the possibility of pregnancy in any female of childbearing age.[3,29]
  - When is the expected date of confinement? To estimate this date, count back 3 months from the first day of the last known menstrual period and add 7 days.
  - Previous pregnancy history? Vaginal or cesarean deliveries?
  - What problems or complications have occurred during this or other pregnancies?
  - Is there a possibility of more than one fetus?
  - Is there vaginal bleeding?
  - Are uterine contractions or abdominal pain present?
  - Is there fetal activity?
  - Consider the possibility of interpersonal violence

H: Head-to-Toe Assessment

Inspect for the following:

- The shape and contour of the abdomen: A change in shape may indicate concealed hemorrhage or uterine rupture.
- Signs of fetal movement.
- Vaginal bleeding or the presence of amniotic fluid around the perineum.
  - The patient may describe having had a sudden gush of fluid. This may be an indication of a spontaneous bladder void or premature rupture of the amniotic membranes.
- Crowning or any abnormal fetal presentation at the vaginal opening.
  - Prolapse of the cord is rare. If present, relieve cord compression immediately. If positioning the mother to relieve pressure on the cord is contraindicated, manual displacement of the presenting part of the cord may be needed.

Auscultate for the following:

- Fetal heart tones and rate.
- The pregnant patient, owing to her increase in circulating blood volume, can better compensate for blood loss. Fetal distress may be the first indication of maternal shock.
- Fetal heart rate is an indicator of the well-being of both the mother and the fetus. The normal range for fetal heart rate is between 120 and 160 beats/minute. Fetal heart tones may be heard using a Doppler ultrasound by 10 weeks' gestation.[8]
- Continuous fetal monitoring (cardiotocography) is recommended for all pregnant patients of more than 20 weeks' gestation to assess fetal well-being and should be performed by a clinician with appropriate education and competency. An abnormal fetal heart rate may also serve as an early warning of impending maternal decompensation.[20,29]

Palpate for the following:

- The height of the fundus.
  - Fundal height is an indicator of gestational age.[24] The fundus is measured in centimeters from the symphysis pubis to the top of the fundus and

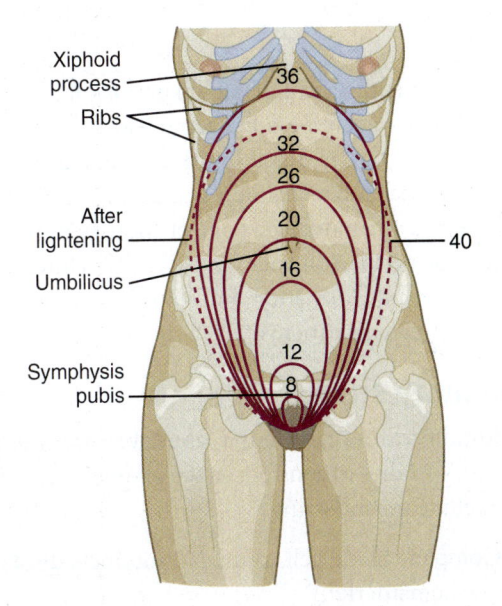

Figure 16-2 *Uterine size and location reflecting gestational age.*

approximates the number of weeks' gestation. The fundal height reaches the symphysis at 12 weeks, the umbilicus at 20 weeks, and the costal margin at 36 weeks (**Figure 16-2**).
- Fundal height may be elevated with a concealed intrauterine bleed from placental abruption.[23]
- Tenderness or contractions of the uterus or abdomen.
- Fetal parts outside the uterus.

Interventions

Maternal stabilization is the priority with a pregnant trauma patient, so the initial interventions are focused on resuscitation of the mother. Interventions specific to the pregnant trauma patient include the following:

- Obtain early obstetric consultation in all cases of injury in pregnant patients.[18,19,38] A multidisciplinary team approach is recommended in which team members have defined roles and follow established protocols.[18,19,38] It is essential that a healthcare provider experienced in the interpretation of fetal monitoring be present to assist in the care of the patient.
- If obstetric services are not available, arrange for a transfer to a trauma center with obstetrical capability.[8]
  - A CT scan may demonstrate abruptio placentae.[8]
  - Keep the patient positioned on the left side if possible.
  - Vaginal drainage should be evaluated for pH. Vaginal fluid with a pH of > 4.5 is suggestive of amniotic fluid. However, the presence of blood alters the pH, producing inaccurate results.[18]
- A surgical laparotomy alone is not an indication for a cesarean section.[24] During a laparotomy, the uterus should be handled with care.
- Continue fetal monitoring for a minimum of 6 hours for any viable pregnancy, and up to 24 hours in the case of abnormal findings.[6,30,38]
- Pain can be controlled with narcotics in any trimester. Consider the effect that narcotics may have on the fetus if delivery is anticipated while medications are still in the maternal system.[6]
- Tetanus vaccination is safe to administer during pregnancy.[3,8]
- Cautious administration of bicarbonate is warranted because rapid correction of maternal acidosis may reduce compensatory hyperventilation.[3]

Reevaluation

Reevaluation measures include diagnostic procedures, ultrasound, laboratory studies, diagnostic peritoneal lavage (DPL), and some additional adjuncts.

Diagnostic Procedures

Patients and members of the healthcare team are often concerned about possible adverse effects of radiation on the fetus.[24] Exposure to less than 5 rad has not been associated with an increase in fetal anomalies or pregnancy loss (**Table 16-2**).[3,14,24] There should be no delay of radiological evaluation because of concerns regarding fetal

TABLE 16-2 Estimated Fetal Exposure for Various Radiographic Studies

Examination Type	Estimated Fetal Dose per Examination (rad)
Plain Radiograph	
Cervical spine	.0001
Chest (two views)	.001
Abdominal	.01–.3
Upper or lower extremity	< 0.0001
CT Scans	
Head	0.0001–.001
Chest	0.001–.066
Abdominopelvic	.13–3.5

Data from Committee on Obstetric Practice. (2017). Committee opinion no. 723: Guidelines for diagnostic imaging during pregnancy and lactation. *Obstetrics & Gynecology, 130*(4), e210–e216. https://doi.org/10.1097/aog.0000000000002355

exposure.[3,24] Even so, it is important to shield the fetus for all radiographic films or CT studies, except for those of the pelvis or lumbar spine.[3] Consider a consultation with the radiologist to assist in calculating the estimated radiation dose to the fetus when multiple diagnostic radiographs are performed.[3] The risk of radiation to the fetus depends on the gestational age and the amount of radiation.[24] Imaging procedures not associated with ionizing radiation are recommended instead of radiographs whenever possible.[24] Magnetic resonance imaging is generally considered safe in pregnancy and may be needed for certain injuries (e.g., spinal cord injury).[6]

Diagnostic Peritoneal Lavage

Although rarely done, DPL can be safe in pregnant trauma patients when other imaging options are not available.[6] Insert a gastric tube and urinary catheter before the procedure. If a DPL is performed, place the catheter above the umbilicus using the open technique.[8]

CT Scan

Head CT should be performed when appropriate.[3] Diagnostic imaging is not contraindicated in pregnancy and may demonstrate obstetrical complications such as placental abruption or uterine rupture. A contrast-enhanced CT scan has high sensitivity for the identification placental abruptions and performs better than an ultrasound.[22]

FAST Exam

FAST can be useful in evaluation of intrabdominal hemorrhage, with no harmful effect from radiation.[3] The sensitivity of a FAST exam in detecting intraperitoneal fluid in a pregnant patient approaches 83%.[3] The FAST exam is less accurate in pregnant patients, although serial FAST exams may improve accuracy.[45] Obstetrical ultrasonography should be done along with the FAST exam in cases of significant maternal injury.[3]

Ultrasound

Ultrasound involves the use of sound waves and is not a source of ionizing radiation. Uterine views are being incorporated with the FAST exam at some trauma facilities to screen for pregnancy in patients who cannot communicate or do not know if they are pregnant. An ultrasound may detect placenta abruption in only 25–60% of cases.[19] A more comprehensive ultrasound (fetal FAST) may be performed by the obstetric team during the secondary survey to determine the following[30]:

- Gestational age
- Placenta presentation
- Cardiac activity: normal, abnormal, absent
- Placental location

REBOA

Resuscitative endovascular balloon occlusion of the aorta (REBOA) can benefit hemorrhaging patients by preserving perfusion proximal and limiting bleeding from sites distal to endovascular balloon occlusion.[26] REBOA has been used as a hemorrhage control strategy in the management of peripartum hemorrhage.[5,26,40] However, the risk of thrombus formation and injury to vasculature is higher in pregnant patients.[26]

Laboratory Studies

In addition to routine trauma laboratory studies, other laboratory studies to consider in the pregnant trauma patient include the following[23]:

- Complete blood cell count will routinely display a low hematocrit.[8,18]
- Prothrombin time and partial thromboplastin time, fibrinogen, and serial coagulation studies.
- If available, thromboelastography or thromboelastometry should be performed with known or suspected hemorrhage.[18]
- Beta human chorionic gonadotropin.
  - It is recommended that all female patients of childbearing age have a pregnancy test and be shielded for radiologic imaging whenever possible.[18,29] A serum beta human chorionic gonadotropin test can confirm pregnancy in as little as 1 to 2 weeks after conception and in urine in 2 to 4 weeks after conception.[8]
- Kleihauer–Betke test.
  - The Kleihauer–Betke (KB) test identifies fetal hemoglobin in maternal blood, signaling fetal hemorrhage, which most often results from a separation of the placenta from the mother.[18] The utility of this test is not clear because it can produce false positives and false negatives; it may be most helpful for Rh-negative women.[18,30]
  - Fetomaternal hemorrhage has many causes, including malformation, twin-to-twin transfusion, monoamniotic monochorionic twins, fetal death, placenta previa, abruption, tumors, umbilical vein thrombosis, maternal trauma, amniocentesis, hypertension, and substance abuse (cocaine).[32]
  - While a positive KB test indicates fetomaternal hemorrhage, a negative test does not exclude minor fetomaternal bleeding, which is capable of isoimmunization of the Rh-negative mother.[3,8]
  - The KB test can assist in determining the need to administer Rh immune globulin to prevent maternal alloimmunization when the mother is Rh

negative and the fetus is Rh positive.[39] It may be used to determine the correct dosage of Rh immune globulin.[24,38] A standard 300 mcg dose of Rho(D) immune globulin (RhoGAM) will protect up to 30 mL of fetal blood maternal exposure.[45] RhoGAM should be administered within 72 hours in pregnant trauma patients who are Rh negative and at risk of fetal–maternal hemorrhage.[45]

Additional Reevaluation Measures

Some additional diagnostics and interventions include the following:

- Pelvic examination. This should be done by a skilled obstetrical clinician.
  - The cervix is assessed to determine whether the cervical os is closed and the membranes are intact. If not, there is a risk for preterm delivery, and the patient may need to be admitted.
  - Because of the potential for causing or exacerbating bleeding, repeat pelvic exams should be avoided.
- Provide psychosocial support and realistic reassurance related to the well-being of the fetus; allay maternal and family concerns related to fetal safety during diagnostic procedures.
- Screen the patient for intimate partner violence.[29,30]

Reevaluation and Post-Resuscitation Care

In addition to those assessments described in Chapter 4, reevaluation of the pregnant trauma patient includes the following steps:

- Monitor the vaginal blood loss.
- Measure and record fundal height every 30 minutes.
- Monitor the fetal heart rate and activity, and assess uterine activity.
  - Use cardiotocographic monitoring for a minimum of 6 hours in all women of greater than 20 weeks' gestation who experience trauma.[8] This monitoring is commonly initiated in the emergency department by a clinical with the appropriate education and competency and continued in the labor and delivery or inpatient area.

Definitive Care or Transport

Prepare the patient for hospital admission, operative intervention, or transfer as indicated. Patients who are discharged should receive instructions for follow-up with an obstetrician, management of injuries, community resources, and injury prevention teaching (e.g., seatbelt use, alcohol and substance abuse, and interpersonal violence risks).[18,29]

Summary

The consequences of trauma during pregnancy may include the following:

- Maternal or fetal injury
- Preterm labor and delivery
- Maternal or fetal hemorrhage
- Abruptio placentae
- Uterine rupture
- Maternal or fetal death

The pregnant trauma patient presents the team with unique challenges and responsibilities related to assessing and managing two patients—the mother and the fetus. The resuscitation priorities for the injured pregnant patient are identical to those of any injured patient. Fetal well-being is dependent on adequate blood flow to the uterus and placenta; therefore, the best chance for fetal survival is optimal resuscitation of the mother.

References

1. Adan, A., Nafday, A., Beyer A., Odom, M., Theyyunni, N., & Ward, K. (2019). Use of tandem perimortem cesarean section and open-chest cardiac massage in the resuscitation of peripartum cardiomyopathy cardiac arrest. *Annals of Emergency Medicine, 74*(6), 772–774. https://doi.org/10.1016/j.annemergmed.2019.03.012
2. Agency for Healthcare Research and Quality. (2015). *Intimate partner violence screening.* https://www.ahrq.gov/ncepcr/tools/healthier-pregnancy/fact-sheets/partner-violence.html#:~:text=IPV%20can%20have%20direct%20and,fetal%20alcohol%20syndrome%2C%20and%20others
3. Aggarwal, R., Soni, K., & Trikha, A. (2018). Initial management of a pregnant woman with trauma. *Journal of Obstetric Anesthesia and Critical Care, 8*(2), 66–72. https://doi.org/10.4103/joacc.JOACC_4_18
4. Alhusen, J. L., Ray, E., Sharps, P., & Bullock, L. (2015). Intimate partner violence during pregnancy: Maternal and neonatal outcomes. *Journal of Women's Health, 24*(1), 100–106. https://doi.org/10.1089/jwh.2014.4872
5. Allenson, K., & Moore, L. (2019). REBOA enables operative management of the peripartum trauma patient in hemorrhagic shock. *Journal of Endovascular Resuscitation and Trauma Management, 3*(1), 42–44. https://doi.org/10.26676/jevtm.v3i1.78
6. American College of Emergency Physicians. (n.d.). *Trauma in the obstetric patient: A bedside tool.* https://www.acep.org/by-medical-focus/trauma/trauma-in-the-obstetric-patient-a-bedside-tool/#sm.00001qaywj7yeld1xy3qntc0x7jmp

7. American College of Obstetricians and Gynecologists Committee on Obstetric Practice. (2020). *Hospital-based triage of obstetric patients* (Committee Opinion No. 667). https://www.acog.org/clinical/clinical-guidance/committee-opinion/articles/2016/07/hospital-based-triage-of-obstetric-patients
8. American College of Surgeons. (2018). Trauma in pregnancy and intimate partner violence. In *Advanced trauma life support: Student course manual* (10th ed., pp. 226–239).
9. American Heart Association. (2020). Part 3: Cardiac arrest associated with pregnancy. In *Advanced cardiac life support provider manual* (pp. 144–149).
10. Ananth, C. V., & Kinzler, W. L. (2022). Acute placental abruption: Pathophysiology, clinical features, diagnosis, and consequences. *UpToDate*. Retrieved September 9, 2022, from https://www.uptodate.com/contents/acute-placental-abruption-pathophysiology-clinical-features-diagnosis-and-consequences
11. Battaloglu, E., & Porter, K. (2017). Management of pregnancy and obstetric complications in prehospital trauma care: Faculty of prehospital care consensus guidelines. *Emergency Medicine Journal*, 34(5), 318–325. https://doi.org/10.1136/emermed-2016-205978
12. Bermans, B. L. (2022). Maternal adaptations to pregnancy: Musculoskeletal changes and pain. *UpToDate*. Retrieved August 6, 2021, from https://www.uptodate.com/contents/maternal-adaptations-to-pregnancy-musculoskeletal-changes-and-pain
13. Bryant, M., Roy, S., Lurcell, L., Porras, K., Spencer, A., & Udekwu, P. (2019). Trauma in pregnancy: The relationship of trauma activation level and obstetric outcomes. *The American Surgeon*, 85(7), 772–777. https://doi.org/10.1177%2F000313481908500742
14. Committee on Obstetric Practice. (2017). Committee Opinion No. 723: Guidelines for diagnostic imaging during pregnancy and lactation. *Obstetrics & Gynecology*, 130(4), e210–e216. https://doi.org/10.1097/aog.0000000000002355
15. Deshpande, N., Kucirka, L., Smith, R., & Oxford, C. (2017). Pregnant trauma victims experience nearly 2-fold higher mortality compared to their nonpregnant counterparts. *American Journal of Obstetrics & Gynecology*, 217(5), 590.e1–590.e9. doi:10.1016/j.ajog.2017.08.004
16. Durga, P., Padhy, S., & Bardaa, A. (2019). Challenges of cardiopulmonary resuscitation during pregnancy. *Indian Journal of Cardiovascular Disease in Women*, 4(1), 32–39. https://doi.org/10.1055/s-0039-1692304
17. Gonzalez, M. G., Wei, R. M., Hatch, K. D., Gries, L. M., & Hill, M. G. (2019). A novel treatment for massive hemorrhage after maternal trauma in pregnancy. *American Journal of Perinatology Reports*, 9(1), e27–e29. https://doi.org/10.1055/s-0039-1678735
18. Harvey, C. K., & Dawson, M. F. (2020). Trauma in pregnancy. In K. A. McQuillan & M. B. Flynn Makic (Eds.), *Trauma nursing: From resuscitation through rehabilitation* (5th ed., pp. 639–676). Elsevier.
19. Huls, C., & Detlefs, C. (2018). Trauma in pregnancy. *Seminars in Perinatology*, 42, 13–20. https://doi.org/10.1053/j.semperi.2017.11.004
20. Irving, T., Menon, R., & Ciantar, E. (2021). Trauma during pregnancy. *British Journal of Anesthesia Education*, 21(1), 10–19. https://www.ncbi.nlm.nih.gov/pmc/articles/PMC7808026/
21. Jain, V., Chari, R., Maslovitz, S., Farine, D., Maternal Fetal Medicine Committee, Bujold, E., Gagnon, R., Basso, M., Bos, H., Brown, R., Cooper, S., Gouin, K., McLeod, N. L., Menticoglou, S., Mundle, W., Pylypjuk, C., Roggensack, A., & Sanderson, F. (2015). Guidelines for the management of a pregnant trauma patient. *Journal of Obstetrics and Gynaecology Canada [Journal d'obstetrique et gynecologie du Canada]*, 37(6), 553–574. https://doi.org/10.1016/s1701-2163(15)30232-2
22. Jha, P., Melendres, G., Bijan, B., Ormsby, E., Chu, L., Li, C., & McGanan, J. (2017). Trauma in pregnant women: Assessing detection of post-traumatic placental abruption on contrast-enhanced CT versus ultrasound. *Abdominal Radiology*, 42, 1062–1067. https://doi.org/10.1007/s00261-016-0970-x
23. Jordan, K. S. (2018). Obstetric and gynecologic emergencies. In V. Sweet (Ed.), *Emergency nursing core curriculum* (7th ed., pp. 366–386). Elsevier.
24. Krywko, D. M., Toy, F. K., Mahan, M. E., & Kiel, J. (2022). Pregnancy trauma. *StatPearls*. StatPearls Publishing. https://www.ncbi.nlm.nih.gov/books/NBK430926/
25. Lee, A., Sheen, J., & Richards, S. (2018). Intrapartum maternal cardiac arrest: A simulation case for multidisciplinary providers. *MedEdPORTAL*, 14, Article 10768. https://doi.org/10.15766/mep_2374-8265.10768
26. Lee, L., Potnuru, P., Stephens, C., & Pivalizza, E. (2021). Current approaches to resuscitative endovascular balloon occlusion of the aorta use in trauma and obstetrics. *Advances in Anesthesia*, 39, 17–33. https://doi.org/10.1016/j.aan.2021.07.002
27. Lentz, S., Grossman, A., Koyfman, A., & Long, B. (2020). High-risk airway management in the emergency department: Diseases and approaches, part II. *The Journal of Emergency Medicine*, 59(4), 573–585. doi:10.1016/j.jemermed.2020.05.009
28. Levi, M. M., & Schmaeier, A. H. (2022). Disseminated intravascular coagulation (DIC) workup. *Medscape*. Retrieved September 3, 2022, from https://emedicine.medscape.com/article/199627-workup
29. Lucia, A., & Dantoni, S. E. (2016). Trauma management of the pregnant patient. *Critical Care Clinics*, 32(1), 109–117. https://doi.org/10.1016/j.ccc.2015.08.008
30. MacArthur, B., Foley, M., Gray, I., & Sisley, A. (2019). Trauma in pregnancy: A comprehensive approach to the mother and fetus. *American Journal of Obstetrics & Gynecology*, 220(5), 465–468.E1. https://doi.org/10.1016/j.ajog.2019.01.209
31. McMurtry Baird, S., Braun, B., & Wolf, L. (2020). *Emergency care for patients during pregnancy and the postpartum period* [Joint consensus statement]. Emergency Nurses Association, Association of Women's Health, Obstetric and Neonatal Nurses. https://opqic.org/wp-content/uploads/2020/11/ENA-AWHONN-Consensus-Statement-Final-11.18.2020.pdf
32. Marciano, A., Di Luca, L., Maranella, E., Conte, E., Di Natale, C., Pannone, V., & Di Fabio, S. (2018). How to manage fetomaternal hemorrhage: Description of five cases and literature

review. *Journal of Pediatric and Neonatal Individualized Medicine, 7*(1), Article e070101. https://doi.org/10.7363/070101

33. Maxwell, B. G., Greenlaw, A., Smith W. J., Barbosa, R, R., Ropp, K. M., & Lundeberg, M. R. (2020). Pregnant trauma patients may be at increased risk of mortality compared to non-pregnant women of reproductive age: Trends and outcomes over 10 years at a level I trauma center. *Women's Health, 16*. Article 1745506520933021. https://doi.org/10.1177/1745506520933021

34. Mulder, M., Quiroz, H., Yang, W., Lasko, D., Perez, E., Proctor, K., Sola, J., & Thorson, C. (2020). The unborn fetus: The unrecognized victim of trauma during pregnancy. *Journal of Pediatric Surgery, 55*, 938–943. https://doi:10.1016/j.jpedsurg.2020.01.047

35. Muraoka, J., Otsuka, T., Yamauchi, A., & Terao, K. (2019). Uterine trauma and intrauterine fetal death caused by seatbelt injury. *Case Reports in Obstetrics and Gynecology*. Article 5262349. https://doi.org/10.1155/2019/5262349

36. Owattanapanich, N., Lewis, M. R., Benjamin, E. R., Wong, M. D., & Demetriades, D. (2020). Motor vehicle crashes in pregnancy: Maternal and fetal outcomes. *Journal of the American College of Surgeons, 231*(4), e242. https://doi.org/10.1016/j.jamcollsurg.2020.08.648

37. Panchal, A., Bartos, J., Cabanas, J., Donnino, M., Drennan, I., Hirsh, K., Kudenchuk, P., Kurz, M., Lavanonas, E., Morley, P., O'Neil, J., Reberdy, M., Rittenberger, J., Rodriguez, A., Sawyer, K., Berg, K., & Adult Basic and Advanced Life Support Writing Group. (2019). Part 3: Adult basic and advanced life support: 2020 American Heart Association Guidelines for Cardiopulmonary Resuscitation and Emergency Cardiovascular Care. *Circulation, 142*(16 Suppl. 2), S366–S468. https://doi.org/10.1161/cir.0000000000000916

38. Pearce, C., & Martin, S. R. (2016). Trauma and considerations unique to pregnancy. *Obstetrics & Gynecology Clinics of North America, 43*(4), 791–808. https://doi.org/10.1016/j.ogc.2016.07.008

39. Ravishankar, S., Migliori, A., Struminsky, J., Has, P., Sung, C. J., & He, M. (2017). Placental findings in feto-maternal hemorrhage in livebirth and stillbirth. *Pathology–Research and Practice, 213*(4), 301–304. https://doi.org/10.1016/j.prp.2017.02.005

40. Smith, K., & Bryce, S. (2020). Managing the pregnant trauma patient in the emergency department. *EB Medicine, 22*(10), 1–36. https://www.ebmedicine.net/topics/ob-gyn/pregnancy-trauma

41. Stadtlander, L. (2018). *Pregnancy and intimate partner violence*. School of Psychology Publication. Article 125. Walden University. https://scholarworks.waldenu.edu/cgi/viewcontent.cgi?article=1875&context=facpubs. (Reprinted from "Pregnancy and intimate partner violence," 2018, *International Journal of Childbirth Education, 33*[4], 28–31)

42. Stortroen, N., Tubog, T., & Shaffer, S. (2020). Prophylactic tranexamic acid in high-risk patients undergoing cesarean delivery: A systematic review and meta-analysis of randomized controlled trials. *AANA Journal, 88*(4), 273–281. https://www.aana.com/docs/default-source/aana-journal-web-documents-1/stortroen-r4db321ecc579453fb1b1332fd2f95e5a.pdf?sfvrsn=b84bd022_10

43. Tibbott, J., Di Carlofelice, M., Menon, R., & Ciantar, E. (2021). Trauma and pregnancy. *The Obstetrician & Gynaecologist, 23*(4), 258–264. https://doi.org/10.1111/tog.12769

44. Wallace, M., Gillispie-Bell, V., Cruz, K., Davis, K., & Vilda, D. (2021). Homicide during pregnancy and the postpartum period in the United States, 2018–2019. *Obstetrics & Gynecology, 138*(5), 762–769. https://www.ncbi.nlm.nih.gov/pmc/articles/PMC9134264/pdf/nihms-1804550.pdf

45. Wilkerson, R., Annous, Y., & Hasbini, Y. (2020, August 17). Plus one: Care of the pregnant trauma patient. *EM Resident*. https://www.emra.org/emresident/article/pregnant-trauma-patient/

CHAPTER 17

Interpersonal Violence

Sara Daykin, DNP, RN, CNEcl, TCRN, CPEN

OBJECTIVES

Upon completion of this chapter, the learner will be able to:
1. Identify types of interpersonal violence.
2. Discuss assessment priorities for the patient experiencing interpersonal violence.
3. Describe trauma-informed care principles for the patient who has experienced interpersonal violence.

Introduction

Understanding the prevalence and outcomes of interpersonal violence, as well as its global impact, is integral to providing care to the patient who has experienced trauma. In 2021, the World Health Organization (WHO) estimated that 1 in 3 women globally have experienced physical and/or sexual violence in their lifetime. The Centers for Disease Control and Prevention (CDC) states that nearly 1 in 4 men in the United States have experienced some sort of contact sexual violence by an intimate partner.[12] The National Coalition Against Domestic Violence[47] published data showing that more than 10 million men and women are abused by their intimate partner each year and that intimate partner violence (IPV) increased by 42% from 2016 to 2018. This equates to about 20 people per minute who experience physical abuse or interpersonal violence. This does not account for those who are not physically injured but suffer emotionally or financially.

Patients seeking healthcare services following acts of violence constitute a public health epidemic.[30] People experiencing interpersonal violence often seek treatment in the emergency department (ED) for their injuries but rarely report the actual mechanism of injury for fear of retribution from their abuser or stigma from the community. Approximately 30,000 patients die in the ED each year from injuries.[13] Interpersonal violence and nonfatal injuries can lead to psychological, physical, and financial problems. Research demonstrates that the economic cost of injury is approximately $4.2 trillion, which includes medical care and wages related to loss of work.[54]

Interpersonal violence is the intentional use of physical power or force, actual or threatened, against a person or community. It is specifically violence against family members, intimate partners, children, friends, acquaintances, and strangers. Interpersonal violence includes child maltreatment, youth violence, IPV, sexual violence, and elder abuse. It is violence against men, women, and those who do not identify with either group. It is youth gang violence. This type of violence has significant lifelong health and social consequences.

Interpersonal violence carries a risk of death, injury, psychological damage, and, in children, delayed development. Cultural considerations may influence the type of interpersonal violence that occurs, although violence occurs across all cultures and environments.[76] The International Association for Forensic Nursing (IAFN) and the Emergency Nurses Association (ENA) have stated the need for a safe and private environment in which those who have experienced interpersonal violence can receive nonjudgmental support for their individual care choices.[6]

Caring for this vulnerable population requires incorporating forensic nursing principles and trauma-informed care, which include timely patient centered care, appropriate medico-legal documentation, the collection and preservation of evidence, and appropriate referral options. It begins with education and awareness, recognition of patterns of injuries, and documentation for and reporting to appropriate jurisdictional law enforcement agencies as directed by local laws and facility policies. Such care involves an interdisciplinary trauma team whose members understand how to apply the trauma-informed framework.[11]

Epidemiology

There are two distinct categories of interpersonal violence[76]:

- *Family and intimate-partner violence* typically occurs within a family unit or between partners. It includes child maltreatment and elder maltreatment.
- *Community violence* occurs between people who may be strangers or acquainted but who are not related. It includes youth violence, random violence, rape or sexual violence, and institutional violence in schools, workplaces, prisons, and care facilities.

Some types of violence classified as family/intimate-partner violence or community violence have similarities and may fall under both categories (**Figure 17-1**).[74] For example, sex trafficking (under community violence) can involve a stranger or an intimate partner or child. Sexual assault can be perpetrated by an intimate partner or a stranger. These crimes are similar in the use of power and control by the perpetrator as a method of abuse. Psychological coercion, physical assaults, isolation, and other abusive power strategies are used by perpetrators to gain control over the other person.[55]

Risk Factors

Interpersonal violence is seen across all cultures and environments. However, some characteristics place certain people at higher risk for being subjected to this type of violence. **Table 17-1** lists some of the individual, relational,

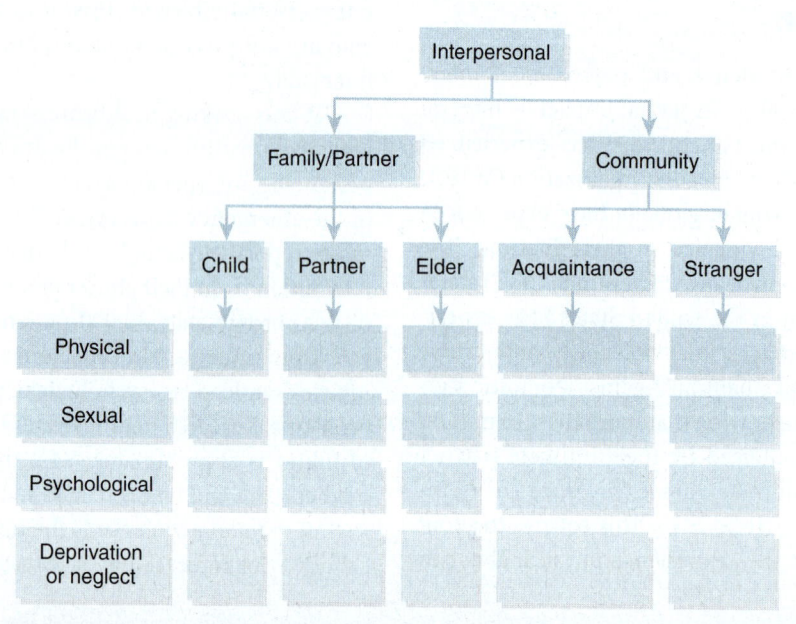

Figure 17-1 *Typology of interpersonal violence.*
Reproduced from World Health Organization. (n.d). The VPA approach. https://www.who.int/groups/violence-prevention-alliance/approach

TABLE 17-1 Interpersonal Violence Risk Factors

Individual	Interpersonal Relationship	Community and Social	Society or Macro-Level Factors
Personal attitude and beliefs that tolerate IPV Age Youth due to immaturity Adolescent dating population Pregnancy, childbirth, postpartum Gender Women age 12–25 years Vulnerable persons Linguistic isolation Minority ethnic status Cultural beliefs such as patriarchal gender beliefs, collectivism, power distance Prior abuse history Poverty or inadequate resources	Relationship with peers involving dominance and control Family violence Exposure to interpersonal violence as a child Human trafficking Runaways Rural area Inadequate support by family, including migration Labor trafficking	Social vulnerability Poverty Lack of access to services or transportation Crowded housing Schools with economic disadvantage and lack of safety Children in foster care Children involved in human trafficking	Gender inequality Belief in traditional gender roles and norms

Antisocial personality traits
Substance use disorders
Heavy alcohol use
Behavioral health disorders
Special populations
People covered by the Americans with Disabilities Act, such deaf and blind individuals
Lesbian, gay, bisexual, transgender, queer, or questioning individuals
Institutionalized individuals:
    Nursing homes
    Assisted living facilities
    Correctional facilities/juvenile system
Isolation
Unemployment
Homeless
Lack of education
Marginalized persons
	Relationship with partners
	Marital conflict
	Unstable marriages
	Divorce
	Separation
	Financial stress
	One partner displaying dominance and control in the relationship
		Workplaces
		Low economic social situations
		Neighborhoods
		Poverty
		Overcrowding
		Weak community response to IPV
			Religious or cultural beliefs
			Society norms
			Economic or social policies

IPV = intimate-partner violence.

Data from Washington State Department of Social and Health Services. (n.d.). *Types and signs of abuse.* https://www.dshs.wa.gov/altsa/home-and-community-services/types-and-signs-abuse; Beal, J. A. (2017). Healthcare of the transgender youth still inadequate . . . still at risk. *Journal of Maternal/Child Nursing, 42*(5), 296. https://doi.org/10.1097/NMC.0000000000000362; Macias-Konstantopoulos, W., & Ma, Z. B. (2017). Physical health of human trafficking survivors: Unmet essentials. In M. Chisolm-Straker & H. Stoklosa (Eds.), *Human trafficking is a public health issue* (pp. 185–210). Springer. https://doi.org/10.1007/978-3-319-47824-1_11; Mills, T. J. (2019). Elder abuse. *Medscape.* Retrieved January 25, 2022, from https://emedicine.medscape.com/article/805727-overview; National Coalition Against Domestic Violence. (n.d.). *Statistics.* https://www.ncadv.org/statistics; Tracy, E. E., & Macias-Konstantopoulos, M. (2021). Human trafficking: Identification and evaluation in the health care setting. *UpToDate.* Retrieved January 25, 2022, from https://www.uptodate.com/contents/human-trafficking-identification-and-evaluation-in-the-health-care-setting community, and societal risk factors that are associated with greater risk (it is not all inclusive). Anything that can make an individual vulnerable increases the individual risk.[5,35,39,63,69] Trauma team members will want to maintain a high index of suspicion for identifying interpersonal violence in high-risk populations.[24,52,74]

Patterns of Abusive Behavior

The Power and Control Wheel (**Figure 17-2**), developed by Domestic Abuse Intervention Programs is a powerful tool for understanding the full picture of the types and patterns of abusive behavior.[44]

The Power and Control Wheel describes behaviors that abusers use to gain power and control over another person.[46] Power and control can even result from infrequent assault. The threat of future violence is enough to enable the abuser to exert control.

Types of Interpersonal Violence

The term "interpersonal violence" is often used in place of "intimate partner violence." However, these terms are not synonymous. "Interpersonal violence" is a broader term that includes multiple aspects of violence, including intimate-partner violence, child maltreatment, and sexual assault.[20] To understand interpersonal violence, it is useful to consider the various types. Many survivors of abuse have experienced more than one type of abuse.[77]

Child Maltreatment

Child maltreatment is the neglect or abuse of a person younger than 18 years. It involves emotional or physical abuse, negligence, commercial exploitation, or other abusive or exploitative behaviors.[9,42] Many children are not only survivors of abuse but also witness their sibling or parent experiencing abuse. Often there is an overlap

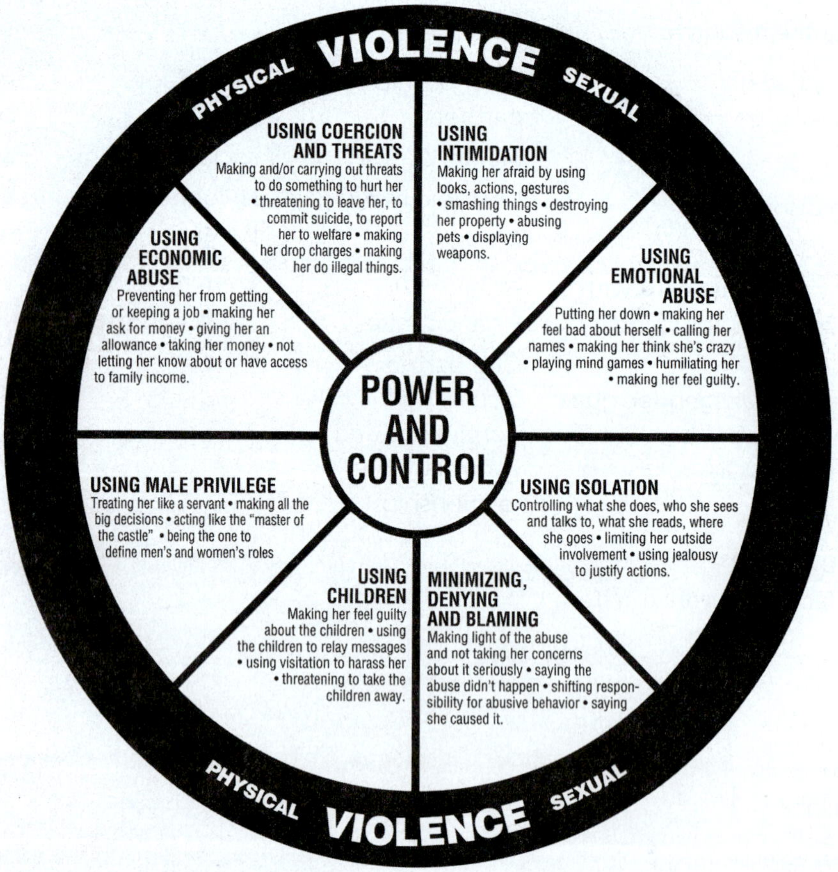

Figure 17-2 *The Power and Control Wheel.*

All too often the 200+ women's voices whose words and experiences are contained in and create that wheel, are forgotten; often, people think it is just a tool created by professionals... and though that is true... it is not the whole story. Please visit the wheel gallery here: https://www.theduluthmodel.org/wheel-gallery/, watch some videos about the wheel here: https://www.theduluthmodel.org/wheels/, and find a quick explanation about aspects of the wheel here: https://www.theduluthmodel.org/wheels/faqs-about-the-wheels/

DOMESTIC ABUSE INTERVENTION PROGRAMS. 202 East Superior Street Duluth, MN 55802. 218-722-2781. www.theduluthmodel.org

between witnessing and surviving abuse. The impact of witnessing abuse of another is also considered a form of child maltreatment.

Child abuse and neglect can be defined as any act or patterns of acts that are committed or omitted by parent or a caregiver (teacher, coach, clergy, or person of authority over a child) that result in harm, threat of harm, or potential for harm to a child.[9] Acts of commission are intentional or deliberate words or actions that can cause harm, threat of harm, or potential harm, even if harm was not the intended consequence. Physical abuse, psychological abuse, and sexual abuse are examples of acts of commission. Acts of omission, or child neglect, are the failure to protect the child from harm or the potential for harm, and/or failure to provide for the child's needs as defined by what is normal and reasonable.[64] Examples include physical neglect, emotional neglect, educational neglect, inadequate supervision, exposure to violent environments, or medical and dental neglect.[59] In 2019, there were 618,000 reported incidents of child maltreatment in the United States, including 1,750 child deaths from maltreatment.[3,65] The majority of reported cases are related to neglect. It is often incorrectly assumed that a man in the child's life is the perpetrator. However, data show that the majority of perpetrators were mothers or women in the child's life.[65]

See Chapter 13, "The Pediatric Trauma Patient," for additional physical signs of child maltreatment.

Intimate Partner Violence

Commonly referred to as domestic violence, intimate partner violence is a public health problem that affects more than 10 million people annually.[47] IPV is the willful intimidation, physical assault, battery, sexual assault, and/or other abusive behavior as part of a systematic pattern of power and control perpetrated by one intimate partner against another. It includes physical or sexual violence, threats, and emotional/psychological abuse, financial control, or intimidation by a current or former intimate partner. The frequency and severity of IPV vary dramatically and can escalate with each incident.[9] In the United States, 1 in 3 women and 1 in 4 men have experienced some form of physical violence by an intimate partner, and it may begin at a young age.[46] When IPV is experienced by those under 18 years of age, it is called teen dating violence, and it affects millions of teens every year. As the violence escalates, it often results in physical injury and even death. The mental health impact for survivors can include post-traumatic stress disorder (PTSD) and depression and may be lifelong.[9]

On a global scale, it is estimated that approximately 27% of women aged 15–49 years have experienced IPV, and 38% of murdered women were killed by their intimate partner.[77]

Physical Assault/Abuse

Women between 18 and 24 years of age experience IPV most often.[47] Physical abuse is most often inflicted by dating partners rather than spouses.[47] Approximately 25% of women and 10% of men experience some form of IPV in their lifetime.[47]

People who experience abuse often incur injuries to the head, neck, or face. Types of physical violence cover a wide range of actions, such as pushing, slapping, punching, biting, strangulation, and striking with an object such as a belt.

Strangulation is the application of external pressure to the neck that causes obstruction of blood vessels and/or the airway, resulting in decreased oxygen delivery to the brain.[71] It is classified as fatal strangulation when death results and nonfatal strangulation when it does not.[71] The different methods of strangulation include the following[19,71]:

- Manual: The hands are used to apply pressure to the neck.
- Ligature: An object, such as a scarf, is used to apply pressure to the neck.
- Chokehold (headlock): The arm is placed around the neck and pressure applied.
- Hanging: An object, such as a rope, is used to suspend the person above the ground by the neck, cutting off air and blood supply.

Nonfatal strangulation is a form of severe violence, *even when external signs of injury are minimal or nonexistent*; nonfatal strangulation significantly increases the risk of future homicide.[19,37] Research reveals a 7.5-fold increased likelihood of homicide when previous episodes of nonfatal strangulation by an intimate partner have occurred.[19,37] Those who experience strangulation often do not use the term "strangulation" when describing the event; instead, they often use words such as "choked," "suffocated," "headlock," or "throttling."[19] Nonfatal strangulation is often repetitive, and people who have experienced this abuse frequently do not seek medical treatment. Perpetrators use this type of violence to subdue, exert dominance, and create intense fear.[71] A computed tomography (CT) angiogram is considered the standard of care when evaluating for injury related to nonfatal strangulation.[81]

Having a partner with an alcohol use disorder and/or a mental health condition is a major risk factor for IPV. A person whose partner misuses alcohol is 3.6 times more likely to be assaulted by their partner than a person whose partner does not.[73] The consumption of alcohol during a dispute is likely to decrease inhibitions and increase impulsivity, thereby creating an opportunity for an argument to escalate into a physical altercation. Drinking may or may not be the cause of the violence, but alcohol use disorder could introduce more tension into the relationship; this can lead to aggression and violence, particularly if a weapon is in the home.[21,60]

IPV can lead to death—1 in 3 female homicides and 1 in 20 male homicides are perpetrated by intimate partners.[47]

Sexual Assault

Sexual assault is any sexual contact—including rape, attempted rape, fondling, or any sexual touching—that is unwanted and not consensual or that forces the person to perform sexual acts.[2] Rape is penetration, without consent, of the vagina or anus with a body part or object.[2,4] The term "sexual assault" can apply to anyone of any age or gender and to those who do not identify with a gender; it also includes incest and drug-facilitated sexual assault. In the United States, approximately 26% of women and 3.8% of men have been raped or experienced attempted rape at some point in their life.[4] More than half of people raped in the United States are raped by an acquaintance: 56.1% of females and 57.3% of males.[4] This number markedly increases with children: 93% knew their attacker.[57] Women and girls who are raped are most often raped as a child or young adult, with more than 80% of female rape victims reporting that they were first raped before age 25. Almost half were raped as a minor.[4] Sexual assault in more likely to be perpetrated by an intimate partner than an acquaintance or stranger.[48] People who experience both physical and sexual abuse are more likely to be killed by their abuser than those who suffer one type of abuse.[48] Just over one-third of people raped ever report the crime to law enforcement.[48]

Interpersonal Violence During Pregnancy

IPV is a global phenomenon and in some areas is more common than the health conditions pregnant women are routinely screened for, such as gestational diabetes.[17] In this vulnerable population, IPV is known to begin or, if already present, to escalate during pregnancy.[16,17,32] A number of physical, emotional, social, and economic changes can add stressors during a time of intense personal and relationship transition. The prevalence of physical and sexual abuse among pregnant women is also affected by marital status and whether the pregnancy was intended and planned by the woman or the partner.[16]

IPV during pregnancy is a significant public health issue and is associated with adverse pregnancy outcomes and negative consequences for both mother and child.[7,16,17] Pregnant women who experience IPV are twice as likely to delay prenatal care and more likely to experience adverse outcomes, including low birth weight, preterm delivery, and placental abruption. There is also increased risk of miscarriage/abortion, fetal injury, and perinatal maternal death due to injuries sustained during an assault.[1] The leading causes of death during pregnancy in the United States are homicide, suicide, and drug overdose.[7]

Pregnant women who experience IPV are vulnerable to adverse mental health consequences, including depression, anxiety disorders, PTSD, and suicidal ideation. It is important to screen all people for interpersonal violence, especially pregnant patients who are high risk for IPV. Care of the pregnant trauma patient presents a unique opportunity for providers to build a relationship based on trust; doing so may increase the likelihood for detection of IPV, enabling mitigation of the negative consequences for both mother and child (**Figure 17-3**).[75] For many women, especially those experiencing IPV, pregnancy is the only time when they maintain regular contact with healthcare providers. Trauma nurses should have a high index of suspicion for IPV in pregnant patients with traumatic injuries.

For more information on physical assessment of the pregnant trauma patient, see Chapter 16, "The Pregnant Trauma Patient."

Drug-Facilitated Sexual Assault

Drug-facilitated sexual assault (DFSA) is associated with the inability of a patient to consent to a sexual act because of incapacitation from drugs and/or alcohol, whether self-administered or covertly given to an unsuspecting individual. Substances used in DFSA include, but are not limited to, alcohol, flunitrazepam, gamma-hydroxybutyrate acid, ketamine, tetrahydrozoline, phenobarbital, and promethazine.[66,72] Other substances, such as marijuana, benzodiazepines, cocaine, heroin, and amphetamines, can also be associated with sexual violence. Some of these substances can go undetected when added to food or drink. The effects of these drugs include sedation and amnesia, and a person may not be able to resist the assault or may not be aware that a sexual act has occurred.[66,72] More than half of sexual assault cases involve the administration of a chemical.[58]

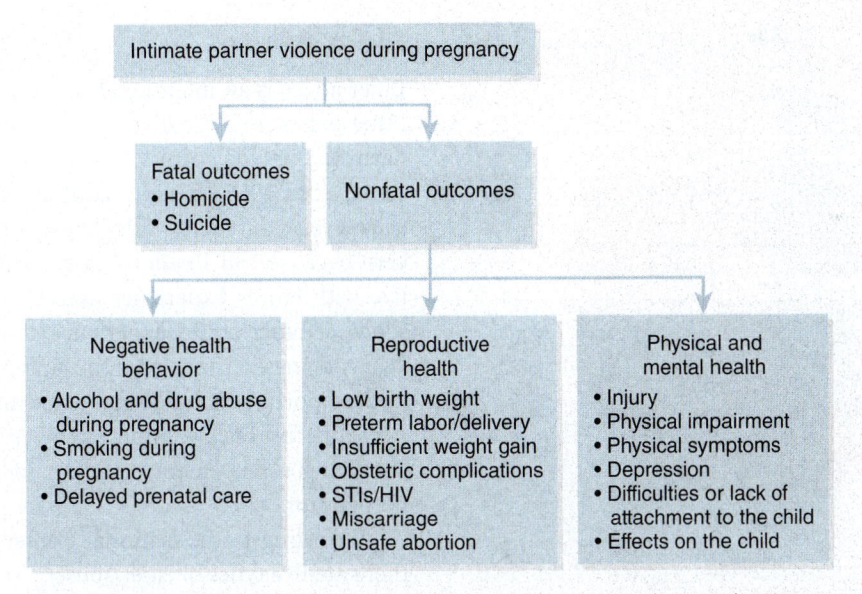

Figure 17-3 Health outcomes of intimate partner violence during pregnancy.
Reproduced from World Health Organization. (2011). Intimate partner violence during pregnancy information sheet. http://apps.who.int/iris/bitstream/handle/10665/70764/WHO_RHR_11.35_eng.pdf;sequence=1

Lesbian, Gay, Bisexual, Transgender, Asexual, and Questioning Populations

Research focused on the lesbian, gay, bisexual, transgender, queer (questioning), intersex, asexual, and agender (LGBTQ+) populations has increased considerably in the past decade. The prevalence of IPV among LGBTQ+ individuals may be as high as or higher than that of the general population, and those assaulted encounter the same barriers to seeking assistance.[5] Additional barriers unique to this population include legal definitions of IPV that exclude LGBTQ+ individuals and couples, lack of resources, and personal conflict over "outing" themselves and their partner. Healthcare providers who are not knowledgeable about LGBTQ+ considerations for care can be a barrier as well. This lack of knowledge about, or comfort level with, how to address LGBTQ+ issues can make it difficult for patients to seek help. For more information on specific care of the LGBTQ+ patient, see Chapter 12, "The LGBTQ+ Trauma Patient."

Human Trafficking

Human trafficking is often described as modern-day slavery; it is a crime of exploitation of a person for forced sex or labor.[53] Human trafficking is a complex public health problem that spans the globe. Sex trafficking is the recruitment, harboring, provision, transportation, soliciting, patronizing, or obtaining a person for commercial sex acts that involves coercion or force.[53] Labor trafficking is the harboring, recruitment, provision, transportation, or obtaining of a person for labor services by using force, coercion, and fraud for involuntary servitude, debt bondage, slavery, or peonage.[63] An estimated 40 million people experience this type of modern-day slavery globally. International labor organizations estimate that 19 million people are exploited in a variety of private industry, governmental, and rebel groups. The exact incidence and prevalence are unknown because of the inherently hidden nature of human trafficking, underreporting by survivors, variations in severity of activities, multiple definitions, and lack of standardized tracking databases.[63]

IPV and human trafficking can occur simultaneously to the same person. The perpetrator may have an intimate relationship with the individual and may traffic family members or their own children.

Three-fourths of people being trafficking are women and girls, and 25% are children. In 2016, 1 in 6 runaways reported by the U.S. National Center for Missing and Exploited Children were likely to be sex trafficked, with food and safety used to further control the runaway.[24,55,78]

Emergency nurses should understand that IPV and human trafficking survivors will not usually self-identify, but they are among the most vulnerable patient populations receiving care. The use of a validated tool can help raise awareness in the healthcare setting.[63] **Figure 17-4** provides additional context for understanding human trafficking.[56]

Age
- Unknown 1,575
- Minor 2,762
- Adult 6,204

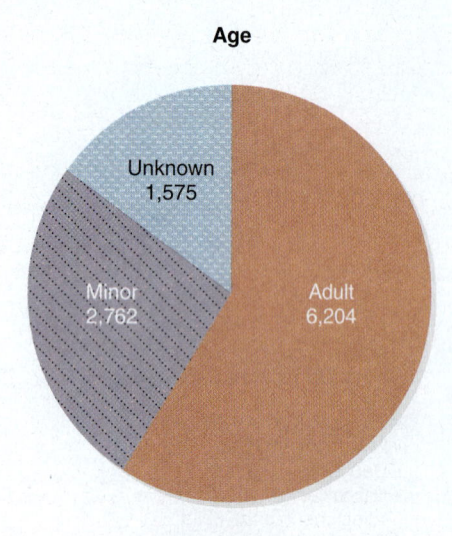

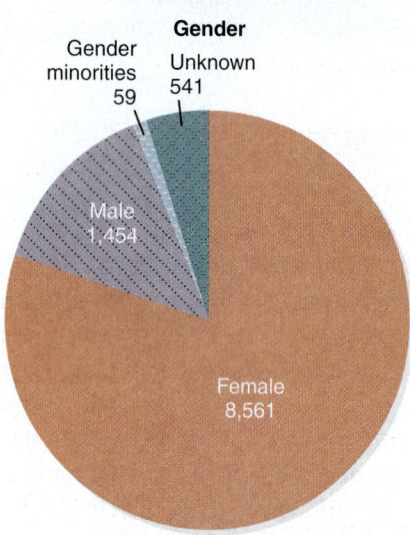

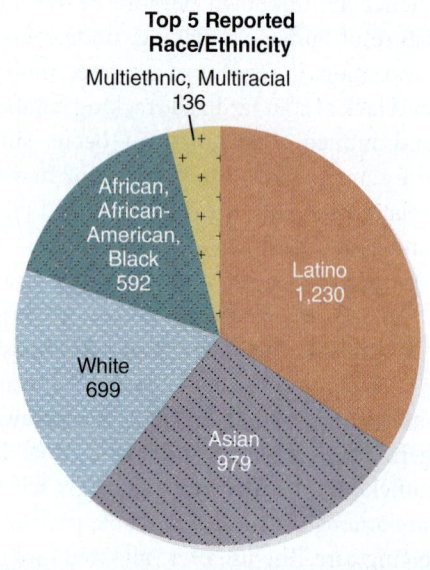

Gender
- Gender minorities 59
- Unknown 541
- Male 1,454
- Female 8,561

Top 5 Reported Race/Ethnicity
- Multiethnic, Multiracial 136
- African, African-American, Black 592
- Latino 1,230
- Asian 979
- White 699

Figure 17-4 *Data from the National Human Trafficking Hotline, 2020.*

Data from Polaris. (2021). Polaris analysis of 2020 data from the National Human Trafficking Hotline. https://polarisproject.org/wp-content/uploads/2022/01/Polaris-Analysis-of-2020-Data-from-the-National-Human-Trafficking-Hotline.pdf

Elder Abuse

Elder abuse is an intentional act, or failure to act, by another person or a caregiver that creates or causes a risk of harm to the older adult. According to the Older Americans Act of 1965, an older adult is an individual who is age 60 years or older.[10] Elder abuse is a public health concern because 1 in 10 adults older than the age of 60 who live with family experience abuse.[10] Hundreds of thousands of older adults experience abuse or neglect each year, yet these crimes often go unreported. Reasons for underreporting include dementia, culture, language barriers, distrust of law enforcement, fear of losing a present living arrangement, and fear of retribution by the perpetrator.[18,39,45]

According to the National Center on Elder Abuse,[45] there are five types of elder abuse:

- Physical abuse
- Sexual abuse
- Emotional abuse
- Neglect
- Financial abuse

Abandonment is sometimes also discussed as a sixth form of elder abuse, and it is discussed as such here, but some consider it a subtype of neglect.

Physical injuries may be the result of a single incident or multiple incidents. Injuries can range from minor, in the form of minor scratches and bruises, to serious, as in broken bones, head injuries, lasting disabilities, and death.[25,39]

For more information on how to care for the injuries incurred due to elder abuse and specific age-related care, refer to Chapter 15, "The Older Trauma Patient."

Emotional (Psychological) Abuse

Emotional abuse is the deliberate attempt to destroy or impair a person's self-esteem, competence, or perception of events. It includes verbal and nonverbal insults, humiliation, isolation, and gaslighting. This type of abuse can be focused on any age group and has lasting psychological impact on the survivor. All forms of abuse include some level of emotional abuse.[10] Persistent or unexplained change in a person's behavior may be the result of emotional abuse.

Neglect

Neglect is the failure to provide for a person's basic needs, including food, shelter, clothing, education, or medical care. It is one of the most common forms of child and elder maltreatment. Physical signs may be nonspecific, and healthcare providers may have to rely on behavioral indicators to identify an abusive situation. Neglect is often hard to identify or substantiate. However, it is estimated that approximately 5% of elder abuse in the United States is neglect.[61]

Emotional Neglect

Unlike emotional abuse, emotional neglect occurs when caregivers withhold love and nurturing behavior and fail to meet the person's emotional and developmental needs, including psychological care. It is usually seen in children but may also be present in the elderly population. Fear and passivity can accompany this type of neglect. It requires careful listening and sensitive probing to uncover. This type of abuse can lead to feelings of depression, hopelessness, and helplessness in individuals.[41] Additionally, caregivers may fail to seek necessary care for an individual with emotional or behavioral problems.

Physical Neglect

Physical neglect is the failure to prevent harm to a person or to provide for that person's basic needs, such as healthcare, food, shelter, and supervision.[52] It may involve an older adult or child who is unable to care for themselves and is left unattended. It may also include failure to provide proper nutrition, to ensure seasonally appropriate clothing, or to follow up with necessary medical or dental care. If there is an expectation of care and that care is not provided by a caregiver or facility, it is neglect. Consideration should be given to the family circumstances and what is considered culturally and socially acceptable, as well as what is legally required.

Abandonment

Abandonment occurs when a person who has assumed responsibility for providing care purposefully and permanently deserts the caregiving needs of that individual without arranging sufficient care for the duration of the absence. The individual can be a child, elderly person, a person with disabilities, or any sort of dependent. Signs of abandonment can include poor hygiene, malnourishment, dehydration, or unattended health problems. Individuals are commonly abandoned at a hospital, a nursing facility, or even a public place.[45] This is deliberate and done with malintent and should not be confused with a mother using safe haven laws to turn over their child. Many jurisdictions have their own safe haven laws specifying age limitations and where the infant can be surrendered.[15]

Financial Abuse

Financial abuse takes many forms. It can include the restriction or control of funds currently available or those expected in the future in the manner of trusts or inheritance. Financial exploitation commonly involves trusted persons in the life of the person being abused,[43] but scams and frauds committed by strangers are also common. Such frauds and scams are often perpetrated on the elderly. Financial abuse can be a form of maintaining power and control over the person being abused, and it is also common in the elderly and those being trafficked.[51]

Tools for Identification of At-Risk individuals

Multiple validated tools are available to assist with identification of abuse and neglect in both children and adults. Some tools are simple questions, and others are longer interviews. Such tools can highlight the majority of those at risk. If tools are not utilized routinely, some patients at risk will not be identified. The use of a screening tool is encouraged and is recommended in the IAFN and ENA joint statement[6] to identify those who require a lengthier discussion, interview, or evaluation.

Initial Assessment for Interpersonal Violence

The initial assessment of a trauma patient specifically affected by interpersonal violence includes a trauma-informed care approach, starting from the time of initial notification through preparation and triage, including all interactions with the patient and family (**Box 17-1**).[62] Trauma-informed care recognizes the distress and vulnerability of patients who may also have experienced current or past trauma. It focuses on assuring the patient that they are safe, autonomous, and in a place to start the healing process.

Safe Practice

Violence against healthcare workers is at an all-time high worldwide, and trauma team members face safety concerns when caring for patients because of the prevalence of violence. It is estimated that 82% of nurses experience workplace violence in their career.[70] Staff are entitled to be safe in their work environment. Having a security plan, and being ready to implement it, is an important aspect of trauma care. Identifying and addressing gaps in knowledge or skill in the implementation of the security plan is vital for the protection of staff and patients. Based on the circumstances involved in the activation of the security plan, staff

BOX 17-1 Trauma-Informed Care

Communicating with survivors of interpersonal violence to provide trauma-informed care requires the following[23,62]:

- Providing clear explanations of the plan of care, including what to expect in the screening and assessment process.
- Approaching the patient in a matter-of-fact, yet supportive, manner. Be sensitive to how the patient might hear what you have to say in response to personal disclosures. Patients who have been traumatized may be reactive to benign or well-intended questions.
- Respecting the patient's personal space. Survivors may have a particular sensitivity about their bodies, personal space, and boundaries.
- Not touching the patient without discussion or consent. This includes touching a hand or a shoulder.
- Being aware of your own emotional responses to hearing a patient's traumatic history. Hearing about the victim's experience may be very painful and can elicit strong emotions or even the provider's own trauma response. The patient may perceive your reaction as disinterest, disgust, or some other inaccurate interpretation.
- Eliciting only the information necessary. Given the lack of a therapeutic relationship in which to process the information safely, pursuing details of trauma can cause retraumatization.
- Giving the patient as much personal control as possible during the assessment:
  - Explaining the purpose of the interview and its stress-inducing potential, and clarifying that the patient has the right to refuse to answer any and all questions.
  - Providing the option of being interviewed by someone of the gender with which the patient is most comfortable.
  - Avoiding phrases that imply judgment, such as asking about their responses to an attack.
  - Giving the patient time to process their reactions.

Data from Fischer, K. R., Bakes, K. M., Corbin, T. J., Fein, J. A., Harris, E., J., James, T. L., & Melzer-Lange, M. D. (2019). Trauma-informed care for violently injured patients in the emergency department. *Annals of Emergency Medicine, 73*(2), 193–202. https://doi.org/10.1016/j.annemergmed.2018.10.018; Substance Abuse and Mental Health Services Administration. (2014). *Trauma-informed care in behavioral health services.* Treatment Improvement Protocol (TIP) Series 57, HHS Publication No. (SMA) 13-4801. U.S. Department of Health & Human Services. https://store.samhsa.gov/sites/default/files/d7/priv/sma14-4816.pdf

BOX 17-2 Personal Response

Healthcare providers can find negligence, abuse, or intentional injury to vulnerable patient populations extremely difficult to manage, both professionally and personally. In these circumstances, a professional approach may conflict with the emotions the trauma nurse is experiencing. It is recommended that staff identify and evaluate their personal emotions, beliefs, values, and past experiences to determine how these perceptions may affect their attitude toward, and care of, these patients.[33,62]

Data from Jimenez-Herrera, M. F., Llaurado-Serra, M., Acebedo-Urdiales, S., Bazo-Hernandez, L., Font-Jimenez, I., & Axelsson, C. (2020). Emotions and feelings in critical and emergency caring situations: A qualitative study. *BMC Nursing, 19*, Article 60. https://doi.org/10.1186/s12912-020-00438-6; Substance Abuse and Mental Health Services Administration. (2014). *Trauma-informed care in behavioral health services.* Treatment Improvement Protocol (TIP) Series 57, HHS Publication No. (SMA) 13-4801. U.S. Department of Health & Human Services. https://store.samhsa.gov/sites/default/files/d7/priv/sma14-4816.pdf

may benefit from debriefings or employee counseling. Additionally, when caring for people who have experienced interpersonal violence, staff may experience a personal response that may be difficult to manage (**Box 17-2**). See Chapter 18, "Psychosocial Aspects of Trauma Care," for additional information.

Special Considerations for the Care of Patients with Physical Abuse

Special considerations for care of patients with injuries from physical abuse are highlighted in this section. Please review the relevant chapters for specific injuries.

H: History

A thorough history may reveal the following elements of concern:

- Unreasonable delay in seeking medical attention
- Previous ED visits or hospitalization for an injury or a medical condition that might have been prevented with appropriate care
- Vague, unclear, or changing account of how the injury occurred
- Patient is accompanied by another person who acts controlling in attitude or speaks for the patient
- Poor hygiene and/or inappropriate attire

> **RED FLAG**
>
> Red flags to consider for possible human trafficking include the following[55,63]:
>
> - The patient arrives at the ED without control of their own identification or without identification.
> - The person bringing the patient to the ED does not speak the same language as the patient and appears unrelated.
> - The patient who is trafficked may be branded or tattooed with specific symbols, such as a dollar sign ($), the trafficker's name, a number identifier, or a gang name.
> - A patient has a history of multiple abortions and/or sexually transmitted infections.
> - The patient is a migrant worker.[31]
> - Workplace injuries involve lack of proper protective gear, working long hours, or heavy physical activities with limited availability of food or drink.
> - The patient's pain is consistent with repetitive use injuries. Factory workers and sex workers may have back pain, musculoskeletal complaints, and abdominal pain.
> - Runaway children are at risk for sex trafficking; estimates from 2016 suggest that 1 out of 6 runaways are endangered and may be exploited. Of those exploited runaway children, 86% are estimated to have run away from foster care or social services care.[55]

> **RED FLAG**
>
> Red flags to consider for child neglect and abuse include the following[38,52,79]:
>
> - Malnourished, failure to thrive (weight below the 5th percentile), and child's physical appearance inappropriate for age
> - Inappropriate reaction to injury for developmental age—for example, infants, toddlers, or children failing to cry with pain
> - Deficits or delays in emotional and intellectual development, especially language
> - Use of self-soothing behaviors such as finger sucking, biting, scratching, or rocking by an older child
> - A child who arrives at the ED with immunizations incomplete or unknown, suggesting neglect or that the person accompanying the child may not be the primary caregiver
> - No explanation for the injury, discrepancy between the caregiver's and the patient's accounts, or explanation inconsistent with identified injuries
> - History of previous injuries, ingestions, or exposures to toxic substances
> - History of being left alone, abandoned, or with inadequate supervision
> - Excessive absenteeism from school or other social events/programs
> - Isolation from friends and other family members
> - Substance misuse
> - Delinquency or repeated encounters with law enforcement
> - Child in foster care
> - Child in an environment characterized by IPV directed at a parent or caregiver—such behavior also puts the child at risk for abuse and is considered a form of child maltreatment

- Multiple sexually transmitted infections
- Multiple pregnancies and/or abortions
- Malnourishment or chronic dehydration
- Inactivity or extreme passiveness
- Untreated medical conditions such as dental caries and periodontal disease

H: Head-to-Toe Assessment

When assessing the patient with suspected physical abuse, inconsistencies between the injury history and the injuries sustained should alert the trauma team to the possibility of abuse as the cause. Examples of the behaviors and injuries are discussed in the following sections.

Head Injuries

Certain types of head injuries can indicate interpersonal violence. For example, skull fractures; intracranial or extracranial bleeds; spotty balding (from hair pulling); retinal hemorrhage or other eye injuries, such as a dislocated lens or corneal laceration; and dental injuries all can indicate interpersonal violence. Abusive head trauma is a serious form of child maltreatment that occurs when the child has sustained sudden shaking or other impact injuries. A head injury in an adult that is inconsistent with the history may also be suspicious of abusive head trauma.

See also Chapter 7, "Head Trauma."

Strangulation

Strangulation occurs when external pressure is placed on the neck, leading to reduced blood flow to the brain and/or airway closure. Occlusion of the jugular veins results in venous congestion and intracranial pressure. Carotid artery obstruction stops blood flow and impedes oxygen delivery to the brain. Pressure on the carotid sinus can cause acute bradycardia and/or cardiac arrest.

Strangulation can result in injuries to the soft tissues of the neck, esophagus, larynx, trachea, and cervical spine and the laryngeal and facial nerves.[22,28,37] Nonfatal strangulation may result in minimal or no external signs of injury. A CT angiogram is considered the standard of care when evaluating for injury related to nonfatal strangulation.

Other assessment findings include the following:

- Dysphonia, dysphagia, odynophagia, or dyspnea
- Neck and mastoid—ligature marks, edema, abrasions, erythema, contusions
- Petechiae in/on the eyelids, periorbital region, face, scalp, neck, ears, or soft palate, or under the tongue
- Subconjunctival or scleral hemorrhage
- Neurologic findings—ptosis, facial droop, unilateral weakness, loss of sensation, paralysis, or seizure
- Lung injuries—aspiration pneumonia, pulmonary edema

Bruises

Bruises, or ecchymosis, may be seen in cases of interpersonal violence. These intentionally inflicted injuries have distinguishing characteristics that can raise the index of suspicion for maltreatment:

- Unexplained bruises or welts
- Multiple or symmetric bruises or marks
- Bruises and welts to the face, mouth, neck, chest, abdomen, back, flank, thighs, or anogenital area
- Bruises and welts with patterns descriptive of an object, such as a looped cord, belt buckle, boot tread, wire hanger, or hand or pinch marks (patterned injury)
- Bruises in various stages of healing (patterns of injury)

Burns

Correlation of the severity and pattern of the burn injury with the history provides a basis for the identification of inflicted burns.

- Burns to the lips or tongue, especially if surrounded by bruising. This may indicate forcing hot liquids.
- Burns to the rectum or perineum.
- Bilateral burns, such as a stocking-type (on the lower extremities) or glove-type (on the upper extremities) burn, with sharp lines of demarcation; these indicate that the person was held down in hot liquid. In contrast, an accidental burn usually has irregular borders and splash burns.
- Sharp lines of demarcation, limited injury to the protected area, and uniform burn depth.
- Burns in the shape of an object such as a cigar or cigarette, cigarette lighter, iron, heating grate, or stove coils.

See Chapter 11, "Surface and Burn Trauma," for specific care of injury.

Bite Injuries

Assess bite injuries for specific patterns:

- Ovoid patterns of bruising, abrasions, or lacerations may be indicative of a bite mark, triggering the need for the patient to be screened and evaluated for interpersonal violence.
- Clenched-fist injuries, resulting from a clenched fist striking the teeth of another person, are treated as potential bite marks. Because of the site of injury (the knuckles) and the velocity, there is a higher risk of injury to bone, joint, tendon, or cartilage.
- Bite wounds involving marked tissue destruction have an increased risk for transmission of infection through blood and body fluids.
- Bite marks should be swabbed as part of collection of evidence.

Skeletal Injuries

Fractures resulting from physical abuse may be single or multiple, recent or old, or a combination of fractures involving both multiple numbers and sites. One of the more commonly injured bones from child abuse is the metaphysis of the humerus, whose fracture is caused by the individual being grasped by the arm and pulled, swung, or jerked. In this injury, a piece of the bone is broken from the growth plate by shearing forces. This should not be confused with nursemaid's elbow, which is not an abuse injury. Other types of suspicious fractures include bilateral or symmetric fractures; transverse, oblique, and spiral shaft fractures in those who are not mobile; rib fractures; scapular or sternal fractures; dislocations; multiple fractures in various bones; and fractures in different stages of healing. Seventy-seven percent of children presenting with rib fractures have been found to be abused.[40]

Abdominal Injuries

Abdominal injuries that may be indicative of interpersonal violence include intestinal perforation, hemorrhage, and laceration; abdominal contusion; or hematoma of the organs of the abdomen and retroperitoneum, including the liver, spleen, and kidney due to blunt force trauma. Concurrent findings such as abdominal distention, vomiting, abdominal pain, bruising, fever, hematuria, and shock (septic and hypovolemic) may also be signs of abuse.

Abdominal injuries are commonly seen in the pregnant population. Injuries from sexual violence include genital and rectal trauma, as well as vaginal infections. Such injuries should raise concern for the safety of the patient and the ability to return to a safe environment.

See Chapter 9, "Abdominal and Pelvic Trauma," for specific care.

Psychosocial Impact: Trauma-Informed Care Framework

It is essential to recognize the profound long-term psychological, biological, neurologic, physical, and/or interpersonal adverse effects that can occur after a traumatic event or series of events. The trauma-informed care framework encourages emergency nurses to approach all patients as potential abuse survivors in order to diminish the retraumatization that the emergency visit may trigger. It involves identifying survivor strengths and resilience, assisting survivor recovery and healing, and working collaboratively with the survivor to develop short- and long-term care plans that support healthy coping mechanisms. How questions are worded can be important. They should not sound like blaming. Asking for clarification or more detail versus "why" will support the patient and provide trauma-informed care.[26]

Each survivor needs to, and has a right to, feel safe during care; this will encourage active participation in their recovery. Each patient should be approached with respect, patience, and empathy. On a practical level, this means sharing information, sharing control, respecting boundaries, and encouraging mutual learning to understand healing stages (refer to Box 17-1). These practices demonstrate awareness and understanding of interpersonal violence and help both the survivor and the nurse initiate and engage in the recovery process.

Diagnostic Procedures

Diagnostic procedures include the following:

- Imaging studies: Full-body radiographic films are used to determine whether evidence of previously healed fractures or other injuries exists. If fractures are suspected or confirmed, document these findings with at least two views. CT is used to detect intracranial or extracranial injuries such as skull fractures, hemorrhage, or hematoma. CT scans can also document injuries to the solid and hollow abdominal organs. For strangulation injuries, a CT angiogram can detect damage to the carotid and vertebral arteries, and bony structures.[22]
- Laboratory studies: Laboratory studies include a toxicology screen of the patient's blood and urine if there is a suspicion of ingestion or exposure to toxic substances, use of alcohol, or overmedication. Blood and urine are the best samples for collection because the substance used may have been metabolized and be present only in the urine. A urine or blood pregnancy test should be performed on pregnancy-capable trauma survivors. If excessive bruising is discovered, complete blood count, platelet count, and coagulation studies can rule out bleeding disorders.

Considerations for the Care of Patients Who Have Experienced Sexual Violence: National Protocol for Sexual Assault Medical Forensic Examinations

Nurses need to review and understand their facility's protocol, including legal jurisdiction policies and procedures regarding chain of custody in medico-legal forensic examinations.[15] It is important for the trauma nurse to offer a medical forensic evaluation if the patient has disclosed being sexually assaulted or is concerned that they may have been sexually assaulted. Based on national protocols,[67,68] sexual assault medical forensic examinations can be performed up to 5 days after the assault, even if the patient has brushed their teeth, showered, urinated, defecated, and/or changed clothes. Forensic technology advancements have enabled the extension of post–sexual assault forensic examinations up to 9 days in some situations with living persons.[49] The nurse must obtain informed consent for a medical forensic evaluation, which is separate from consent for medical treatment. Often, additional consent may be needed to obtain blood and urine specimens in suspected drug-facilitated sexual assault patients. It is important to follow the facility's policies regarding consent. If the act was not one that requires mandated reporting, the patient can defer or decline the medical forensic exam or reporting to the authorities without available medical treatment being affected.[67] Pediatric forensic evaluations have slight variations from adult examinations, and each nurse should identify the needs of each patient as an individual.[49]

Additional Considerations

Additional considerations include the following:

- Use a safe, private room for the primary patient consultation and initial law enforcement interviews.
- Offer a waiting area for family members and friends, and provide childcare if possible.
- Assess and respond to safety concerns, such as threats to the patient or staff.
- Follow facility and jurisdictional procedures, while respecting patients and maximizing evidence collection and preservation.

Triage considerations include the following:

- Given the time-sensitive nature of the situation, treatment required, the possibility of severe psychological distress, and recognition that waiting to be examined may cause loss of evidence and undue secondary trauma, patients who experience sexual assault are assigned a minimum triage category of Emergency Severity Index level 2 or its equivalent in other triage systems. They are considered a priority for care.
- Make all efforts to bring the patient immediately to a private room.
- Triage nurses should be mindful of their questioning techniques. As patients arrive, assess for any life-threatening injuries that require immediate intervention, and ask when the assault occurred. Incorporate therapeutic communication techniques, such as active listening and observation skills, to decrease unintentional distress during the interaction. Communicate that it is not their fault, and convey concern for their health, safety, and well-being; trauma-informed care is critical at this time.[23]
- Notify specially trained medical forensic examiners if available and according to facility policy.

Healthcare professionals with specialized training in providing comprehensive medical forensic care to patients who have been sexually assaulted should care for these patients whenever possible. Specialized training includes trauma-informed care, crisis intervention, injury identification, forensic evidence collection and preservation, photo and written documentation, legal reporting, and chain-of-custody requirements. If the facility does not use medical forensic examiners, the emergency nurse will likely assist in the medical forensic examination (**Appendix 17-1**). Specialized medical forensic providers may include the following professionals:

- Sexual Assault Nurse Examiners (SANEs) are registered nurses with specialized education and training to provide comprehensive care to patients after a sexual assault. They fulfill the didactic and clinical training requirements to competently perform medical forensic examinations.[29,80]
- Registered nurses are certified as SANE-Adult and Adolescent (SANE-A) and/or SANE-Pediatric (SANE-P) through the International Association of Forensic Nurses.[27,80]
- Registered nurses may fulfill the clinical requirements that qualify them as a Forensic Nurse Examiner (FNE), enabling them to collect forensic evidence in a variety of situations, not just cases of sexual assault.
- Sexual Assault Forensic Examiners (SAFE) are physicians or physician assistants who have specialized education and training in caring for patients following sexual assault.
- Medical forensic care extends to patients who experience other forms of violence or trauma, such as interpersonal violence, human trafficking, occupational injuries, elder and child abuse, death investigation, mass casualties, and disaster response. Legal nurse consulting and working in correctional facilities are other examples of forensic nurse examiner roles.
- Advocates assist with safety and resource planning and community advocacy for patients who have experienced sexual assault and rape.[50,80]

History includes a detailed description of the incident. Be objective, and use direct quotes. This record should include the following elements:

- Date, time, and place of the incident
- Events surrounding the incident
- Information regarding all acts committed by the suspect, including verbal and physical threats, weapons or restraints used, sites of penetration and/or ejaculation, and the use or nonuse of a condom or lubricant, if known
- Injuries associated with the incident

- Activities by the patient following the incident, such as bathing or showering, wound care, drinking, eating, urination, defecation, and/or changing clothes

Additional obstetric and gynecologic history includes the following:

- Gravida and para status
- Date of last menstrual period
- Current method of birth control and compliance with method
- Time of last consensual intercourse (oral, vaginal, anal) and condom usage

If drug-facilitated sexual assault is suspected, the history may include the following:

- The patient may report having awakened in strange surroundings with disheveled clothing, unclear memory, or a feeling of being sexually violated.
- If some memory of the event remains, the patient may describe feeling paralyzed or powerless, or a disassociation of mind and body.
- The patient may report similar symptoms to the feeling of alcohol intoxication, although the severity may not match the amount consumed.
- The patient may report the sudden onset of symptoms such as drowsiness, lack of coordination, confusion, impaired memory, or complete lack of memory (amnesia) within 15–20 minutes of consuming a drink.

Mandated Reporting

A mandated reporter is required by law to report suspected maltreatment or abuse of a child, an older adult, or an adult with a disability.[45,65] This designation may be applied to many professionals, including healthcare and law enforcement professionals, teachers, clergy, and others. Nurses are mandated reporters in most jurisdictions. As such, they are responsible for screening the patient, assessing the patient for signs of maltreatment or abuse, and reporting their suspicions to social services and/or law enforcement. Nurses are mandated reporters of child abuse or neglect in 47 U.S. states, the District of Columbia, the Northern Mariana Islands, Guam, American Samoa, Puerto Rico, and the U.S. Virgin Islands.[65] Mandatory reporting for abuse of an older adult or an adult with disabilities varies widely by region.[45]

Nurses must follow jurisdictional requirements and facility policies for reporting the assault and/or abuse of a child, older adult, or an adult with a disability. Jurisdictions frequently amend laws, and it is incumbent upon the nurse to be knowledgeable about the legal requirements in their region of practice. If children are in the care of a patient who experienced interpersonal violence or IPV, reporting may also be required. Many areas have adopted legislation to require reporting for suspected child abuse, elder abuse, IPV, and human trafficking.

Danger and Lethality Assessment

Recognizing a survivor of IPV is not always easy. In fact, such abuse is often missed. The sequelae of a missed opportunity to offer the patient resources could place the patient back into a high-risk environment. The Danger Assessment is a lethality screening tool with an accompanying referral protocol that prompts appropriate action based on the results of the screening process.[34] The goal of the Danger Assessment is to prevent IPV homicides, serious injury, and reassault through the identification and utilization of IPV support services. Different versions of the tool are available for people in same-sex relationships, immigrants, and different languages.

The Lethality Assessment tool is a shortened version used by law enforcement. A Danger Assessment for clinicians is another shortened version useful in the ED.[36] These assessments are tools to support decision making and help identify IPV. Patients have the choice to use resources offered but are not required to do so.

Rehabilitation

Persons who experience violence or are exposed to interpersonal violence may be affected long term. If a person's psychological traumatic history and related symptoms go undetected, providers may deliver care and resources for disorders that only partially explain the patient's presentation and distress. Providers should screen all patients for assault, abuse, and/or neglect as a part of routine care. Universal screening for trauma history and trauma-related symptoms can help identify individuals at risk of developing more pervasive symptoms of traumatic stress. Screening, early identification, and intervention serve as a prevention strategy.[62]

All staff need to incorporate trauma-informed care into the care provided to these patients (**Figure 17-5**).[76] PTSD and other trauma-related disorders can affect a patient's healthcare experience and change how they interact in the healthcare environment. The nurse should eliminate, when possible, any practice that is potentially harmful, including seclusion and restraint use; interactions that are shaming, minimizing, discrediting, or that ignore the patient's response; labeling intense feelings as pathological; treatment planning without collaboration; and providing medical interventions without privacy.[8]

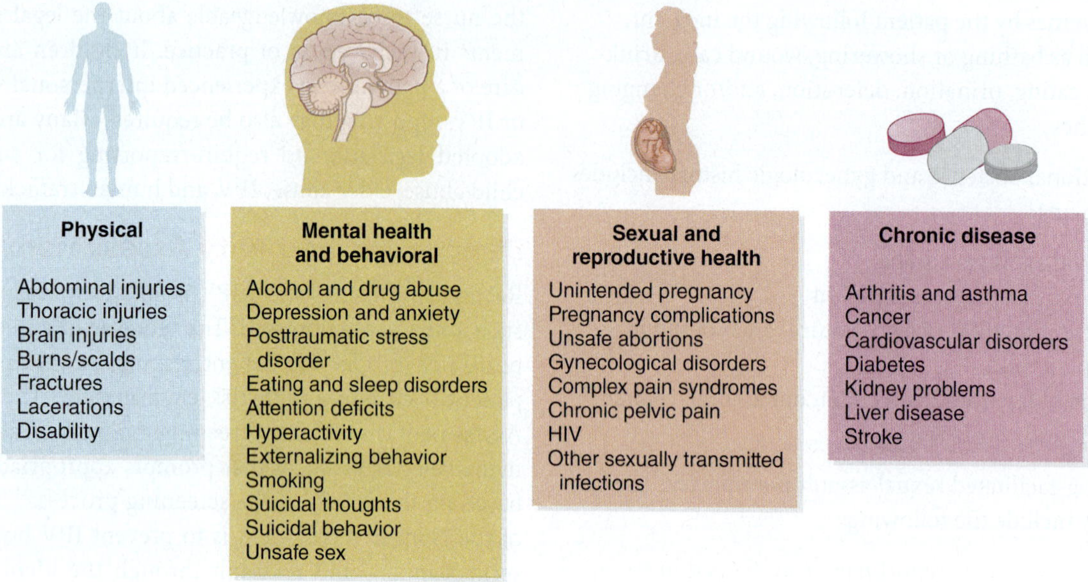

Physical	Mental health and behavioral	Sexual and reproductive health	Chronic disease
Abdominal injuries Thoracic injuries Brain injuries Burns/scalds Fractures Lacerations Disability	Alcohol and drug abuse Depression and anxiety Posttraumatic stress disorder Eating and sleep disorders Attention deficits Hyperactivity Externalizing behavior Smoking Suicidal thoughts Suicidal behavior Unsafe sex	Unintended pregnancy Pregnancy complications Unsafe abortions Gynecological disorders Complex pain syndromes Chronic pelvic pain HIV Other sexually transmitted infections	Arthritis and asthma Cancer Cardiovascular disorders Diabetes Kidney problems Liver disease Stroke

Figure 17-5 *Behavior and health consequences of violence.*

Reproduced from World Health Organization. (2014). *Global status report on violence prevention.* Retrieved January 12, 2022, from https://apps.who.int/iris/bitstream/handle/10665/145086/9789241564793_eng.pdf;sequence=1

Nurses need to be aware that interpersonal violence inflicts a wide range of emotions, from anger and rage to terror and withdrawal. Should these responses develop, ensure patients are referred to appropriate follow-up counseling. Patient discharge teaching should be provided from a trauma-informed framework. Innovative programs that utilize neurofeedback, meditation, yoga, sports, and drama to help recovery are available. Refer to **Appendix 17-2** and **Appendix 17-3** for a small sample of available resources.

Prevention

Identification of patients who have experienced interpersonal violence is fundamental to the provision of care and improved health outcomes. Many national and international professional nursing and physician organizations recommend screening for child maltreatment and abuse of older adults and adults with a disability. Screening should be conducted and the appropriate actions taken according to facility policy.

Prevention of interpersonal violence focuses on healthy relationships across the life span. The causes of interpersonal violence are complex and multifaceted, and they include individual, familial, community, cultural, and societal factors. Collaboration is essential to include diverse professional perspectives, as well as increased community awareness and participation, to address interpersonal violence within communities. This approach should include law enforcement professionals, nurses, physicians, social workers, advocacy groups, and academic–community collaborative groups. A collaborative response increases efficacy by building comprehensive, well-coordinated policies and procedures that maximize community resources.[14]

Preventive measures also include distribution of educational materials that discuss interpersonal violence, including IPV or domestic violence, child and adult maltreatment and abuse, sexual assault, and human trafficking. ED waiting rooms, treatment rooms, and restrooms are excellent areas for placement of materials that educate about this public health epidemic.

Nurses can also become active participants in policy and legislative processes to support and develop prevention programs that address forming healthy relationships and prevention of interpersonal violence. The ENA and IAFN have developed a joint position statement that provides suggestions for nurses regarding interpersonal violence prevention and documentation.[6] As reported by the World Health Organization and the Centers for Disease Control and Prevention, a growing body of research demonstrates that interpersonal violence can be prevented and its consequences mitigated on a national and international level. Prevention programs and survivor services, along with national action plans, policies, and laws to support prevention and response efforts, can begin to address the gaps that are still seen in violence prevention and mitigation in countries around the world.[76]

Summary

Interpersonal violence is a complex, multifaceted problem that has many contributing factors. The public health consequences—both physical and psychological—are far-reaching. Interpersonal violence occurs across all ages, cultures, genders, ethnicities, and economic classes. Patients who have experienced interpersonal violence require special considerations to support their physical and mental health and continued safety, in addition to high-quality trauma care. Trauma nurses should utilize a patient-centered and trauma-informed framework of care that addresses the patient's physical, medico-legal, cultural, and psychosocial needs, thereby helping to facilitate their recovery. Recognition and education are the first steps toward care and advocacy for what may often be hidden situations involving interpersonal violence.

Trauma nurses are in a unique position to bring about change, not only by effectively and empathetically caring for patients who have experienced interpersonal violence, but also by advocating for action plans; policies for prevention; and resources at the local, national, and global levels.

References

1. Alhusen, J. L., Ray, E., Sharps, P., & Bullock, L. (2015). Intimate partner violence during pregnancy: Maternal and neonatal outcomes. *Journal of Women's Health, 24*(1), 100–106. https://doi.org/10.1089/jwh.2014.4872
2. American College of Obstetricians and Gynecologists. (2019). *Sexual assault* (Committee Opinion No. 777). https://www.acog.org/clinical/clinical-guidance/committee-opinion/articles/2019/04/sexual-assault
3. American Society for the Positive Care of Children. (2018). *Child maltreatment statistics in the U.S.* https://americanspcc.org/child-abuse-statistics/
4. Basile, K. C., Smith, S. G., Kresnow, M., Khatiwada, S., & Leemis, R. W. (2022). *The National Intimate Partner and Sexual Violence Survey 2016/2017 report on sexual violence.* https://www.cdc.gov/violenceprevention/pdf/nisvs/nisvsreportonsexualviolence.pdf
5. Beal, J. A. (2017). Healthcare of the transgender youth still inadequate . . . still at risk. *Journal of Maternal/Child Nursing, 42*(5), 296. https://doi.org/10.1097/NMC.0000000000000362
6. Bush, K., & Nash, K. (2018). *Intimate partner violence* [Joint position statement]. Emergency Nurses Association and International Association of Forensic Nurses. https://www.forensicnurses.org/wp-content/uploads/2021/11/intimate_partner_violence_jo.pdf
7. Campbell, J., Matoff-Stepp, S., Velez, M. L., Hunter-Cox, H., & Laughon, K. (2021). Pregnancy-associated deaths from homicide, suicide, and drug overdose: Review of research and the intersection with intimate partner violence. *Journal of Women's Health, 30*(2), 236–244. https://doi.org/10.1089/jwh.2020.8875
8. Cannon, L M., Coolidge, E. M., LeGierse, J., Moskowitz, Y., Buckley, C., Chapin, E., Warren, M., & Kuzma, E. (2020). Trauma-informed education: Creating and pilot testing a nursing curriculum on trauma-informed care. *Nurse Education Today, 85*, Article 104245. https://doi.org/10.1016/j.nedt.2019.104256
9. Centers for Disease Control and Prevention. (n.d.). *Fast facts: Preventing child abuse & neglect.* https://www.cdc.gov/violenceprevention/childabuseandneglect/fastfact.html?CDC_AA_refVal=https%3A%2F%2Fwww.cdc.gov%2Fviolenceprevention%2Fchildabuseandneglect%2Fdefinitions.html
10. Centers for Disease Control and Prevention. (n.d.) *Fast facts: Preventing elder abuse.* https://www.cdc.gov/violenceprevention/elderabuse/fastfact.html
11. Centers for Disease Control and Prevention. (n.d.). *Infographic: 6 guiding principles to a trauma-informed approach.* https://www.cdc.gov/cpr/infographics/6_principles_trauma_info.htm
12. Centers for Disease Control and Prevention. (n.d.). *Intimate partner violence, sexual violence, and stalking among men.* https://www.cdc.gov/violenceprevention/intimatepartnerviolence/men-ipvsvandstalking.html
13. Centers for Disease Control and Prevention. (n.d.). *The economics of injury and violence prevention.* https://www.cdc.gov/injury/features/health-econ-cost-of-injury/index.html
14. Centers for Disease Control and Prevention. (2017). *Preventing intimate partner violence across the lifespan: A technical package of programs, policies, and practices.* https://www.cdc.gov/violenceprevention/pdf/ipv-technicalpackages.pdf
15. Child Welfare Information Gateway. (2021). *Links to state and tribal child welfare law and policy.* U.S. Department of Health and Human Services, Children's Bureau. https://www.childwelfare.gov/topics/systemwide/laws-policies/statutes/resources/
16. Cizmeli, C., Lobel, M., Harland, K., & Saftlas, S. (2018). Stability and changes in types of intimate partner violence across pore-pregnancy, pregnancy, and the postpartum period. *Women's Reproductive Health, 5*(3), 153–169. https://doi.org/10.1080/23293691.2018.1490084
17. Clarke, S., Richmond, R., Black, E., Fry, H, Obol, J. H., & Worth, H. (2019). Intimate partner violence in pregnancy: A cross-sectional study from post-conflict norther Uganda. *British Medical Journal, 9*, Article e027541. https://doi.org/10.1136/bmjopen-2018-027541
18. Colwell, C. (2021). Geriatric trauma: Initial evaluation and management. *UpToDate.* Retrieved August 2, 2022, from https://www.uptodate.com/contents/geriatric-trauma-initial-evaluation-and-management
19. DeBoos, J. (2019). Review article: Non-fatal strangulation: Hidden injuries, hidden risks. *Emergency Medicine Australasia, 31*(3), 302–308. https://doi.org/10.1111/1742-6723.13243
20. De Marchis, E. H., McCaw, B., Fleegler, E. W., Cohen, A. J., Lindau, S. T., Huebschmann, A. G., Tung, E. L.,

Hessler, D. M., & Gottlieb, L. M. (2021). *American Journal of Preventive Medicine, 61*(3), 439–444. https://doi.org/10.1016/j.amepre.2021.02.010

21. Diez, C., Kurland, R. P., Rothman, E. F., Bair-Merritt, M., Fleegler, E., Xuan, Z., & Siegel, M. (2017). State intimate partner violence-related firearm laws and intimate partner homicide rates in the United States, 1991–2015. *Annals of Internal Medicine, 167,* 536–543. https://doi.org/10.7326/M16-2849

22. Dunn, R. J., Sukhija, K., & Lopez, R. A. (2022, June 22). Strangulation injuries. *StatPearls.* StatPearls Publishing. https://www.ncbi.nlm.nih.gov/books/NBK459192/

23. Fischer, K. R., Bakes, K. M., Corbin, T. J., Fein, J. A., Harris, E., J., James, T. L., & Melzer-Lange, M. D. (2019). Trauma-informed care for violently injured patients in the emergency department. *Annals of Emergency Medicine, 73*(2), 193–202. https://doi.org/10.1016/j.annemergmed.2018.10.018

24. Greenbaum, V. J., Dodd, M., & McCracken, C. (2018). A short screening tool to identify victims of child sex trafficking in the health care setting. *Pediatric Emergency Care, 34*(1), 33–37. https://doi.org/10.1097/PEC.0000000000000602

25. Halphen, J. M., & Dyer, C. B. (2021). Elder abuse, self-neglect, and related phenomena. *UpToDate.* Retrieved May 23, 2022, from https://www.uptodate.com/contents/elder-abuse-self-neglect-and-related-phenomena/print

26. International Association of Chiefs of Police. (2017). *Successful trauma informed victim interviewing.* https://www.theiacp.org/sites/default/files/2020-06/Final%20Design%20Successful%20Trauma%20Informed%20Victim%20Interviewing.pdf

27. International Association of Forensic Nurses. (n.d.). *Areas of forensic nursing practice.* https://www.forensicnurses.org/page/AreasFNPractice

28. International Association of Forensic Nurses. (n.d.). *Non-fatal strangulation documentation toolkit.* https://www.forensicnurses.org/page/STAssessment

29. International Association of Forensic Nurses. (2018). *Sexual assault nurse examiner (SANE) education guidelines.* https://www.forensicnurses.org/wp-content/uploads/2022/03/SANE_EdGuidelines_2022_Updated_Resources_-2.pdf

30. International Association of Forensic Nurses. (2022). *Violence is a public health and healthcare issue.* https://www.forensicnurses.org/wp-content/uploads/2022/05/Violence-is-a-Health-Issue-2022.pdf

31. International Labour Office. (2017). *Global estimates of modern slavery: Forced labour and forced marriage.* http://www.ilo.org/global/publications/books/WCMS_575479/lang--en/index.htm

32. Irving, T., Menon, R., & Ciantar, E. (2021). Trauma during pregnancy. *BJA Education, 21*(1), 10–19. https://doi.org/10.1016/j.bjae.2020.08.005

33. Jimenez-Herrera, M. F., Llaurado-Serra, M., Acebedo-Urdiales, S., Bazo-Hernandez, L., Font-Jimenez, I., & Axelsson, C. (2020). Emotions and feelings in critical and emergency caring situations: A qualitative study. *BMC Nursing, 19,* Article 60. https://doi.org/10.1186/s12912-020-00438-6

34. Johns Hopkins University School of Nursing. (2019). *Danger Assessment.* https://www.dangerassessment.org

35. Macias-Konstantopoulos, W., & Ma, Z. B. (2017). Physical health of human trafficking survivors: Unmet essentials. In M. Chisolm-Straker & H. Stoklosa (Eds.), *Human trafficking is a public health issue* (pp. 185–210). https://doi.org/10.1007/978-3-319-47824-1_11

36. Messing, J. T., Campbell, J. C., & Snider, C. (2017). Validation and adaptation of the Danger Assessment-5: A brief intimate partner violence risk assessment. *Journal of Advanced Nursing, 73,* 3220–3230. https://doi.org/10.1111/jan.13459

37. Messing, J. T., Patch, M., Wilson, J. S., Kelen, G. D., & Campbell, J. (2018). Differentiating among attempted, completed, and multiple nonfatal strangulation in women experiencing intimate partner violence. *Women's Health Issues, 28*(1), 104–111. https://doi.org/10.1016/j.whi.2017.10.002

38. Mikton, C. R., Tanaka, M., Tomlinson, M., Streiner, D. L., Tonmyr, L., Lee, B. X., & MacMillan, H. (2017). Global research priorities for interpersonal violence prevention: A modified Delphi study. *Bulletin of the World Health Organization, 95*(1), 36–48. https://doi.org/10.2471/BLT.16.172965

39. Mills, T. J. (2019). Elder abuse. *Medscape.* Retrieved February 15, 2022, from https://emedicine.medscape.com/article/805727-overview

40. Mitchell, I. C., Norat, B. J., Auerbach, M., Bressler, C. J., Como, J. J., Escobar, M. A., Flynn-O'Brien, K. T., Lindberg, D. M., Nickoles, T., Rosado, N., Weeks, K. & Maguire, S. (2021). *Academic Emergency Medicine, 28*(1), 5–8. https://doi.org/10.1111/acem.14122

41. Musetti, A., Grazia, V., Manari, T., Terrone, G., & Corsano, P. (2021), Linking childhood emotional neglect to adolescents' parent-related loneliness: Self-other differentiation and emotional detachment from parents as mediators. *Child Abuse & Neglect, 122.* https://www.sciencedirect.com/science/article/abs/pii/S0145213421004075

42. Nagle, J. (2020). Child maltreatment. In D. Brecher (Ed.), *Emergency nursing pediatric course: Provider manual* (5th ed., pp. 129–141). Jones & Bartlett Learning.

43. National Adult Protective Services Association. (n.d.). *Resources regarding financial exploitation.* https://www.napsa-now.org/additional-resources-for-financial-exploitation/

44. National Center on Domestic and Sexual Violence. (2020). *Power and Control Wheel.* http://www.ncdsv.org/images/powercontrolwheelnoshading.pdf

45. National Center on Elder Abuse. (n.d.). *Research, statistics, and data.* https://ncea.acl.gov/What-We-Do/Research/Statistics-and-Data.aspx

46. National Coalition Against Domestic Violence. (n.d.). *Dynamics of abuse.* https://ncadv.org/dynamics-of-abuse

47. National Coalition Against Domestic Violence. (n.d.). *Statistics.* https://www.ncadv.org/statistics

48. National Coalition Against Domestic Violence. (2017). *Domestic violence & sexual assault.* https://assets.speakcdn.com/assets/2497/sexual_assault_dv.pdf

49. National Institute of Justice. (2017). *National best practices for sexual assault kits: Multidisciplinary approach.* U.S. Department of Justice, Office of Justice Programs. https://www.ncjrs.gov/pdffiles1/nij/250384.pdf

50. National Institute of Justice. (2017, July 11). *The most important features for an effective sexual assault response team*. U.S. Department of Justice, Office of Justice Programs. https://nij.gov/topics/crime/rape-sexual-violence/Pages/important-features-for-sart.aspx
51. National Network to End Domestic Violence. (2017). *About financial abuse*. https://nnedv.org/content/about-financial-abuse/
52. Nielson, M. H. (2018). Abuse and neglect. In V. Sweet (Ed.), *Emergency nursing core curriculum* (7th ed., pp. 36–46). Elsevier.
53. Office for Victims of Crime. (n.d.). *Human trafficking*. U.S. Department of Justice, Office of Justice Programs. https://ovc.ncjrs.gov/humantrafficking/
54. Peterson, C., Miller, G. F., Barnett, S., & Florence, C. (2021). Economic cost of injury—United States, 2019. *Morbidity and Mortality Weekly Report, 70*(48), 1655–1659. https://doi.org/10.15585/mmwr.mm7048a1
55. Polaris. (n.d.). *Human trafficking: The facts*. https://polarisproject.org/human-trafficking/facts
56. Polaris. (2021). *Polaris analysis of 2020 data from the National Human Trafficking Hotline*. https://polarisproject.org/wp-content/uploads/2022/01/Polaris-Analysis-of-2020-Data-from-the-National-Human-Trafficking-Hotline.pdf
57. Rape, Abuse & Incest National Network. (n.d.). *Child sexual abuse*. https://www.rainn.org/articles/child-sexual-abuse
58. Richer, L. A., Fields, L., Bell, S., Heppner, J., Dodge, J., Boccellari, A., & Shumway, M. (2015). Characterizing drug-facilitated sexual assault subtypes and treatment engagement of victims at a hospital-based rape treatment center. *Journal of Interpersonal Violence, 32*(10), 1524–1542. https://doi.org/10.1177%2F0886260515589567
59. Rodrigues, J. L., Lima, A. P., Nagata, J. Y., Rigo, L., Cericato, G. O., Franco, A., & Paranhos, L. R. (2016). Domestic violence against children detected and managed in the routine of dentistry: A systematic review. *Science Direct, 43*, 34–41. https://doi.org/10.1016/j.jflm.2016.07.006
60. Sontate, K. V., Kamaluddin, M. R., Mohamed, I. N., Mohamed, R. M., Shaikh, M. F., Kamal, H., & Kumar, J. (2021). Alcohol, aggression, and violence: From public health to neuroscience. *Frontiers in Psychology, 12*, Article 699726. https://doi.org/10.3389/fpsyg.2021.699726
61. Stodolska, A., Parnicka, A., Tobiasz-Adamczyk, B., & Grodzicki, T. (2020). Exploring elder neglect: New theoretical perspectives and diagnostic challenges. *The Gerontologist, 60*(6), e438–e448. https://doi.org/10.1093/geront/gnz059
62. Substance Abuse and Mental Health Services Administration. (2014). *Trauma-informed care in behavioral health services*. Treatment Improvement Protocol (TIP) Series 57, HHS Publication No. (SMA) 13-4801. U.S. Department of Health & Human Services. https://store.samhsa.gov/sites/default/files/d7/priv/sma14-4816.pdf
63. Tracy, E. E., & Macias-Konstantopoulos, M. (2021). Human trafficking: Identification and evaluation in the health care setting. *UpToDate*. Retrieved January 25, 2022, from https://www.uptodate.com/contents/human-trafficking-identification-and-evaluation-in-the-health-care-setting
64. U.S. Department of Health and Human Services, Administration for Children and Families, Administration on Children, Youth and Families, Children's Bureau. (2018). *Child maltreatment 2016*. https://americanspcc.org/wp-content/uploads/2018/03/2016-Child-Maltreatment.pdf
65. U.S. Department of Health & Human Services. (2022). *Child maltreatment 2020*. https://www.acf.hhs.gov/sites/default/files/documents/cb/child-maltreatment-report-2020_0.pdf
66. U.S. Department of Justice, Drug Enforcement Administration. (2017). *Drug-facilitated sexual assault*. https://www.dea.gov/sites/default/files/2018-07/DFSA_0.PDF
67. U.S. Department of Justice, Office of Violence Against Women. (2013). *A national protocol for sexual assault forensic examinations: Adults/adolescents* (2nd ed.). https://www.ncjrs.gov/pdffiles1/ovw/241903.pdf
68. U.S. Department of Justice, Office of Violence Against Women. (2016). *A national protocol for sexual abuse medical forensic examinations: Pediatric*. https://www.justice.gov/ovw/file/846856/download
69. Washington State Department of Social and Health Services. (n.d.). *Types and signs of abuse*. https://www.dshs.wa.gov/altsa/home-and-community-services/types-and-signs-abuse
70. Watson, A., Jafari, M., & Seifi, A. (2020). The persistent pandemic of violence against health care workers. *The American Journal of Managed Care, 26*(12), e377–e379. https://doi.org/10.37765/ajmc.2020.88543
71. White, C., Martin, G., Schofield, A. M., & Majeed-Ariss, R. (2021). "I thought he was going to kill me": Analysis of 204 case files of adults reporting non-fatal strangulation as part of a sexual assault over a 3-year period. *Journal of Forensic and Legal Medicine, 79*, Article 102128. https://doi.org/10.1016/j.jflm.2021.102128
72. Wiemann, C. M., & Miller, E. (2022). Date rape: Identification and management. *UpToDate*. Retrieved October 2, 2022, from https://www.uptodate.com/contents/date-rape-identification-and-management
73. Wong, J. Y., Choi, A. W., Fong, D. Y., Choi, E. P., Wong, J. K., So, F. L., Lau, C. L., & Kam, C. (2016). A comparison of intimate partner violence and associated physical injuries between cohabitating and married women: A 5-year medical chart review. *BMC Public Health, 16*, Article 1207. https://doi.org/10.1186/s12889-016-3879-y
74. World Health Organization. (n.d.). *The VPA approach: Definition and typology of violence*. https://www.who.int/groups/violence-prevention-alliance/approach#:~:text=Definition%20and%20typology%20of%20violence&text=%22the%20intentional%20use%20of%20physical,%2C%20maldevelopment%2C%20or%20deprivation.%22
75. World Health Organization. (2011). *Intimate partner violence during pregnancy* [Information sheet]. http://apps.who.int/iris/bitstream/handle/10665/70764/WHO_RHR_11.35_eng.pdf;jsessionid=4EC5CBA17EF2F2F32A53A1D7E44BD05C?sequence=1
76. World Health Organization. (2014). *Global status report on violence prevention 2014*. http://apps.who.int/iris/bitstream/10665/145086/1/9789241564793_eng.pdf?ua=1&ua=1

77. World Health Organization. (2021, June 9). *Violence against women.* https://www.who.int/news-room/fact-sheets/detail/violence-against-women
78. Wyatt, T. R., & Sinutko, J. (2018). Hidden in plain sight: A guide to human trafficking for home healthcare clinicians. *Home Healthcare Now, 36*(5), 282–288. https://doi.org/10.1097/nhh.0000000000000731
79. Zijlstra, E., Esselink, G., Moors, M. L., LoFoWong, S., Hutschemaekers, G., & Lagro-Janssen, A. (2017). Vulnerability and revictimization: Victim characteristics in a Dutch assault center. *Journal of Forensic and Legal Medicine, 52,* 199–207. https://doi.org/10.1016/j.jflm.2017.08.003
80. Zilkens, R. R., Smith, D. A., Kelly, M. C., Mukhtar, A., Semmens, J. B., & Philips, M. A. (2017). Sexual assault and general body injuries: A detailed cross-sectional Australian study of 1163 women. *Forensic Science International, 279,* 112–120. https://doi.org/10.1016/j.forsciint.2017.08.001
81. Zuberi, O. S., Dixon, T., Richardson, A., Gandhe, A., Hadi, M., & Joshi, J. (2019). CT angiograms of the neck in strangulation victims: Incidence of positive findings at a level one trauma center over a 7-year period. *Emergency Radiology, 26*(5), 485–492. https://doi.org/10.1007/s10140-019-01690-3

APPENDIX 17-1
Forensic Evidence Collection: Maintain Chain of Custody Preservation

Evidence protection and collection[2-4] can be an essential aspect of the care provided to the patient who has experienced interpersonal violence. Consideration is given to the patient's potential life-threatening injuries, their emotional response, and their rights. Complete the forensic examination only after the patient's immediate life threats are treated and the patient is stabilized. Consider the following points when collecting evidence:

- Patients are cautioned not to wash, change clothes, urinate, defecate, smoke, drink, or eat until initially evaluated by examiners, unless necessary for treating acute medical needs. If the patient did any of these prior to examination, include what and when in documentation.
- Clothing:
  - When cutting to remove the patient's clothing, avoid any areas that appear to be cut or torn by a weapon or projectile, that are stained, or that have debris, such as gunshot residue.
  - Dry and store each item of patient clothing in a separate paper bag. Plastic bags are not recommended for evidence collection because moisture can cause fungal growth, rendering evidence useless.
- Carefully assess all skin surfaces, and ask the patient about areas that were hurt or injured.
- Use body diagrams to identify and describe each injury in detail, using correct terminology and direct quotes.
  - Because direct quotes are an important aspect of clear and complete documentation, certain terms used by the patient may not reflect medical terminology.
  - Documentation includes explanation of the agreed-on terminology for clarification.
- Forensic photography of injuries:
  - Many jurisdictions have policies regarding who is qualified to take forensic photographs. Follow the organizational guidelines for forensic photography.
  - Obtain photographs whenever possible before medical treatment.
  - Obtain consent.
  - Use good lighting.
  - Include a patient identifier (date of birth, medical record label) in the photograph.
  - Take a distance shot of the whole body; take a picture at midrange and a close-up of the injury.
  - Include a measuring device, such as a ruler or scale (the American Board of Forensic Odontology scale is recommended).
  - Photograph bite marks for dental forensic analysis.
- Specimen collection:
  - Swabs
    - Moisten the swab with sterile water.
    - Swab the following by rolling the moistened swab across the skin:
      - Potential areas of retained body fluids, including sites of kissing or licking
      - Bite marks
      - Vagina, vaginal vault, and external genitalia
      - Penis
      - Anus
    - Label all swabs for the specific site, including the date, patient's name, and name of collector.
    - Allow the swab to dry completely.
    - Scrape under the fingernails (in some jurisdictions, swabbing may be preferred).
  - Comb the patient's hair, both head hair and pubic hair. This step can help investigators differentiate between strands of the patient's hair and that of the perpetrator.
  - Use evidence tape to seal and sign or initial each receptacle once sealed.
  - Place all properly sealed biohazard evidence (sexual assault kit) in a locked refrigerator area.
  - The key to the locked evidence refrigerator should be locked in a secure area.
    - A log should be maintained that documents chain of custody until evidence is transferred to law enforcement.
    - The name and title of the person who placed the forensic evidence in the locked refrigerator should be noted, along with date and time.
    - In the same log, document transfer of chain of evidence information with the name, badge number, and law enforcement agency of the person picking up the evidence, along with the date and time collected.

Additional considerations for the patient presenting to the ED following sexual violence include the following:

- Provide emotional support; incorporate the trauma-informed care framework principles.[1]
- Interpersonal violence and human trafficking survivors often develop PTSD, depression, anxiety, and suicidal ideation.
- Contact a survivor advocate to provide services to the patient, if not done already.
- Follow jurisdictional and organizational policies regarding reporting.
- Complete medico-legal documentation, to include a description of the events, body maps, diagrams, and photos (as required or allowed). Use direct quotes as appropriate. Do not allow the evidentiary chain of custody to be broken.
- Provide emergency contraceptive prophylaxis.
- Provide sexually transmitted infection prophylaxis, including human immunodeficiency virus prophylaxis.
  - Adhere to the current CDC guidelines.
  - Refer to facility protocols.
- Arrange for follow-up care to address any new infections or other medical issues, monitor both physical and psychological effects of the incident and treatment, and arrange posttrauma counseling or other treatments as may be appropriate for the patient's situation.

References

1. Fischer, K. R., Bakes, K. M., Corbin, T. J., Fein, J. A., Harris, E. J., James, T. L., & Melzer-Lange, M. D. (2019). *Annals of Emergency Medicine, 73*(2), 193–202. https://doi.org/10.1016/j.annemergmed.2018.10.018
2. National Institute of Justice. (2017). *National best practices for sexual assault kits: A multidisciplinary approach.* U.S. Department of Justice, Office of Justice Programs. https://www.ncjrs.gov/pdffiles1/nij/250384.pdf
3. U.S. Department of Justice, Office of Violence Against Women. (2013). *A national protocol for sexual assault forensic examinations: Adults/adolescents* (2nd ed.). https://www.ncjrs.gov/pdffiles1/ovw/241903.pdf
4. U.S. Department of Justice, Office of Violence Against Women. (2016). *A national protocol for sexual abuse medical forensic examinations: Pediatric.* https://www.justice.gov/ovw/file/846856/download

APPENDIX 17-2
IPV and Human Trafficking: Resources for the Community

Organization	Phone Number/Website
CDC Facebook page on violence prevention	www.facebook.com/vetoviolence
National Domestic Violence Hotline	www.ndvh.org 1-800-799-SAFE (7233), 1-800-787-3224 TTY
National Coalition Against Domestic Violence	www.ncadv.org
National Sexual Violence Resource Center	www.nsvrc.org
Futures Without Violence (formerly Family Violence Prevention Fund)	www.futureswithoutviolence.org
Department of Homeland Security: Human Trafficking	www.dhs.gov/topic/human-trafficking
Human Trafficking—HEAL (Health, Education, Advocacy, and Linkage)	https://healtrafficking.org
Polaris Project	www.polarisproject.org
National Resource Center on Domestic Violence	www.nrcdv.org
National Human Trafficking Hotline	www.humantraffickinghotline.org Forced sex? Text "BeFree" to 233-733 or call 1-888-373-7888
National Adult Protective Services Association	www.napsa-now.org
National Center on Elder Abuse	https://ncea.acl.gov 1-800-677-1116
Love Is Respect: National Dating Abuse Helpline	www.loveisrespect.org
National Domestic Violence Hotline	www.thehotline.org

APPENDIX 17-3

IPV and Human Trafficking: Resources for the Healthcare Worker

Organization	Phone Number/Website
National Child Traumatic Stress Network	www.nctsn.org
National Protocol for Sexual Assault Medical Forensic Examinations, Adult/Adolescent (2013): SAFE Protocol	www.ncjrs.gov/pdffiles1/ovw/241903.pdf
U.S. Department of Justice (2017): National Best Practices for Sexual Assault Kits: A Multidisciplinary Approach	www.ncjrs.gov/pdffiles1/nij/250384.pdf
Healthcare Toolbox: Healthcare Providers' Guide to Traumatic Stress in the Ill or Injured Child: After the ABCs, Consider the DEF (Distress, Emotional Support, Family) Protocol for Trauma-Informed Care	www.healthcaretoolbox.org
SOAR free online human trafficking training resources	https://nhttac.acf.hhs.gov/soar/soar-for-individuals/soar-online
Recognizing and Responding to Human Trafficking in a Healthcare Context	https://humantraffickinghotline.org/sites/default/files/Recognizing%20and%20Responding%20to%20Human%20Trafficking%20in%20a%20Healthcare%20Context_pdf.pdf
Nation Human Trafficking Hotline Data Report	https://humantraffickinghotline.org/sites/default/files/2016%20National%20Report.pdf
Alliance 8.7	www.alliance87.org
2017 Global Estimates of Modern Slavery: Forced Labour and Forced Marriage	www.ilo.org/global/publications/books/WCMS_575479/lang--en/index.htm
Substance Abuse and Mental Health Services Administration (SAMHSA): a free in-depth trauma-informed treatment care protocol in behavioral health services that trauma nurses can obtain	https://store.samhsa.gov/product/SAMHSA-s-Concept-of-Trauma-and-Guidance-for-a-Trauma-Informed-Approach/SMA14-4884
International Association of Forensic Nurses	www.forensicnurses.org
World Health Organization: Strengthening Health Systems to Respond to Women Subjected to Intimate-Partner Violence or Sexual Violence: A Manual for Health Managers	https://apps.who.int/iris/bitstream/handle/10665/259489/9789241513005-eng.pdf?sequence=1&isAllowed=y
Hate Crimes Bureau of Justice Statistics, 2005–2019	https://bjs.ojp.gov/sites/g/files/xyckuh236/files/media/document/hcv0519_1.pdf
Human Trafficking Data Collection Activities, 2021	https://bjs.ojp.gov/content/pub/pdf/htdca21.pdf
Danger Assessment for Clinicians	www.dangerassessment.org

CHAPTER 18

Psychosocial Aspects of Trauma Care

Candice M. Palmisano, MSN, RN, ACGNS-BC, CEN, MICN, CPN, CCRN, VA-BC

> **OBJECTIVES**
>
> Upon completion of this chapter, the learner will be able to:
> 1. Identify risk factors for the development of traumatic stress disorders.
> 2. Discuss the purpose and application of trauma-informed care.
> 3. Discuss the causes of and interventions for compassion fatigue, secondary traumatic stress, and burnout.

Introduction

Patients who experience a traumatic injury are at risk for suffering long-term physical consequences associated with the injuries. In addition, patients and their families may experience lasting psychological, emotional, and spiritual effects as a result of trauma.

Caring is at the heart of nursing practice, and evidence suggests that repeated exposure to traumatic situations can have lasting effects on nurses, with potential physical, psychological, emotional, social, and behavioral consequences.[14,32,57] Nurses who routinely work with severely injured and traumatized patients may experience psychological harm, which may pose a threat for both the nurse and patient.[32] Moreover, nurses may experience organizational violence, which can accumulate over time, contributing to burnout, posttraumatic stress disorder (PTSD), and less than optimal patient care. Nurses may ultimately exit the profession if interventions are not provided.[110]

While treating life-threatening physical injuries remains the priority, focusing on the psychological aspects of trauma care by completing a thoughtful assessment and planning and implementing psychosocial interventions can significantly affect recovery. Approximately 20–40% of injured trauma survivors experience acute and chronic stress and depressive disorders. Suicidal ideation and alcohol and substance misuse are also common.[22,35]

Responses to Trauma

A traumatic event can be characterized as dangerous, frightening, unpredictable, violent, an actual or perceived threat of serious injury or death, or actual or threatened sexual violence.[26,60] Although individual responses to traumatic events vary, support and guidance are needed for patients and their families as they work through the process of coping with trauma.

Common responses to trauma include the following[28,73,106]:

- Irritability and angry or aggressive outbursts
- Being easily startled
- Disrupted sleep and eating patterns
- Impaired ability to concentrate or make decisions
- Memory loss
- Feelings of being on guard, overwhelmed, or anxious
- Feeling lost
- Changes in behaviors
- Excessive silence
- Withdrawal
- Conflict in and strain on relationships
- Physical reactions, such as increased heart rate, diaphoresis, headache, chest pain, nausea, lightheadedness, dizziness, and tremors

The following factors can affect the level of distress experienced by the patient and their family[17,28]:

- The nature of the injury or traumatic event, including the following:
  - Intensity
  - Inescapability
  - Uncontrollability
  - Unexpectedness
  - Prolonged exposure
- Characteristics of the individual exposed to the event, including the following:
  - Previous exposure to trauma
  - History of behavioral health conditions
  - Substance use disorder or substance misuse
  - Support systems
  - Cultural factors
- The reaction or response, including the following:
  - Coping mechanisms
  - Defense mechanisms
  - Availability of resources and access to medical care

Each individual is unique in their response; these factors can influence the experience of injury, loss, and difficult news in the emergency care setting, leading to reactions that can range from stoic acceptance to a tearful response, anger, or even violent outbursts.

Psychosocial Nursing Care of the Trauma Patient

The psychosocial assessment begins after life-threatening injuries have been identified and stabilized. See Chapter 4, "Initial Assessment," for the systematic approach to care of the trauma patient. The purpose of the psychosocial assessment and appropriate interventions is to provide trauma-informed care (TIC) through understanding the correlation between the present injury and past psychosocial or trauma history. The aim of TIC is to prevent re-traumatization by recognizing the impact of previously experienced trauma.[19,45] The importance of patient–caregiver interactions cannot be overstated; the patient's perception of a healthcare provider's compassion during a crisis can help reduce the likelihood of developing PTSD.[67]

The six guiding principles to a trauma-informed approach follow[29,95]:

- Safety: Ensure physical and psychological safety
- Trustworthiness and transparency: Care is transparent, which builds and maintains trust and rapport with the patient
- Peer support (peer is defined as an individual with experiences of trauma): Assists with building trust and collaboration
- Collaboration and mutuality: Partnering and leveling of power differences between staff and patients
- Empowerment, voice, and choice: Empowerment for staff and patients
- Cultural issues: Eliminating cultural stereotypes and biases

Adverse Childhood Experiences

Adverse childhood experiences (ACEs), stressful and traumatic events that occur during childhood, have significant long-term impact on health and well-being. ACEs can include sexual, physical, or emotional abuse; neglect; or witnessing violence.[77,89] ACEs are associated with lifelong psychologic and physical consequences related to stress, including heart disease, stroke, chronic lung disease, or diabetes later in life.[89]

Children who have experienced adverse events, including violence or abuse, may not feel safe even when in a safe environment; they will require reassurance and patience because they may exhibit heightened levels of anxiety and emotional distress.[71] The traumatic event that brings a child to an ED can become an ACE; in addition, the painful and frightening experience of care in the ED, potentially worsened by the loud, confusing, and often chaotic environment, can itself become an ACE. To improve the outcomes of injured children experiencing trauma, it is of the utmost importance that a trauma-informed approach be employed when caring for them.[13]

Secondary Survey

As is typical, the secondary survey begins with obtaining history and proceeds to the head-to-toe assessment.

H: History

A thorough psychosocial history can improve care. Areas to assess include the following:

- Circumstances leading up to the event
- The patient's recollection of the event
- Any previously diagnosed stress disorders or mental health issues, including substance use
- Violence risk (intimate partner violence)
- Coping skills
- Resources that may be needed to cope with the effects of the events

H: Head-to-Toe Assessment

Complete all necessary assessments to rule out a physiologic cause for behavioral signs and symptoms. Many signs and symptoms can have either physiologic or emotional causes, and these can be difficult to differentiate. They include the following[28]:

- Physical: Nausea, vomiting, lightheadedness, dizziness, gastrointestinal distress, pain, tachycardia, jumpiness, tremors, sleep disturbances, headaches, fatigue, hyperventilation, palpitations, myalgias, hyperarousal, or startling easily
- Emotional: Shock, feeling lost, fear of harm to self and/or loved ones, numbness, depression, disbelief, volatile emotions, or feeling nothing
- Cognitive: Inability to concentrate, impaired decision-making, distraction, lack of focus, intrusive memories, feeling disoriented, memory loss
- Behavioral: Withdrawal, excessive silence, irritability, suspicion, inappropriate humor, altered eating patterns, increased substance use or misuse, increased smoking, change in sexual desire or behavior

Interventions

Repeated reassessments can guide evidence-based interventions that may help lessen symptoms. TIC provides a framework to help prevent traumatic stress responses and avoid retraumatization in injured patients.[20] A TIC approach includes the following[20,95]:

- Recognize the widespread impact of trauma exposure
- Identify how trauma may impact patients, family, and staff in the system
- Apply knowledge to practice and institutional policies
- Prevent retraumatization

Trauma-informed services within an institution benefit the patient, family, and staff in many ways. These include improved communication, assessments, screening, and interventions for people who have sustained traumatic injury, as well as the staff who care for them.[95]

To provide TIC, begin by assuring patients that they are safe and being cared for. Present a calm and soothing demeanor to facilitate coping as you support the patient and family emotionally and psychologically. The **RESPOND** mnemonic provides the nurse with an outline for the patient and family following a traumatic event:

- **R**eassure the patient and family that they are safe and well cared for.
- **E**stablish rapport with the patient and family; introduce yourself and the trauma team. Create a connection between the patient and key trauma team members.
- **S**upport the patient through the initial aftermath of the trauma. Help the patient contact family or friends. Assign a primary support person from the trauma team or department. Involve the hospital chaplain, bereavement team, and/or other appropriate resources. Encourage a member of the support team to remain with the patient or family when possible.
  - Patients or family members may prefer to have a social worker, trusted friend, or advisor from the community fill the role of support.
  - Some patients may wish to be alone or to involve others only after the extent of injury is known. It is important to respect the patient's wishes.
- **P**lan care and manage **p**ain.
  - Explain the plan of care to the patient and family succinctly, clearly, and in simple language.
  - Explain the reasons for diagnostic procedures and the process used to evaluate the extent of injury.
  - Set expectations for changes in the plan of care as a result of assessment or diagnostic findings.
  - Include the patient and family in the planning of care whenever possible.
  - Update the patient and family regularly and keep them apprised of what to expect next in the plan of care.
  - Explain the pain assessment tool and regularly assess the patient's level of pain, the response to medication, and the need for additional analgesia.
- **O**ffer hope.
  - While the nurse should not offer false hope regarding the extent of injury or the likelihood of

survival, it is essential to provide reassurance and support to the patient and family with open, compassionate communication.
- With the patient's consent, update family members regularly and as changes occur.
- **N**ever deliver news of death or disability to the patient or family by yourself. See the BREAKS protocol for additional information (**Box 18-1**).[16,70]
- **D**etermine the patient's needs.
  - Encourage the patient and family to express their feelings and needs following a traumatic event.
  - Determine the patient's decisions for confidentiality and sharing information with family.
  - Allow the patient and family to express fear, anger, vulnerability, and other emotions in response to the event.
  - Consider the use of a tool to screen for acute stress disorder (ASD) and PTSD. Advocate for early interventions.

> **NOTE**
>
> The RESPOND Mnemonic
>
> - R: Reassure.
> - E: Establish rapport.
> - S: Support the patient.
> - P: Plan care; manage pain.
> - O: Offer hope.
> - N: Never deliver news of death or disability to the patient or the family by yourself.
> - D: Determine the patient's needs.

> **BOX 18-1** BREAKS Protocol for Delivering Bad News
>
> - **Background**
>   Know the patient's background, clinical history, and family or support person.
> - **Rapport**
>   Build rapport, and allow time and space to understand the patient's concerns.
> - **Explore**
>   Determine the patient's understanding, and start from what the patient knows about the illness.
> - **Announce**
>   Preface the bad news with a warning; use nonmedical language. Avoid long explanations or stories of other patients. Give no more than three pieces of information at a time.
> - **Kindle**
>   Address emotions as they arise. Ask the patient to recount what you said. Be aware of denial.
> - **Summarize**
>   Summarize the bad news and the patient's concerns. Provide a written summary for the patient. Ensure patient safety (e.g., suicidality, ability to safely drive home) and provide follow-up options (e.g., on-call physician, help line, office appointment).
>
> Data from Berkey, F. J., Wiedemer, J. P., & Vithalani, N. D. (2018). Delivering bad or life-altering news. *American Family Physician, 98*(2), 99–104; Narayanan, V., Bista, B., & Koshy, C. (2010). BREAKS protocol for breaking bad news. *Indian Journal of Palliative Care, 16*(2), 61–65.

Nurses are often involved in sharing difficult information or when family members are informed that a patient has died. Occasionally, nurses may need to deliver this information themselves if this is in accordance with facility policies and protocols. Being as prepared as possible and using a tool such as the BREAKS protocol (Box 18-1) may assist the nurse in having difficult conversations or delivering bad news to a patient or family.[70]

Selected Psychosocial Trauma Reactions

This section highlights selected psychosocial conditions that can occur as a result of trauma.

Acute Stress Reaction

An acute stress reaction is caused by a traumatic event and can evoke feelings of fear, hopelessness, sadness, and/or other signs of psychological distress.[7,44] A stress reaction is considered a normal response to an abnormal event that causes physical and mental stress.[7] The stress reaction may have a rapid onset and is typically short-lived, resolving within hours or days.[7,44,100] An acute stress reaction may be experienced by the injured patient, as well as family members, and may occur in the absence of any preexisting behavioral health issues.[100] Distress and symptoms that interfere with relationships, work, or daily functioning may transition into a traumatic stress disorder.[7,44,46]

Crisis

A crisis can occur following an extraordinary or traumatic event and is defined as an overwhelming state.

It can happen to anyone, in any place, and at any time.[96,108] In a crisis, strong reactions can overwhelm the individual's normal coping mechanisms, and the person may be unable to function normally because of distress.[72,108,112] Patients may become anxious or disorganized, and they may panic or try to escape. They may also revert to less functional behaviors, such as violence or substance misuse, and/or they may experience depression or other psychological symptoms.[72] Applying the basic principles of crisis assessment and intervention is essential (**Table 18-1**).[96,108,112]

Traumatic Stress Disorders

Traumatic stress disorders, including ASD and PTSD, make up a constellation of conditions related to witnessing or experiencing a traumatic event(s).[105] Early recognition of and intervention for traumatic stress disorders is essential for optimal recovery, emphasizing the importance of the nursing assessment and screening during the acute care phase.[1,75] Evidence suggests that early interventions for traumatic stress may mitigate suffering.[75]

Acute Stress Disorder

According to the American Psychological Association,[7] ASD is a disabling psychological condition in which symptoms can begin immediately after the traumatic event.[5,44] Many symptoms of ASD are similar to, or the same as, PTSD, with time as the differentiating factor. ASD symptoms persist for at least 3 days and resolve within 30 days of the trauma.[7,100] The *Diagnostic and Statistical Manual of Mental Disorders, Fifth Edition* (DSM-5)[4] identifies five categories of symptoms[21,44,100]:

- Intrusion symptoms: Distressing memories of the event, repetitive dreams of the event, enactment (flashbacks), and intense distress when reminded of the event
- Negative mood: Unable to feel love, be happy, or feel successful
- Dissociative symptoms: Sense of detachment from self and emotions, dissociative amnesia
- Avoidance symptoms: Avoiding thoughts and feelings about, and memories of, the event; avoidance of external reminders
- Arousal symptoms: Sleep disturbances, irritability, and rage attacks with minimal or no provocation; hyper-alert, distracted, unusually strong reflexive reaction to sudden events

It is estimated that up to 20% of patients who have experienced a traumatic event will develop ASD.[21] Between 40% and 80% of people who are diagnosed with ASD subsequently develop PTSD, underscoring the need for early

TABLE 18-1 Assessment and Interventions for Patients in Crisis

Assessment	Intervention
Assess for the patient's perception of what happened. Assess mental status and risk for harm to self or others.	Ensure patient safety. Provide one-to-one observation if the patient is at risk for suicide. Remove any potentially harmful items. Provide reassurance and support. Communicate regularly to relay information throughout the ED stay.
Determine past and present medical history, including medications. Screen for the presence of substances that may alter behavior.	Use a calm and empathetic manner.
Assess for family and social issues.	Establish rapport and trust. Enable expression of feelings.
Ask about previous successful coping mechanisms. Inquire about existing support systems.	Focus on problem-solving. Offer simple, basic choices to promote decision-making. Facilitate patient involvement in the plan of care. Monitor for therapeutic communication with visitors and encourage a supportive person to stay with the patient.

Data from Substance Abuse and Mental Health Services. (2020). *National guidelines for behavioral health crisis care – A best practice toolkit knowledge information transformation*. https://www.samhsa.gov/sites/default/files/national-guidelines-for-behavioral-health-crisis-care-02242020.pdf; Wang, D., & Gupta, V. (2022). Crisis intervention. *StatPearls*. StatPearls Publishing. https://www.ncbi.nlm.nih.gov/books/NBK559081/; Zhang, L., Ahou, J., & Li, L. (2015). Crisis intervention in the acute stage after trauma. *International Journal of Emergency Mental Health and Human Resilience, 17*(4), 714–716. https://www.ncbi.nlm.nih.gov/books/NBK559081/

recognition and intervention.[21] However, many people who develop PTSD were not previously diagnosed with ASD.[21,105] Screening for stress reactions and disorders is a part of the post-resuscitative acute care phase and the post–acute care phase.

Posttraumatic Stress Disorder

Similar to ASD, PTSD is the result of a traumatic event, either experienced or witnessed; the individual believes that there is a threat to life and safety and experiences fear, terror, or helplessness.[6] Symptoms must persist for more than 30 days and result in impairment severe enough to interfere with daily activities, relationships, and work.[73] In addition, symptoms of PTSD may negatively affect recovery and overall quality of life, possibly contributing to long-term disability.[93,107] PTSD is a chronic disorder and often coexists with other mental health conditions, including major depression (48%), suicidal ideation, anxiety, panic disorders, and alcohol dependence.[65,66,80] The DSM-5 identifies four categories of symptom clusters, with a total of 20 symptoms[4,65,66]:

- Intrusion symptoms: Recurrent involuntary, intrusive thoughts regarding the traumatic event; distressing nightmares that may be repetitive; dissociative reactions and flashbacks; intense distress with event reminders; marked physiological response, such as tachycardia and increased blood pressure, when reminded of the event.
- Avoidance: Persistent avoidance of memories or thoughts associated with the event; efforts to avoid people, activities, places, or any external event reminders.
- Negative mood changes: Loss of recall of the event; distorted negative beliefs about self; distorted thinking that leads to blame of self or others; negative emotions such as fear or shame; decreased interest in activities that previously had been enjoyable; feeling detached from others; unable to feel love, be happy, or feel satisfied.
- Changes in arousal and reactivity: Irritable or aggressive with minimal or no provocation; reckless, self-destructive behavior; hyper-alert; unusually strong reflexive reaction to sudden events; sleep disturbances; difficulty concentrating.

Screening Tools

The American College of Surgeons recommends using an established protocol for the screening and referral process for patients at risk for mental health psychological sequelae related to trauma.[2] A number of evidence-based screening tools are available to assist in identifying individuals at risk for, or those experiencing symptoms of, a stress disorder. Screening tools that are efficient and brief may be more successful.[100] Three such tools are the Primary Care PTSD Screen for DSM-5[79]; the DEPITAC tool[62]; and the Injured Trauma Survivor Screen (Table 18-2).[53,54,76]

The Primary Care PTSD Screen for DSM-5 consists of a screening question ("Have you ever experienced this kind of event?") that, if answered affirmatively, is followed by five questions that correlate to the diagnostic criteria for ASD and PTSD.[79] The questions are as follows:

In the past month, have you. . .

- Had nightmares about the event(s) or thought about the event(s) when you did not want to?
- Tried hard not to think about the event(s) or gone out of your way to avoid situations that remind you of the event(s)?
- Been constantly on guard, watchful, or easily startled?
- Felt numb or detached from people, activities, or your surroundings?
- Felt guilty or unable to stop blaming yourself or others for the event(s) or any problems the events may have caused?

Generally, a score of 4 or more Yes answers indicates probable PTSD, although the cut point may be lower in some cases.

The DEPITAC (French acronym for screening/trauma/motor vehicle crash) screening questionnaire is a 10-question screening tool that predicts PTSD diagnosis one year after admission to the orthopedic trauma unit following a motor vehicle accident. However, it was reported that this questionnaire could be reduced to two items plus two elements of the patient's medical record, yielding a quick list of four questions[62]:

- Was there another person who was injured or died during the accident?
- Did you feel that you were about to die?
- How many children do you have?
- How long did you stay in the trauma area?

The Injured Trauma Survivor Screen (Table 18-2) was designed for use in the acute care setting and assesses the risk for PTSD and depression.[53,54,76] The tool has nine questions: four specific to PTSD, four specific to depression, and one that applies to both. Two or more Yes answers constitute a finding of probable PTSD or depression.

A positive finding while screening, regardless of the tool used, may warrant further psychological or neuropsychological evaluation and treatment.

TABLE 18-2 Injured Trauma Survivor Screen (ITSS)

Before This Injury		PTSD	DEP
Have you ever taken medication for, or been given, a mental health diagnosis?		– 1	0
Has there ever been a time in your life when, for more than 2 weeks, you have been bothered by feeling down or hopeless or lost all interest in things you usually enjoyed?		– 1	0
When You Were Injured or Right Afterward			
Did you think you were going to die?		1 0	1 0
Do you think this was done to you intentionally?		1 0	–
Since Your Injury			
Have you felt emotionally detached from your loved ones?		–	1 0
Do you find yourself crying and are unsure why?		–	1 0
Have you felt more restless, tense, or jumpy than usual?		1 0	–
Have you found yourself unable to stop worrying?		1 0	–
Do you find yourself thinking that the world is unsafe and that people are not to be trusted?		1 0	–
Total			

Yes = 1, No = 2
PTSD total ≥ 2 is positive for PTSD risk.
DEP total ≥ 2 is positive for depression risk.

Data from Hunt, J. C., Herrera-Hernandez, E., Brandolino, A., Jazinski-Chambers, K., Maher, K., Jackson, B., Smith, R. N., Lape, D., Cook, M., Berner, C., Schramm, A. T., Brasel, K. J., deMoya, M. A., & DeRoon-Cassini, T. A. (2021). Validation of the injured trauma survivor screen: An American Association for the Surgery of Trauma multi-institutional trial. *Journal of Trauma and Acute Care Surgery, 90*(5), 797–806; Hunt, J. C., Sapp, M., Walker, C., Warren, A. M., Brasel, K., & DeRoon-Cassini, T. A. (2017). Utility of the injured trauma survivor screen to predict PTSD and depression during hospital admission. *Journal of Trauma and Acute Care Surgery, 82*(1), 93–101; Petrucci, C. M., Villasenor, S., Brown, W. G., & Peters, R. M. (2022). Traumatic stress and depression risk screening at an ACS verified trauma center. *Journal of Trauma Nursing, 29*(3), 142–151.

Fear and Anxiety

Fear is the neurophysiological condition exhibited through the fight or flight response to a real or perceived current or imminent danger.[30] Anxiety is related to fear; however, it is anticipatory in nature, regarding future events or situations perceived as threatening.[30] After experiencing a traumatic event, patients may be fearful and/or anxious, demonstrating various degrees of uneasiness, distress, and worry. Patients or their family members may also exhibit irritability, restlessness, or difficulty concentrating, or they may experience tachycardia, palpitations, or tachypnea.[30] The nurse can help to mitigate these emotions by creating a safe environment and providing appropriate interventions (Table 18-1). The provision of clear information delivered in a thoughtful, concise manner to patients and families can increase perception of control and diminish fear and anxiety.[41]

Grief, Bereavement, and Mourning

Grief, bereavement, and mourning are not static events but processes that are influenced by personality, family, culture, religion, the circumstances involving the loss, the manner of death, and the relationship to the deceased person.[69,87] While the terms "bereavement," "mourning," and "grief" are often used interchangeably, each is a unique concept[69,86,87]:

- Grief: Natural and personal; an emotional and physiologic response to loss or anticipated loss
- Mourning: The individualized outward expression of grief and loss; involves adaptation to and acceptance of the finality of the loss
- Bereavement: The state of loss and the period of grief and mourning

Grief, in response to an actual or anticipated loss, can affect emotions, behaviors, and thoughts (Table 18-3).[24,69]

TABLE 18-3 Human Responses Following Grief

Dimension of Grief	Behaviors
Somatic expression	Physical complaints, such as pain, nausea, and headache
	Loss of appetite
	Overeating or weight gain
	Restlessness, sleep disturbances, fatigue
Cognitive expression	Preoccupation with the loss
	Fear and loneliness
	Low self-esteem
	Inability to concentrate or remember
	Helplessness and hopelessness
	Situations seeming unreal
Affective expression	Anxiety
	Guilt, resentment, and aggression
	Depression and despair
	Loneliness
	Anger
	Defensiveness or self-blame
Behavioral expression	Agitation
	Fatigue
	Crying
	Difficulty sleeping
	Social withdrawal

Note. Most common sign of grief in children

Data from Cancer.Net. (n.d.) *Understanding grief and loss.* https://www.cancer.net/coping-with-cancer/managing-emotions/grief-and-loss/understanding-grief-and-loss; Mughal, S., Azhar, Y., Mahon, M. M., & Siddiqui, W. J. (2022, May 22). Grief reaction. *StatPearls.* StatPearls Publishing. https://www.ncbi.nlm.nih.gov/books/NBK507832/#:~:text=Grief%20is%20a%20person's%20emotional,and%20mourning%20after%20a%20loss

Mourning is the expression of grief. Although commonly associated with the death of a loved one, grief and mourning can also occur from other meaningful losses[25,27,87]:

- Material: Loss of a home or other objects that have meaning to a person (sentimental value)
- Intrapsychic or spiritual: Loss of an aspect of one's self-image, or focus on possibilities of what might have been
- Relationship: Loss of the ability to have shared experiences and the physical presence of a person
- Functional: Loss of body function or parts (such as quadriplegia or limb amputation) or loss of sight
- Role: Loss of a specific role or the ability to perform a role

Grief Assessment

The experience of grief has physical, emotional, cognitive, behavioral, and spiritual dimensions.[69,87] While grief may be considered a universal, shared emotion, not all patients or family members experience it in the same way. Observations of reactions can guide the nurse in planning interventions on behalf of the patient and family (Table 18-3). A number of factors can influence how an individual processes grief, and a person's ability to adapt may be complex and depend on their life history.[74]

Cultural Considerations of Grief

Response to loss and death also has cultural variations and factors, in addition to individual responses.[43,88] Beliefs, attitudes, and practices are deeply personal, and sensitivity to a patient and family's cultural background, beliefs, values, and practices is foundational to nursing practice. Cultural humility enables understanding of the complexity of identities and reflects a lifelong commitment to self-reflection and redressing power imbalances when dealing with patients, families, and communities.[48] Cultural humility is different from cultural competence in that the focus of cultural humility is relationship-based and honoring of another's values, beliefs, and customs.[94]

Grief Interventions

Grief is a normal response when loss is experienced, and the goal for the patient and/or family is to facilitate healthy grieving. Many interventions for patients experiencing stress, fear, worry, and crisis are applicable to the patient experiencing grief. It is important to offer the patient or family the option of spiritual interventions and resources that are appropriate to each individual's unique responses to grief and aligned with their wishes. Questions related to these interventions include the following:

- Does the patient have preferred rites or rituals?
- Is there a spiritual leader or family member who can be contacted?
- Can these needs be facilitated within the emergency setting?

Immediate considerations and interventions can include the following:

- Facilitating family presence at the bedside
- Providing spiritual support
- Supporting person/friend/community member to be with them
- Social work support

Support can also be provided as the patient or family prepares to leave the ED. A grief discharge packet that includes pamphlets and phone numbers of local support groups or resources, as well as a follow-up phone call the next day, may help to identify needs or questions that arise after discharge. TIC assists in the process of grief and may diminish the likelihood of sequelae, including complicated grief and stress disorders.[20]

Additional Psychosocial Care Considerations

Providing resources for support of patients who have experienced injury is a fundamental step in the process of recovery. Clear policies and procedures should serve to support patients and their family by addressing the following needs:

- Communication and provision of interpreter services
- Family-centered care
- Family presence during resuscitation and invasive procedures

Communication and Interpreter Services

Approximately 20% of adults in the United States speak a language other than English.[58] When a language barrier exists, the use of medically trained interpreters is necessary for accurate medical information to be communicated. In the United States, the Office of Minority Health issues standards for culturally and linguistically appropriate care. It requires healthcare organizations to provide interpreters in a timely manner, and the service must be available during all hours of operation.[104] The Affordable Care Act places restrictions on family members functioning as interpreters, particularly if they are under 18 years of age.[91]

Communication interventions include the following:

- Determining the patient's preferred language for communication
- Identifying family or friends designated to receive important medical information if the patient cannot speak for themselves
- Speaking slowly and clearly to patients and families and making time for questions when delivering clinical findings or discussing the plan of care
- Using a professional interpreter
- Avoiding the use of friends or family members as interpreters; they may attempt to protect the patient instead of simply translating.
- Following organization policy regarding the use of interpreters

Hearing-impaired persons also may require an interpreter to address communication barriers.[91]

Family-Centered Care

Family-centered care and patient involvement in care are essential components of appropriate, safe, and timely healthcare in the trauma setting. This approach is grounded in partnership and collaboration between patients, families, and healthcare providers.[56] The Institute for Patient- and Family-Centered Care provides four core concepts for family-centered care[56]:

- Dignity and respect: Listen to and honor patient and family choices.
- Information sharing: Timely provision to the patient and family of complete, unbiased, accurate information to enable the making of informed decisions.
- Participation: Patients and family should be encouraged to participate in care and decision-making.
- Collaboration: Collaboration between the healthcare team, leadership, and patients and families in policy development, implementation, research, and delivery of care.

The Institute for Patient- and Family-Centered Care suggests that hospitals review and revise visitor policies, changing the focus from "visitor" to "partner" (**Table 18-4**).[55] It is essential that patients have necessary support, and the definition of "family" should include the people the patient considers family members.[55]

Family Presence During Resuscitation and Invasive Procedures

Family presence during resuscitation (FPDR) and invasive procedures in a high-acuity setting such as the ED and the intensive care unit is more likely to be a positive experience when facilities have clear policies and procedures in place that support such a practice.[38,78,99] Evidence indicates that many patients prefer to have family members present during invasive procedures or resuscitation for emotional support, with an expectation of decreased

TABLE 18-4 Guide for Being PARTNERS with Family

Mnemonic	Description
P	**P**resent yourself, and explain that you will work together.
A	**A**sk the patient and care partners to participate in decision-making when possible.
R	**R**eassure patients and care partners that their input is valued.
T	**T**rust the shared goal: Optimal care and outcome for the patient.
N	**N**urture relations with the care team.
E	**E**ncourage input and shared decision-making when possible.
R	**R**eview plans of care and discharge plans so that preferences and goals are recognized.
S	**S**upport participation of care partners as team members.

Data from Institute for Patient- and Family-Centered Care. (n.d.). *Better together pocket guide for staff.* https://www.ipfcc.org/bestpractices/IPFCC_Better_Together_Staff_Pocket_Print.pdf

pain, anxiety, and fear.[38] Family presence also promotes timely information sharing, eliminating the emotions associated with waiting while in a separate area such as a waiting room.[99] Each situation is unique and should be managed by asking the family member and/or patient if they would like to be present, and each institution should develop culturally relevant policies and procedures.[38]

Psychosocial Aspects of Caring for Agitated Patients and Families

The ED often serves as a safety net for many who, for a variety of reasons, have limited access to healthcare. Each ED is a microcosm of the community it serves, and staff in this setting may be exposed to difficult or even violent behavior. This behavior may be demonstrated by patients or family members under the influence of drugs or alcohol, or those with psychiatric disorders, poor coping mechanisms, or ineffective communication patterns. The ED is often the primary entry to the hospital, with public access 24 hours a day. Patients and families experiencing stress may exhibit escalating behaviors such as agitation, inappropriate communication, hostility, and threatened or actual physical violence. Workplace violence in the emergency setting is a global phenomenon.[98] Education regarding the best approach to take with patients and families, de-escalation techniques, and care of the psychiatric or agitated patient can help the nurse control difficult situations.[37] It is also important to implement a safety response for situations that may become out of control.

Preventing Escalation

Some techniques for preventing escalation include the following:

- Minimize chaos whenever possible.
- Have one point-of-contact person for message clarity.
- Talk to families in a designated, quiet, private area.
- Limit environmental stimuli when possible.
- Promote clear communication with support.
- Assess the need for, and try to provide, personal space.
- Sit and talk on the same level.
- Promote and assist with contacting other family members or support persons.
- Assess the need for spiritual support.
- Make multidisciplinary referrals for support.
- Provide comfort measures such as food, drink, and a quiet room.
- Observe verbal and nonverbal cues because they may indicate patient or family member needs.

De-escalation

If tension and frustration lead to escalating behaviors, take the following steps:

- Notify public safety personnel to stand by.
- Attempt to remain calm and nonjudgmental.
- Speak in a calm, quiet voice.
- Listen actively and observe the individual's nonverbal behavior.
- Maintain an exit route; place yourself between the patient or family and the door.
- Set limits and offer realistic choices if possible.

Mitigating Violence

Clinical and safety considerations in the management of violent behavior may include the following:

- Minimize stimulation in the environment.
- Use a low voice, and speak calmly and slowly to the patient and family. Avoid a condescending tone.

- Facilitate a safe environment for patients, families, and staff.
- For a patient who is violent, consider the following:
  - Assess for a physiologic cause of the behavior.
    - Obtain a point-of-care glucose level to assess for hypoglycemia.
    - Assess for oxygen desaturation and other signs that could suggest hypoxemia.
    - Anticipate diagnostics, such as a computed tomography scan, to assess for neurologic injury.
    - Obtain a toxicology screen to determine substance use.
  - If a reversal agent such as naloxone was administered, anticipate the possibility of aggressive behavior.
  - Administer medications as ordered, with support from other staff.
  - If restraints are necessary, follow organizational policies and procedures regarding their application, as well as monitoring, patient assessments, and documentation requirements.
- If assaulted, ensure safety for you and other staff, seek treatment, and report the incident according to organizational policies and procedures. Consider counseling.

Ethical Considerations in Trauma

The nurse will encounter ethical dilemmas in practice and may also experience moral distress. Moral distress is pervasive in nursing practice; it is the recognition of what is the right thing to do in a given situation but being unable to do so because of external constraints, such as organizational restraints.[3] The American Nurses Association provides a Nursing Code of Ethics, which includes nine nonnegotiable provisions of ethical behavior. The Emergency Nurses Association has provided interpretive statements to provide further guidance for emergency nurses.[36] This standard of practice describes the nurse's role as an advocate for all patients and families despite any personal beliefs or values.

Providers have an ethical, legal, and moral duty to provide care and ensure the safety of vulnerable patients, respect the wishes and dignity of the patient or family, determine decision-making authority, and adhere to legal precedent.[3,36] It is imperative that nurses be familiar with both implied and informed consent. With informed consent, providers have a duty to disclose the risks of, benefits of, and alternatives to suggested medical care. Implied consent may be presumed in instances in which a patient or their decision-maker is unable to authorize informed consent. It is not uncommon for injured patients to present to the hospital with conditions that prevent them from exercising self-determination and providing informed consent. National and regional laws and regulations determine the requirements regarding implied consent for emergency care, consent for nonemergent care, and when a surrogate decision maker is required, as in the case of a minor or incapacitated adult.

Advance Directives

Advance directives are legal documents intended to inform others of a person's wishes regarding healthcare options and what they do and do not want.[12,52] These documents may not be available when a patient arrives in the ED. If the patient is alert, ask about any particular wishes related to care. If the patient is not alert, ask the family or legal guardian to provide a copy of any advance directives. If there are no advance directives and the patient is not alert, follow organizational policy for care.

Nurses must be familiar with legal statutes and regulations, as well as organizational policies, that relate to consent and advance directives. Advance directives include living wills and a healthcare power of attorney or proxy. They can include directives such as the following[12,52]:

- Do not intubate
- Do not resuscitate (DNR)
- Do not defibrillate
- Do not hospitalize
- Comfort care only
- Physician orders for life-sustaining treatment (POLST)

Documents and forms can vary, so it is important to be familiar with the documents used and to understand the implications of each directive. Advance directives are often signed in the context of a medical illness, and the patient or proxy may wish them to be revoked in the event of a traumatic injury.[12,52] Clear explanations will help the patient or proxy decide whether the original criterion in the advance directive is still relevant in the current situation. Consider the following examples of the patient's right to choose and the patient's right to be informed.

Patient's Right to Choose

An 80-year-old pedestrian is hit by a motor vehicle and sustains a fractured femur. She has a history of hypertension and heart failure, and the family brought a signed DNR order from a past hospitalization. The patient is currently living independently in her own home. What is the responsibility of the trauma team in this situation?

Discussion

Autonomy is one of the foundational ethical principles in healthcare and provides patients with the right to make their own decisions regarding their healthcare options.[51,52] The nurse should examine the hospital policy regarding the use of DNR orders and the circumstances in which they are legally binding. An order from a previous hospitalization may not be applicable to future hospitalizations. In this scenario, the trauma team should educate the patient regarding the meaning of advance directives and ensure that the patient understands the implications of advance directives within the context of the injury and surgery. With the patient's health history, extubation following surgery may be difficult and carry some risk. It is important to discuss with the patient what will be involved during recovery and rehabilitation and to explain that chances for recovery may be very good. The patient and family need to consider all risks and benefits to make decisions for care with this hospitalization.

Right to Be Fully Informed

The concept of the right to be fully informed is perhaps best explained through a case. An 89-year patient arrives at the ED following a fall at ground level. The options for treatment for the injury sustained is a surgical repair or conservative treatment. The patient's daughter states that she wishes for the conservative treatment option and requests that the staff not discuss it with patient because it would be upsetting. The patient is alert, oriented, and able to communicate. What is the responsibility of the trauma team in this situation?

Discussion

Unless there is documentation giving the daughter healthcare power of attorney *and* the patient is unable to make decisions, the daughter is not legally able to make decisions for the patient. In this instance, the patient is alert and oriented and, therefore, has the right to know all the treatment options. The patient may include the daughter in the decision-making process if she chooses to, but the patient must be fully informed.

Organ and Tissue Donation

When death is inevitable, some families may receive comfort from the ability to donate their loved one's organs or tissues. Sensitivity and respect are vital when approaching families with this request, and who approaches the family is typically determined by organizational policy, statutes, or regulations and may vary from one location to another.

Organ procurement organizations (OPOs) determine whether the patient meets the potential donor qualifications and whether the patient is medically suitable for donation. OPOs are not-for-profit and follow strict federal regulations in the procurement process.[11] Additionally, OPOs help organizations develop policies and procedures regarding organ donation and provide education to healthcare professionals.[11] The process of organ or tissue donation and recovery is a collaborative team effort between the OPO and the patient care team.

Psychosocial Care of the Nurse

The nature of trauma care exposes the nurse to suffering. This exposure has been compounded by the suffering and stressors associated with the COVID-19 pandemic in the emergency and critical setting.[23] Repeated exposure to suffering or trauma can lead to compassion fatigue (CF) or secondary traumatic stress (STS).[10,14,59] Although different, both CF and STS affect the nurse's ability to deliver high-quality, empathetic care. STS and burnout are often considered components of CF.[10,14,57,59] Emergency nurses commonly go from one tragic event to the next without any opportunity to process the previous event or for any kind of self-care.[102]

Compassion Fatigue

Emergency departments (EDs) are fast-paced, high-stress environments with frequent staff exposure to death and suffering.[61,85] Compassion is defined as sympathy for another's pain or distress and a desire to help alleviate it. The definition of CF in the literature has a multitude of variations. However, most include some element of emotional, physical, and spiritual exhaustion after long-term exposure to people who are suffering.[50,64] CF can result in work-related, physical, and emotional symptoms (**Table 18-5**).[63,85,90]

Moral Injury

The ED can be a chaotic and challenging environment, and moral injury can result when team members cannot provide the high-quality care and healing they have been trained to perform.[49] Moral injury results from circumstances that violate a person's beliefs. This is not uncommon in healthcare; the nurse may struggle to provide the care the patient needs, being prevented from doing so because of circumstances beyond the provider's control,[34] such as in the case of decisions related to life and death or resource allocation. Emotional responses to moral injury include cynicism, grief, guilt, remorse, and anger. Symptoms associated with moral injury include depression, self-harm, aggression toward others, social isolation, and flashbacks.[49] Nurses who experience moral injury may need assistance and emotional support.

TABLE 18-5 Symptoms of Compassion Fatigue

Work-Related	Physical	Emotional
Avoidance or dread of working with certain patients or patient types	Chronic fatigue	Chronic worry
	Headaches	Depression
Reduced ability to feel empathy toward patients or families	Digestive problems: diarrhea, constipation, upset stomach	Moral distress, stress-related illness
Errors in judgment	Muscle tension	Anxiety
Impaired focus	Sleep disturbances: inability to sleep, insomnia, too much sleep	Irritability
Chronic tardiness		Anger and resentment
Frequent use of sick days	Cardiac symptoms: chest pain/pressure, palpitations, tachycardia	Detached or disinterested
Decreased sense of purpose	Frequent and lingering illness	

Data from Lombardo, B. L. (2011). Compassion fatigue: A nurse's primer. *The Online Journal of Issues in Nursing, 16*(1). https://ojin.nursingworld.org/table-of-contents/volume-16-2011/number-1-january-2011/compassion-fatigue-a-nurses-primer/; Salmond, E., Salmond, S., Ames, M., Kamienski, M., & Holly, C. (2019). Experiences of compassion fatigue in direct care nurses: A qualitative systematic review. *JBI Database System Reviews and Implementation Reports, 17*(5), 682–753; Sorenson, C., Bolick, B., Wright, K., & Hamilton, R. (2017). An evolutionary concept analysis of compassion fatigue. *Journal of Nursing Scholarship, 49*(5), 557–563.

Secondary Traumatic Stress

STS occurs as a result of witnessing or providing care for those who are suffering physically or emotionally.[42,59,83] Overall, approximately 18–33% of nurses have experienced symptoms consistent with STS. Such symptoms are similar to PTSD symptoms.[42,83] Symptoms can be clustered into three categories: intrusion, avoidance, and arousal (**Table 18-6**).[31,83] Nurses who develop STS may also experience depression, anxiety, increased work-related stress, and absenteeism.[18]

Burnout

Burnout is also considered a component of CF.[59] It occurs over time, with a gradual onset, building to a stress response. Burnout is a global phenomenon and results from chronic exposure to emotional or psychological stressors at work.[23,84] It is not unique to healthcare providers, but when occurring in these professionals, it may manifest as emotional exhaustion, patient depersonalization, a negative attitude toward patients, cynicism, and diminished feelings of personal and work accomplishments.[23,84] Burnout symptoms may be organized into three categories:

- Emotional exhaustion
- Depersonalization or distancing oneself from work and others
- Decreased sense of accomplishment (loss of joy in the practice of the profession)

Burnout is associated with difficulty managing work-related stress and feelings of helplessness and

TABLE 18-6 Secondary Traumatic Stress Symptoms

Category	Symptoms
Intrusion	Recurring thoughts about patients
	Dreams about work and patients
	Sense of reliving the disturbing events over and over
Avoidance	Avoiding certain patients
	Staying away from people and crowded places
	Inability to remember patient information
	Emotionless
	Disconnected from others
	Inactive
Arousal	Sleep disturbances
	Irritability
	Inability to focus
	Nervousness and agitation

Data from Columbo, L., Emanuel, F., & Zito, M. (2019). Secondary traumatic stress: Relationship with symptoms, exhaustion, and emotions among cemetery workers. *Frontiers in Psychology, 10*, Article 633. https://doi.org/10.3389%2Ffpsyg.2019.00633; Robinson, L. K., Sterling, L., Jackson, J., Gentry, E., Araujo, F., LaFond, C., Jacobson, K. C., & Lee, R. (2022). A secondary traumatic stress reduction program in emergency room nurses. *SAGE Open Nursing, 8*. https://doi.org/10.1177/23779608221094530

TABLE 18-7 Burnout Symptoms

Burnout Component	Symptoms
Emotional exhaustion	Headache
	Fatigue
	Gastrointestinal complaints
	Muscle strain and tightness
	Increased blood pressure
	Respiratory symptoms
	Sleep disorders
Depersonalization	Anxiety
	Irritability
	Sadness and despair
	Hopelessness
Personal accomplishment	Absenteeism
	Frustration
	Thinking about quitting
	Inefficiency on the job
	Decreased satisfaction with the job
	Lack of dedication to the job

Data from Arimon-Pages, E., Fernandez-Ortega, P., Fabrellas-Padres, N., Castro-Garcia, A. M., & Canela-Soler, J. (2022). Dealing with emotional vulnerability and anxiety in nurses from high-risk units–A multicenter study. *International Journal of Environmental Research and Public Health, 19*(9), Article 5569. https://doi.org/10.3390%2Fijerph19095569; Berg, G. M., Harshbarger, J. L., Ahlers-Schmidt, C. R., & Lippoldt, D. (2016). Exploring compassion fatigue and burnout syndrome in a trauma team: A qualitative study. *Journal of Trauma Nursing, 23*(1), 3–10. https://doi.org/10.1097/jtn.0000000000000172; Lee, H. J., Lee, M., & Jang, S. J. (2021). Compassion satisfaction, secondary traumatic stress, and burnout among nurses working in trauma centers: A cross-sectional study. *International Journal of Environmental Research and Public Health, 18*(14), Article 7228. https://doi.org/10.3390/ijerph18147228

professional inadequacy (**Table 18-7**).[10,15,61] A nurse experiencing burnout may be judgmental of patients or may be easily irritated by patients and colleagues. The nurse with burnout may be easily overwhelmed by routine or ordinary work conditions. It is estimated that 35–45% of nurses are affected by burnout. Burnout is associated with negative consequences for the nurse's well-being.[23,84]

Vicarious Trauma

Vicarious trauma is a result of an empathic response while in a therapeutic relationship with someone who has experienced, or is experiencing, a traumatic event. This results in the caregiver also experiencing some aspects of the trauma.[57,68,82] Vicarious trauma is often associated with the "cost of caring" and may be referred to as CF, STS, or burnout.[57,68] Vicarious trauma can result in a change in the caregiver's world view, spirituality, or relationships, as well as symptoms similar to those of PTSD.[82]

Social Media

Social networking as an outlet for debriefing after an emotionally distressing shift or event may be tempting. However, the nurse should recognize the risks involved and ensure compliance with institutional policies, as well as legal and ethical responsibilities, for social networking, confidentiality, and professionalism. The Emergency Nurses Association's position statement for social networking outlines the ethical responsibility of an emergency nurse as it relates to following institutional policies regarding code of conduct when using a social media platform.[39]

Workplace Violence

Workplace violence in the ED is highly prevalent and underreported.[37,81] Emergency nurses are particularly vulnerable, with approximately 70% reporting being hit or kicked while working.[40] Research indicates that as many as 80% of nurses have been verbally abused in the previous year.[92] Workplace violence can result in feelings of anger, a sense of feeling unsafe and fearful, and decreased job satisfaction. Additionally, workplace violence increases burnout, development of stress disorders, and absenteeism, and contributes to staff turnover.[37,92]

The Emergency Nurses Association, in an effort to mitigate workplace violence, promotes a comprehensive approach that includes practical measures to prevent, respond to, and report occurrences, with a recognition that mitigation requires a zero-tolerance environment for workplace violence.[37]

Critical Incidents

A critical incident is a traumatic event that elicits unusually strong emotional reactions or responses to the event by healthcare team members, which in turn may adversely affect workplace morale. Care for children and adults who have been injured as a result of interpersonal violence, pediatric resuscitation, and caring for a dying colleague are examples of possible critical incidents. Additional stressors may be acute, chronic, or cumulative in effect, resulting in changes in both the personal and professional lives of nurses. **Table 18-8** lists common reactions to a traumatic event such as a critical incident.[28]

TABLE 18-8   Common Responses to a Traumatic Event

Cognitive	Emotional	Physical	Behavioral
Poor concentration	Shock	Nausea	Suspicion
Confusion	Numbness	Light-headedness	Irritability
Disorientation	Disbelief	Dizziness	Arguments with friends and loved ones
Indecisiveness	Anger or short-temperedness	Loss of appetite	Withdrawal
Shortened attention span	Anxiety or fear	Gastrointestinal problems	Substance misuse
Memory loss	Feeling overwhelmed	Skin rashes	Excessive silence
Unwanted thoughts and images	Depression	Rapid heart rate	Inappropriate humor
Difficulty making decisions	Fear of harm to self and/or loved ones	Tremors	Increased/decreased eating
Nightmares	Feeling nothing	Headaches	Change in sexual desire or functioning
	Feeling abandoned	Grinding of teeth	Increased smoking
	Uncertainty of feelings	Fatigue	
	Volatile emotions	Worsening of chronic health problems	
		Poor sleep	
		Pain	
		Hyperarousal	
		Jumpiness	

Reproduced from Centers for Disease Control and Prevention. (n.d.). *Helping patients cope with a traumatic event.* https://www.cdc.gov/masstrauma/factsheets/professionals/coping_professional.pdf

Approach to the Care of the Trauma Team

Healthy work environments are essential to and critical for nurses' longevity, as well as optimal patient care.[103]

Assessment Tools

Use of the Professional Quality of Life (ProQOL) scale (**Appendix 18-1**) and the Maslach Burnout Inventory (MBI) instrument is discussed here.

The ProQOL

The Professional Quality of Life: Compassion Satisfaction and Fatigue (Version 5) tool is a 30-item instrument used to score responses related to burnout, STS, and compassion satisfaction. This tool has been useful in identifying nurses' response to traumatic events, their ability to cope, and the possible need for intervention. Support, interventions, and programs may be needed to promote recovery from the traumatic events for the individual nurse and the entire department.

Maslach Burnout Inventory

The MBI is used to measure a person's level of burnout by dividing elements of burnout into six categories[33]:

- Workload: Addressing both quality and quantity
- Control: Having autonomy at work and influence over one's own practice
- Reward: Being recognized by others and having internal job satisfaction
- Sense of community: Being engaged at work and having a supportive work environment
- Fairness: Feeling that decisions are made equitably and fairly
- Values: Having purpose and enthusiasm for the work

Research consistently validates that multiple variables contribute to burnout, including long shifts, high workload, low staffing, negative nurse–physician relations, poor leadership, negative team relationships, low schedule flexibility, time pressure, and high job and psychological demands.[33] The results from this tool can be used to develop strategies for preventing the emotional exhaustion, depersonalization, and lack of a sense accomplishment associated with burnout.

Support and Strategies for the Trauma Team

Support and strategies for the trauma team include developing resilience, promoting self-awareness, and using critical incident stress management.

Developing Resilience

Resilience comprises a unique set of attributes or protective behaviors that may buffer an individual from the detrimental effects of acute and chronic stress. The literature emphasizes that development of personal and professional resilience enables coping with the effects of stress and achieving a positive work experience.[47]

Examples of attributes that contribute to resilience include the following[47]:

- Hardiness
- Coping skills
- Self-efficacy
- Optimism
- Patience
- Tolerance
- Faith
- Adaptability
- Self-esteem
- Sense of humor

The American Psychological Association has outlined additional factors associated with resiliency based on learned behaviors[8]:

- The power to make realistic plans and take steps to carry them out
- A positive self-view and confidence in one's strengths and abilities
- Learned communication skills and problem-solving
- The self-control to manage strong feelings and impulses

Box 18-2 describes ways to build resilience.

BOX 18-2 Ways to Build Resilience

Ways to build resilience include the following[8]:

- **Build connections.** Prioritizing relationships and connecting with people who are empathetic and understanding can help remind you that you are not alone. Finding trustworthy and compassionate individuals will reinforce that you are not alone in challenging situations. Be with people who will support you and validate your feelings.
- **Foster wellness.** Take care of your body. Positive lifestyle factors such as getting regular exercise, adequate sleep, and proper nutrition, and staying hydrated can strengthen you and decrease the effects of anxiety and depression. Practice mindfulness through yoga, meditation, or prayer. Avoid negative outlets; do not mask pain with drugs, alcohol, and other substances.
- **Find purpose.** Helping others can empower you and improve resiliency.
- **Move toward your goals.** Develop some realistic goals. Do something regularly—even if it seems like a small accomplishment—that enables you to move toward your goals. Instead of focusing on tasks that seem unachievable, ask yourself, "What's one thing I know I can accomplish today that helps me move in the direction I want to go?"
- **Take decisive actions.** Act on adverse situations as much as you can. Take decisive actions, rather than detaching completely from problems and stresses and wishing they would just go away.
- **Look for opportunities for self-discovery.** People often learn something about themselves and may find that they have grown in some respect because of their struggle with loss. Many people who have experienced tragedies and hardship have reported better relationships, greater sense of strength even while feeling vulnerable, increased sense of self-worth, a more developed spirituality, and heightened appreciation for life.
- **Nurture a positive view of yourself.** Developing confidence in your ability to solve problems and trusting your instincts help build resilience.
- **Keep things in perspective.** Even when facing very painful events, try to consider the stressful situation in a broader context and keep a long-term perspective. Avoid blowing the event out of proportion.
- **Maintain a hopeful outlook.** An optimistic outlook enables you to expect that good things will happen in your life. Try visualizing what you want rather than worrying about what you fear.

Data from American Psychological Association. (2020). *Building your resilience*. https://www.apa.org/topics/resilience/building-your-resilience

Promoting Self-Awareness

Awareness of loss of caring and a negative attitude can prevent the development of CF and burnout, including the potentially negative mental, emotional, and physical effects of these conditions. A formal mentorship program within the department or referral to a program through a professional organization are ways to provide this support.

Management of Stress in Healthcare Providers

In addition to the areas already discussed, critical incident stress debriefing is widely used but is not without controversy. There is no clear consensus in the literature regarding efficacy, and some evidence of possible harm exists.[9,111] Eye movement desensitization and reprocessing therapy has been used as a first-line treatment for military veterans with PTSD.[109] One study of individuals who experienced workplace violence demonstrated eye movement desensitization and reprocessing to be more effective than critical incident stress debriefing following a critical incident.[97]

Overall, support following a critical incident or other traumatic event is not a one-size-fits-all process, and the needs of the individual, as well as the team, must be considered. Many options are available to nurses to manage their stress. It is important to find what works best for each individual so they can continue to provide care to others.

Emerging Trends and Resources

As more is learned about the lasting secondary effects of trauma, new resources for patients, families, and providers have emerged.

As noted earlier, awareness of the approach of TIC and interventions is growing. In addition, hospitals and providers may develop programs on their own or partner with others, such as the American Trauma Society's Trauma Survivor Network, to adopt practices and access resources that promote recovery.[101] The Trauma Survivor Network assists trauma survivors in connecting with other survivors and families and enhancing their survivor and self-management skills, and provides education to healthcare providers and hospital-based peer support.[101]

Summary

Provision of competent, safe, and compassionate psychosocial nursing care to those suffering sudden, unexpected injury or death remains a cornerstone of emergency and trauma nursing. Understanding the human response to trauma can be key in offering support and guidance to patients and families, and it plays an important role in the development of assessment skills for nurses to use not only with patients and families, but also with colleagues and themselves.

Trauma nurses work in a highly stressful environment that often includes exposure to severely injured and dying patients, emotionally intense situations, or violence. Secondary traumatic stress and burnout can be a predictable consequence of that exposure, so it is essential that nurses be aware of and recognize the potential for these conditions to develop. It is important to realize that compassion fatigue is a predictable, treatable, and preventable consequence of working with suffering people.[61,85] The nurse can use awareness, information, education, and selected interventions to ameliorate the symptoms and limit maladaptive consequences of acute, chronic, and continual exposure.

References

1. Agarwal, T. M., Muneer, M., Asim, M., Awad, M., Afzal, Y., Al-Thani, H., Alhassan, A., Mollazehi, M., & El-Menyar, A. (2020). Psychological trauma in different mechanisms of traumatic injury: A hospital-based cross-sectional study. *PLOS ONE, 15*(11), Article e0242849. https://doi.org/10.1371/journal.pone.0242849

2. American College of Surgeons. (2022). *Resources for optimal care of the injured patient (2022 standards)*. https://www.facs.org/quality-programs/trauma/quality/verification-review-and-consultation-program/standards/

3. American Nurses Association. (2017). *Exploring moral resilience toward a culture of ethical practice.* https://www.nursingworld.org/~4907b6/globalassets/docs/ana/ana-call-to-action--exploring-moral-resilience-final.pdf

4. American Psychiatric Association. (2013). Trauma- and stressor-related disorders. In *Diagnostic and statistical manual of mental disorders* (5th ed., pp. 265–290).

5. American Psychological Association. (n.d.). Acute stress disorder (ASD). In *APA dictionary of psychology*. Retrieved October 28, 2022, from https://dictionary.apa.org/acute-stress-disorder

6. American Psychological Association. (n.d.). Posttraumatic stress disorder (PTSD). In *APA dictionary of psychology*. Retrieved October 28, 2022, from https://dictionary.apa.org/posttraumatic-stress-disorder

7. American Psychological Association. (2019). *How to cope with traumatic stress.* https://www.apa.org/topics/trauma/stress

8. American Psychological Association. (2020). *Building your resilience.* https://www.apa.org/topics/resilience/building-your-resilience

9. American Red Cross Advisory Council on First Aid, Aquatics, Safety, and Preparedness. (2010). *Critical incident stress*

debriefing [Scientific review]. https://www.redcross.org/content/dam/redcross/Health-Safety-Services/scientific-advisory-council/Scientific%20Advisory%20Council%20SCIENTIFIC%20REVIEW%20-%20Critical%20Incident%20Stress%20Debriefing.pdf

10. Arimon-Pages, E., Fernandez-Ortega, P., Fabrellas-Padres, N., Castro-Garcia, A. M., & Canela-Soler, J. (2022). Dealing with emotional vulnerability and anxiety in nurses from high-risk units—A multicenter study. *International Journal of Environmental Research and Public Health, 19*(9), Article 5569. https://doi.org/10.3390%2Fijerph19095569

11. Association of Organ Procurement Organizations. (n.d.). *OPO services.* https://aopo.org/opo-services/

12. Baker, E. F., & Marco, C. (2020). Advance directives in the emergency department. *Journal of the American College of Emergency Physicians Open, 1*(3). https://doi.org/10.1002%2Femp2.12021

13. Bartlett, J. D., Griffin, J. L., Spinazzola, J., Fraser, J. G., Norona, C. R., Bodian, R., Todd, M., Montagna, C., & Barto, B. (2018). The impact of a statewide trauma-informed care initiative in child welfare on the well-being of children and youth with complex trauma. *Children and Youth Services Review, 84,* 110–117. https://doi.org/10.1016/j.childyouth.2017.11.015

14. Beres, K. E., Zajac, L. M., Mason, H., Krenke, K., & Costa, D. K. (2022). Addressing compassion fatigue in trauma emergency and intensive care setting: A pilot study. *Journal of Trauma Nursing, 29*(4), 210–217. https://doi.org/10.1097/jtn.0000000000000663

15. Berg, G. M., Harshbarger, J. L., Ahlers-Schmidt, C. R., & Lippoldt, D. (2016). Exploring compassion fatigue and burnout syndrome in a trauma team: A qualitative study. *Journal of Trauma Nursing, 23*(1), 3–10. https://doi.org/10.1097/jtn.0000000000000172

16. Berkey, F. B., Wiedemer, J. P., & Vithalani, N. D. (2018). Delivering bad or life-altering news. *American Family Physician, 98*(2), 99–104. https://www.aafp.org/pubs/afp/issues/2018/0715/p99.html

17. Birur, B., Moore, N. C., & Davis, L. L. (2017). An evidence-based review of early intervention and prevention of posttraumatic stress disorder. *Community Mental Health Journal, 53*(2), 183–201. https://doi.org/10.1007/s10597-016-0047-x

18. Bock, C., Heitland, I., Zimmermann, T., Winter, L., & Kahl, K. G. (2020). Secondary traumatic stress, mental state, and work ability in nurses—Results of a psychological risk assessment at a university hospital. *Frontiers in Psychiatry, 11,* Article 298. https://doi.org/10.3389/fpsyt.2020.00298

19. Brown, T., Ashworth, H., Bass, M., Rittenberg, E., Levy-Carrick, N., Grossman, S., Lewis-O'Connor, A., & Stoklosa, H. (2022). Trauma-informed care interventions in emergency medicine: A systematic review. *Western Journal of Emergency Medicine, 23*(2), 334–344. https://doi.org/10.5811/westjem.2022.1.53674

20. Bruce, M. M., Kassam-Adams, N., Rogers, M., Anderson, K. M., Sluys, K. P. & Richmond, T. S. (2018). Trauma provider's knowledge, views, and practice of trauma-informed care. *Journal of Trauma Nursing, 25*(2), 131–138. https://doi.org/10.1097/jtn.0000000000000356

21. Bryant, R. (2019). Acute stress disorder in adults: Epidemiology, pathogenesis, clinical manifestations, course, and diagnosis. *UpToDate.* Retrieved October, 28, 2022, from https://www.uptodate.com/contents/acute-stress-disorder-in-adults-epidemiology-pathogenesis-clinical-manifestations-course-and-diagnosis

22. Bulger, E., Johnson, P., Parker, L., Moloney, K. E., Roberts, M., K., Vaziri, N., Seo, S., Nehra, D., Thomas, P., & Zatzick. D. (2022). Nationwide survey of trauma center screening and intervention practices for posttraumatic stress disorder, firearm violence, mental health, and substance use disorders. *Journal of the American College of Surgeons, 234*(3), 274–287. https://doi.org/10.1097/xcs.0000000000000064

23. Butera, S., Brasseur, N., Filion, N., Bruyneel, A., & Smith, P. (2021). Prevalence and associated factors of burnout risk among intensive care and emergency nurses before and during the Coronavirus disease 2019 pandemic: A cross-sectional study in Belgium. *Journal of Emergency Nursing, 47*(6), 879–891. https://doi.org/10.1016/j.jen.2021.08.007

24. Cancer.Net. (n.d.) *Understanding grief and loss.* https://www.cancer.net/coping-with-cancer/managing-emotions/grief-and-loss/understanding-grief-and-loss

25. Carmassi, C., Shear, K. M., Corsi, M., Bertelloni, C. A., Dell'Oste, V., & Dell'Osso, L. (2020). Mania following bereavement: State of the art and clinical evidence. *Frontiers in Psychiatry, 11*(366), 1–7. https://doi.org/10.3389/fpsyt.2020.00366

26. Centers for Disease Control and Prevention. (n.d.). *Coping with a traumatic event.* https://www.cdc.gov/masstrauma/factsheets/public/coping.pdf

27. Centers for Disease Control and Prevention. (n.d.). *Grief and loss.* https://www.cdc.gov/mentalhealth/stress-coping/grief-loss/index.html

28. Centers for Disease Control and Prevention. (n.d.). *Helping patients cope with a traumatic event.* https://www.cdc.gov/masstrauma/factsheets/professionals/coping_professional.pdf

29. Centers for Disease Control and Prevention. (n.d.). *Infographic: 6 guiding principles to a trauma-informed approach.* https://www.cdc.gov/cpr/infographics/6_principles_trauma_info.htm

30. Chand, S. P., & Marwaha, R. (2022, May 8). Anxiety. *StatPearls.* StatPearls Publishing. https://www.ncbi.nlm.nih.gov/books/NBK470361/

31. Columbo, L., Emanuel, F., & Zito, M. (2019). Secondary traumatic stress: Relationship with symptoms, exhaustion, and emotions among cemetery workers. *Frontiers in Psychology, 10,* Article 633. https://doi.org/10.3389/fpsyg.2019.00633

32. Costa, D. K., & Moss, M. (2018). The cost of caring: Emotion, burnout, and psychological distress in critical care clinicians. *Annals of the American Thoracic Society, 15*(7), 787–790. https://doi.org/10.1513%2FAnnalsATS.201804-269PS

33. Dall'Ora, C., Ball, J., Reinius, M., & Griffiths, P. (2020). Burnout in nursing: A theoretical review. *Human Resources for Health, 18,* Article 41. https://doi.org/10.1186/s12960-020-00469-9

34. Dean, W., Talbot, S., & Dean, A. (2019). Reframing clinician distress: Moral injury not burnout. *Federal Practitioner*, *36*(9), 400–402. https://www.ncbi.nlm.nih.gov/pmc/articles/PMC6752815/
35. DeRoon-Cassini, T. A., Hunt, J. C., Geier, T. J., Warren, A. M., Ruggiero, K. J., Scott, K., George, J., Halling, M., Jurkovich, G., Fakhry, S., Zatzick, D., & Brasel, K. J. (2019). Screening and treating hospitalized trauma survivors for PTSD and depression. *Journal of Trauma and Acute Care Surgery*, *87*(2), 440–450. https://doi.org/10.1097/ta.0000000000002370
36. Emergency Nurses Association. (2017). *Nursing code of ethics: Provisions and interpretative statements for emergency nurses* [Code of ethics]. https://enau.ena.org/Users/LearningActivity/LearningActivityDetail.aspx?LearningActivityID=o1cZArcv0vSJ9aLQ%2f5ktBg%3d%3d
37. Emergency Nurses Association. (2019). *Violence and its impact on the emergency nurse* [Position statement]. https://enau.ena.org/Users/LearningActivity/LearningActivityDetail.aspx?LearningActivityID=T8vaf5Sal5Y38QrdhzvpIQ%3D%3D&tab=4
38. Emergency Nurses Association. (2021). *Family presence during invasive procedures and resuscitation* [Clinical practice guideline]. https://enau.ena.org/Users/LearningActivity/LearningActivityDetail.aspx?LearningActivityID=r56E4fVaVAdDXzfXsYFmGA%3D%3D&tab=4
39. Emergency Nurses Association. (2022). *Position statement social networking by emergency nurses*. https://enau.ena.org/Users/LearningActivity/LearningActivityDetail.aspx?LearningActivityID=Ycxe55vQNJ9SeIjtVYKRXg%3D%3D&tab=4
40. Emergency Nurses Association. (2022). *Workplace violence*. https://www.ena.org/quality-and-safety/workplace-violence#:~:text=No%20Silence%20on%20ED%20Violence,kicked%20while%20on%20the%20job.
41. Emergency Nurses Association & International Association of Forensic Nurses. (2022). *Adult and adolescent sexual assault patients in the emergency care setting* [Joint position statement]. https://enau.ena.org/Users/LearningActivity/LearningActivityDetail.aspx?LearningActivityID=5E4DR2UsItvFqlG1So5fKg%3D%3D&tab=4
42. Epstein, E. G., Haizlip, J., Liaschenko, J., Zhao, D., Bennett, R., & Marshall, M. F. (2020). Moral distress, mattering, and secondary traumatic stress in provider burnout: A call for moral community. *AACN Advanced Critical Care*, *31*(2), 146–157. https://doi.org/10.4037/aacnacc2020285
43. Falzarano, F., Winoker, H., Burke, R. V., Mendoza, J. A., Munoz, F., Tergas, A., Maciejewski, P. K., & Pregerson, H. G. (2022). Grief and bereavement in the Latino/a community: A literature synthesis and directions for future research. *Health Equity*, *6*(1). https://doi.org/10.1089/heq.2022.0031
44. Fanai, M., & Khan, M. A. (2022, July 17). Acute stress disorder. *StatPearls*. StatPearls Publishing. https://www.ncbi.nlm.nih.gov/books/NBK560815/
45. Fleishman, J., Kamsky, H., & Sundborg, S. (2019). Trauma-informed nursing practice. *The Online Journal of Issues in Nursing*, *24*(2), Article 3. https://doi.org/10.3912/OJIN.Vol24No02Man03
46. Garfin, D. R., Thompson, R. R., & Holman, A. (2018). Acute stress and subsequent health outcomes: A systematic review. *Journal of Psychosomatic Research*, *112*, 107–113. https://doi.org/10.1016/j.jpsychores.2018.05.017
47. Grafton, E., Gillespie, B., & Henderson, S. (2010). Resilience: The power within. *Oncology Nursing Forum*, *37*(6), 698–705. https://doi.org/10.1188/10.onf.698-705
48. Green-Moton, E., & Minkler, M. (2020). Cultural competence or cultural humility? Moving beyond the debate. *Health Promotion Practice*, *21*(1), 142–145. https://doi.org/10.1177/1524839919884912
49. Griffin, B. J., Purcell, N., Burkman, K., Litz, B. T., Bryan, C. J., Schmitz, M., Villierme, C., Walsh, J., & Maguen, S. (2019). Moral injury: An integrative review. *Journal of Traumatic Stress*, *32*(3), 350–362. https://doi.org/10.1002/jts.22362
50. Gustafsson, T., & Hemberg, J. (2021). Compassion fatigue as bruises in the soul: A qualitative study on nurses. *Nursing Ethics*, *29*(1), 157–170. https://doi.org/10.1177/09697330211003215
51. Haddad, L. M., & Geiger, R. A. (2022, August 22). Nursing ethical considerations. *StatPearls*. StatPearls Publishing. https://www.ncbi.nlm.nih.gov/books/NBK526054/
52. House, S. A., School, C., & Ogilive, W. A. (2022, April 30). Advance directives. *StatPearls*. StatPearls Publishing. https://www.ncbi.nlm.nih.gov/books/NBK459133/
53. Hunt, J. C., Herrera-Hernandez, E., Brandolino, A., Jazinski-Chambers, K., Maher, K., Jackson, B., Smith, R. N., Lape, D., Cook, M., Berner, C., Schramm, A. T., Brasel, K. J., deMoya, M. A., & DeRoon-Cassini, T. (2021). *Journal of Trauma and Acute Care Surgery*, *90*(5), 797–806. https://doi.org/10.1097/ta.0000000000003079
54. Hunt, J. C., Sapp, M., Walker, C., Warren, A. M., Brasel, K., & DeRoon-Cassini, T. A. (2017). Utility of the injured trauma survivor screen to predict PTSD and depression during hospital admission. *Journal of Trauma and Acute Care Surgery*, *82*(1), 93–101. https://doi.org/10.1097/ta.0000000000001306
55. Institute for Patient- and Family-Centered Care. (n.d.). *Better together pocket guide for staff*. https://www.ipfcc.org/bestpractices/IPFCC_Better_Together_Staff_Pocket_Print.pdf
56. Institute for Patient- and Family-Centered Care. (n.d.). *Patient- and family-centered care*. https://www.ipfcc.org/about/pfcc.html
57. Isobel, S., & Thomas, M. (2022). Vicarious trauma and nursing: An integrative review. *International Journal of Mental Health Nursing*, *31*(2), 247–259. https://doi.org/10.1111/inm.12953
58. Karliner, L. S. (2018). When patients and providers speak different languages. *Patient Safety Network*. Agency for Healthcare Research and Quality. https://psnet.ahrq.gov/web-mm/when-patients-and-providers-speak-different-languages
59. Kellogg, M. (2020). Secondary traumatic stress in nursing. *Advances in Nursing Science*, *44*(2), 157–170. https://doi.org/10.1097/ans.0000000000000338
60. Kleber, R. J. (2019). Trauma and public mental health: A focused review. *Frontiers in Psychiatry*, *10*, Article 451. https://doi.org/10.3389/fpsyt.2019.00451
61. Lee, H. J., Lee, M., & Jang, S. J. (2021). Compassion satisfaction, secondary traumatic stress, and burnout among nurses

working in trauma centers: A cross-sectional study. *International Journal of Environmental Research and Public Health, 18*(14), Article 7228. https://doi.org/10.3390/ijerph18147228

62. Leroy, A., Cotentin, O., Labreuche, J., Mascarel, P., De Pourtales, M., Molenda, S., Paget, V., Lemogne, C., Bougerol, T., Gregory, T., Chantelot, C., Demarty, A., Meyer, S., Warembourg, F., Duhem, S., & Guillaume, V. (2022). Four questions nurses can ask to predict PTSD 1 year after a motor vehicle crash. *Journal of Trauma Nursing, 29*(2), 70–79. https://doi.org/10.1097/jtn.0000000000000638

63. Lombardo, B. L. (2011). Compassion fatigue: A nurse's primer. *The Online Journal of Issues in Nursing, 16*(1), Article 3. https://doi.org/10.3912/OJIN.Vol16No01Man03

64. Ma, H., Huang, S. Q., We, B., & Zhong, Y. (2022). Compassion fatigue, burnout, compassion satisfaction and depression among physicians and nurses: A cross-sectional study. *British Medical Journal Open, 12*(4), Article e055941. https://doi.org/10.1136/bmjopen-2021-055941

65. Mann, S. K., & Marwaha, R. (2022, February 7). Posttraumatic stress disorder. *StatPearls.* StatPearls Publishing. https://www.ncbi.nlm.nih.gov/books/NBK559129/

66. Miao, X. R., Chen, Q. B., Wei, K., Tao, K. M., & Lu, Z. J. (2018). Posttraumatic stress disorder: From diagnosis to prevention. *Military Medical Research, 5*(32), 1–7. https://doi.org/10.1186%2Fs40779-018-0179-0

67. Moss, J., Roberts, M. B., Shea, L., Jones, C. W., Kilgannon, H., Edmondson, D. E., Trzeciak, S., & Robers, B. W. (2019). Healthcare provider compassion is associated with lower PTSD symptoms among patients with life-threatening medical emergencies: A prospective cohort study. *Intensive Care Medicine, 45*(6), 815–822. https://doi.org/10.1007/s00134-019-05601-5

68. Muehlhausen, B. L. (2021). Spirituality and vicarious trauma among trauma clinicians: A qualitative study. *Journal of Trauma Nursing, 28*(6), 367–377. https://doi.org/10.1097/JTN.0000000000000616

69. Mughal, S., Azhar, Y., Mahon, M. M., & Siddiqui, W. J. (2022, May 22). Grief reaction. *StatPearls.* StatPearls Publishing. https://www.ncbi.nlm.nih.gov/books/NBK507832/#:~:text=Grief%20is%20a%20person's%20emotional,and%20mourning%20after%20a%20loss

70. Narayanan, V., Bista, B., & Koshy, C. (2010). "BREAKS" protocol for breaking bad news. *Indian Journal of Palliative Care, 16*(2), 61–65. https://www.ncbi.nlm.nih.gov/pmc/articles/PMC3144432/

71. National Child Traumatic Stress Network. (n.d.). *About child trauma.* https://www.nctsn.org/what-is-child-trauma/about-child-trauma

72. National Geographic Area Coordination Centers. (2015). *Reactions to crisis and trauma.* https://gacc.nifc.gov/swcc/management_admin/cism/documents/2015/reactions.pdf

73. National Institute of Mental Health. (n.d.). *Post-traumatic stress disorder.* https://www.nimh.nih.gov/health/publications/post-traumatic-stress-disorder-ptsd

74. O'Connor, M. F. (2019). Grief: A brief history of research on how body, mind, and brain adapt. *Psychosomatic Medicine, 81*(8), 731–738. https://doi.org/10.1097/psy.0000000000000717

75. Papini, S., Pisner, D., Shumake, J., Powers, M. B., Beevers, C. G., Rainey, E. E., Smits, J. A., & Warren, A. M. (2018). Ensemble machine learning of posttraumatic stress disorder screen status after emergency room hospitalization. *Journal of Anxiety Disorders, 60,* 35–42. https://doi.org/10.1016%2Fj.janxdis.2018.10.004

76. Petrucci, C. M., Villasenor, S., Brown, W. G., & Peters, R. M. (2022). Traumatic stress and depression risk screening at an ACS verified trauma center. *Journal of Trauma Nursing, 29*(3), 142–151. https://doi.org/10.1097/jtn.0000000000000640

77. Ports, K. A., Tang, S., Treves-Kagan, S., & Rostad, W. (2021). Breaking the cycle of adverse childhood experiences (ACEs): Economic position moderates the relationship between mother and child ACE scores among Black and Hispanic families. *Children and Youth Services Review, 127,* Article 106067. https://doi.org/10.1016/j.childyouth.2021.106067

78. Powers, K., & Reeve, C. L. (2020). Family presence during resuscitation: Medical-surgical nurses' perceptions, self-confidence, and use of invitations. *American Journal of Nursing, 120*(11), 28–38. https://doi.org/10.1097/01.naj.0000721244.16344.ee

79. Prins, A., Bovin, M. J., Kimerling, R., Kaloupek, D. G., Marx, B. P., Pless Kaiser, A., & Schnurr, P. P. (2015). *Primary care PTSD screen for DSM-5 (PC-PTSD-5).* https://www.ptsd.va.gov/professional/assessment/documents/pc-ptsd5-screen.pdf

80. Qassem, T., Aly-ElGabry, D., Alzarouni, A., Abdel-Aziz, K., & Arnone, D. (2021). Psychiatric co-morbidities in post-traumatic stress disorder. Detailed findings from the adult psychiatric morbidity survey in the English population. *Psychiatric Quarterly, 92,* 321–330. https://doi.org/10.1007/s11126-020-09797-4

81. Querin, L. B., Dallaghan, B., & Shenvi, C. (2022). A qualitative study of resident physician and health care worker experiences of verbal and physical abuse in the emergency department. *Annals of Emergency Medicine, 79*(4), 391–396. https://doi.org/10.1016/j.annemergmed.2021.04.019

82. Roberts, C., Darroch, F., Giles, A., & van Bruggen, R. (2022). You're carrying so many people's stories: Vicarious trauma among fly-in and fly-out mental health service providers in Canada. *International Journal of Qualitative Studies in Health and Well-Being, 17*(1), Article 2040089. https://doi.org/10.1080%2F17482631.2022.2040089

83. Robinson, L. K., Sterling, L., Jackson, J., Gentry, E., Araujo, F., LaFond, C., Jacobson, K. C., & Lee, R. (2022). A secondary traumatic stress reduction program in emergency room nurses. *SAGE Open Nursing, 8.* https://doi.org/10.1177%2F23779608221094530

84. Rushton, C. H., & Pappas, S. (2020). Systems to address burnout and support well-being: Implications for intensive care nurses. *AACN Advanced Critical Care, 31*(2), 141–145. https://doi.org/10.4037/aacnacc2020771

85. Salmond, E., Salmond, S., Ames, M., Kamienski, M., & Holly, C. (2019). Experiences of compassion fatigue in direct care nurses: A qualitative systematic review. *JBI Database Systematic Reviews and Implementation Reports, 17*(5), 682–753. https://doi.org/10.11124/jbisrir-2017-003818

86. Shear, M. K., Reynolds, C. F., Simon, N. M., & Zisook, S. (2021). Bereavement and grief in adults: Clinical features. *UpToDate.*

Retrieved January 12, 2023, from https://www.uptodate.com/contents/bereavement-and-grief-in-adults-clinical-features

87. Shear, M. K., Reynolds, C. F., Simon, N. M., & Zisook, S. (2021). Bereavement and grief in adults: Management. *UpToDate*. Retrieved January 12, 2023, from https://www.uptodate.com/contents/bereavement-and-grief-in-adults-management

88. Smid, G. E., Groen, S., de la Rie, S. M., Kooper, S., & Boelen, P. A. (2018). Toward cultural assessment of grief and grief-related psychopathology. *Psychiatric Services, 69*(10), 1050–1052. https://doi.org/10.1176/appi.ps.201700422

89. Soares, S., Richa, V., Kelly-Irving, M., Stringhini, S., & Fraga, S. (2021). Adverse childhood event and health biomarkers: A systematic review. *Frontiers in Public Health, 9*, Article 649825. https://doi.org/10.3389/fpubh.2021.649825

90. Sorenson, C., Bolick B., Wright, K., & Hamilton, R. (2017). An evolutionary concept analysis of compassion fatigue. *Journal of Nursing Scholarship, 49*(5), 557–563. https://doi.org/10.1111/jnu.12312

91. Squires, A. (2018). Strategies for overcoming language barriers in healthcare. *Nurse Management, 49*(4), 20–27. https://doi.org/10.1097/01.numa.0000531166.24481.15

92. Stafford, S., Avsar, P., Nugent, L., O'Connor, T., Moore, Z., Patton, D., & Watson, C. (2022). What is the impact of patient violence in the emergency department on emergency nurses' intention to leave? *Journal of Nursing Management, 30*(6), 1852–1860. https://doi.org/10.1111/jonm.13728

93. Stevens, S. K., Timmer-Murillo, S. C., Tomas, C. W., Boals, A., Larson, C. L., DeRoon-Cassini, T., & Larsen, S. E. (2022). Event centrality and posttraumatic stress symptoms after traumatic injury: A longitudinal investigation. *Journal of Traumatic Stress, 35*(6), 1734–1743. https://doi.org/10.1002/jts.22877

94. Stubbe, D. E. (2020). Practicing cultural competence and cultural humility in the care of diverse patients. *Focus, 18*(1), 49–51. https://doi.org/10.1176%2Fappi.focus.20190041

95. Substance Abuse and Mental Health Services Administration. (2014). *SAMHSA's concept of trauma and guidance for a trauma-informed approach.* https://ncsacw.acf.hhs.gov/userfiles/files/SAMHSA_Trauma.pdf

96. Substance Abuse and Mental Health Services Administration. (2020). *National guidelines for behavioral health crisis care—A best practice toolkit knowledge information transformation.* https://www.samhsa.gov/sites/default/files/national-guidelines-for-behavioral-health-crisis-care-02242020.pdf

97. Tarquinio, C., Rotonda, C., Houlle, W. A., Montel, S., Rydberg, J. A., Minary, L., Dellucci, H., Tarquinio, P., Fayard, A., & Alla, F. (2016). Early psychological preventive intervention for workplace violence: A randomized controlled explorative and comparative study between EMDR-recent event and critical incident stress debriefing. *Issues in Mental Health Nursing, 37*(11), 787–799.

98. Timmons, F., Catania, G., Zanini, M., Ottonello, G., Napolitano, F., Musio, M. E., & Bagnasco, A. (2022). Nursing management of emergency department violence—Can we do more? *Journal of Clinical Nursing.* Advance online publication. https://doi.org/10.1111/jocn.16211

99. Toronto, C. E., & LaRocco, S. A. (2019). Family perception of and experience with family presence during cardiopulmonary resuscitation: An integrative review. *Journal of Clinical Nursing, 28*, 32–46. https://doi.org/10.1111/jocn.14649

100. Traumadissociation.com. (n.d.). *Acute stress disorder.* http://traumadissociation.com/acutestressdisorder.html

101. Trauma Survivor Network. (2022). *Who we are.* http://traumasurvivorsnetwork.org/pages/who-we-are

102. Trudgill, D. I., Gorey, K. M., & Donnelly, E. A. (2020). Prevalent posttraumatic stress disorder among emergency department personnel: Rapid systematic review. *Humanities & Social Sciences Communications, 7*, Article 89. https://doi.org/10.1057/s41599-020-00584-x

103. Ulrich, B., Barden, C., Cassidy, L., & Varn-Davis, N. (2019). Critical care nurse work environments 2018: Findings and implications. *Critical Care Nurse, 39*(2), 67–84. https://doi.org/10.4037/ccn2019605

104. U.S. Department of Health and Human Services Office of Minority Health. (n.d.). *CLAS, cultural competency, and cultural humility.* https://www.minorityhealth.hhs.gov/Assets/PDF/TCH%20Resource%20Library_CLAS%20CLC%20CH.pdf

105. U.S. Department of Veterans Affairs. (n.d.). *Acute stress disorder.* https://www.ptsd.va.gov/professional/treat/essentials/acute_stress_disorder.asp

106. U.S. Department of Veterans Affairs. (n.d.). *Common reactions after trauma.* https://www.ptsd.va.gov/understand/isitptsd/common_reactions.asp

107. Van der Vlegel, M., Polinder, S., Toet, H., Panneman, M., Geraerds, A. J., & Haagsma, J. A. (2022). Anxiety, depression and post-traumatic stress symptoms among injury patients and the association with outcome after injury. *European Journal of Psychotraumatology, 13*(1). https://doi.org/10.1080%2F20008198.2021.2023422

108. Wang, D., & Gupta, V. (2022, April 28). Crisis intervention. *StatPearls.* StatPearls Publishing. https://www.ncbi.nlm.nih.gov/books/NBK559081/

109. Wininger, B. (2022). Posttraumatic stress disorder. In F. F. Ferri (Ed.), *Ferri's clinical advisor* (pp. 1241–1243). Elsevier.

110. Wolf, L. A., Delao, A. M., Perhats, C., Clark, P. R.., Edwards, C., & Frankenberg, W. D. (2020). Traumatic stress in emergency nurses: Does your work environment feel like a war zone? *International Emergency Nursing, 52*, Article 100895. https://doi.org/10.1016/j.ienj.2020.100895

111. World Health Organization. (2012). *Psychological debriefing in people exposed to a recent traumatic event.* https://www.who.int/teams/mental-health-and-substance-use/treatment-care/mental-health-gap-action-programme/evidence-centre/other-significant-emotional-and-medical-unexplained-somatic-complaints/psychological-debriefing-in-people-exposed-to-a-recent-traumatic-event

112. Zhang, L., Ahou, J., & Li, L. (2015). Crisis intervention in the acute stage after trauma. *International Journal of Emergency Mental Health and Human Resilience, 17*(4), 714–716. https://www.omicsonline.org/open-access/crisis-intervention-in-the-acute-stage-after-trauma-1522-4821-1000299.pdf

CHAPTER 19

Disaster Management

Cindy Joseph, BSN, RN, CPEN

OBJECTIVES

Upon completion of this chapter, the learner will be able to:
1. Discuss the four phases of disaster management and their role in emergency preparedness.
2. Identify types of illnesses or injuries associated with natural and human-made disasters.
3. Compare conventional triage to mass-casualty triage.

Introduction

At the end of March 2020, the wildfires of Australia had burned more than 46 million acres and caused over $100 billion in damage. This devastation earned the Australian bushfire season the name "Black Summer." This natural disaster was considered the costliest in Australian history.[74] Following on the heels of this natural disaster was the pandemic of COVID-19. The year 2020 was known in the United States as a "billion-dollar" year for weather and climate disasters. That year, the United States experienced 22 separate disasters: 7 tropical cyclones, 13 severe storms, 1 drought, and 1 wildfire. The previous record was set in 2017, with 16 disasters.[51] As of September, 31 international natural disasters have been documented in 2022 by the National Aeronautics and Space Administration, including flooding in Bangladesh, Brazil, Ecuador, Gambia, Honduras, India, Nigeria, Pakistan, Russia, and South Africa.[50] The number of human-made disasters related to a variety of causes, including violence and transportation, is less clearly documented, but these disasters also increase traumatic injury and may disrupt the provision of patient care.

Disaster Defined

The International Federation of Red Cross and Red Crescent Societies defines a disaster as serious disruption in the functioning of a community that exceeds its ability to cope using its own resources.[36] The International Disaster Database defines a disaster as a "situation or event, which overwhelms local capacity, necessitating a request to national or international level for external assistance."[25] Both definitions describe disaster as a situation in which the demand for support exceeds the normal available resources.

It is important to note that every disaster is unique and can stress a system at various levels. A multiple casualty incident (MCI) typically occurs much more frequently than disasters and may have substantial impact at the local level, but it does not typically exceed resources beyond the health system. An example is a multiple-vehicle pileup on a highway. The healthcare system may be strained, but it is not overwhelmed, and community resources are not exceeded. By contrast, a mass-casualty event (MCE) is one that has casualties that exceed the resources at the local level and often affects the community.[2(ApD)]

Given the diversity of disaster definitions and types, it is important to understand the flexibility and adaptability necessary to respond appropriately. A small community hospital with limited healthcare resources could define a school bus crash as a disaster, whereas an urban facility would be more likely to have the resources to accommodate all patients.

Disasters are either natural or human-made.[68] Although most disasters are natural, the world appears to be facing an increased incidence of human-made disasters. This increase has shifted the focus for disaster management to a more integrated response effort and more resilient infrastructure.[52,63]

The all-hazards approach to emergency management acknowledges that the specific type of disaster that may strike is uncertain; considering the different threats and potential hazards that might be encountered is necessary. An organization's emergency management plan should include a hazard vulnerability analysis that identifies specific threats and vulnerabilities that may be present, and provides strategies for prevention, deterrence, or minimization of possible impacts.[52]

Emergency management is typically organized into an ongoing four-phase process known as the disaster life cycle. These four phases are mitigation, preparedness, response, and recovery (**Figure 19-1**).[52]

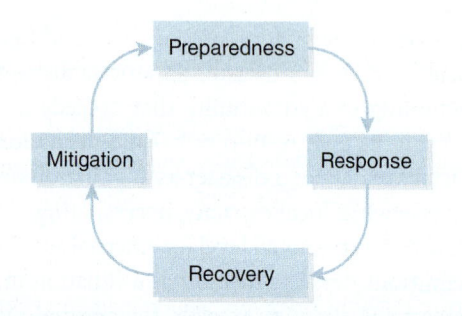

Figure 19-1 *The disaster life cycle.*
Reproduced from National Earthquake Hazards Reduction Program. (n.d.). *Earthquake coordinators web site.* Federal Emergency Management Agency. https://training.fema.gov/emiweb/earthquake/neh0101220.htm

Mitigation

Mitigation is an attempt to help reduce or avoid loss of life and property. It emanates from a foundation of knowledge based on lessons learned from past events. Findings from real events and drills are key elements that drive the mitigation process. Information obtained during these processes can help identify areas of needed improvement and inadequacies in the processes or plans currently in place. Identifying such elements can minimize the impact of an anticipated event, should one occur.[79]

A hazard vulnerability analysis (HVA) and risk assessment is a systematic process of identifying the hazards and risks that have the highest probability of adversely affecting the healthcare facility and the community.[70] The HVA may identify a wide range of natural and human-caused hazards, each of which is scored based on its potential to affect the facility, the preparedness of the facility, and the available external resources. By using this tool, the facility can focus on the highest-risk hazards and determine what actions could be taken to prevent or lessen their impact. For example, an HVA might identify a weather-related vulnerability such as flooding that would likely result in water leaks or loss, electrical outages, loss of use of areas, and loss of supplies to water damage. Steps to mitigate those effects might involve regular inspections by maintenance personnel for leak-prone areas throughout the facility, a plan for alternative sources of water, creation of a defined process for generator use, and identification of alternative locations to store supplies and materials. The procedures and processes identified for mitigation are the components that should drive the development of an emergency operations plan.

The goal of the mitigation phase is not to prevent the disaster. Instead, infrastructure mitigation efforts are intended to minimize the impact on lives and property.

Preparedness

Preparedness is built upon the premise that not all disasters can be prevented. To be ready for the situations identified in an HVA, hospitals should have properly maintained emergency operations, and all staff should be familiar with the hospital incident command system. The goal of preparedness is to improve safety and resilience through drills, education, and obtaining and maintaining equipment.[17]

Hospital Disaster Preparedness Plans

After the outbreak of COVID-19, most healthcare systems and governing bodies had to reassess their HVA with regard to infectious disease outbreaks and pandemic preparedness. Hospitals include six critical areas in planning and demonstrate preparedness for them through drills[72,73]:

- Staff responsibilities
- Patient clinical and support activities
- Communication
- Resources and assets
- Safety and security
- Utilities

The hospital emergency operations plan should encompass unit-based response plans and expand outward to include coordination with the community.[12] Disaster plans should include the reallocation of supplies/equipment and system process changes as necessary. In addition, when preparing for a disaster, it is vital to assess the resiliency of the system and how well it is prepared to respond to a disaster. During an infectious disease outbreak, health facilities and/or systems may benefit from assessing 10 categories[48]:

- Capacity and capabilities
- Critical infrastructure and transportation
- Financial considerations
- Barriers to accessing healthcare
- Communication and partnerships
- Leadership and command structure
- Surge capacity
- Risk communication
- Workforce
- Infection control

Disaster exercises vary in complexity, from simple tabletop to full-scale exercises. There are seven types of exercises, which are divided into discussion- and operations-based scenarios. Discussion-based exercises focus on plans and policies, including developing new ones and familiarizing staff with them. Examples of these exercises are seminars, workshops, tabletop exercises, and games. Operations-based exercises focus on validating existing plans, identifying gaps, and clarifying roles, and they include drills, functional exercises, and full-scale exercises.[27] The most challenging endeavor is a full-scale exercise, which often takes months to plan and requires the participation of multiple organizations at one time.[27]

Regardless of the type of exercise, it should serve the following purposes[62]:

- Enhancing the participant's knowledge of their role and responsibility
- Improving the performance of the team response from previous exercises
- Improving likelihood of an efficient response when a disaster occurs
- Meeting predetermined measurable objectives

Incident Command System

The Incident Command System (ICS) is a standardized tool used to manage the response during a disaster. The ICS was originally developed following severe wildfires in California, during which confusion and improper use of resources occurred from a lack of organized coordination accompanied by communication failures. The U.S. Department of Homeland Security was created following the 2001 terrorist attacks in the United States. This department subsequently developed the National Incident Management System, of which the incident command system is a key component.[29]

Hospitals in the United States, as well as many elsewhere, have implemented a form of ICS called the Hospital Incident Command System (HICS).[7,10,28,37] Using HICS enables hospitals to standardize the management of an incident within an organizational structure. Nurses must be knowledgeable regarding facility policies, procedures, role delineation, responsibilities, and terminology associated with their disaster response and HICS.

Response

Of the four phases of emergency management, "response" is the one that most often comes to mind. Often the disaster that occurs is not one that was anticipated or even considered on the HVA. The attacks on the barracks of American and French service members in Beirut, Lebanon, in 1983 and the attacks of September 11, 2001, were almost completely unprecedented when they occurred (**Box 19-1**). Regardless of the disaster type, the response is always one that the trauma nurse hopes to be prepared for but wishes they never have to exercise their training for in real time.

Patient Surge

Surge capacity is the ability to respond to and care for an influx of patients.[7] Anticipating and preparing for surges in patient volumes during a mass casualty incident constitute an integral component of disaster preparedness. Managing this surge may include placing patients in different areas of the hospital or discharging them. Inpatients may be included, as well as emergency department (ED) patients. The degree of surge is dictated by the circumstances surrounding the event and the event itself. An example is the mass shooting that occurred in Las Vegas in 2017; 58 people were killed and 422 injured. This incident caused a rapid surge at local hospitals, which carried on for several hours.[7,42] The influx of a large number of patients can quickly overwhelm a system that may already be operating at low staffing levels and with high patient-to-staff ratios.

BOX 19-1 Unanticipated Disasters

The Attack in Beirut

"From a terrorist perspective, the true genius of this attack is that the objective and the means of attack were beyond the *imagination* of those responsible for Marine security."

—Department of Defense Commission on Beirut International Airport (BIA) Terrorist Act of 23 October 1983. (1983). *Report of the DOD Commission on Beirut International Airport Terrorist Act, October 23, 1983* (p. 123). https://irp.fas.org/threat/beirut-1983.pdf

The Attack on the World Trade Center

"As we detail in our report, this was a failure of policy, management, capability, and, above all, a failure of *imagination*."

—Thomas Kean, Chair of the 9/11 Commission, 2004

Crisis Standards of Care

Crisis standards of care have been defined to help guide recommendations for healthcare systems facing situations in response to a disaster. The definition of crisis standards of care is a "substantial change in usual healthcare operations and the level of care it is possible to deliver, which is made necessary by a pervasive (e.g., pandemic influenza) or catastrophic (e.g., earthquake, hurricane) disaster."[34(p3)] This definition removes the focus from individual care and places it on a population-based model. This enables healthcare systems to better assign resource allocations. Furthermore, there is a psychological component to crisis standards of care; during a disaster, healthcare providers may experience moral distress because of an inability to fulfill patient care duties because of factors outside their control (e.g., lack of supplies, short staffing, fatigue). Providing caregivers with standards of care that are based on a disaster model rather than an individual care model helps support their emotional and mental state while they provide the best care possible under the circumstances.[32] Often there is little or no warning before a disaster, which underscores the importance of preparing staff to respond effectively and efficiently when a disaster does arise.

NOTE
CDC Mass Casualty Predictor

The CDC published a mass casualty predictor formula:

Total Expected Casualties = # of casualties arriving in a 1-hour window multiplied by 2.

Approximately 50% of acute casualties may arrive at closest medical facilities within 60 minutes, and 50–80% may arrive within 90 minutes. Most arrive within 1–4 hours.[9]

Disaster Triage

Although triage is an essential cornerstone of disaster management, it can be one of the greatest challenges a nurse might encounter. Nurses must forgo their typical triage assessment based on individual care to support the goal of disaster triage, which is "the greatest good for the greatest number."[2(ApDp289)] This approach is contrary to the philosophy that is frequently at the heart of nursing, in which the sickest patients receive the highest priority, and heroic efforts are put forth to resuscitate them. In a disaster, the sickest patients may consume too many resources and divert resources away from the larger group of patients who have a better chance of survival.

Disaster triage algorithms were created to quickly identify patients who are most likely to survive and those who are not. These tools are meant to interpret physiological conditions with very little assessment. These algorithms assess and sort patients based on their condition as determined by specific parameters, while considering available resources (**Appendix 19-1**).

The concept of triage has been around since the Napoleonic era.[49] However, there is not a universally accepted algorithm or tool to guide clinicians in this process. Multiple triage algorithms have been developed for disaster triage, including Simple Triage and Rapid Treatment (START) (Appendix 19-1A); JumpSTART, a pediatric version of START (Appendix 19-1B); Sort–Assess–Lifesaving Interventions–Treatment and/or Transport (SALT) (Appendix 19-1C); Fire Department of New York modified START (FDNY-START) (Appendix 19-1E); Modified Physiological Triage Tool (MPTT); and the Amberg-Schwandorf Algorithm for Primary Triage (ASAV). Common characteristics of disaster triage algorithms and tools include speed, accuracy, impartiality, and consistency between prehospital and hospital application.[39] Appendix 19-1F provides a comparison of the main disaster triage systems presently in use.

Most tools and algorithms prioritize patients using a color-coded system (e.g., black, red, yellow, and green) to represent the urgency of care required. Some systems have additional colors, such as orange and gray. Nurses must be thoroughly familiar with the tool used in their geographic location.[39]

Communicable disease outbreaks may also require disaster triage. The Susceptible–Exposed–Infectious–Removed–Vaccinated (SEIRV) (Appendix 19-1D) method can be used during outbreaks.[46] While biological events are similar to other MCEs, additional considerations include exposure, duration of the symptom-free period, and infectiousness of the pathogen. The benefit of the SEIRV model includes the ability to manage patients while controlling possible transmission to asymptomatic patients.

Primary triage occurs at first contact with the patient after the incident, in either the field or the ED. A patient triaged in the field may need the primary triage performed again after arrival in the ED because their condition may have changed. After the primary triage, a secondary triage is completed. This is typically performed at a casualty clearing area after the initial sorting but can also be done in the hospital setting. Three considerations can help determine who receives treatment first: task, time, and treaters (**Table 19-1**).[33] There is variation in disaster triage methods, and it is essential that the nurse be familiar with the tool their system has adopted and be ready to immediately implement it if necessary. The transition from the daily process of ED triage to a disaster model is not easy; practice and training before an incident will assist in making that transition as seamless as possible.

Evacuation

The United Nations Office for Disaster Risk Reduction defines evacuation as "moving people and assets temporarily to safer places before, during or after the occurrence of a hazardous event in order to protect them."[78] A hospital evacuation may be necessary because of the threat or occurrence of an internal or external disaster.[6] In the United States, approximately 150 hospitals were evacuated between 2000 and 2017.[64] The Netherlands had 67 hospital evacuations between 1990 and 2020, increasing significantly over time.[6] Hospital evacuations due to a disaster are a global phenomenon; it is estimated that in some areas of the world, more than 50% of healthcare facilities are in geographical areas that are at high risk for natural disasters.[40]

Hospital evacuations are a complex process, and it is essential for evacuation planning to be part of every hospital's emergency preparedness plan.[64] Effective and thorough planning is necessary to limit morbidity and mortality during a disaster requiring hospital evacuation; this may include a partial evacuation that involves movement vertically or horizontally to other areas within the facility.[40] Consideration must be afforded to the type of disaster that could be encountered; the response to a hurricane, for example, would be different from that of a bomb threat. Questions to consider when developing an evacuation plan might include the following[82]:

- How is the decision made whether to evacuate or shelter-in-place?
- What process is in place for the patient who can be discharged versus being transferred?
- How will it be determined which patients are evacuated first?
- How will the treatment/care needs of the patients be maintained during the evacuation?
- How are staff assigned responsibilities?
- What interfacility transport methods will be used?

The evacuation process should be clearly defined and include the sequence of evacuation based on the physical structure and possible disaster situations. Depending on the circumstances, including the location and acuity of patients, it might be more appropriate to evacuate from the top floors moving downward, or in the opposite direction. During an evacuation, it is of the utmost importance to maintain accurate tracking of patient movement. This enables staff to record which patients went to other areas within the facility or community, as well as their locations. Accurate tracking facilitates the continuity of care and the ability to inform families and visitors of the current patient location. If the disaster overwhelms the community, additional governmental resources may be available.

Shelter-in-Place

In a shelter-in-place situation, staff and patients are moved to a safe location inside the facility for a portion

TABLE 19-1 Secondary Triage Criteria

Criterion	Description
Task	What interventions are required for the patient's care, and what resources does this involve?
Time	How much time is required for the needed interventions versus competing priorities (e.g., chest tube vs. exploratory laparotomy vs. major vascular repair)?
Treaters	How much expertise is required for the interventions versus competing priorities (e.g., emergency physician vs. vascular surgeon)?

Modified from Hick, J. L., Nelson, J., Fildes, J., Kuhls, D., Eastman, A., & Dries, D. (2020). Triage, trauma, and today's mass violence events. *Journal of the American College of Surgeons, 230*(2), 251–256. https://doi.org/10.1016/j.jamcollsurg.2019.10.011

or duration of the disaster. A shelter-in-place can be activated for a variety of reasons, including a hazardous material exposure, earthquake, hurricane, environmental threats such as civil unrest or rioting, or an active shooter. To shelter-in-place, individuals retreat to an interior location until the threat is resolved and the "all clear" signal is sent. Some areas of refuge may have locking mechanisms to ensure security in the event of an active shooter within the building.[43] Trauma nurses should familiarize themselves with area of refuge locations in case a shelter-in-place is activated.

Children in Disasters

Children represent approximately 22% of the U.S. population and are frequently involved when disasters occur.[19,26] Unfortunately, disaster planning at all levels, including local, state, and national, is typically insufficient to meet their needs during a disaster.[22] Research suggests that fewer than 50% of hospitals have disaster plans that directly incorporate pediatric considerations.[21] Compounding this challenge is the variable availability of pediatric specialty–trained staff, pediatric-sized equipment, pediatric-focused systems, and available space to address pediatric-specific cases.

Pediatric considerations should be incorporated into all phases of disaster planning, including preparedness, response, recovery, and mitigation.[71] Children have unique needs and characteristics that make them a vulnerable population.[22,26] Their anatomy and physiology differ from those of adults. For example, compared with adults, children have a larger occiput, larger tongue, higher respiratory rates, and higher metabolic rates, as well as a variable range of cognitive development. It is important to incorporate these special considerations of children into disaster drills and emergency response plans.[24] For more information, refer to Chapter 13, "The Pediatric Trauma Patient."

Recovery

Disasters have significant impact on communities and their infrastructure long after the response phase has ended. In the recovery phase, a continuity of operations plan for healthcare organizations is essential in ensuring financial and operational recovery once the acute phase of a disaster has resolved. Within the trauma and emergency services realm, operational ability in the aftermath of a disaster needs to be maintained because regular patient volume will continue. The emergency response plan addresses the immediate needs for minimal operation, such as repair of damage to the facility, restoration of services, restocking of supplies, and accounting for any equipment damaged or lost during the event. Continuity of operations, by contrast, focuses on restoration of the facility to its normal day-to-day function. This is important, not just to restart clinical operations but also for logistical and financial accounting. Many organizations have a business continuity plan.[35]

Mass-Fatality Incidents

Traditional emergency management plans focus on the preservation of life and property. However, these plans must also consider the possibility of a mass-fatality disaster. While emergency responders, hospitals, and law enforcement routinely train for multiple- and mass-casualty incidents, not all practice responses to disasters in which many or all of the victims suffer fatal injuries.[47] Incidents with a large number of fatalities have implications for triage. They can overwhelm a system's resources in the same manner as a large number of sick and injured patients. The remains of victims will need to be recovered and stored for identification and for later investigation by a medical examiner or coroner. Incidents in which remains are highly fragmented can be challenging because identification may be possible only with DNA testing.[30] Preparedness for mass-fatality incidents is especially important given that the severity and frequency of civilian mass-shooting incidents are on the rise. Social services, the coroner's office, and local mortuary services should be involved in the planning and response phases of a mass-fatality incident. Federal government resources, such as a disaster mortuary operational response team (DMORT), can provide tracking and a variety of funeral services when the number of fatalities exceeds the capacity of local resources to handle them. Additional information on DMORT resources can be found by researching the National Disaster Medical System under the Department of Health and Human Services.[60]

Family Reunification

Immediately following an incident in which multiple people were separated, injured, or killed, people will quickly travel to where they believe their loved one is located or where believe they can obtain information.[69] Reunification of families can seem overwhelming, and the nurse should anticipate that family members and victims will come to the ED requesting assistance, adding to the congestion and crowding in the department. Family members typically have four basic questions in these situations[69]:

- Was their loved one involved?
- What is the location, and condition, of the victim?
- Where are the personal effects of the victim?
- What are the available resources such as food, clothing, and shelter?

Not all people presenting to the ED will have a medical issue; many victims of a disaster may present with a social or psychological need. Children may have lost or been separated from their caregiver, and elderly or unconscious people may not have identification. There will likely be a sense of heightened anxiety and helplessness as people try to find their loved one. This can be exacerbated by delays in identification of victims, ongoing threats, as in a lockdown situation, delayed scene evacuation, and communication difficulties among responders, receiving facilities, and other agencies.[69] Additionally, consideration must be given to unique community needs, such as culture and language.

Family information centers (FICs) staffed with support personnel are useful tools to deal with this cohort of victims and should be included throughout the response and recovery phase of an event. To minimize overcrowding, setup of a FIC is most beneficial when it is located away from the ED. FICs, typically organized by the facility's social work and spiritual care departments, can provide family members with resources for family reunification, spiritual care, bereavement, and childcare.[44]

Psychological Triage

Disasters may also produce psychological trauma to members of the community and professional responders who were a part of the incident. Early identification of psychological needs can facilitate a return to adaptive function after the event and can identify people at risk for serious mental health outcomes, enabling intervention before the trauma becomes a permanent part of their lives.[14] The PsySTART mental health triage is a method that can be used to assess individuals by measuring their exposure to severe traumatic events after a disaster and prioritizing crisis intervention resources.[65] Examples of serious traumatic events include death of an immediate family member, a friend, or pet; a situation in which there was a direct threat to the individual's life; witnessing loss of life; a missing family member; loss of the home; or a child isolated from all caretakers. These severe events would trigger crisis intervention resources, clinical providers, and trauma-focused cognitive behavioral therapy. Moderate risk categories include family members separated but accounted for, history of mental health needs, having been decontaminated after an exposure, or health concerns related to a possible exposure; such risks would trigger secondary screening and monitoring as a part of a community unit (i.e., schools). Low-risk individuals are those without any identified risk factors; they would be connected with community resources as needed.

Long after patients have been treated for physical injuries related to a disaster, the psychological effects may persist among both patients and healthcare professionals. If trauma nurses are aware of the risk factors associated with traumatic events, they will be in a position to assist traumatized patients and any colleagues who were affected.[61] See Chapter 18, "Psychosocial Aspects of Trauma Care," for additional information.

> **NOTE**
>
> **Pitfalls of Recovery**
>
> The pitfalls of recovery may include the following:
>
> - Not conducting postevent analysis and critique
> - Not including mental health in planning
> - Missing the HVAs at the local level
> - Not identifying the opportunities for improvement from a previous disaster
> - Not identifying the value in the local assets
>
> Data from Armstrong, J., Berg, B., Doucet, J., Ginzburg, E., Greenhalgh, D., Gross, R., Jawa, R., Murdock, A., O'Neill, P., Reynolds, C., Shatz, D., Upperman, J., Weireter, Jr., L., & Young, D. (2018). *Disaster Management and Emergency Preparedness (DMEP) Manual* (2nd ed.). American College of Surgeons.

Types of Disasters

Types of disasters include natural and human-made.

Natural Disasters

It is important to recognize the potential for high-risk natural disasters in the community and their effects on healthcare facilities. Natural disasters include floods, hurricanes, wildfires, severe temperatures, landslides, volcanoes, and earthquakes.[15] As part of the mitigation and preparedness phases, specific planning considerations unique to each type of natural hazard are considered. Additionally, the potential for the consequences of one disaster to overlap with another concurrent hazard must be recognized. For example, a large-scale wildfire may be contained, but severe rain may follow, causing mudslides and flooding. The trauma nurse can expect the nearby hospital to incur a loss of power, ventilation issues, and possible staffing shortages due to road closures, all while a surge of patients continue to seek medical care.

Natural disasters can be costly, and the recovery process may affect the healthcare facility. For example, Puerto Rico was struck by Hurricane Maria in September 2017 and suffered substantial damage as a result. Puerto Rico was a major supplier of intravenous normal saline to healthcare facilities. In the aftermath of the hurricane, the Puerto Rican suppliers' operations were curtailed, and consequently, hospitals were faced with shortages of saline.[66]

The year 2021 was, to date, the most expensive year for natural disasters within the United States (**Figure 19-2**).[51] **Table 19-2** outlines the various types of injuries that can result from the different kinds of natural disasters.

Earthquake

Between 1998 and 2017, there were almost 750,000 deaths across the globe due to earthquakes.[83] Certain areas of the world are more prone to earthquakes, which are a shifting in the earth's tectonic plates that results in shaking of the planet's surface. In the United States, California and Alaska are well-known seismically active regions; Alaska is home to 11% of the world's recorded earthquakes, including the second largest earthquake ever recorded.[81]

Earthquakes occur suddenly and can vary in magnitude but have the potential to cause widespread damage and destruction. The extent of destruction is determined by magnitude, intensity, duration, time of day of the event, local geology, and local building design and construction.[83] Infrastructure such as roads, water resources, and public utilities can be damaged and become unstable when an earthquake strikes, creating additional challenges. Healthcare facilities may be rendered unusable because of damage from the earthquake or after-effects such as fire, landslide, tsunami, or building collapse. Evacuation plans may need to be implemented with no notice.[41] Earthquake-prone regions often have extensive planning and mitigation efforts in place to prepare for an earthquake. However, earthquakes can happen anywhere.

Hurricane

Hurricanes are large but slow-moving tropical cyclones that have sustained winds of 74 miles per hour or greater. They most often form around the Atlantic Coast and Gulf of Mexico, but other geographic locations are also susceptible to their effects. Hurricanes are dangerous not only because of their winds, but also because of the accompanying storm surge and heavy flooding.[5]

Potential short- and long-term hurricane consequences include changes in the social, physical, and biochemical environment; pollutants and contaminants; infrastructure damage; limitations to healthcare access and worsening of chronic medical conditions; and unintentional injuries such as drowning, heat stress, and infectious disease outbreaks.[80]

Tornado

Tornadoes are a worldwide phenomenon that can occur with little to no warning. While tornado warnings and

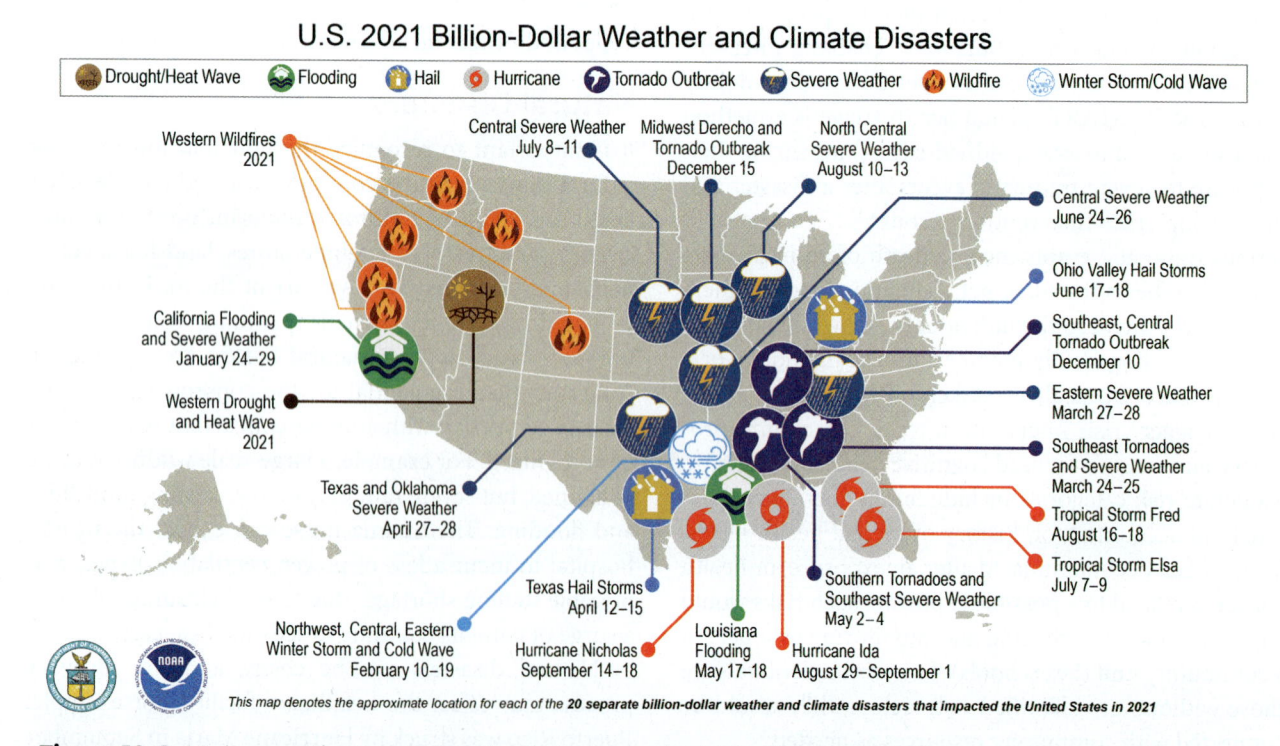

Figure 19-2 *Major weather and climate disasters in the United States, 2021.*

Reproduced from National Centers for Environmental Information. (2022). *U.S. 2021 billion-dollar weather and climate disasters*. National Oceanic and Atmospheric Administration. https://www.climate.gov/news-features/blogs/beyond-data/2021-us-billion-dollar-weather-and-climate-disasters-historical

TABLE 19-2 Natural Disasters and Associated Risks and Injuries

Disaster	Risk and Injury
Hurricanes	Waterborne infections (drinking water that is contaminated with toxins and sewage)
	Wound infections
	Orthopedic injuries
	Hypothermia
	Mosquito-borne infections
	Crush injuries
Tornadoes	Lacerations
	Abrasions
	Crush injuries
	Compound fractures
Floods	Hypothermia
	Blunt trauma from debris
	Lacerations
Earthquakes	Crush injuries to pelvis, chest, and legs (especially at night due to people sleeping and debris falling)
	Lacerations
	Head trauma (especially during the day)

watches have become more accurate in recent years, the exact timing and location of a tornado remain unpredictable; tornadoes often occur with very little lead time.[58] Although more common in the Midwestern area of the United States, tornadoes have occurred in all 50 states.[54] Tornadoes occur all over the world; Bangladesh and Argentina have the highest incidence of tornadoes outside the United States. The Enhanced Fujita (EF) Scale is used to classify the strength of a tornado. This is based on the amount of damage the tornado creates, and the wind speed is determined from that damage. An EF5 tornado is estimated to have a 3-second wind gust between 262 and 317 miles per hour.[53]

Flood

Flooding may occur from many causes, including heavy rain, snow, coastal storms, and damage to dams or diversionary systems. More than 50% of all deaths during a flood occur from driving a vehicle into floodwater, followed by people walking into moving water. As little as 6 inches of moving water can create enough force to cause someone walking to fall and even potentially carry a vehicle away. Standing water can pose a risk when waded through; toxins, sewage, sharp debris, and electrical charges from downed power lines may be in the water.[55]

Burn Mass-Casualty Incident

Wildfires are natural disasters caused when vegetation burns uncontrollably. During the 2019–2020 Australian wildfires, it was estimated that 400 megatons of carbon dioxide and significant amounts of nitrous oxide were released into the atmosphere. Nitrous oxide can cause children to develop lung disease, such as asthma.[56] In addition, the inhalation of pollutants caused by wildfires can exacerbate bronchitis, chronic obstructive pulmonary disease, and cardiovascular disease and cause increased hospitalizations and mortality.[8]

Along with inhalation of toxins, burn injuries are a concern with any type of thermal exposure. Burn injuries vary in severity based on the extent of the burn and the nature of the fire. Early anticipation for transfer to a burn center is important, and initial care always includes stopping the burning process. In 2020 in the United States, there were only 133 burn centers, which would be problematic in the case of a burn mass-casualty incident.[38] This small number of burn centers makes bed availability a challenge, and nurses should be prepared to care for patients with these injuries.

Human-Made Disasters

Human-made disasters occur suddenly, and their impact is difficult to predict, requiring a heightened sense of awareness. These disasters can be intentional or unintentional and include industrial incidents, shootings, acts of terrorism, or mass violence.

Active Shooter

The frequency of active shooter events is steadily increasing, with a staggering number of casualties. In many of the recent shooting events, there has been an increase in the number of fatal wounds occurring as a result. As mentioned earlier in this chapter, the 2017 mass shooting in Las Vegas in 2017 killed 58 people and injured 422.[7,42]

An active shooter event occurs unexpectedly and rapidly. Anticipation of the type of injuries most likely to be encountered and anticipating necessary interventions help decrease mortality. The trauma nurse should be alert to the possibility of major vascular injuries, hidden blood loss, and the potential for fatal injuries. The most common causes of death are wounds to the brain, lung, and heart.[45]

Preventable death can occur in active shooter events related to uncontrolled hemorrhage. For example, at one active shooter event, 90% of the victims had an extremity wound, but none of the patients had tourniquets or any pressure dressing applied before arrival at the hospital. It was estimated that 32% of the those who died had potentially survivable injuries.[67]

Chemical, Biological, Radiological, Nuclear, and Explosives Countermeasures

The U.S. Department of Homeland Security reports that reliable chemical, biologic, radiologic, nuclear, and explosive (CBRNE) countermeasures can be used to "protect life, health, property, and commerce."[76] If a CBRNE agent is involved, immediate identification of the specific agent is not as important as immediate recognition of, response to, and treatment of any unusual symptoms presenting across various age groups and populations.

Decontamination

Decontamination is defined as "any action that reduces, removes, neutralizes or inactivates contamination."[23(p2)] Decontamination in the event of a hazardous exposure during a disaster is crucial to ensure the safety of emergency personnel and to minimize cross-contamination to other people.

Decontamination is typically performed in the field. However, many victims may not wait for emergency response personnel to receive field decontamination and instead transport themselves to the hospital.[11] Rapid identification of patients presenting to the hospital who may have bypassed scene decontamination is essential. Immediate decontamination according to facility protocols is initiated, with only basic lifesaving interventions conducted in the hot or warm zones to minimize delays in the decontamination process. An example of a typical decontamination design is seen in **Figure 19-3**. Each step in the process of decontamination is outlined in **Table 19-3**.[18]

Personal Protective Equipment

Emergency responders have a variety of personal protective equipment (PPE) available to protect them from different types of hazards. Such equipment includes fully encapsulating suits that provide splash protection and respiratory protection at various levels. Correct use of PPE requires ongoing training and, at some levels, certification for use.

Disasters may bring a number of hazards, including infectious, radioactive, or chemical events. Identifying the specific hazardous substance is important but not required. If the substance is unknown, the trauma nurse should increase their index of suspicion and potentially increase their level of PPE until a determination can be made. Staff should be familiar with proper donning and doffing of PPE as part of the decontamination response. Adhering to the donning and doffing sequence is critical to ensuring maximal protection from exposure to hazards brought into the facility. The use of a trained observer provides an extra safeguard. Such an individual monitors compliance with PPE protocols, guides and corrects any deviations from the appropriate process, and assists trauma nurses in properly protecting themselves.

Chemical Agents

Chemical exposures have the potential to harm multiple people simultaneously and can be intentional or unintentional. Chemical agents can be lethal, with a very short window for effective treatment. Chemicals are classified according to their effect on health or the environment.[13]

The *2020 Emergency Response Guidebook* can be used to quickly identify the class of materials involved in an incident.[77] The *National Institute for Occupational Safety and Health (NIOSH) Pocket Guide to Chemical Hazards* has general information on several hundred chemicals.[75] These guides include contact information for manufacturers and specialists on chemical agents. Additional resources regarding specific chemical agents include the Poison Control Center and Safety Data Sheets, which are required by the Occupational Safety and Health Administration (OSHA) to be available at all worksites that

> **NOTE**
>
> **Exposure versus Contamination**
>
> **Exposure** is contact with a substance by ingestion, inhalation, or direct contact and can be acute, intermediate, or chronic.[1] A person can be exposed but not necessarily contaminated; exposure does not require decontamination, nor is it transmittable.
>
> **Contamination** is the entry of a contaminant into the body. It can be internal, through ingestion, inhalation, or exposure through an open wound, or external, through contact with the skin, hair, or eyes.[23] Decontamination is necessary with chemical, biological, and external radiologic contamination to prevent further harm and to reduce the risk of transmission.

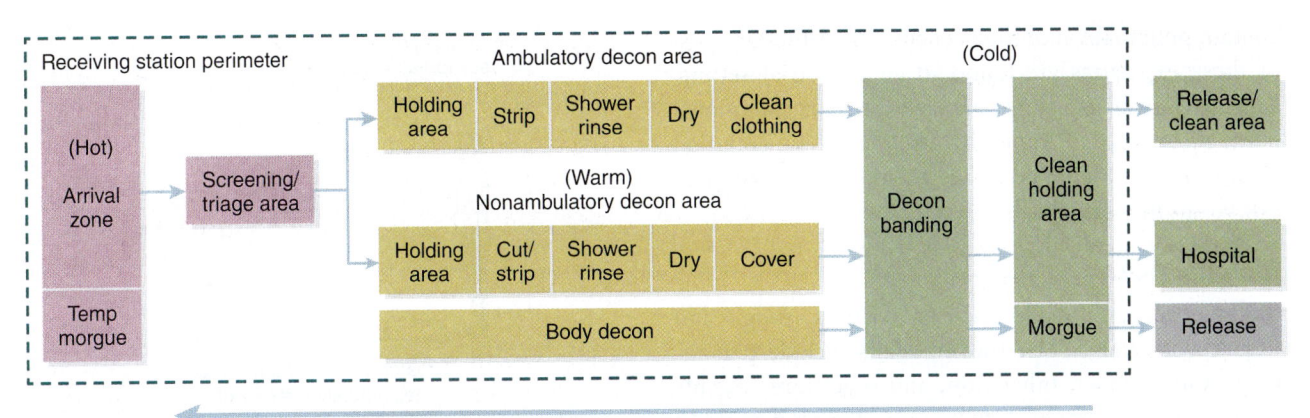

Figure 19-3 *Example decontamination design.*

TABLE 19-3	Primary Response Incident Scene Management (PRISM) Processes	
Best Practice	**Description**	**Rationale**
Evacuation	Casualties should be evacuated from the scene of a hazardous chemical release.	Self-evacuation halts continued exposure or worsened contamination.
Disrobe	Remove all clothing, jewelry, and other inanimate objects on each person as soon as possible and before showering. Avoid removing clothing over the head. Cut clothing if necessary.	Limits transfer of contaminants to skin and prevents secondary contamination through off-gassing from clothing. Eliminates 90% or more of contaminants after an incident.
Improvised decontamination	Can be dry or wet; the victim immediately wipes or rinses off the skin.	Removes visible contamination from exposed skin rapidly after the incident, further decreasing ongoing exposure. Using a cloth or sponge can increase removal of the contaminant by 20%.
Gross decontamination	The use of standard equipment to grossly decontaminate a large number of victims with copious water. Large-diameter water discharges from fire apparatus or hydrants can be used.	Using copious amounts of water from a fire truck ladder pipe system, decontamination corridor, or decontamination trailer is an effective way to remove remaining contaminants from skin.
Active drying	Victims use a dry towel or other material following any form of wet decontamination.	Dry towels remove small portions of contaminants that may remain following other forms of decontamination.
Technical decontamination	Thorough manual decontamination focused on reducing contamination to an acceptable level. This is the step at which soap should be used if determined to be necessary.	A more time-consuming and in-depth process that is used to decontaminate victims to a higher degree or those who are not ambulatory.

Data from Chilcott, R. P., & Amlôt, R. (Eds). (2015). Strategic guidance for mass casualty disrobe and decontamination. In *Primary Response Incident Scene Management (PRISM) guidance for chemical incidents* (Vol. 2). https://www.medicalcountermeasures.gov/media/36872/prism-volume-1.pdf

contain potentially hazardous chemicals. Although most of these exposures are found in an industrial setting, some chemical exposures are acquired for intentional harm by terrorists.[4] **Appendix 19-2** lists these common chemical agents and describes their known signs and symptoms in more detail.

Biologic Agents

Biologic agents include bacteria, viruses, fungi, and toxins. Potential disease transmissions include person-to-person, contact, inhalation, and ingestions. Agents used as a weapon are likely to be aerosolized but could be transmitted by person to person via ingestion or personal contact. Bioterrorism attacks can be directed against people, animals, or plants, not just causing death but also destroying crops and killing livestock.[31]

The release of these agents might not be immediately recognized because of the delay between exposure to the agent and illness onset. In many cases, presenting symptoms can closely resemble those that occur naturally.[41] Indications of intentional release of a biologic agent include an unusual geographic clustering of illness and an unusual age distribution for common diseases. Biologic agents that could cause a communicable disease disaster include anthrax, botulism, plague, tularemia, and smallpox; these are discussed in more detail in **Appendix 19-3**. Most biologic agents are found naturally. Others have been eradicated and are found only in secure labs.

Radiologic/Nuclear Events

Ionizing radiation is electromagnetic energy, or energy containing particles emitted from a source. In a living thing, it causes damage to cells by denaturation of DNA. The two major types of ionizing radiation are electromagnetic (gamma and x-rays) and particle (alpha and beta particles). Differentiating between patients who are only exposed versus those who are contaminated is an important component of victim management during a radiologic event. A contamination occurs when a radioisotope is released into the environment and is ingested, inhaled, or deposited onto a patient's body surface.

Three basic elements determine the amount of exposure: time, distance, and shielding (**Figure 19-4**). The risk of acute radiation illness is minimized by a shorter duration of exposure, a greater distance from the nucleus of the explosion, and a greater amount of shielding between the person and the explosion. Symptoms of acute radiation syndrome include nausea, vomiting, headache, and diarrhea, which, depending on duration and other factors, can progress to include poor appetite, fatigue, fever, and skin damage.[16] **Appendix 19-4** describes specific acute radiation syndromes in detail,

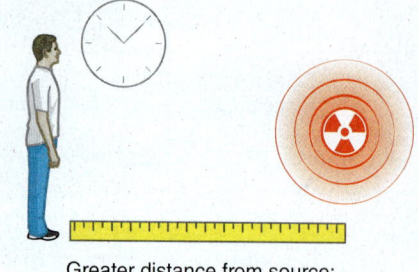

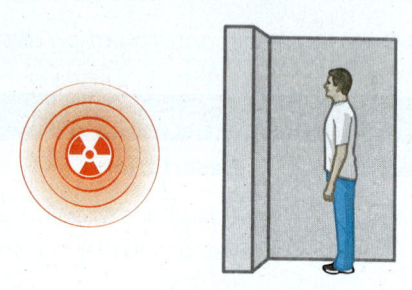

Figure 19-4 *Determinants of radiation exposure.*

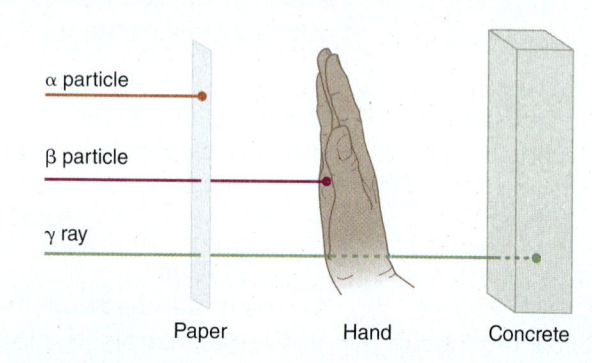

Figure 19-5 *Penetrating abilities of various types of radiation.*

while **Figure 19-5** illustrates the penetrating ability of various types of radiation.

Radiologic and nuclear events are not isolated to radiation exposure; the trauma nurse should anticipate concurrent thermal and blast injuries.

Explosives

Explosions, whether intentional or unintentional, are the most likely disaster to occur in any community. Intentional acts may involve bombs, acts of terrorism, and improvised explosive devices, and unintentional explosions include events such as industrial and transportation-related incidents. In mass-casualty situations, explosions cause a blast wave that can affect victims over a wide area. This overpressurization shock wave can cause multiple levels of injury. See Chapter 3, "Biomechanics and Mechanism of Injury," for additional information.

Most explosives involved in a mass-casualty situation can cause life-threatening hemorrhage on a large scale. Research has shown that the faster this hemorrhage is controlled, the greater the chance of survivability. Bystanders are often present before the arrival of first responders and can quickly provide interventions such as tourniquets or wound packing. The "Stop the Bleed" campaign combines both interventions in training laypersons how to stop profuse bleeding and save lives using direct pressure, wound packing, or a commercial tourniquet.[3] See Chapter 10, "Spinal and Musculoskeletal Trauma," for more information on tourniquet application.

Emerging Trends

Emergency management agencies are including new strategies for disaster management and response. Communication methodologies are expanding to include mass notifications within hospitals, school systems, and communities. Social media have features to disseminate and gather information related to disasters. As an event is unfolding, emergency management professionals are embracing opportunities to disseminate information and correct inaccuracies through social media technology.[59]

Communities and schools are participating in active shooter drills with increasing frequency to familiarize individuals with the options-based response (run–hide–fight) when a lockdown is simply not enough.

Cybersecurity is assuming a crucial role in preparing for disasters; cyberterrorism can compound disruptions that occur during a disaster or can be the disaster itself. Phishing attacks, ransomware, and malware can disrupt infrastructure on a global scale, paralyzing governments, businesses, and organizations. Healthcare systems worldwide are at risk for cyberattacks, which are a potential risk to patient safety.[20,57]

Summary

Disasters, which can happen any place at any time, continue to occur frequently, affecting more and more people. Although most disasters are natural, it is important to be aware of and familiar with human-made disasters. Understanding the hospital's emergency operations plan and the mitigation, preparedness, response, and recovery phases of disaster management is foundational during a disaster, enabling the greatest care possible for the greatest number of people.

Finally, it is important to understand the implications of personal preparedness in one's own response to a disaster. If the nurse is experiencing concerns about the welfare of their own family or has suffered a personal loss related to the disaster, it is possible that the nurse may not be able to perform the duties required. Personal preparedness can include establishing communication methods with family and stores of emergency supplies for at least 3 days. Ready.gov has multiple resources available for setting up a personal preparedness plan.

References

1. Agency for Toxic Substances and Disease Registry. (n.d.). Exposure. In *Glossary of terms*. U.S. Department of Health and Human Services. https://www.atsdr.cdc.gov/glossary.html#G-D-
2. American College of Surgeons. (2018). *Advanced trauma life support: Student course manual* (10th ed.).
3. American College of Surgeons. (2022). *Our story*. Stop the Bleed. https://www.stopthebleed.org/our-story
4. Armstrong, J., Berg, B., Doucet, J., Ginzburg, E., Greenhalgh, D., Gross, R., Jawa, R., Murdock, A., O'Neill, P., Reynolds, C., Shatz, D., Upperman, J., Weireter, Jr., L., & Young, D. (2018). *Disaster management and emergency preparedness (DMEP) manual* (2nd ed.). American College of Surgeons.
5. Atlantic Oceanographic and Meteorological Laboratory. (2021, June 1). *Hurricanes: Frequently asked questions*. National Oceanic and Atmospheric Administration. https://www.aoml.noaa.gov/hrd-faq/
6. Barton, D. G., Fijten, M., Gaakeer, M. I., Klokman, V. W., Mortelmans, L. J., van Osch, F., Peters, N. A., Wijnands, J. J., Tan, E. C., & Boin, A. (2022). Three decades of hospital evacuations in the Netherlands: A scoping review. *International Journal of Disaster Risk Reduction, 81*. https://doi.org/10.1016/j.ijdrr.2022.103252
7. Binkley, J. M., & Kemp, K. M. (2022). Mobilization of resources and emergency response on the national scale. *Surgery Clinics of North America, 102*(1), 169–180. https://www.ncbi.nlm.nih.gov/pmc/articles/PMC8598287/pdf/main.pdf
8. Black, C., Tesfaigzi, Y., Bassein, J. A., & Miller, L. A. (2017). Wildfire smoke exposure and human health: Significant gaps in research for a growing public health issue. *Environmental Toxicology and Pharmacology, 55*, 186–195. https://doi.org/10.1016%2Fj.etap.2017.08.022
9. California Department of Public Health. (2016). *15 'til 50 . . . mass casualty incident guide for healthcare entities*. http://cdphready.org/wp-content/uploads/2016/01/15-til-50-MCI-Guide.pdf
10. California Emergency Medical Services Authority. (2016, May). *Hospital Incident Command System: Current guidebook and appendices*. http://www.emsa.ca.gov/disaster-medical-services-division-hospital-incident-command-system/

11. Carter, H., Amlot, R., Williams., R., Rubin, G. J., & Drury, J. (2016). Mass casualty decontamination in a chemical or radiological/nuclear incident: Further guiding principles. *PLOS Currents Disasters, 15*(8). https://www.ncbi.nlm.nih.gov/pmc/articles/PMC4648544/
12. Center for Medicare and Medicaid Services. (2021, April 16). Emergency preparedness for all provider and certified supplier types: Interpretive guidance. In *State operations manual*. https://www.cms.gov/Regulations-and-Guidance/Guidance/Manuals/Downloads/som107ap_z_emergprep.pdf
13. Centers for Disease Control and Prevention. (n.d.). *Chemical emergencies*. https://emergency.cdc.gov/chemical/overview.asp
14. Centers for Disease Control and Prevention. (n.d.). *Coping with a disaster or traumatic event*. https://www.emergency.cdc.gov/coping/index.asp
15. Centers for Disease Control and Prevention. (n.d.). *National disasters and severe weather*. https://www.cdc.gov/disasters/index.html
16. Centers for Disease Control and Prevention. (2017). *A brochure for physicians: Acute radiation syndrome*. https://emergency.cdc.gov/radiation/pdf/ars.pdf
17. Chartoff, S. T., Kropp, A. M., & Roman, P. (2021, September 5). Disaster planning. *StatPearls*. StatPearls Publishing. https://www.ncbi.nlm.nih.gov/books/NBK470570/
18. Chilcott, R. P., & Amlôt, R. (Eds.). (2015). Strategic guidance for mass casualty disrobe and decontamination. In *Primary Response Incident Scene Management (PRISM) guidance for chemical incidents* (Vol. 2). https://www.medicalcountermeasures.gov/media/36872/prism-volume-1.pdf
19. Childstats Forum on Child and Family Statistics. (n.d.). *Children as a percentage of the population*. Federal Interagency Forum on Child and Family Statistics. https://www.childstats.gov/americaschildren/tables/pop2.asp
20. Choi, S., & Johnson, M. E. (2017, June 26–27). *Do hospital data breaches reduce patient care quality?* [Paper presentation]. 16th Workshop on the Economics of Information Security, La Jolla, CA, United States. https://arxiv.org/pdf/1904.02058.pdf
21. Chung, S., Charney, R., Biddinger, P., & Krupa, R. (Eds.). (2018). *Family reunification following disasters: A planning tool for health care facilities*. American Academy of Pediatrics. https://downloads.aap.org/AAP/PDF/AAP%20Reunification%20Toolkit.pdf
22. Chung, S., Gardner, A. H., Schonfeld, D. J., Franks, J. L., So, M., Dziuban, E. J., & Peacock, G. (2018). Addressing children's needs in disasters: A regional pediatric tabletop exercise. *Disaster Medicine and Public Health Preparedness, 12*(5), 582–586. https://doi.org/10.1017%2Fdmp.2017.137
23. Collins, S., James, T., Carter, H., Symons, C., Southworth, F., Foxall, K., Marczylo, T., & Amlot, R. (2021). Mass casualty decontamination for chemical incidents: Research outcomes and future priorities. *International Journal of Environmental Research and Public Health, 18*(6), Article 3079. https://doi.org/10.3390%2Fijerph18063079
24. Dziuban, E. J., Peacock, G., & Frogel, M. (2017). A child's health is the public's health: Progress and gaps in addressing pediatric needs in public health emergencies. *American Journal of Public Health, 107*(S2), S134–S137. https://doi.org/10.2105/AJPH.2017.303950
25. EM-DAT, The International Disaster Database. (n.d.). Disaster. *EM-DAT glossary*. https://www.emdat.be/Glossary
26. Emergency Medical Services for Children. (2022, August). *Checklist of essential pediatric domains and considerations for every hospital's disaster policies (Pilot)*. https://media.emscimprovement.center/documents/EIICDisasterChecklist_Current081822.pdf
27. Emergency Preparedness. (n.d.). *Types of exercises*. California Hospital Association. https://www.calhospitalprepare.org/post/types-exercises
28. Farcas, A., Ko, J., Chan, J., Malik, S., Nono, L., & Ciampas, G. (2021). Use of incident command system for disaster preparedness: A model for an emergency department COVID-19 response. *Disaster Medicine and Public Health Preparedness, 15*(3), e31–e36. https://doi.org/10.1017%2Fdmp.2020.210
29. Federal Emergency Management Agency. (2022, September 26). *National Incident Management System*. https://www.fema.gov/national-incident-management-system
30. Gadd, C., & Jones, C. (2018). Accidents and ethics: A visual-narrative approach. *Emergency Nurse, 25*(9), 35–41. https://doi.org/10.7748/en.2018.e1727
31. Hayoun, M. A., & King, K. C. (2022, July 1). Biologic warfare agent toxicity. *StatPearls*. StatPearls Publishing. https://www.ncbi.nlm.nih.gov/books/NBK441942/
32. Hertelendy, A. J., Ciottone, G. R., Mitchell, C. L., Gutberg, J., & Burkle, F. M. (2021). Crisis standards of care in a pandemic: Navigating the ethical, clinical, psychological and policy-making maelstrom. *International Journal for Quality in Health, 33*(1), Article mzaa094. https://doi.org/10.1093/intqhc/mzaa094
33. Hick, J. L., Nelson, J., Fildes, J., Kuhls, D., Eastman, A., & Dries, D. (2020). Triage, trauma, and today's mass violence events. *Journal of the American College of Surgeons, 230*(2), 251–256. https://doi.org/10.1016/j.jamcollsurg.2019.10.011
34. Institute of Medicine. (2009). *Guidance for establishing crisis standards of care for use in disaster situations: A letter report*. The National Academies Press. https://doi.org/10.17226/12749
35. Institute of Medicine. (2015). *Healthy, resilient, and sustainable communities after disasters: Strategies, opportunities, and planning for recovery*. The National Academies Press. https://doi.org/10.17226/18996
36. International Federation of Red Cross and Red Crescent Societies. (n.d.). *What is a disaster?* http://www.ifrc.org/en/what-we-do/disaster-management/about-disasters/what-is-a-disaster/
37. Kaye, A. D., Cornett, E. M., Kallurkar, A., Colontonio, M. M., Chandler, D., Mosieri, C., Brondeel, K. C., Kikkeri, S., Edinoff, A., Fitz-Gerald, M. J., Ghali, G. E., Liu, H., Urman, R. D., & Fox, C. J. (2021). Framework for creating an incident command center during crises. *Best Practice & Research: Clinical Anaesthesiology 35*(3), 377–388. https://doi.org/10.1016%2Fj.bpa.2020.11.008

38. Kearns, R. D., Bettencourt, A. P., Hickerson, W. L., Palmieri, T. L., Biddinger, P. D., Ryan, C. M., & Jeng, J. C. (2020). Actionable, revised (v.3), and amplified American Burn Association triage tables for mass casualties: A civilian defense guideline. *Journal of Burn Care & Research, 41*(4), 770–779. https://doi.org/10.1093/jbcr/iraa050

39. Khorram-Manesh, A., Nordling, J., Carlström, E., Goniewicz, K., Faccincani, R., & Burkle, F. M. (2021). A translational triage research development tool: Standardizing prehospital triage decision-making systems in mass casualty incidents. *Scandinavian Journal of Trauma, Resuscitation and Emergency Medicine, 29*(1), Article 119. https://doi.org/10.1186/s13049-021-00932-z

40. Khorram-Manesh, A., Phattharapornjaroen, P., Mortelmans, L. J., Goniewicz, K., Verheul, M., Sorensen, J. L., Pereira, I., Ricklin, M. E., Raccincani, R., Dark, P. M, Carlstrom, E., Marzaleh, M. A., Peyravi, M. R., Sultan, M. A., Santamaria, E., Comandante, J. D., & Burkle, F. (2022). Current perspectives and concerns facing hospital evacuation: The results of a pilot study and literature review. *Disaster Medicine and Public Health Preparedness, 16*(2), 650–658. https://doi.org/10.1017/dmp.2020.391

41. Kwo, J., & Johnson, D. W. (2018). Disaster medicine, bioterrorism, and Ebola. In P. E. Parsons, J. P. Wiener-Kronish, R. D. Stapleton, & L. Berra (Eds.), *Critical care secrets* (6th ed., pp. 457–464). Elsevier.

42. Lake, C. K. (2018). *A day like no other: A case study of the Las Vegas mass shooting*. Nevada Hospital Association. https://nvha.net/a-day-like-no-other-case-study-of-the-las-vegas-mass-shooting/

43. Los Angeles County Emergency Medical Services Agency. (2012). Part I: Guidance. In *Evacuation and shelter in place guidance for healthcare facilities* (pp. 1–28). https://www.calhospitalprepare.org/sites/main/files/file-attachments/evac_sip_1.pdf

44. Los Angeles County Emergency Medical Services Agency. (2017). *Family information center: Planning guide for healthcare entities*. https://www.calhospitalprepare.org/sites/main/files/file-attachments/fic_planning_guide_final_062813_v62_0.pdf

45. Maghami, S., Hendrix, C., Matecki, M., Mahendran, K., Amdur, R., Mitchell, R., Diaz, F., Estroff, J., Smith, E. R., Shapiro, G., & Sarani, B. (2020). Comparison of the causes of death and wounding patterns in urban firearm-related violence and civilian public mass shooting events. *The Journal of Trauma and Acute Care Surgery, 88*(2), 310–313. https://doi.org/10.1097/TA.0000000000002470

46. Meng, X., Cai, Z., Si, S., & Duan, D. (2021). Analysis of epidemic vaccination strategies on heterogeneous networks: Based on SEIRV model and evolutionary game. *Applied Mathematics and Computation, 403*, Article 126172. https://doi.org/10.1016/j.amc.2021.126172

47. Merrill, J. A., Orr, M., Chen, D. Y., Zhi, Q., & Gershon, R. R. (2016). Are we ready for mass fatality incidents? Preparedness of the U.S. mass fatality infrastructure. *Disaster Medicine and Public Health Preparedness, 10*(1), 87–97. https://doi.org/10.1017/dmp.2015.135

48. Meyer, D., Bishai, D., Ravi, S. J., Rashid, H., Mahmood, S. S., Toner, E., & Nuzzo, J. B. (2020). A checklist to improve health system resilience to infectious disease outbreaks and natural hazards. *BMJ Global Health, 5*(8), Article e002429. https://doi.org/10.1136/bmjgh-2020-002429

49. Nakao, H., Ukai, I., & Kotani, J. (2017). A review of the history of the origin of triage from a disaster medicine perspective. *Acute Medicine & Surgery, 4*(4), 379–384. https://doi.org/10.1002%2Fams2.293

50. National Aeronautics and Space Administration. (n.d.). *International disaster charter activations*. https://eol.jsc.nasa.gov/ESRS/Disasters/ShowIDCTracking.pl

51. National Centers for Environmental Information. (2022). *U.S. billion-dollar weather and climate disasters*. National Oceanic and Atmospheric Administration. https://doi.org/10.25921/stkw-7w73

52. National Earthquake Hazards Reduction Program. (n.d.). *Earthquake coordinators web site*. Federal Emergency Management Agency. https://training.fema.gov/emiweb/earthquake/neh0101220.htm

53. National Severe Storms Laboratory. (n.d.). *Tornado basics*. National Oceanic and Atmospheric Administration. https://www.nssl.noaa.gov/education/svrwx101/tornadoes/

54. National Weather Service. (n.d.). *Tornado safety*. https://www.weather.gov/safety/tornado

55. National Weather Service. (n.d.). *Turn around don't drown*. U.S. Department of Commerce, National Oceanic and Atmospheric Administration. https://www.weather.gov/safety/flood-turn-around-dont-drown

56. Nguyen, H. D., Azzi, M., White, S., Salter, D., Trieu, T., Morgan, G., Rahman, M., Watt, S., Riley, M., Chang, L. T., Barthelemy, X., Fuchs, D., Lieschke, K., & Nguyen, H. (2021). The summer 2019–2020 wildfires in East Coast Australia and their impacts on air quality and health in New South Wales, Australia. *International Journal of Environmental Research and Public Health, 18*(7), Article 3538. https://doi.org/10.3390/ijerph18073538

57. Niki, O., Saira, G., Arvind, S., & Mike, D. (2022). Cyber-attacks are a permanent and substantial threat to health systems: Education must reflect that. *Digital Health, 8*. https://doi.org/10.1177/20552076221104665

58. Occupational Safety and Health Administration. (n.d.) *Tornado preparedness and response*. U.S. Department of Labor. https://www.osha.gov/tornado

59. Page-Tan, C. (2021). The role of social media in disaster recovery following Hurricane Harvey. *Journal of Homeland Security and Emergency Management, 18*(1), 93–123. https://doi.org/10.1515/jhsem-2018-0054

60. Public Health Emergency. (n.d.). *Disaster mortuary operational response teams*. U.S. Department of Health and Human Services. https://www.phe.gov/Preparedness/responders/ndms/ndms-teams/Pages/dmort.aspx

61. Raveis, V. H., VanDevanter, N., Kovner, C. T., & Gershon, R. (2017). Enabling a disaster-resilient workforce: Attending to individual stress and collective trauma. *Journal of Nursing Scholarship, 49*, 653–660. https://doi.org/10.1111/jnu.12340

62. Ready. (2021, October 12). *Exercises.* U.S. Department of Homeland Security. https://www.ready.gov/exercises
63. Ready. (2021, February 19). *Planning.* U.S. Department of Homeland Security. https://www.ready.gov/planning
64. Sahebi, A., Jahangiri, K., Alibabaei, A., & Khorasani-Zavareh, D. (2021). Factors influencing hospital emergency evacuation during fire: A systematic literature review. *International Journal of Preventive Medicine, 12,* Article 147. https://www.ncbi.nlm.nih.gov/pmc/articles/PMC8631117/
65. Schreiber, M. (2018). *PsySTART® emergency mental health triage systems for disasters and public health emergencies.* https://www.myctb.org/wst/HELPERS/Emergency%20Preparedness%20Documents/PsySTART_Overview.pdf
66. Scutti, S. (2018, January 17). IV bags in short supply across U.S. after Hurricane Maria. *CNN.* https://www.cnn.com/2018/01/16/health/iv-bag-shortage/index.html
67. Smith, E. R., Shapiro, G., & Sarani, B. (2018). Fatal wounding pattern and causes of potentially preventable death following the Pulse Night Club shooting event. *Prehospital Emergency Care, 22*(6), 662–668. https://doi.org/10.1080/10903127.2018.1459980
68. Substance Abuse and Mental Health Services Administration. (2022). *Types of disasters.* https://www.samhsa.gov/find-help/disaster-distress-helpline/disaster-types
69. Technical Resources, Assistance Center, and Information Exchange. (2018, August). *Tips for healthcare facilities: Assisting families and loved ones after a mass casualty incident.* U.S. Department of Health and Human Services, Administration for Strategic Preparedness and Response. https://files.asprtracie.hhs.gov/documents/aspr-tracie-family-assistance-center-fact-sheet.pdf
70. Technical Resources, Assistance Center, and Information Exchange. (2019, April). *Topic collection: Hazard vulnerability/risk assessment.* U.S. Department of Health and Human Services, Administration for Strategic Preparedness and Response. https://asprtracie.hhs.gov/technical-resources/3/hazard-vulnerability-risk-assessment/
71. Technical Resources, Assistance Center, and Information Exchange. (2022). *Topic collection: Pediatric/children.* U.S. Department of Health and Human Services, Administration for Strategic Preparedness and Response. https://asprtracie.hhs.gov/technical-resources/31/pediatric-children/0#trauma-care-and-triage
72. The Joint Commission. (2020). *Emergency management—Emergency response requirements during the COVID-19 public health emergency.* https://www.jointcommission.org/standards/standard-faqs/hospital-and-hospital-clinics/emergency-management-em/000002335/
73. The Joint Commission. (2021). *Emergency management standards: Supporting collaboration and planning.* https://www.jointcommission.org/-/media/tjc/documents/standards/r3-reports/final-r3-report-emergency-management.pdf
74. Tin, D., Hertelendy, A. J., & Ciottone, G. R. (2021). What we learned from the 2019–2020 Australian Bushfire disaster: Making counter-terrorism medicine a strategic preparedness priority. *The American Journal of Emergency Medicine, 46,* 742–743. https://doi.org/10.1016/j.ajem.2020.09.069
75. U.S. Department of Health and Human Services. (2007). *NIOSH pocket guide to chemical hazards* (DHHS Publication No. 2005-149). https://www.cdc.gov/niosh/docs/2005-149/pdfs/2005-149.pdf
76. U.S. Department of Homeland Security. (2022, January 18). *Science and technology: National strategy for chemical, biological, radiological, nuclear, and explosives standards.* https://www.dhs.gov/national-strategy-chemical-biological-radiological-nuclear-and-explosives-cbrne-standards
77. U.S. Department of Transportation. (2020). *Emergency response guidebook.* Skyhorse. https://www.phmsa.dot.gov/sites/phmsa.dot.gov/files/2020-08/ERG2020-WEB.pdf
78. United Nations Office for Disaster Risk Reduction. (n.d.). *Evacuation.* https://www.undrr.org/terminology/evacuation
79. United Nations Office for Disaster Risk Reduction. (n.d.). *Understanding disaster risk.* https://www.preventionweb.net/understanding-disaster-risk
80. Waddell, S. L., Jayaweera, D. T., Mirsaeidi, M., Beier, J. C., & Kumar, N. (2021). Perspectives on the health effects of hurricanes: A review and challenges. *International Journal of Environmental Research and Public Health, 18*(5), Article 2756. https://doi.org/10.3390%2Fijerph18052756
81. Wilkey, R. (2013, September 5). Alaskan earthquake could destroy California coast: U.S. Geological Survey. *HuffPost.* https://www.huffingtonpost.com/2013/09/05/alaska-earthquake-california_n_3875015.html
82. Wisconsin Department of Health Services Health Care Preparedness Program. (2020, June). *CMS emergency preparedness rule workbook: Hospitals.* https://www.dhs.wisconsin.gov/publications/p01948b.pdf
83. World Health Organization. (n.d.). *Earthquakes.* https://www.who.int/health-topics/earthquakes#tab=tab_1

APPENDIX 19-1
Triage Methods

A. START Adult Triage

Simple Triage and Rapid Treatment (START) triage is a quick and rapid method to identify and sort patients in a situation in which the number of patients overwhelms current resources available. Patients are sorted in a manner that enables the trauma nurse to provide the most good to the greatest number of patients.[6]

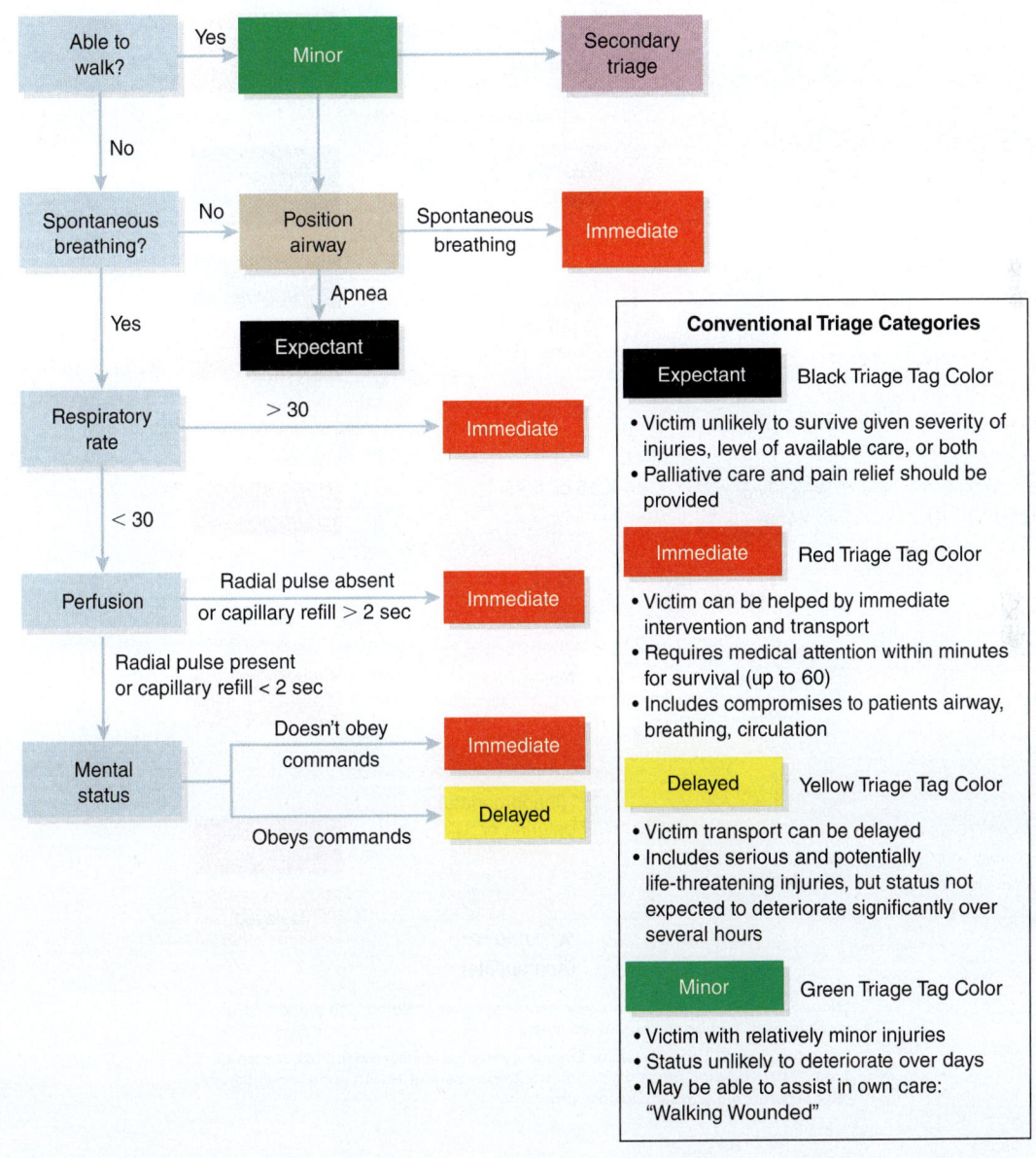

Conventional Triage Categories

Expectant — Black Triage Tag Color
- Victim unlikely to survive given severity of injuries, level of available care, or both
- Palliative care and pain relief should be provided

Immediate — Red Triage Tag Color
- Victim can be helped by immediate intervention and transport
- Requires medical attention within minutes for survival (up to 60)
- Includes compromises to patients airway, breathing, circulation

Delayed — Yellow Triage Tag Color
- Victim transport can be delayed
- Includes serious and potentially life-threatening injuries, but status not expected to deteriorate significantly over several hours

Minor — Green Triage Tag Color
- Victim with relatively minor injuries
- Status unlikely to deteriorate over days
- May be able to assist in own care: "Walking Wounded"

Reproduced from Chemical Hazards Emergency Medical Management. (2022, September 1). *START adult triage algorithm*. U.S. Department of Health and Human Services. https://chemm.hhs.gov/startadult.htm

B. JumpSTART Pediatric Multiple Casualty Incident Triage

JumpSTART is a modified version of START triage that considers the differences in the pediatric population. JumpSTART provides for limited interventions to the nonbreathing patient that are appropriate for the pediatric population, but the overall premise is the same as that of the START triage algorithm.[5]

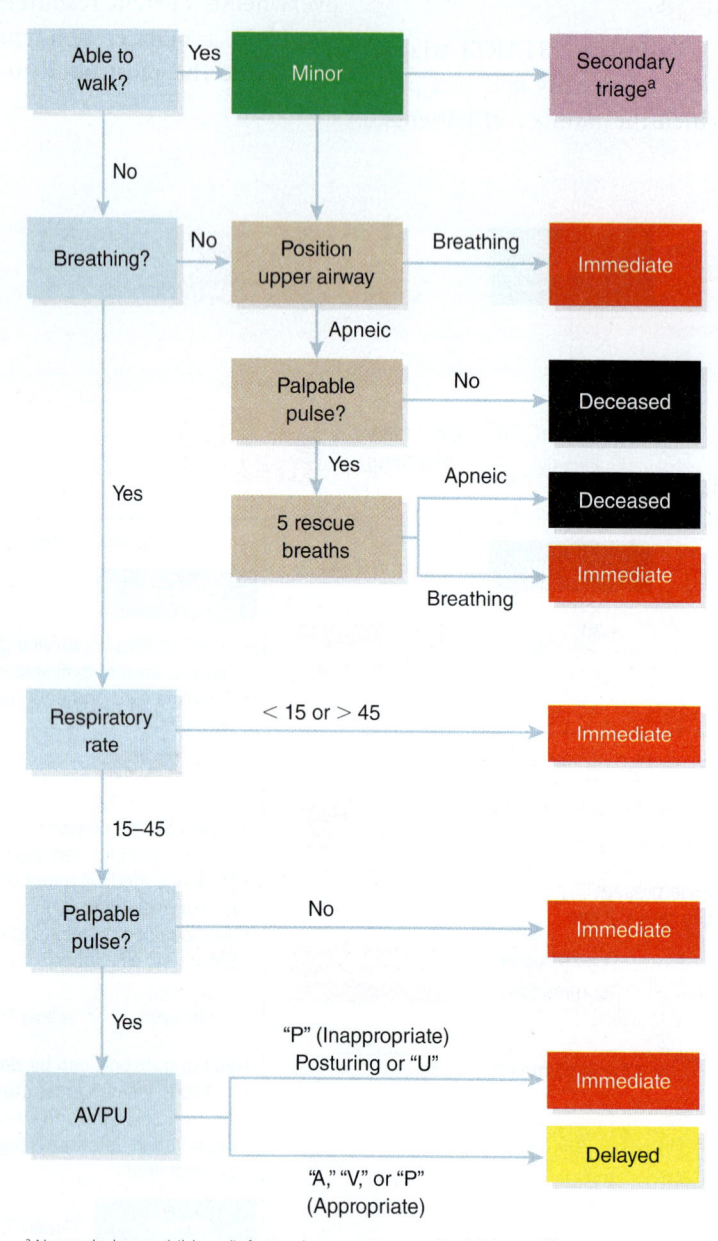

[a] Nonambulatory children (infants who cannot yet walk, children with preexisting conditions) are evaluated beginning with breathing.[3]

Reproduced from Chemical Hazards Emergency Medical Management. (2022, September 1). *JumpSTART pediatric triage algorithm.* U.S. Department of Health and Human Services. https://chemm.hhs.gov/startpediatric.htm

C. SALT Triage

Sort–Assess–Lifesaving Interventions–Treatment and/or Transport (SALT) uses a sorting method similar to that of START triage to sort and assess victims, provide limited lifesaving interventions, and then prioritize treatment and transportation.[2,4] SALT has been found to be more accurate than START for identifying higher priority patients, but healthcare systems have been slow to adopt this method. Trauma nurses should be aware of the standard used by their healthcare facility.

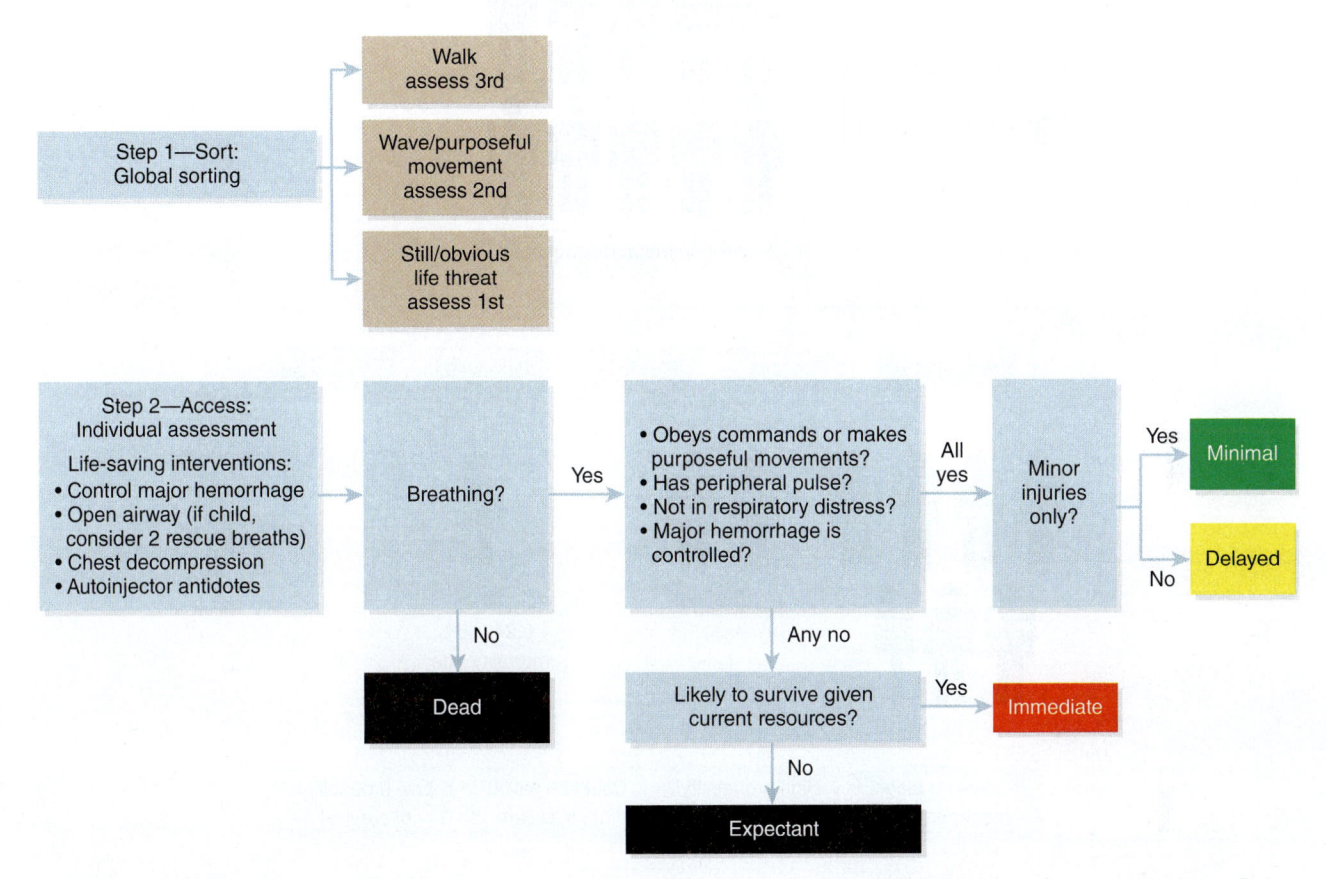

Step 1—Sort: Global sorting
- Walk → assess 3rd
- Wave/purposeful movement → assess 2nd
- Still/obvious life threat → assess 1st

Step 2—Access: Individual assessment

Life-saving interventions:
- Control major hemorrhage
- Open airway (if child, consider 2 rescue breaths)
- Chest decompression
- Autoinjector antidotes

Breathing?
- No → Dead
- Yes →
  - Obeys commands or makes purposeful movements?
  - Has peripheral pulse?
  - Not in respiratory distress?
  - Major hemorrhage is controlled?
    - Any no → Likely to survive given current resources?
      - Yes → Immediate
      - No → Expectant
    - All yes → Minor injuries only?
      - Yes → Minimal
      - No → Delayed

Reproduced from SALT Mass Casualty Triage: Concept Endorsed by the American College of Emergency Physicians, American College of Surgeons Committee on Trauma, American Trauma Society, National Association of EMS Physicians, National Disaster Life Support Education Consortium, and State and Territorial Injury Prevention Directors Association. (2008). *Disaster Medicine and Public Health Preparedness, 2*(4), 245–246. doi:10.1097/DMP.0b013e31818d191e

D. SEIRV Triage

Susceptible–Exposed–Infectious–Removed–Vaccinated (SEIRV) is a triage sorting method that can be used to sort patients during a biological or pandemic-like event.[1]

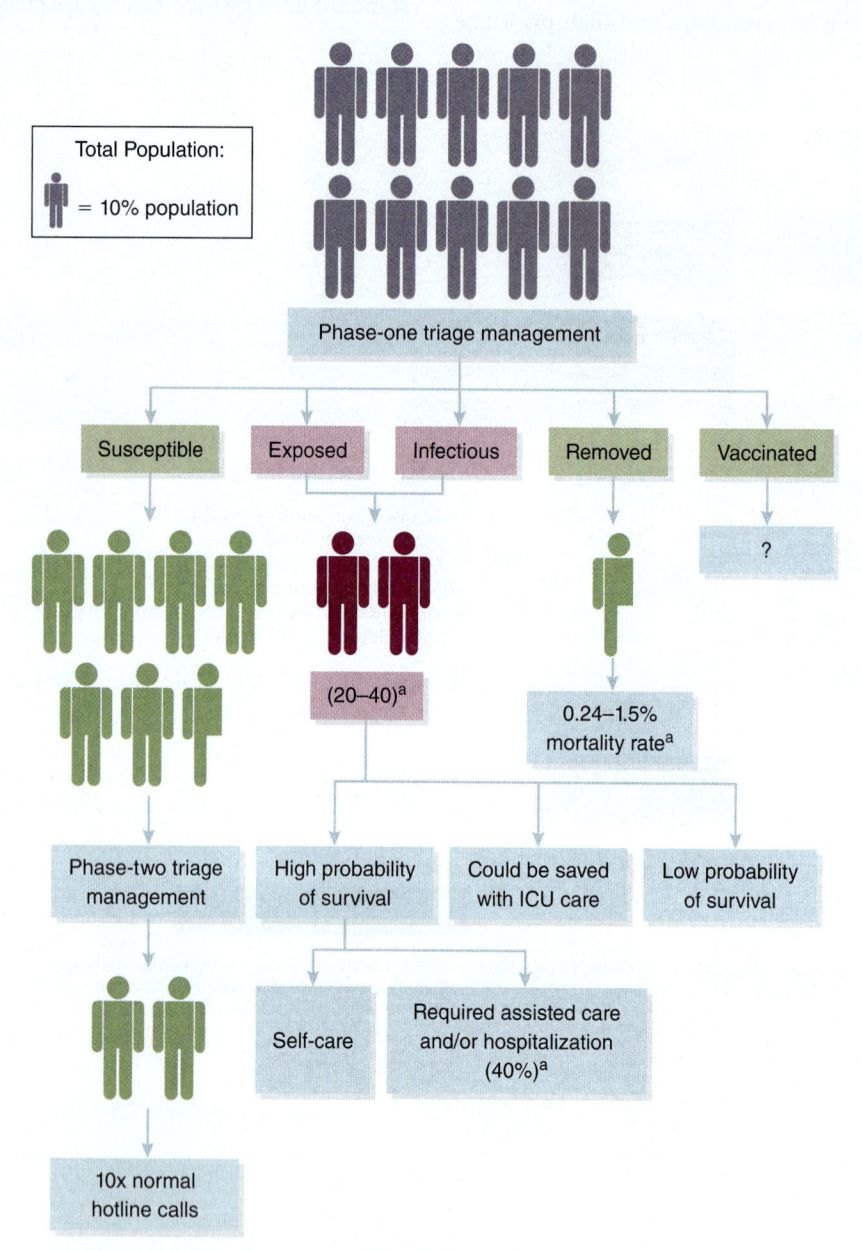

[a] Percentages based on influenza and severe acute respiratory syndrome outbreak data.

Reproduced from Burkle, F. M. (2006). Population-based triage management in response to surge-capacity requirements during a large-scale bioevent disaster. *Journal of Academic Emergency Medicine, 13*(11), 1118–1129. https://doi.org/10.1197/j.aem.2006.06.040

E. FDNY-START Triage

The Fire Department of New York City uses a modified version of the START triage algorithm that includes an Orange (urgent) category between Immediate and Delayed indicating patients who need urgent, but not immediate, transport.[3]

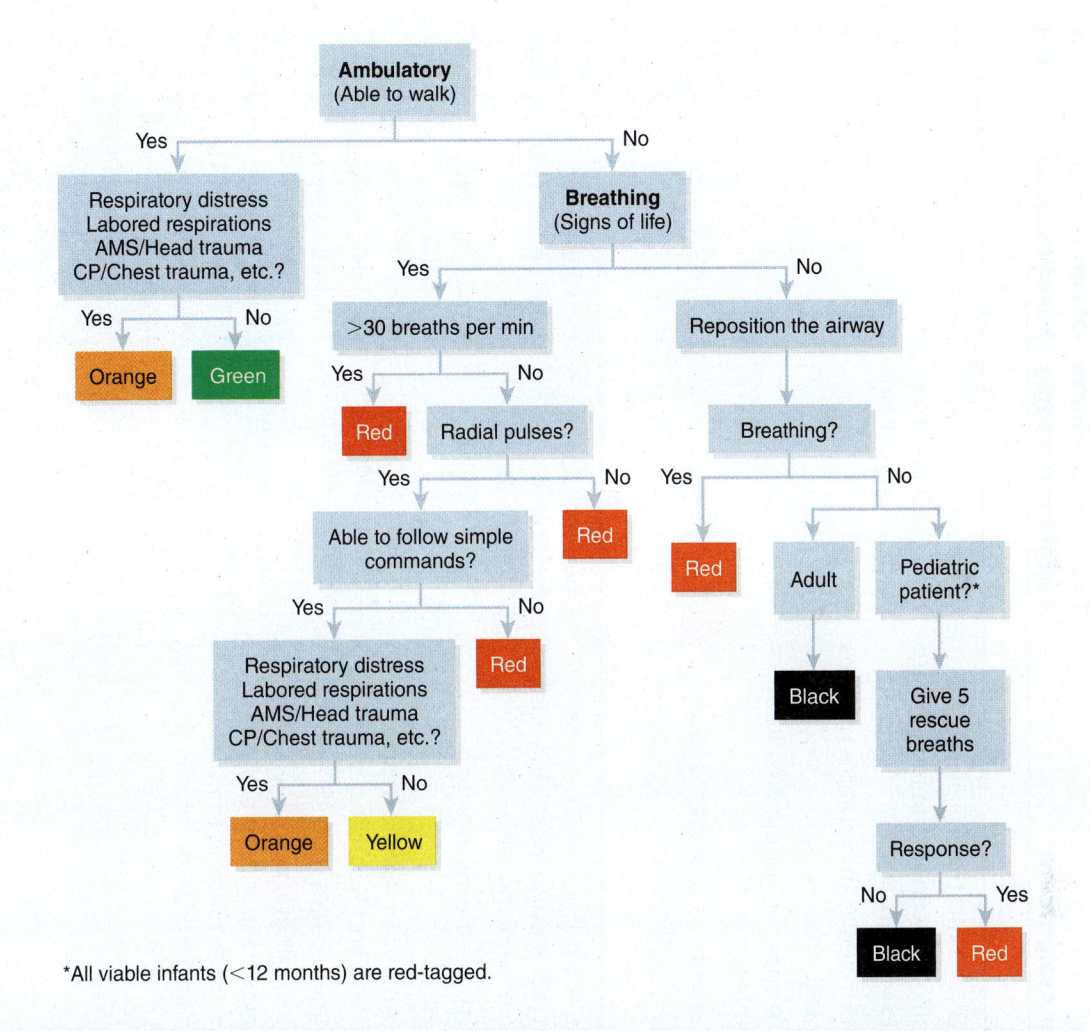

*All viable infants (<12 months) are red-tagged.

F. Triage Comparison

Triage System	Sorting Categories	Criteria for Assignment	Treatments Prior to Assigning Category	Observations/ Miscellaneous	Countries That Use the System
Simple Triage and Rapid Treatment (START)	Immediate: Red Delayed: Yellow Walking Wounded: Green Deceased: Black	Immediate: RR > 30 breaths/minute, capillary refill > 2 seconds/no radial pulse, cannot follow commands Walking wounded: Can move themselves to a separated zone Deceased: Apneic or apneic despite airway opening Delayed: Patients who don't meet any of the other criteria	Open an airway with head tilt-chin lift or jaw thrust, one attempt		United States, Canada, Australia, Israeli-occupied territories
JumpSTART	Immediate: Red Delayed: Yellow Minor: Green Deceased: Black	Immediate: RR <15 or > 45 breaths/minute, no radial pulse, posturing with stimulation or unresponsive Minor: Can move themselves to a separated zone Deceased: Apneic or apneic despite airway opening and 5 assisted breaths Delayed: Patients with a RR 15–45 breaths/minute, palpable radial pulse and alert, responding to verbal stimulation or responding to painful stimulation appropriately, unable to walk	Open the airway and deliver 5 breaths if not spontaneously breathing Reassess those who are deceased immediately after Immediate and delayed patients are treated	Developed for patients 1–8 years old Similar structure to START but for pediatric patients Pediatric patients might be taken to green zone by others and will need to be assessed for appropriateness Modification made for children who are not ambulatory	

Sieve Triage

Priority 1 (immediate): Red Priority 2 (urgent): Yellow Priority 3 (delayed): Green Priority 3: Walking injured Dead: White or black	Priority 1: Not walking with RR < 10 or > 29 breaths/minute or capillary refill > 2 sec Priority 2: Not walking with RR 10–29 breaths/minute and capillary refill < 2 seconds Dead: Not breathing after airway adjusted	Open airway	Heart rate of > 120 beats/minute can be used in place of capillary refill in situations of cold temperatures or poor lighting. Does not include mental status in decision-making	Parts of Europe, United Kingdom, Australia

CareFlight

Immediate: Red Urgent: Yellow Delayed: Green Unsalvageable: Black	Delayed: Walks Unsalvageable: Apneic despite open airway Immediate: Unable to follow commands but has a palpable radial pulse Urgent: Can follow commands and has a palpable radial pulse but is unable to walk	Open airway	No respiratory rate included in decision-making Can be applied to pediatrics	United States

FDNY-START

Immediate: Red Orange: Urgent transfer Delayed: Yellow Walking Wounded: Green Deceased: Black	Immediate: RR > 30, capillary refill > 2 seconds, no radial pulse, cannot follow commands Urgent transfer: Walked to green zone or met Delayed criteria but found to have respiratory distress, labored respirations, altered mental status, head trauma, chest pain and/or chest trauma Walking wounded: Can move themselves to a separated zone Deceased: Apneic or apneic despite airway opening Delayed: Patients who don't meet any of the other criteria	Reposition airway For pediatrics, give 5 bag-mask ventilations	Similar to START Combines START and JumpSTART Uses an orange category for further assessment and prioritization	United States

(continues)

Triage System	Sorting Categories	Criteria for Assignment	Treatments Prior to Assigning Category	Observations/ Miscellaneous	Countries That Use the System
Pediatric Triage Tape	Immediate: Red Urgent: Yellow Delayed: Green Dead: White	Immediate: Abnormally slow or fast respiratory rate or abnormally slow or fast pulse rate Urgent: Not walking, with capillary refill < 2 seconds Delayed: Child who is walking or an infant who is alert and moving all four extremities Dead: Apneic	Does not breathe after airway is opened	Uses a tape to show parameters for the patient Adapted from the Sieve triage	
Sort, Assess, Lifesaving Interventions, Treatment/Transport (SALT)	Immediate: Red Delayed: Yellow Minimal/"Walking Wounded": Green Expectant: Gray Dead: Black Contaminated: Orange	Immediate: Patient has no radial pulse, is in respiratory distress, has uncontrolled hemorrhage, and/or is unable to follow commands. Delayed: Patient has a radial pulse, is not in respiratory distress, does not have uncontrolled hemorrhage, and is able to follow commands but may have a significant injury such as long bone fracture Minimal: Meets criteria for Delayed but with minor injuries Expectant: Patient meets Immediate criteria but is unlikely to survive based on provider judgment Dead: Apneic after opening airway on adult, apneic after 2 rescue breaths for pediatric	Open an airway with head tilt-chin lift or jaw thrust, one attempt Give pediatric patient 2 bag-mask ventilations if not breathing after opening airway May apply a tourniquet if uncontrolled hemorrhage Needle decompression if suspected tension pneumothorax Administer antidote autoinjector if known exposure	Incorporates both adult and pediatric Does not require counting, but rather yes/no answers Incorporates CBRNE into treatments	United States

CBRNE = chemical, biologic, radiologic, nuclear, and explosive.

References

1. Burkle, F. M. (2006). Population-based triage management in response to surge-capacity requirements during a large-scale bioevent disaster. *Journal of Academic Emergency Medicine, 13*(11), 1118–1129. https://doi.org/10.1197/j.aem.2006.06.040
2. Federal Interagency Committee on Emergency Medical Services. (2014). *National implementation of the model uniform core criteria for mass casualty incident triage: A report of the ICEMS.* https://www.ems.gov/pdf/National_Implementation_Model_Uniform_Core_Criteria_Mass_Casualty_Incident_Triage_Mar2014.pdf
3. Regional Emergency Medical Advisory Committee of New York City. (2018). *Modified START triage.* https://www.nycremsco.org/wp-content/uploads/2018/02/2018-01-REMAC-Advisory-Modified-START-Triage.pdf
4. U.S. Department of Health & Human Services. (2022, September 1). Chemical Hazards Emergency Medical Management. *SALT mass casualty triage algorithm.* https://chemm.hhs.gov/salttriage.htm
5. U.S. Department of Health and Human Services. (2022, September 1). *JumpSTART pediatric triage algorithm.* Chemical Hazards Emergency Medical Management. https://chemm.hhs.gov/startpediatric.htm
6. U.S. Department of Health and Human Services. (2022, September 1). *START adult triage algorithm.* Chemical Hazards Emergency Medical Management. https://chemm.hhs.gov/startadult.htm

APPENDIX 19-2
Chemical Agents

Agent	Signs and Symptoms	Decontamination and Treatment
Nerve Agents		
Tabun (GA) Sarin (GB) Soman (GD) Cyclosarin (GF) V agents (VX)	Exposure results in a cholinergic toxidrome. Acronym DUMBBELLS: 　D: Diarrhea 　U: Urination 　M: Miosis (small pupils) 　B: Bradycardia 　E: Emesis 　L: Lacrimation 　L: Lethargy 　S: Salivation	Remove contaminated clothing Flush with soap and water Treat with atropine, 2-PAM, Mark I kit/DuoDote autoinjector
Vesicants (Blister Agents)		
Sulfur mustard (HD) Nitrogen mustard (HN)	Acts first as a cellular irritant, then as a cellular poison Conjunctivitis, reddened skin, blisters, nasal irritation, inflammation of throat and lungs Usually not fatal	Remove contaminated clothing Flush with soap and water Supportive care (no antidote)
Lewisite (L)	Immediate pain with blisters later Readily absorbed through skin and moist tissue	
Pulmonary Agents		
Phosgene oxime (CX)	Cough, burning, and immediate pain, with blisters later Necrosis equivalent to full- and partial-thickness burns	Leave area of exposure and get to fresh air Remove clothing and double-bag it in plastic bags to contain off-gassing
Chlorine	Coughing; chest tightness; burning sensation to nose, throat, and eyes; watery eyes; blurry vision; nausea and vomiting; shortness of breath or difficulty breathing; burning pain, redness, or blisters on skin	Flush with soap and water, irrigate eyes if affected

Agent	Signs and Symptoms	Decontamination and Treatment
Chemical Asphyxiants (Blood Agents)		
Hydrogen cyanide (AC) Cyanogen chloride (CK) Arsine (SA)	Cherry-red skin or approximately 30% cyanosis May appear to be gasping for air Seizures before death Effect is similar to asphyxiation but is more sudden	Remove contaminated clothing Decontaminate patient's skin with a soap and water solution

Data from Centers for Disease Control and Prevention. (2016). *Emergency preparedness and response: Chemical emergencies.* https://emergency.cdc.gov/chemical/index.asp

APPENDIX 19-3
Biologic Agents

Agent	Symptoms	Transmission	Treatment
Anthrax (*Bacillus anthracis*) Incubation usually less than 7 days but can be up to 60 days	Cutaneous: Intense itching with raised bump initially; progresses to ulcerated blister with necrotic center and scabs Inhalation: Initially, nonspecific flulike illness characterized by fever, myalgia, headache, nonproductive cough, and mild chest discomfort; followed by marked high fever, dyspnea, stridor, cyanosis, and shock	Person-to-person spread extremely unlikely	Multiple antibiotics, including doxycycline, ciprofloxacin, fluoroquinolones, and others; effective for both types
Botulism (*Clostridium botulinum*) Incubation usually 12–36 hours (range of 6 hours to 2 weeks)	Double vision, blurred vision, drooping eyelids, slurred speech, difficulty swallowing, and dry mouth	Not spread person-to-person	Antitoxin effective if diagnosed early; supportive care
Plague (*Yersinia pestis*) Incubation usually 2–4 days	Fever, chills, headache, severe debilitation, rapidly developing shortness of breath, and chest pain	Person-to-person (airborne and droplet precautions recommended)	Early treatment is crucial Streptomycin, doxycycline; gentamicin when streptomycin is not available
Smallpox (*Variola major*) Incubation usually 7–17 days	Initially, high fever, fatigue, headache, and backaches Rash usually develops 2–3 days after onset of symptoms; rash appears first on the mouth, face, and extremities, then spreads inward to the trunk of the body	Person-to-person (airborne and droplet precautions recommended)	Supportive therapy; antibiotics to treat secondary infections
Tularemia (*Francisella tularensis*) Incubation usually 3–5 days	Insect bite: Slow-healing sore and swollen lymph nodes Inhalation: High fever, chills, headache, fatigue, cough, and chest pain Ingestion: Sore throat, abdominal pain, diarrhea, and vomiting	Not spread person-to-person	Streptomycin; gentamicin also effective

Agent	Symptoms	Transmission	Treatment
Viral hemorrhagic fevers (VHF) Incubation usually 4–21 days	Fever, fatigue, dizziness, muscle aches, loss of strength, and exhaustion Severe cases often show signs of bleeding under the skin, in internal organs, or from body orifices Severely ill patients may also experience shock, nervous system malfunction, coma, delirium, and seizures Some types of VHF are associated with renal failure	Person-to-person (Follow the CDC's infection control recommendations)	Antibiotics for secondary infections, blood transfusions and supportive care; some types respond to antiviral medication

Data from Centers for Disease Control and Prevention. (2017). *Emergency preparedness and response: Bioterrorism agents/diseases.* https://emergency.cdc.gov/agent/agentlist-category.asp

APPENDIX 19-4
Acute Radiation Syndromes

Syndrome	Dose[a]	Prodromal	Latent Stage	Manifest Illness Stage	Recovery
Hematopoietic (bone marrow)	> 0.7 Gy (> 70 rads) (mild symptoms may occur from exposure as low as 0.3 Gy or 30 rads)	Symptoms are anorexia, nausea, and vomiting Onset occurs 1 hour to 2 days after exposure Stage lasts for minutes to days	Stem cells in bone marrow are dying, although the patient may appear and feel well Stage lasts 1–6 weeks	Symptoms are anorexia, fever, and malaise Drop in all blood cell counts occurs for several weeks Primary cause of death is infection and hemorrhage Survival decreases with increasing dose Most deaths occur within a few months after exposure	In most cases, bone marrow cells will begin to repopulate the marrow There should be full recovery for a large percentage of patients from a few weeks up to 2 years after exposure Death may occur for some patients at 1.2 Gy (120 rads) The LD50/60[b] is about 2.5–5 Gy (250–500 rads)
GI	> 10 Gy (> 1,000 rads) (some symptoms may occur from exposure as low as 6 Gy or 600 rads)	Symptoms are anorexia, severe nausea, vomiting, cramps, and diarrhea Onset occurs within a few hours after exposure Stage lasts about 2 days	Stem cells in bone marrow and cells lining the GI tract are dying, although the patient may appear and feel well Stage lasts less than 1 week	Symptoms are malaise, anorexia, severe diarrhea, fever, dehydration, and electrolyte imbalance Death is due to infection, dehydration, and electrolyte imbalance Death occurs within 2 weeks of exposure	The LD100[c] is about 10 Gy (1,000 rads)

Appendix 19-4 Acute Radiation Syndromes

Syndrome	Dose[a]	Prodromal	Latent Stage	Manifest Illness Stage	Recovery
CV/CNS	> 50 Gy (5,000 rads) (some symptoms may occur from exposure as low as 20 Gy or 2,000 rads)	Symptoms are extreme nervousness and confusion; severe nausea, vomiting, and watery diarrhea; loss of consciousness; and burning sensations of the skin Onset occurs within minutes of exposure Stage lasts for minutes to hours	Patient may return to partial functionality Stage may last for hours but often is shorter	Symptoms include return of watery diarrhea, convulsions, and coma Onset occurs 5–6 hours after exposure Death occurs within 3 days of exposure	No recovery is expected

LD = lethal dose; GI = gastrointestinal; CV = cardiovascular; CNS = central nervous system.

[a] The absorbed doses quoted here are "gamma equivalent" values. Neutrons or protons generally produce the same effects as gamma radiation, beta radiation, or radiographs, but at lower doses. If the patient has been exposed to neutrons or protons, consult radiation experts on how to interpret the dose. [b] The LD50/60 is the dose that can kill 50% of the exposed population in 60 days. [c] The LD100 is the dose that can kill 100% of the exposed population.

Reproduced from Centers for Disease Control and Prevention. (2017). *A brochure for physicians: Acute radiation syndrome.* https://stacks.cdc.gov/view/cdc/50897

CHAPTER 20

Transition of Care for the Trauma Patient

Michael Bailey, PhD, MSN/Ed, RN, CCRN-K, NPD-BC

OBJECTIVES

Upon completion of this chapter, the learner will be able to:

1. Describe trauma patient characteristics that may require specialized or a higher level of care.
2. Recognize national and regional laws and regulations that are in place to protect patients and to facilitate the improvement of outcomes and transport for trauma patients with complex injuries.
3. Examine the risks and benefits of both intrafacility and interfacility trauma transport.
4. Discuss transport modes and qualifications of transport team members.
5. Identify concepts that promote communication for intrafacility and interfacility transport.

Introduction

Patients who experience traumatic injury require rapid assessment and stabilization of life-threatening injuries and transport to a facility capable of providing definitive care. The prehospital team must follow applicable field triage guidelines to ensure that patients are brought to the most appropriate facility with the capability to treat the patient.[3] The American College of Surgeons (ACS) recommends that certain injured patients be transported to a verified trauma center with sufficient resources. Time to treatment is crucial for optimal patient outcomes, particularly the time from injury to definitive care.[4] Timely and definitive care is related to decreased morbidity and mortality from traumatic injury.[4]

As the patient moves through the trauma care continuum, multiple transfers and handoffs occur. These may take place within the hospital (intrafacility) or to a different facility (interfacility). It is essential that each care provider ensures safe transport and provides essential and accurate information to the next care provider using a standardized format. To do so effectively, the trauma nurse needs to be aware of the resources available at their facility as well as local and regional policies, procedures, and laws—particularly those regarding transport.

Care provided in the emergency setting is only one phase of the trauma care continuum. That continuum begins with injury prevention and involves each phase of the patient's progress, from the point of injury through rehabilitation and reintegration into the community.

TABLE 20-1 ACS Committee on Trauma Levels of Trauma Centers

Trauma Center	Description of Trauma Center
Level I	› A regional trauma center is a tertiary care facility. › Capable of providing leadership and total care for every aspect of injury, from prevention to rehabilitation. › Must have adequate depth of resources and personnel. › Commonly a university-based teaching hospital with residency and postgraduate programs. › Research, injury prevention programs, education, and systems planning are essential components. › Has an important role in local trauma system development, regional disaster planning, increasing capacity, and advancing trauma care.
Level II	› Expected to provide initial definitive trauma care for a wide range of injuries and injury severity. › Clinically equivalent to a Level I facility, but capabilities do not include the comprehensive services and specialty care provided by Level I trauma centers. › In many areas without access to a Level I facility, the Level II trauma center will take accountability to provide education, prevention, and community outreach. › May be involved in trauma research, system leadership, and disaster planning.
Level III	› Provides the trauma patient with prompt assessment, resuscitation, stabilization, and emergency surgery as necessary. › Uses accepted trauma triage criteria and ACS transfer guidelines for definitive care of the trauma patient. › Generally does not accept incoming trauma transfers. › Typically serves communities that may not have timely access to a Level I or II trauma center and fulfills a critical role in much of the United States by serving more remote and/or rural populations. › May take accountability to provide education and system leadership in remote areas where patients can be cared for closer to home. › Must have processes in place for the prompt evaluation, initial management, and transfer of patients whose needs might exceed the resources available.

Data from American College of Surgeons. (2022). *Resources for optimal care of the injured patient: 2022 standards.*

Although trauma systems vary from jurisdiction to jurisdiction, the guidelines and standards published by the ACS incorporating injury prevention, acute care, and rehabilitation are widely used.

Trauma nurses are involved in trauma patient transport, both sending and receiving the injured patient, so it is important to understand the trauma system(s) and their classification(s). The ACS Committee on Trauma (ACS-COT) describes capabilities and resources for three levels of trauma centers. Hospitals may apply to the ACS to participate in a rigorous on-site survey and review process through which they can achieve verification by the ACS as a trauma center. A brief description of each trauma center level is provided in **Table 20-1**.[5]

Initial Care and the Emergency Medical Treatment and Active Labor Act

In the United States, the federal Emergency Medical Treatment and Active Labor Act (EMTALA) requires that all patients who present to an emergency department

(ED) receive a medical screening examination, resuscitation, and stabilization of any identified emergency condition, regardless of their ability to pay. If the patient's condition warrants treatment beyond the capabilities and resources of the initial facility and the patient needs to be transferred, EMTALA requires that the following conditions be met before transfer[8]:

- Medical screening examination and necessary stabilizing interventions (within the capacity of the facility)
- Informed consent
- Accepting physician at the receiving facility
- Available bed and resources to deliver appropriate care at the receiving facility
- Patient report provided to the receiving facility
- All available medical records and laboratory, radiographic, and other related information or copies provided to the receiving facility or transferred with the patient
- Appropriate transfer personnel

Although these requirements are only pertinent to those U.S. facilities that receive government funding, they are widely considered the standard of care.

Trauma Patients Who Require Transport

When the patient's care needs exceed the available resources at the initial facility, transport to a facility that can provide the necessary specialized or higher level of care is recommended. In an organized trauma system, severely injured trauma patients are transferred to the closest facility with appropriate resources, preferably a verified trauma center. The ACS has established recommendations to help identify patients most at risk who would benefit from transport to a trauma center. "All trauma centers must have clearly defined transfer protocols that include the types of patients, expected time for initiating and accepting a transfer, and predetermined referral centers for outgoing transfers."[5(p92)] However, each jurisdiction must defer to regional standards and guidelines (see Chapter 1, "Trauma Around the World," and Chapter 2, "Preparing for Trauma," for more information).

Decision to Transport

The decision to transport a patient to a specialized or higher level of care rests solely with the physician responsible for the patient's care at the initial receiving facility. Directly after the primary survey, a reevaluation decision point emphasizes early consideration for patient transfer. At the end of the secondary survey is another reevaluation point, at which all patient assessment findings can be summarized and a determination made regarding need for transfer. Timeliness is key in making this decision. "Subsequent decisions regarding transfer to a facility within a managed care network should be made only after stabilization of the patient's condition and in accordance with the ACS Statement on Managed Care and the Trauma System."[5(p93)] Guidelines for transfer consideration include those presented in **Table 20-2**.[4]

Transport Considerations

Transport considerations include the following:

- Knowledge of facility resources, capabilities, and limitations as they relate to providing the necessary care for that trauma patient.
- Availability of specialty or higher level-of-care trauma centers that can provide definitive care (Level I trauma centers, burn centers, pediatric trauma centers, acute brain and spinal cord injury referral centers, reimplantation centers, high-risk obstetric centers).
- Available transportation services (e.g., ground, air).
- Team configuration, availability, and type of equipment required to accomplish the transport.
- Risks and benefits to the patient (the patient's reaction to transport and/or the mode of transport selected).
- Policies, procedures, protocols, and transfer agreements in place.
- The physician transferring the patient must communicate directly with the physician at the receiving facility.[5]

Once the decision to transport the patient to another facility is made and the patient is accepted by the receiving facility, transportation arrangements are determined, and the sending and receiving physicians collaborate to choose the most appropriate mode of transport. Considerations include the availability of equipment, workspace needs, qualifications of the transport personnel, weather and road conditions or other environmental factors, and the patient's or family's preference. Familiarity with existing procedures, protocols, and interfacility transfer agreements, along with the regulatory requirements pertinent to the jurisdiction, helps to guide the interfacility transfer process.

TABLE 20-2 Guidelines for Considerations of Transfer to Level I or Highest Regional Trauma Center

Primary Survey Findings

- Airway compromise or high risk for airway loss
- Tension pneumothorax
- Hemothorax, open pneumothorax
- Hypoxia, hypoventilation
- Hypotension
- Pelvic fracture
- Vascular injury (expanding hematoma, active bleeding)
- Open fracture
- Abdominal distention/peritonitis
- GCS < 13
- Intoxicated patient who cannot be evaluated
- Evidence of paralysis
- Severe hypothermia

Secondary Survey Findings

- Depressed skull fracture or penetrating injury
- Eye injury
- Open facial fractures or complex lacerations
- Ongoing nasopharyngeal bleeding
- Neck hematoma, crepitus, midline tenderness or deformity
- Multiple rib fractures, flail chest
- Pulmonary contusion
- Widened mediastinum, mediastinal air
- Abdominal rebound or guarding
- Perineal, rectal, or vaginal laceration
- Neurologic deficit
- Complex or multiple fractures or dislocations or bony spine injuries
- Consider other factors, such as age, multiple comorbidities, pregnancy, and burns.

GCS = Glasgow Coma Scale.

Note: It may be appropriate for an injured patient to undergo operative control of ongoing hemorrhage before transfer if a qualified surgeon and operating room resources are promptly available at the referring hospital.

Modified from American College of Surgeons. (2018). *Advanced trauma life support* (10th ed., pp. 243–244).

Modes of Transport

The most frequently used interfacility modes of transport are described in **Table 20-3**.

Transport Team Composition

Transport team composition can be analyzed in terms of whether an intrafacility or interfacility transport is being undertaken.

Intrafacility

Intrafacility transport may involve multiple transfers to various departments: radiology, special procedures, angiography, surgery, inpatient unit, rehabilitation, or other areas within the hospital. Typically, the trauma nurse prepares, coordinates, and carries out these transports. Respiratory therapists, additional nurses, and other personnel may assist. Having an adequate number of personnel with appropriate skills to accomplish the transport is essential.[7,18]

Interfacility

In interfacility transports, the sending physician is responsible for the care of the patient until the patient's arrival at the receiving facility. This physician makes decisions regarding the appropriate level of care and method of transport.

The composition of the transport team used during interfacility transport is determined by the sending physician based on the appropriate method of transport and the required level of care.[4] Depending on the nature and severity of the injuries, personnel trained in critical care or specialized teams may be required.[9] Interfacility transport teams should consist of, at a minimum, two patient care providers and a vehicle operator.[9]

- If ground transportation is used, the transferring facility may send personnel and equipment with the patient.
  - This usually requires a nurse who is experienced in the care of trauma patients, as well as other qualified transport team members.[9]
  - In some instances, specialty trauma centers may send ground transport with their own specially trained personnel.
  - It is important to have facility policies in place before the actual transfer becomes necessary.

TABLE 20-3 Modes of Patient Transportation

Mode of Transport	Benefits	Drawbacks
Ground	› Readily available › May have space for family members › Weather less of a factor › Fewer restrictions on the weight of the team, patient, and equipment	› Longer travel time › Traffic and road conditions › Risk of collision
Helicopter	› Rapid transport within short distances › Improved survival rates when initiated from the field › Usually a dedicated team with advanced skills › Improves access to Level I and II trauma centers for patients in rural areas	› Restricted use in certain weather conditions › Expensive › Risk of crash › Noise and vibration › Physiologic changes from altitude › Space and weight restrictions › Not all hospitals are equipped with a helipad › No clear evidence that the time benefit for interfacility air transport improves patient outcomes
Fixed-wing aircraft	› Able to handle longer distances than a helicopter › May be pressurized	› Prolonged transport times with transition to and from hospital to airfield

Data from American College of Surgeons. (2018). *Advanced trauma life support: Student course manual* (10th ed.); Beaton, A., O'Leary, K., Thorburn, J., Campbell, A., & Christey, G. (2019). Improving patient experience and outcomes following serious injury. *International Journal of Integrated Care, 19*(4), 79. https://doi.org/10.5334/ijic.s3079; Dakessian, A., Bachir, R., & El Sayed, M. J. (2020). Association between trauma center designation levels and survival of patients with motor vehicular transport injuries in the United States. *The Journal of Emergency Medicine, 58*(3), 398–406. https://doi.org/10.1016/j.jemermed.2019.12.029; Dhillon, N. K., Linaval, N. T., Patel, K. A., Colovos, C., Ko, A., Margulies, D. R., Ley, E. J., & Barmparas, G. (2018). Helicopter transport use for trauma patients is decreasing significantly nationwide but remains overutilized. *The American Surgeon, 84*(10), 1630–1634. https://doi.org/10.1177/000313481808401019; Eiding, H., Kongsgaard, U. E., Olasveengen, T. M., & Heyerdahl, F. (2021). Interhospital transport of critically ill patients: A prospective observational study of patient and transport characteristics. *Acta Anaesthesiologica Scandinavica, 66*(2), 248–255. https://doi.org/10.1111/aas.14005; Gotlib Conn, L., Zwaiman, A., DasGupta, T., Hales, B., Watamaniuk, A., & Nathens, A. B. (2018). Trauma patient discharge and care transition experiences: Identifying opportunities for quality improvement in trauma centres. *Injury, 49*(1), 97–103. https://doi.org/10.1016/j.injury.2017.09.028; Gough, B. L., Painter, M. D., Hoffman, A. L., Caplan, R. J., Peters, C. A., & Cipolle, M. D. (2020). Right patient, right place, right time: Field triage and transfer to Level I trauma centers. *The American Surgeon, 86*(5), 400–406. https://doi.org/10.1177/000313482091824; Martín, M., García, M., Silveira, E., Martin-Aragón, S., & Vicedo, T. (2019). Medication errors in the care transition of trauma patients. *European Journal of Clinical Pharmacology, 75*(12), 1739–1746. https://doi.org/10.1007/s00228-019-02757-3; Schneider, A. M., Ewing, J. A., & Cull, J. D. (2020). Helicopter transport of trauma patients improves survival irrespective of transport time. *The American Surgeon, 87*(4), 538–542. https://doi.org/10.1177/0003134820943564; Schumaker, J., Taylor, W., & McGonigle, T. (2019). The emergency, trauma, and transport nursing workforce. *Nursing Management, 50*(12), 20–32. https://doi.org/10.1097/01.numa.0000605152.42445.4b

NOTE

Certification for Transporting Patients

Nurses who specialize in transporting patients may be certified as either a Certified Transport Registered Nurse (CTRN), who specializes in ground transport nursing, or a Certified Flight Registered Nurse (CFRN), who specializes in aeromedical transport.

- Air transportation usually involves a critical care team.
  - Air medical transport teams usually include two clinical care providers in various combinations of roles, plus the pilot.
    - Nurse and paramedic is a common combination.
    - At times, the team may also include a physician and/or a respiratory therapist.[9]
  - Air transport teams are trained for, and qualified to monitor and respond to, altitude-related hazards in addition to caring for traditional trauma conditions and complications.[9]

Risks of Transport

Any transport of trauma patients, whether interfacility or intrafacility, involves risk. It is the responsibility of the team caring for the patient to ensure that the transport is accomplished in a manner that is efficient yet safe for both the patient and the transport team. The trauma nurse anticipates the potential for, and prepares to manage, the following risks of transport:

- Loss of airway patency
- Displaced or obstructed tubes, lines, or catheters
- Dislodged splinting devices
- Need to replace or reinforce dressings
- Deterioration in patient status; change in vital signs or level of consciousness
- Injury to the patient and/or team members

Nursing Considerations for Transport

Multiple factors can affect the outcome of patient transport, so planning is essential. Nursing considerations include assisting with the medical screening examination and required resuscitation and/or stabilizing interventions, within the capabilities of the sending facility. Other considerations that the transferring nurse should anticipate include the following:

- Patient consent
  - Assist with and support the process to ensure that the patient and/or family are aware of the need for, as well as the risks and benefits of, transport; this allows them to make an informed decision regarding transport and sign the consent for transfer.
- Transfer requirements
- Ensure that the sending physician has received acceptance for the transfer from the receiving hospital.
  - Arrange for the transport team.
  - Provide a patient report to the receiving nurse.
  - Send copies of all available medical records and laboratory, radiographic, and other related reports.[9]
- Patient care
  - Ensure definitive airway control.
  - Suction the airway and endotracheal tube as needed.
  - Maintain breathing and provide assisted ventilations.
  - Ensure patency and flow rate of intravenous (IV) infusions.
  - Continually reassess the patient's neurologic status.
  - Secure all monitoring devices and equipment, such as chest tubes.
- Family and patient preparation
  - Explain the logistics of the transport to the patient, family, and assistive staff.
  - Ensure that the family has information regarding where the patient is being taken and directions to that location.
  - Ensure that the family has seen the patient prior to departure, if possible.
- Transport team
  - Give a report to the transporting personnel as necessary.
  - Provide the team with copies of documentation as needed.
- Follow-up
  - Call the receiving facility to notify it of the patient's departure time and the estimated time of arrival.
  - Fax or send electronically any additional laboratory or radiographic reports that become available after the patient has departed.

Equipment for Transport

The trauma nurse caring for the patient is responsible for ensuring the availability of proper equipment needed during transport. Depending on the status of the patient, equipment may include the following:

- Airway equipment
- Suction devices
- Oral airways
- Endotracheal tubes
- Laryngoscope blades and handles
- Supplies to secure the endotracheal tube
- Failed-airway equipment, such as a supraglottic device
- Bag-mask device
- Ventilator
- Medications

- Pain medications
- Sedation agents
- Vasoactive medications
- Resuscitation medications
- IV access supplies
- IV fluids
- Cardiac monitor/defibrillator
- Equipment to monitor vital signs, including oxygen saturation and capnography
- Equipment to perform a needle thoracostomy
- Restraints

Emergency Department Boarding

Once initial assessment and stabilization of the trauma patient has been completed and the decision to transfer the patient to another facility or to admit has been made, it is essential that the patient be moved from the ED to an inpatient unit as quickly as possible for the next phase in the continuum of care.[2,15] If an inpatient bed is not readily available, post-resuscitation care of the trauma patient may be provided in the ED. ED staff may be required to perform inpatient care, or inpatient nursing staff may be redirected to the ED to care for boarding patients. It is important that EDs have policies and procedures in place related to the nursing care of the critically ill trauma patient while they are being held (boarded) in the ED. Such a patient must receive the same standard of care that would be provided on the assigned inpatient unit.

Emerging Trends

ED crowding and boarding may adversely affect patient outcomes, including increased mortality, rates of medical errors, and length of stay.[19] Many organizations have developed performance improvement teams to address the challenges that accompany patient boarding in the ED. Uncovering the root cause of the crowding is imperative to finding solutions. As organizations have struggled with crowding and boarding, some initiatives in these areas have shown promise, including the following:

- Developing an area in the ED designed similarly to a nursing unit, with consistent scheduling of regular non-ED RNs.[19]
- Improving hospital discharge time to drive ED throughput.[16]
- Triaging critical care beds.[19]
- Use of supplemental (float) ED RN staffing to enable one-to-one care of critical patients.
- Implementation of a Senior Streaming Assessment Further Evaluation after Triage (SAFE-T) zone.[20]
- The threat of serious communicable diseases, such as the COVID-19 virus and Ebola virus disease, should be considered during transportation of a patient. Logistical challenges for initiating and maintaining infection control measures during transport need further attention.[1]

Summary

A majority of trauma patients who present to the ED will require transport or patient handoff during their care—whether intrafacility to another department, such as radiology or the inpatient unit, or interfacility to a trauma or specialized center of care. Using a standardized approach to care, communication, and documentation ensures safe and appropriate transitions of care, regardless of how and where patients are being transported. All patient transports must follow the applicable institutional, regional, and federal laws, guidelines, policies, and procedures. The level of trauma care a patient receives should progressively improve as the patient moves from the field to definitive care, and then continue at the same level of care during intrafacility transitions.[4] The goal of trauma teams at the sending and receiving facilities is to provide high-quality, safe care for patients, protecting them from further injury, and to ensure safe practice for the trauma team.

References

1. Air & Surface Transport Nurses Association. (2020). *Transport of patients with serious communicable diseases.* [Position statement]. https://cdn.ymaws.com/www.astna.org/resource/resmgr/newfolder/astna_position_statement_tra.pdf
2. American College of Emergency Physicians. (2017). *Boarding of admitted and intensive care patients in the emergency department.* [Policy statement]. https://www.acep.org/patient-care/policy-statements/boarding-of-admitted-and-intensive-care-patients-in-the-emergency-department/#sm.000irp8m7rz6dnd11bh29rs29mrr4
3. American College of Surgeons. (2014). *Resources for optimal care of the injured patient 2014.* https://www.facs.org/~/media/files/quality%20programs/trauma/vrc%20resources/resources%20for%20optimal%20care.ashx
4. American College of Surgeons. (2018). *Advanced trauma life support* (10th ed.).
5. American College of Surgeons. (2022). *Resources for optimal care of the injured patient: 2022 standards.* https://www.facs.org/quality-programs/trauma/quality/verification-review-and-consultation-program/standards/

6. Beaton, A., O'Leary, K., Thorburn, J., Campbell, A., & Christey, G. (2019). Improving patient experience and outcomes following serious injury. *International Journal of Integrated Care, 19*(4), Article 79. https://doi.org/10.5334/ijic.s3079
7. Blank-Reid, C. (2020). The evolution of trauma systems, trauma centers, and trauma nursing. In K. McQuillan & M. Flynn Makic (Eds.), *Trauma nursing: From resuscitation through rehabilitation* (5th ed., pp. 1–21). Elsevier.
8. Centers for Medicare and Medicaid Services. (2019, July 19). *State operations manual: Appendix V – Interpretive guidelines – Responsibilities of Medicare participating hospitals in emergency cases.* https://www.cms.gov/Regulations-and-Guidance/Guidance/Manuals/Downloads/som107ap_v_emerg.pdf
9. Commission on Accreditation of Medical Transport Systems. (2018, July). *Accreditation standards of the Commission on Accreditation of Medical Transport Systems* (11th ed.). https://www.camts.org/wp-content/uploads/2017/05/CAMTS-11th-Standards-DIGITAL-FREE.pdf
10. Dakessian, A., Bachir, R., & El Sayed, M. J. (2020). Association between trauma center designation levels and survival of patients with motor vehicular transport injuries in the United States. *The Journal of Emergency Medicine, 58*(3), 398–406. https://doi.org/10.1016/j.jemermed.2019.12.029
11. Dhillon, N. K., Linaval, N. T., Patel, K. A., Colovos, C., Ko, A., Margulies, D. R., Ley, E. J., & Barmparas, G. (2018). Helicopter transport use for trauma patients is decreasing significantly nationwide but remains overutilized. *The American Surgeon, 84*(10), 1630–1634. https://doi.org/10.1177/000313481808401019
12. Eiding, H., Kongsgaard, U. E., Olasveengen, T. M., & Heyerdahl, F. (2021). Interhospital transport of critically ill patients: A prospective observational study of patient and transport characteristics. *Acta Anaesthesiologica Scandinavica, 66*(2), 248–255. https://doi.org/10.1111/aas.14005
13. Gotlib Conn, L., Zwaiman, A., DasGupta, T., Hales, B., Watamaniuk, A., & Nathens, A. B. (2018). Trauma patient discharge and care transition experiences: Identifying opportunities for quality improvement in trauma centres. *Injury, 49*(1), 97–103. https://doi.org/10.1016/j.injury.2017.09.028
14. Gough, B. L., Painter, M. D., Hoffman, A. L., Caplan, R. J., Peters, C. A., & Cipolle, M. D. (2020). Right patient, right place, right time: Field triage and transfer to Level I trauma centers. *The American Surgeon, 86*(5), 400–406. https://doi.org/10.1177/0003134820918249
15. Hymel, G., Leskovan, J., Thomas, Z., Greenbaum, J., & Ledrick, D. (2020). Emergency department boarding of non-trauma patients adversely affects trauma patient length of stay. *Cureus, 12*(9), Article e10354. https://doi.org/10.7759/cureus.10354
16. Improta, G., Romano, M., Di Cicco, M., Ferraro, A., Borrelli, A., Verdoliva, C., Triassi, M., & Cesarelli, M. (2018). Lean thinking to improve emergency department throughput at AORN Cardarelli hospital. *BMC Health Services Research, 18*(1). Article 914. https://doi.org/10.1186/s12913-018-3654-0
17. Martín, M., García, M., Silveira, E., Martin-Aragón, S., & Vicedo, T. (2019). Medication errors in the care transition of trauma patients. *European Journal of Clinical Pharmacology, 75*(12), 1739–1746. https://doi.org/10.1007/s00228-019-02757-3
18. McMaster, J., & DiFiore, K. (2020). Performance improvement and patient safety in trauma care. In K. McQuillan & M. Flynn Makic (Eds.), *Trauma nursing: From resuscitation through rehabilitation* (5th ed., pp. 30–48). Elsevier.
19. Mohr, N. M., Wessman, B. T., Bassin, B., Elie-Turenne, M., Ellender, T., Emlet, L. L., Ginsberg, Z., Gunnerson, K., Jones, K. M., Kram, B., Marcolini, E., & Rudy, S. (2020). Boarding of critically ill patients in the emergency department. *Journal of the American College of Emergency Physicians Open, 1*(4), 423–431. https://doi.org/10.1002/emp2.12107
20. Ray, M., & Reinoso, H. (2019). A new process to improve throughput in the emergency department. *The Journal for Nurse Practitioners, 15*(10), e193–e196. https://doi.org/10.1016/j.nurpra.2019.05.016
21. Schneider, A. M., Ewing, J. A., & Cull, J. D. (2020). Helicopter transport of trauma patients improves survival irrespective of transport time. *The American Surgeon, 87*(4), 538–542. https://doi.org/10.1177/0003134820943564
22. Schumaker, J., Taylor, W., & McGonigle, T. (2019). The emergency, trauma, and transport nursing workforce. *Nursing Management, 50*(12), 20–32. https://doi.org/10.1097/01.numa.0000605152.42445.4b

CHAPTER 21

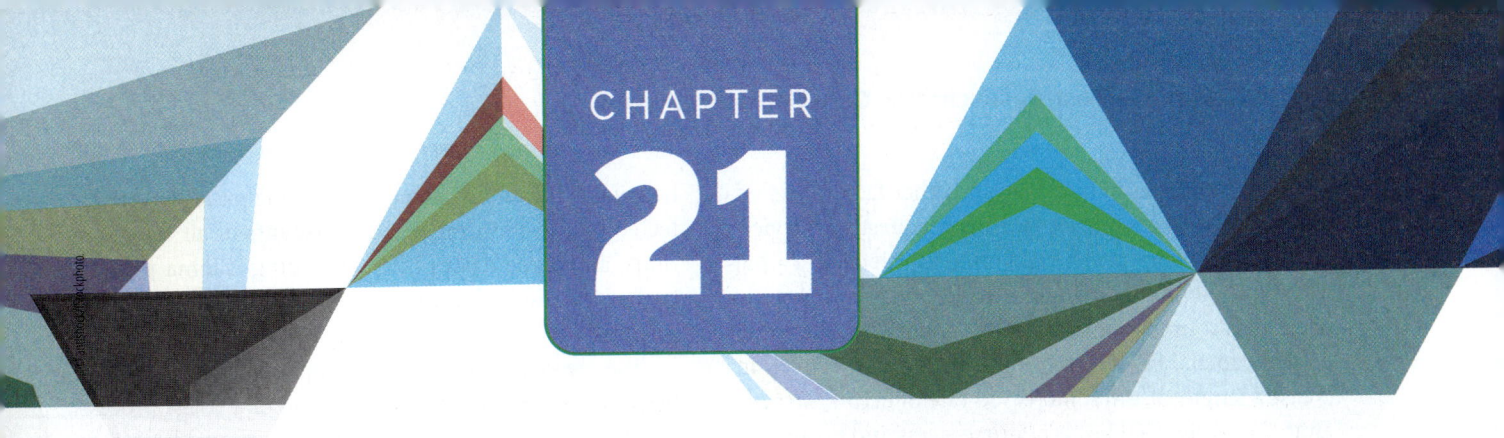

Post-Resuscitation Care Considerations

Steven F. Jacobson, MS, MSN, MBA, RN, CEN, CFRN, CTRN, CPEN, TCRN

OBJECTIVES

Upon completion of this chapter, the learner will be able to:
1. Identify potential consequences of injury and care rendered by anticipating the pathophysiologic changes for the trauma patient during post-resuscitative care.
2. Plan appropriate interventions for the trauma patient during post-resuscitative care.
3. Evaluate the effectiveness of nursing interventions for the trauma patient during post-resuscitative care.

Introduction

Trauma happens quickly, yet the consequences of injury can take hours, months, or years to overcome. Care of the injured patient may begin with activation of emergency medical services or a patient arriving at a hospital emergency department (ED), but the continuum of care for the trauma patient does not end with the initial resuscitation. The goal of trauma care is not only to treat injury to maximize physical recovery and quality of life, but also to involve patients in their care as partners in their treatment plan. This collaboration and ongoing care after the initial resuscitation support the physical and emotional health of the patient and their reintegration into society after the event.

Post-resuscitation care takes place in many environments. Trauma care may begin in the ED or prehospital environment but continues in the intensive care unit (ICU), operating room, medical or surgical unit, rehabilitation unit, and the patient's home after discharge. Multiple disciplines are involved in each step of the process of trauma care, making coordination of care and communication critical. Ideally, the trauma patient will move quickly from the initial assessment and stabilization phase in the ED to definitive care; however, that is not always possible. At times, the trauma patient will remain in the ED past the post-resuscitation phase of care.

Operational Considerations

Trauma care encompasses a broad range of clinical providers as well as administrative and operational needs. ED boarding has led to increased research into the quality of care, costs, and impact of the phenomenon.[68]

Throughput relates to boarding and other factors, including providing timely care to those requesting services, and the right care at the right time. Bottlenecks can affect the ability to provide high-quality, cost-effective care because resources are diverted to tasks other than their primary focus. ED overcrowding has been linked to increased length of stays, increased rate of errors, lost revenue,[65] and elevated levels of nurse stress and burnout.[104]

ED Boarding

Many EDs are designed for the purpose of sorting and implementing rapid diagnostics and interventions to move toward medical stabilization, a process that is uniquely different from that of many inpatient care units. ED overcrowding and boarding admitted patients in the ED are widely associated with poorer patient outcomes, increased hospital length of stay, delayed detection of or missed injuries, and higher rates of mortality.[80] Over the last decade, ED patient volumes have increased by an estimated 30%, and, when coupled with hospital closures, this has created an increase in inpatient boarding in the ED setting.[68]

The trauma patient who is boarded in the ED loses the benefit of specialized nursing care in units where staff are familiar with the post-resuscitation care of injured patients. Instead, the trauma patient continues to receive care from the ED nurse, who has a broad, generalized knowledge base and skill set.[68] Different solutions to this problem are being tried in hospitals around the globe, including the increased use of float/resource nurses or dedicated trauma nurses, increased use of point-of-care testing, clinical decision units, rapid assessment zones, and even attempts at streamlining patient throughput from the computed tomography (CT) scanner directly to the ICU.[105] Ultimately, the issue of ED overcrowding and hospital throughput are complex issues that have not yet been resolved.

Throughput

With increases in ED overcrowding and patient boarding, patients are subjected to longer lengths of stay, which ultimately leads to increased waiting time, increased time to diagnostic imaging, increased pain, and a decrease in patient satisfaction.[62] These delays to disposition have many impacts that range from increased morbidity and mortality[68] to decreased financial reimbursement for care.[101] The imbalance between the healthcare service supply and demand that results in delayed throughput affects more than just patient satisfaction. Patients who are admitted to the hospital but had an ED length of stay greater than 24 hours were at higher risk of mortality within 30 days of their initial presentation to the hospital when compared with patients quickly admitted to the hospital.[31] It was also noted that trauma patients were affected by the boarding of other patients of all classifications, and these delays in transitioning trauma patients to the ICU resulted in an increase in morbidity, including pneumonia.[51]

The need for strategies to improve ED throughput began in the 1950s with the adoption of a triage process, in which crowding and prioritization were addressed by sorting of patients. As this process advanced, it became a nurse-led process of prioritizing patients, often including the ability to initiate standardized diagnostics and interventions based on the triage nurse's assessment of the patient.[62] A more recent strategy is the use of so-called mid-level providers (advanced practice registered nurses, nurse practitioners, physician assistants) in the emergency department, who contribute to the overall quality of patient care in the emergency department.[29] A variety of strategies exist for improving throughput and boarding, but no single intervention can be expected to "fix" the problem of ED overcrowding. The challenges of ED crowding are inextricably tied up with hospital and healthcare system capacity, with four main areas that can be targeted to improve ED overcrowding[65]: smoothing elective admissions, early discharges, weekend discharges, and capacity planning.[94]

The Primary Assessment

Post-resuscitation care reflects the same organized and systematic approach as the initial resuscitation and begins by reevaluating the primary assessment. Frequent, ongoing monitoring can help the nurse to recognize changes in patient condition and to intervene quickly.

Airway

Airway management continues to be the priority in trauma patients during post-resuscitation care. If the patient does not have a definitive airway, continuous monitoring and reassessments will alert the trauma nurse to potential compromise and identify the need for a definitive airway. (See Chapter 5, "Airway and Ventilation," for additional information.) Management of trauma patients includes preventing hypercarbia and maintaining oxygenation, especially in those patients who have sustained a head injury.[6]

Tube Displacement or Obstruction

Endotracheal tubes (ETTs) can easily become displaced or obstructed, particularly during transport to tests or between units.[10] Monitoring for dislodgement or obstruction of an ETT requires diligent observation to ensure that the tube remains properly placed and patent. Use of the DOPE mnemonic can help the trauma nurse to identify these issues; see Chapter 4, "Initial Assessment" for more information. Additional considerations include the following:

- If the patient has a definitive airway, careful and continuous monitoring ensures correct tube placement, adequate oxygenation, and ventilation.
- Informing other providers that an airway was difficult to place can prevent early extubation and enable proper planning and preparation for extubation.
  - Use of a difficult airway identifier, such as an armband or sticker on the ETT, a chart sticker, or a progress note, can communicate this information.

Breathing and Ventilation

Oxygen delivery is guided by monitoring arterial blood gases (ABGs), end-tidal carbon dioxide ($ETCO_2$), and pulse oximetry (SpO_2), along with frequent reassessment of the quality of the patient's respiratory rate and effort, changes in breathing patterns, lung sounds, and overall appearance. Trauma patients may be at higher risk for impaired breathing and inadequate ventilation from many factors.

A variety of injuries and their management impact respiratory effort:

- Traumatic brain injuries (TBIs) with central nervous system depression
- High cervical spinal cord injury—above C3 or C4
- Thoracic injuries (including rib fractures, hemothorax, pneumothorax)
- Prescribed analgesia and sedation

Circulation

Circulation care includes fluid management and hemostatic resuscitation. Ongoing hemorrhage may be subtle or the result of a sudden dislodgement of previously formed clots. Trending vital signs, patient symptoms, and physical examination findings, along with serial hemoglobin and hematocrit values, can identify continued blood loss. It is also necessary to monitor for signs of fluid overload, electrolyte abnormalities, and acid–base imbalances that are common sequelae of aggressive fluid resuscitation. Reassess heart and lung sounds to monitor for volume overload.

Disability (Neurologic Status)

Close attention should be given to the patient with known or suspected neurologic injury because TBIs evolve with time.[28,41] In the patient with a TBI, the CT scan may initially appear normal; radiologic changes may become evident as the injury evolves. Patients with brain injury also require careful monitoring of laboratory values—such as coagulation measures and sodium levels—and careful temperature regulation to avoid hypothermia[99] or fever greater than 38°C (100.4°F).[6,24]

Observe the patient over time for subtle neurologic changes that may identify increasing intracranial pressure (ICP). It is essential to prevent hypoxia and hypotension to lessen the risk of secondary brain injury.[6] Spinal cord injuries may also evolve over time and require the nurse to closely monitor for symptom progression and respiratory compromise.[19,63] See Chapter 7, "Head Trauma," and Chapter 10, "Spinal and Musculoskeletal Trauma," for additional information.

Exposure and Environmental Control

The key exposure and environmental control concerns are hypothermia and hyperthermia. Trauma patients can be at risk of hypothermia because of environmental exposure and injuries, as well as hyperthermia resulting from the nature of their injuries. Hyperthermia syndromes are rare in the initial phase of severe trauma care, but temperature elevation from a systemic inflammatory response may begin early.

Once the trauma patient is successfully resuscitated, their temperature and metabolic rate may increase.[43] This increase is a natural result of stimulation of the immune system, wound healing, tissue remodeling, and functional recovery. Thermoregulation may be impaired in patients with brain injuries, causing fever.[107] Like hypothermia, early fever (i.e., temperature greater than 38.3°C [100.9°F]) is associated with worse outcomes for the trauma patient.[48] While some degree of temperature elevation may be expected, the cause of the hyperthermia should be vigorously investigated because additional treatment may be necessary to address it. Hypothermia will be discussed in more detail as it relates to the trauma triad of death.

Trauma Triad of Death

The *trauma triad of death* is the often lethal combination of processes that may occur in a trauma patient; it is associated with high risk of death. The trio consists of hypothermia, acidosis, and coagulopathy. Outcomes are affected by the severity of the injury and the resuscitative interventions during the course of management.

The resuscitative measures taken to address the triad include damage control surgery, hemostatic resuscitation, and permissive hypotension. They have been associated with improved survival in trauma patients with severe hypovolemia. The triad of death can develop quickly in the hypovolemic trauma patient, and, once established, a vicious cycle ensues that may be difficult to reverse.[69]

Hypothermia

Temperature monitoring is important not just in the immediate resuscitation period; it remains a concern throughout the care of the trauma patient. Interventions include maintaining a warm ambient temperature in the trauma room, implementing warming interventions as needed, and monitoring the patient's temperature to avoid overheating. Prevention of heat loss during transport to other departments is important as well and can be accomplished by using blankets, coverings, or other commercially available devices to cover the patient. Hypothermia, as one third of the trauma triad of death, has the potential to diminish the trauma patient's chance of survival. The following complications can develop in trauma patients who become hypothermic[93]:

- Development of coagulopathy
- Delayed wound healing
- Increased surgical-site infections
- Prolonged hospitalization
- Increased myocardial complications
- Increased blood loss and the need for blood transfusion
- Delayed recovery from anesthesia and increase in postoperative discomfort

Hypothermia in the trauma patient can be a particularly deadly issue. Hypothermia—defined as a core temperature of less than 35°C (95°F)—is highly associated with both early and late mortality in the trauma patient.[18] One of the most serious complications of trauma is the deadly triad of hypothermia, acidosis, and coagulopathy. Because of this risk, prevention of hypothermia is vital to the hypovolemic trauma patient.[18] **Figure 21-1** presents a warming strategy for hypothermic patients.[5]

Targeted temperature management—that is, cooling the patient's core body temperature to between 32°C and 36°C (89.6°F and 96.8°F)—is a common intervention in the post–cardiac arrest patient with return of spontaneous circulation to help preserve neurologic function. Although recommended as part of the 2020 American Heart Association Guidelines for Emergency Cardiovascular Care, prophylactic hypothermia has not been demonstrated to improve outcomes for the trauma patient with severe TBI and should not be used.[102]

Acidosis

Acidosis is a common complication of multiple traumatic injuries. An acidotic environment can affect all body systems because it changes cellular function. Specifically, in the bloodstream, acidosis can affect oxygenation, making it more difficult for hemoglobin to bind with oxygen, thereby decreasing oxygen delivery and cellular ability to use oxygen. Acidosis, in combination with hypothermia, intensifies the adverse effects on coagulation and worsens clotting times.[93] Acidosis can occur via two separate routes: respiratory or metabolic.

Respiratory Acidosis

The respiratory route to acidosis involves the following mechanisms:

- Respiratory acidosis occurs as a result of inadequate ventilation causing retained carbon dioxide (CO_2).
- Hypoventilation in patients with pain, a change in mental status, signs of a developing pneumothorax, or weakening chest muscles, or in those receiving analgesia or sedation, may result in respiratory acidosis.
- Treatment includes improving ventilation by assisting with a bag-mask device, adjusting ventilator settings, or providing pain relief to increase respiratory rate and improve air exchange.

Metabolic Acidosis

The metabolic route to acidosis involves the following mechanisms:

- A by-product of tissue hypoperfusion, metabolic acidosis is associated with hemorrhagic shock in the trauma patient.
- When tissues are deficient in oxygen, cells shift to anaerobic metabolism, which produces lactic acid and leads to acidosis.
- Kidney hypoperfusion leads to the development of acute kidney injury, and the kidney loses its ability to excrete hydrogen ions, resulting in acidosis.
- Acidosis can result in vasodilation, hypotension, and worsened coagulopathy.
- Restoration of tissue perfusion is needed to correct metabolic acidosis. Hypoperfusion may be prevented by hemorrhage control and early balanced resuscitation with blood products and intravenous (IV) fluids.

Monitoring

Acidosis can be detected by monitoring ABGs, serum lactate levels, and base deficit. New, noninvasive technology using near-infrared spectroscopy to monitor tissue oxygen delivery and shock is being used increasingly in EDs and ICUs.[67] See Chapter 6, "Shock," for more information.

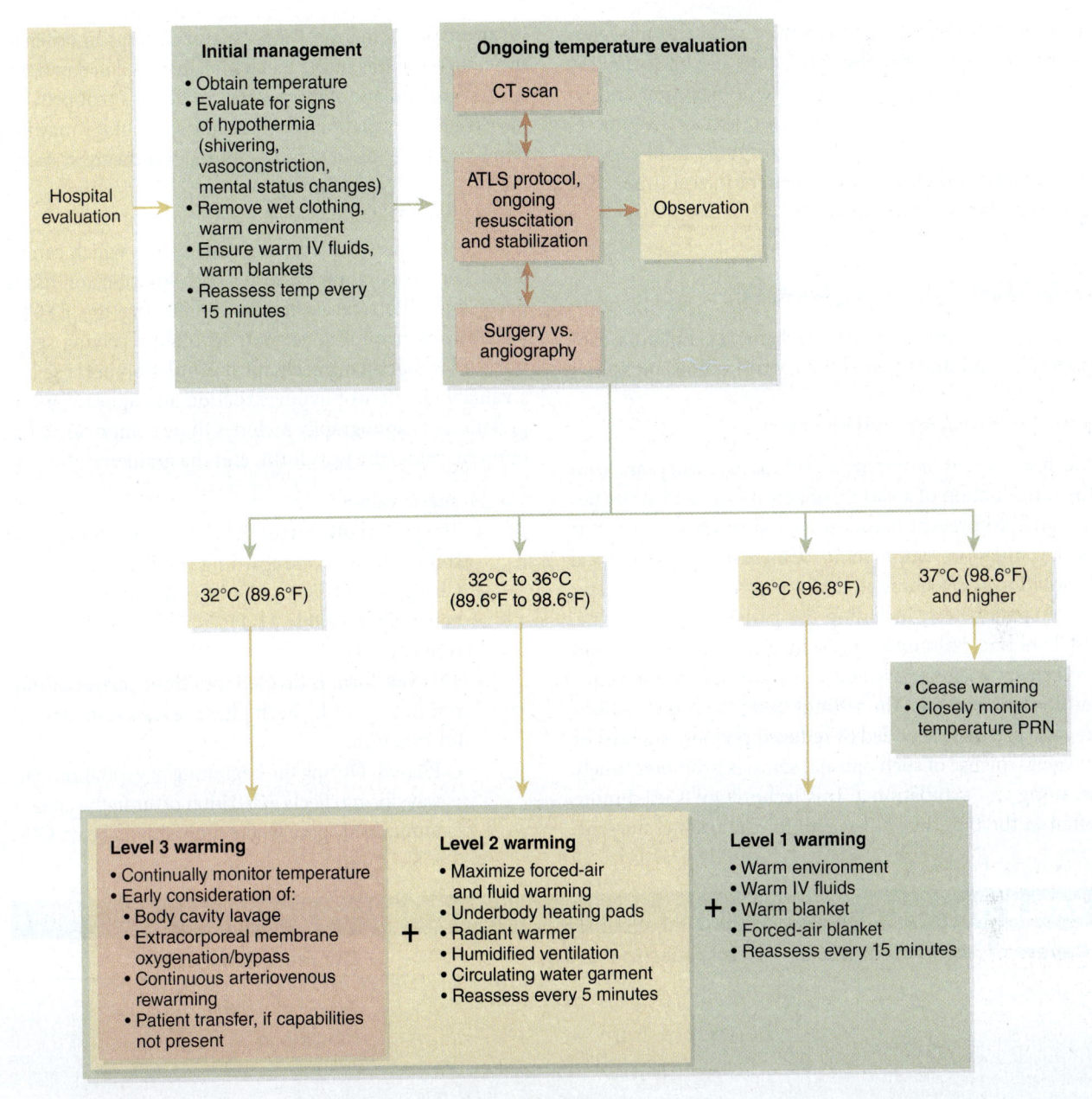

Figure 21-1 *Warming temperature strategies in trauma.*
Reproduced from American College of Surgeons. (2018). Appendix B. *Advanced trauma life support: Student course manual* (10th ed., p. 268).

Coagulopathy

The final component of the trauma triad of death is coagulopathy. Trauma patients may develop coagulopathy because of the combination of injury and overzealous crystalloid resuscitative efforts, or they may have been on anticoagulation therapy before their injury, making the goal of achieving hemostasis more challenging for the trauma team. The trauma nurse should be alert for the possible presence of medications that would impair platelet function, such as aspirin and clopidogrel, or anticoagulant medications, such as warfarin, rivaroxaban, dabigatran, apixaban, and enoxaparin. Patients on oral anticoagulants who suffered trauma were found to have a higher rate of surgical intervention and complications. However, research continues on specific risk factors and individual medications.[22]

Trauma patients with multiple injuries will develop some degree of coagulopathy because of depletion of coagulation factors,[8] which is worsened by hypothermia and acidosis. Mass transfusion protocols with prescribed blood, platelet, and plasma administration and the use of tranexamic acid are linked to improved patient outcomes in adult trauma patients.[3,72] Traditional methods of monitoring clotting ability, including prothrombin/

international normalized ratio and partial thromboplastin time, address only the early steps in clot formation but do not monitor later steps of clot evolution and lysis. Thromboelastography and rotational elastometry are increasingly being used to help guide fluid resuscitation and coagulopathy management in real time.[53] See Chapter 6 for more information.

Monitoring Adjuncts

Monitoring adjuncts include mechanical ventilators, capnography, and measurement of central venous pressure.

Mechanical Ventilators

Mechanical ventilators have advanced in recent years, with the introduction of a variety of new modes and strategies designed to prevent barotrauma and syndromes such as post-ventilation emphysema. Closed-loop mechanical ventilation is a technique that regularly monitors respiratory parameters, including the patient's intrinsic rate, tidal volume, pulmonary resistance and compliance, and oxygen saturation. Based on this information, the ventilator is able to adjust the settings based on preset parameters to provide for added or reduced pressure support or oxygen. The use of such optimal settings promotes timely weaning and extubation.[77] This technology is used more often in the ICU, but it is useful for the trauma nurse to be aware of fluctuations in ventilator settings in order to evaluate the status of the mechanically ventilated patient. As research on and improvement to devices that provide closed-loop ventilation continue, the technology may become more prevalent throughout the healthcare system.

Capnography

ETCO$_2$ measures the level of exhaled CO$_2$, which can be a marker of metabolic acidosis, dehydration, or tissue perfusion.[12] Post resuscitation, monitoring the ETCO$_2$ level can be helpful in patients who are receiving sedation and analgesia or mechanical ventilation because it is a valuable marker of hypoventilation and apnea.[66] Interpretation of capnography includes three components: the numeric value, the waveform, and the gradient.[39,66]

- Numeric value
  - The partial pressure of ETCO$_2$ (PETCO$_2$) reveals some information regarding ventilation.
  - Changes in PETCO$_2$ identify ventilatory issues before SpO$_2$ (**Table 21-1**).[39,58,66,73]
- Waveform
  - The waveform is divided into three phases of the respiratory cycle. Each phase reveals different information.
    - Phase I: During the beginning of expiration, the waveform reflects exhalation of air in the anatomic dead space where there should be no CO$_2$.

TABLE 21-1 Conditions Associated with Changes in PETCO$_2$

Causes of Abnormal PETCO$_2$	Increase in PETCO$_2$	Decreased in PETCO$_2$
Metabolic	Malignant hyperthermia Thyroid storm Severe sepsis	Hypothermia Metabolic acidosis
Circulatory	CO$_2$ rebreathing Treatment of acidosis	Pulmonary embolism Profound hypovolemia/shock Cardiogenic shock
Respiratory	Hypoventilation Chronic obstructive pulmonary disease Asthma	Hyperventilation Intrapulmonary shunt Pulmonary edema
Technical	Exhausted CO$_2$ absorber Contamination of the monitor	Disconnection Blockage in tubing

Data from Eipe, N., & Doherty, D. R. (2010). A review of pediatric capnography. *Journal of Clinical Monitoring and Computing*, 24(4), 261–268. https://doi.org/10.1007/s10877-010-9243-3; Kodali, B. S. (2013). Capnography outside the operating rooms. *Anesthesiology*, 118(1), 192–201. https://doi.org/10.1097/ALN.0b013e318278c8b6; Ortega, R., Connor, C., Kim, S., Djang, R., & Patel, K. (2012). Monitoring ventilation with capnography. *New England Journal of Medicine*, 367(19), e27–e34. https://doi.org/10.1056/NEJMvcm1105237

- Phase II: As CO_2 is exhaled, the waveform rises sharply.
- Phase III: This phase encompasses the majority of the expiratory cycle, where the waveform plateaus. The end of this phase is where the $ETCO_2$ is measured.
- The waveform can reveal a great deal of information to those who know how to interpret it.
  - Loss of waveform indicates a misplaced or occluded ETT or a disconnected circuit.
  - A positive waveform with each compression shows effective cardiopulmonary resuscitation.
  - A change in the shape of the waveform may be an indication of bronchospasm, obstruction, or ventilation/perfusion mismatch.
- $PETCO_2$: $PaCO_2$ gradient
  - A changing gradient can mean hemodynamic instability or decreasing lung compliance.

Post-Resuscitation Care of Selected Injuries and Illnesses

Selected injuries and illnesses covered in this section include the following:

- Rib fractures
- Flail chest
- Pulmonary contusion
- Pneumothorax
- Hemothorax
- Blunt cardiac injury
- Cardiac tamponade
- Diaphragmatic injury
- Deep vein thrombosis
- Venous thromboembolism
- Pulmonary embolism
- Fat embolism
- Acute lung injury/acute respiratory distress syndrome
- Pneumonia and aspiration
- Abdominal trauma
- Shock
- Disseminated intravascular coagulopathy
- Abdominal compartment syndrome
- Rhabdomyolysis
- Systemic inflammatory response syndrome
- Sepsis
- Increased intracranial pressure
- Mental health and substance abuse
- Musculoskeletal trauma

Rib Fractures

Rib fractures are one of the most common thoracic injuries, found in approximately 20% of patients who sustain blunt chest trauma, and are commonly associated with underlying pulmonary contusion or pneumothorax.[36] Rib injury associated with pulmonary contusion is an independent risk factor for the development of pneumonia and increased mortality. Aggressive pain management for trauma patients with rib fractures is recommended to prevent atelectasis and improve functional residual and vital capacity. Effective pain management also promotes mobility, deep breathing, productive coughing, and the ability to clear secretions.[52] Aggressive pain management, in combination with early mobilization and pulmonary toilet (or pulmonary hygiene), is an important strategy to prevent complications of pneumonia and even death in the patient with blunt chest trauma and associated rib fractures. Although the patient will want to take shallow breaths and will be reluctant to cough, such measures are critical in helping to prevent pneumonia. Use of an incentive spirometer can encourage deep breathing—thereby opening atelectatic alveoli and recruiting collapsed airways for gas exchange. Deep breathing has the added benefit of often provoking a cough as mucus in the airways moves and alveoli open. The combination of deep breathing and coughing can be lifesaving for the patient with multiple rib fractures.[16] If a rib fracture has been found in a child younger than 3 years of age, maltreatment should be considered.[103] Children rarely suffer an isolated rib fracture, so careful consideration of and appropriate assessment for other injuries is essential.[103]

Flail Chest

Patients with flail chest may require more aggressive interventions to prevent complications and death.[36] As the number of ribs fractured increases, the risk of severe complications increases.[38] Patients older than age 65 and those with higher Injury Severity Scores are at higher risk. However, the number of rib fractures itself does not predict increased mortality.[64] Open reduction and internal fixation of the rib fractures has also been included as a treatment for flail chest.[36] See Chapter 8, "Thoracic and Neck Trauma," for more information.

Pulmonary Contusion

Pulmonary contusions often occur concomitantly with rib fractures[72] and are associated with respiratory failure that develops over time, rather than immediately following the chest injury. Clinical symptoms—such as respiratory distress with hypoxemia and hypercarbia—peak

72 hours after injury. Management of a pulmonary contusion may change over time as the patient's condition worsens and fluid shifts into the contused area. Significant hypoxia on room air is an indication for elective intubation and ventilation. Management for the patient with pulmonary contusion is largely supportive until the resolution of symptoms occurs, but patients may have long-term respiratory compromise because of fibrosis of the contused area.[81] Pulmonary contusion in children who have experienced thoracic trauma is common because the chest wall is pliable, thereby allowing the kinetic energy to be transferred to the underlying lung.[9] Development of pneumonia or acute respiratory distress syndrome may occur in a large percentage of pediatric patients with pulmonary contusion.[103]

Pneumothorax

Insertion of a chest tube is indicated in many patients with a traumatic pneumothorax, otherwise the pneumothorax may enlarge, increasing the risk of a tension pneumothorax. Positive-pressure mechanical ventilation can worsen pneumothoraces, and left undetected, the pneumothorax can progress to tension pneumothorax. Nurses must be vigilant to assess equality of breath sounds, ventilator airway pressures, and hemodynamic stability for intubated patients to identify pneumothorax development or a worsening condition.[35]

Hemothorax

A hemothorax is usually characterized by decreased or absent lung sounds and hypotension. The initial treatment is aimed at restoration of systemic intravascular blood volume and drainage of blood within the chest cavity. Initial drainage of 1,500 mL in adults, continual blood loss of 200 mL/hr for 2–4 hours or a need to transfuse blood to maintain hemodynamic stability may be an indication for a thoracotomy.[9] In children, "if the immediate blood return of 15 ml/kg, or ongoing losses of 2 to 3 ml/kg/hr for 3 hours or longer, this may indicate further thoracic exploration."[103p227] Autotransfusion may be considered when appropriate.[9]

Blunt Cardiac Injury

Myocardial injury after blunt chest trauma can be a challenge to diagnose. Patients with a blunt cardiac injury will complain of chest discomfort, which might erroneously be attributed to a rib fracture or chest wall contusion. An electrocardiogram (ECG) is performed on any patient suspected of a cardiac injury, and serial ECGs over a period of 4–6 hours can help detect changes in rhythm and conduction or reveal myocardial infarction. Premature ventricular contractions are the most common dysrhythmias in patients with blunt cardiac trauma. The leading cause of death for patients with a blunt cardiac injury is related to the development of lethal arrythmias.[38]

Management of the patient with a suspected blunt cardiac injury starts with monitoring for hemodynamic changes. Patients with preexisting cardiac risk factors, multiple chest injuries, and abnormal ECG findings are commonly admitted and observed on continuous cardiac monitoring for at least the first 24 hours.[9]

Cardiac Tamponade

The assessment findings related to cardiac tamponade due to an atrial rupture may be slow to develop and may not be evident until after the initial trauma survey and resuscitation. Cardiac tamponade from injury causes bleeding and usually presents rapidly, but it also can occur slowly, without complaint or symptoms. Diagnosis for cardiac tamponade can be made with focused assessment with sonography for trauma (FAST). If cardiac tamponade is suspected, patients also need urgent echocardiography, chest radiograph, and ECG. In such a case, the nurse would anticipate that the patient would undergo a pericardiocentesis or an expedited trip to the operating room for a pericardial window, depending on the setting. Inotropic agents and positive pressure ventilation can further impair cardiac filling in patients with cardiac tamponade.[50]

Diaphragmatic Injury

Traumatic diaphragmatic injuries are frequently missed during the initial evaluation of trauma patients. Generally, injuries to the diaphragm are difficult to evaluate with a CT scan and may require surgical intervention for definitive identification of diaphragmatic injury.[32] Diaphragmatic ruptures or tears are more commonly diagnosed when they occur on the left side because the liver may conceal or protect the defect on the right side.[9] Evidence of an elevated diaphragm on a chest radiograph, as well as bowel sounds over the thorax, can indicate a possible diaphragmatic injury and warrants investigation.

Deep Vein Thrombosis

Trauma patients are at substantially increased risk for developing deep vein thrombosis (DVT). When considering DVT, note the classic triad that leads to venous thrombosis:

- Stasis
- Endothelial damage
- Hypercoagulability

Numerous risk factors can influence the development of DVT in the trauma patient, including altered hemodynamics (hypotension), age, obesity, prolonged immobility, existing malignancy, pregnancy, and certain medications.[76] Once the risk is identified, the goal is to limit clot development and prevent pulmonary embolism. Low-molecular-weight heparin (e.g., enoxaparin), compression stockings, and intermittent pneumatic compression devices are also useful in the prevention of DVT.[76]

Venous Thromboembolism

Managing bleeding and blood clotting remains a challenge in the trauma population, and that challenge is only expected to increase as the population ages. Massive transfusion and anticoagulation-reversal guidelines have helped to address the issue of bleeding, and tranexamic acid is a useful tool in preventing clot degradation. Even so, trauma patients remain at increased risk of venous thromboembolism (VTE) formation.

The Caprini score for VTE stratifies risk of VTE in surgical patients and is finding favor in trauma programs to help guide VTE prophylaxis. The Caprini score has been validated for both medical and surgical patients (**Table 21-2**).[27,44,46] It is calculated by adding the scores of all factors present in the patient and is interpreted as follows:

- Score of 0 to 1: Low risk of VTE
- Score of 2: Moderate risk of VTE
- Score of 3 to 4: High risk of VTE
- Score ≥ 5: Highest risk for VTE

TABLE 21-2 Caprini Scale

5 Points	3 Points	2 Points	1 Point
• Stroke[a] • Fracture of the hip, pelvis, or leg • Elective arthroplasty • Acute SCI[a]	• Age greater than 75 years • Prior episodes of VTE • Family history of VTE • Prothrombin 20210A • Factor V Leiden • Lupus anticoagulants • Anticardiolipin antibodies • Elevated blood levels of homocysteine • History of heparin-induced thrombocytopenia • Other congenital or acquired thrombophilia	• Age 61–74 years • Arthroscopic surgery • Laparoscopy or general surgery lasting more than 45 minutes • Cancer • Plaster cast • Bed rest for more than 72 hours • Central venous access	• Age 41–60 years • BMI > 25 kg/m² • Minor surgery • Edema in the lower extremities • Varicose veins • Pregnancy • Postpartum • Oral contraceptives • Hormone therapy • Unexplained or recurrent abortion • Sepsis[a] • Serious lung disease such as pneumonia[a] • Abnormal pulmonary function tests • Acute myocardial infarction • Congestive heart failure[a] • Bed rest • Inflammatory bowel disease

SCI = spinal cord injury; VTE = venous thromboembolism; BMI = body mass index.
[a] Occurring in the last month.
Data from Caprini, J. A. (2005). Thrombosis risk assessment as a guide to quality patient care. *Disease-a-Month, 51*(2–3), 70–78. https://doi.org/10.1016/j.disamonth.2005.02.003

Pulmonary Embolism

Pulmonary embolism (PE) is the third leading cause of death in trauma patients who survive the first 24 hours following initial injury and do not receive DVT prophylaxis. Research has shown that as many as 24% of PEs occur within the first 4 days after injury and may even occur on day 1.[15] Therefore, prevention of venous stasis and early evaluation for signs of a DVT are critical. An acute PE occurs abruptly, and the symptoms exhibited depend on the size of the embolism. Additional considerations include the following:

- PEs can develop early or late; assess the patient who presents even days after the injury for signs of PE.[15]
- Massive PE will cause hemodynamic instability, such as hypotension.
- Pulmonary infarction and ischemia may result from complete disruption of blood flow.
- Massive PE may cause right ventricular failure, hemodynamic instability, and shock, independent of the trauma.[42]

Assessment findings of a PE include the following:

- Abrupt onset of pleuritic chest pain
- Dyspnea
- Hypoxemia (often refractory to supplemental oxygen)
- Hemoptysis
- Cough
- Orthopnea
- Adventitious lung sounds:
  - Wheezing
  - Crackles
- Decreased lung sounds
- Jugular vein distention
- Hypotension
- A feeling of anxiousness

Studies to confirm or exclude a PT include a ventilation–perfusion lung scan, CT pulmonary angiography, magnetic resonance imaging, or pulmonary angiography. CT pulmonary angiography is essentially the gold standard in diagnosing a pulmonary embolus.[15]

Fat Embolism

During manipulation of long bones for fracture fixation, embolic marrow, including lipid microemboli, can become dislodged, resulting in a fat embolism.[82] Nearly all orthopedic patients who have multiple fractures experience intravasation of bone marrow fat. A fat embolism can travel to the pulmonary vasculature, causing obstruction and subsequent ischemia. Most instances of fat embolism syndrome are asymptomatic, but symptomatic patients demonstrate a classic triad presentation:

- Decreased mental status, starting with restlessness and agitation
- Respiratory distress, including dyspnea and hypoxia
- Petechial rash (less common) on the head, neck, anterior thorax, conjunctivae, buccal mucous membranes, and axillae[56]

Presentation can occur as early as 12 hours following injury. However, most fat emboli occur within 24–72 hours after long bone fractures.[91] A helical thoracic CT scan and chest radiographs are the most beneficial imaging for diagnosis. Patchy pulmonary infiltrates or ground glass opacities may be seen on the chest radiograph.[56] ABGs assist in the evaluation and guide treatment of problems with ventilation, acid–base balance, and hypoxia. Fat emboli can contribute to the development of acute respiratory distress syndrome (ARDS). Fat embolism syndrome is often undiagnosed because of the frequency of subclinical presentation.[55] Treatment is supportive, including oxygenation and ventilation and promoting hemodynamic stability.

Acute Lung Injury/Acute Respiratory Distress Syndrome

Acute lung injury (ALI) is a syndrome resulting in alveolar damage or collapse and pulmonary edema that is not attributable to a cardiovascular origin. ALI develops 24–48 hours after injury or onset of illness and is stimulated by the inflammatory process.[21,95] In the trauma patient, ALI can be associated with fluid shifts from the intravascular space to the interstitial space and into the alveoli. ARDS, the most severe form of ALI, was originally known as *shock lung* because of the effects of massive fluid resuscitation with subsequent fluid shift on the lungs. Diagnostic criteria for ALI/ARDS include the following[34,83]:

- Partial pressure of oxygen/fraction of inspired oxygen ratio of less than 200 mm Hg (26.66 kPa) (ARDS) or less than 300 mm Hg (40 kPa) (ALI)
- Pulmonary artery occlusion pressure of 18 mm Hg (2.40 kPa)
- No clinical evidence of left atrial or ventricular dysfunction

Risk factors for ALI/ARDS include the following[34]:

- Aspiration
- Pulmonary contusion or other thoracic trauma
- Fat embolism

- Pulmonary embolism
- Near-drowning
- Inhalation injury
- Nonthoracic trauma
- Massive transfusion
- Oxygen toxicity
- Disseminated intravascular coagulation (DIC)
- Shock
- Pneumonia or sepsis

Treatment for ALI/ARDS includes supportive care and ventilation strategies meant to recruit atelectatic alveoli. Positive end-expiratory pressure (PEEP) ventilation with lower tidal volumes has been shown to reduce airway pressure and barotrauma.

- PEEP decreases intrapulmonary shunting and increases lung compliance.
- At high levels, PEEP can also cause barotrauma, decrease cardiac output, and increase intrathoracic pressure.
- Optimal PEEP is between 10 and 15 mm Hg (1.33 and 2.00 kPa).
- More advanced strategies are generally deferred to after admission in the critical care unit and include prone positioning, high-frequency ventilation, and extracorporeal membrane oxygenation.[71,83]

Pneumonia and Aspiration

Pneumonia occurs in as many as 9–27% of mechanically ventilated trauma patients, with gram-positive organisms being the most frequent cause.[14] Ventilator-associated pneumonia (VAP) develops after more than 48 hours of mechanical ventilation. One of the most critical risk factors for VAP is colonization of the oral cavity by respiratory pathogens. Patients with poor dental hygiene are at higher risk of having distinctive oral bacteria present; when patients develop VAP, the bacteria in their lung secretions may originate from these oral bacteria.[108] VAP is a serious complication in the ICU and is associated with an increased risk of death. A high incidence in trauma patients is believed to be the result of the altered immune function after a major traumatic injury, lung contusions, and aspiration from brain injury.[74]

Symptoms include dyspnea, fever, tachypnea, hemoptysis, crackles, bronchospasm, and increased purulent secretions. Lab values will show worsening hypoxemia and leukocytosis. Imaging will show new or progressive infiltrate on chest radiograph, and respiratory tract samples are useful for diagnosis and antibiotic choices. Blood cultures should also be obtained.[59]

Secretions that adhere to the ETT provide a direct route for bacteria to migrate into the lower airways. Sinus and gastric colonization can also lead to VAP. Although the patient may not develop pneumonia for 48 hours, oral care provided early after intubation, even in the ED, may impact the development of pneumonia.

Comorbidities that can affect the development of pneumonia include the following[84]:

- Obesity
- Hypertension
- Diabetes mellitus
- Congestive heart failure or valvular disease
- Chronic pulmonary disease
- Peripheral vascular disease
- Immunosuppression

Malnutrition VAP prevention bundles may improve outcomes, and include the following:

- Strict hand hygiene for all clinical staff
- Elevating the head of the bed 30–45 degrees to limit the risk of aspiration
- Chlorhexidine oral care to decontaminate the mouth every 6–8 hours
    - Intubated patients can benefit from early chlorhexidine oral care once ETT placement is verified, even in the ED
- Subglottic suctioning
    - Oral secretions pool above the ETT cuff, enabling contaminated fluid to leak down into the lower airway
    - Biofilm forms on the surface of an ETT when bacteria adhere to the tube surface, making aspiration of bacteria into the lungs possible
- Endotracheal suctioning
- Using an inline, closed-system suction device to prevent opening the ETT to contamination is also beneficial[108]

Additional steps in VAP prevention may include interventions such as low-volume tidal-volume ventilation and using the proposed ABCDEF bundle.[47] Following are the ABCDEF bundle components:

- *A: Assess, prevent, and manage pain.* The Pain, Agitation, and Delirium (PAD) guideline released in 2013 and updated in 2018 recognizes that poor pain control is a risk factor for nosocomial infection and prolonged mechanical ventilation. Additionally, inadequate pain control may precipitate delirium.[17,33]
- *B: Both spontaneous awakening trials and spontaneous breathing trials.* Spontaneous awakening and spontaneous breathing trials have been shown to reduce the duration of mechanical ventilation and VAP.[33]

- **C**: *Choice of analgesia and sedation.* While sedation is important in facilitating mechanical ventilation, caution should be used to maintain the lightest level of sedation possible for the patient and to avoid benzodiazepines.[40]
- **D**: *Delirium—assess, prevent, and manage.* Delirium is a frequent consequence of mechanical ventilation, with as many as 81% of ventilated patients experiencing some degree of delirium. It is also associated with prolonged mechanical ventilation, longer length of stay in the ICU, increased morbidity and mortality, and long-term cognitive impairment.[47] Daily monitoring for delirium, promoting uninterrupted sleep at night, early mobilization, and benzodiazepine avoidance are steps that the trauma nurse can take to help prevent delirium in trauma patients.
- **E**: *Exercise and Early mobility.* The PAD guidelines also recommend early exercise and mobility when possible, to help prevent neuromuscular weakness associated with critical illness and mechanical ventilation.[47]
- **F**: *Family engagement and empowerment.* The patient's family can be useful in helping to promote patient well-being and the other components of the ABCDEF bundle. Educating family members about the need to keep the head of bed elevated, behavioral manifestations of pain, and even ways to provide oral care can help both the patient and the family recover from critical illness.

Begin treatment with a broad-spectrum antibiotic as soon as possible, continuing this therapy until an antibiotic can be prescribed that will match the microorganism based on culture result. Timely antibiotic administration can make a difference in overall mortality. Early diagnosis and treatment is important because VAP leads to acute lung injury and ARDS, and carries a high rate of mortality.[108]

Abdominal Trauma

Missed abdominal injuries are often the cause of late mortality in patients who survived the early post-injury period.[61] Additional considerations include limitations of CT and delayed presentation, which may occur hours to days after the initial injury.[61]

Key points for abdominal injury assessment include the following[61]:

- CT can be unreliable imaging and can miss clinically relevant injuries.
- Intra-abdominal injuries can have delayed presentation (hours to days after the initial injury).
- Patients who become unstable, with a suspicion of intra-abdominal injury, should have a diagnostic laparotomy.

Patients with an altered mental status, regardless of cause, are at higher risk for missed abdominal injury. Children are also at higher risk because their developmental stage may not enable an accurate history to be taken.[61]

Awareness of these signs in the patient who seeks care days after the traumatic event or continued, serial assessments can help to identify subtle changes as they develop once the patient has been admitted to the hospital. See Chapter 9, "Abdominal and Pelvic Trauma," for more information.

Splenic Injury

Care of patients with splenic injury has evolved toward nonoperative management based on patient presentation and specific criteria (see Chapter 9 for additional information). It is estimated that up to 80% of patients with splenic injury can be managed nonoperatively.[98] However, possible complications include pseudocysts, pseudoaneurysms, arteriovenous fistulas, and delayed splenic rupture.[13,98] Frequent serial assessments accompanied by serial laboratory evaluation of hemoglobin, hematocrit, and coagulation studies should be performed.[85] Most cases of delayed splenic rupture occur within 21 days of the injury, and patients with splenic injury should be monitored closely for hypotension, tachycardia, and worsening of abdominal pain, including guarding.[85]

Hepatic Injury

Delayed hemorrhage, hepatic abscess, bile leakage, and hepatic artery pseudoaneurysm may develop following initial resuscitation.[54] Bile leakage can cause peritonitis and septic shock[54]; therefore, close monitoring for signs of sepsis or severe sepsis is warranted. Additional laboratory studies to detect these conditions include liver enzymes, bilirubin, and coagulation studies.[54]

Pancreatic Injury

Because of its position in the abdomen, the pancreas can be compressed against the spine with a direct blow during trauma. Pancreatic injuries are rare but can be associated with significant complications, including fistula development and sepsis.[49] Assessment findings with pancreatic injuries may be similar to those found with retroperitoneal hemorrhage, including abdominal pain, nausea and vomiting, diminished or absent bowel sounds, and periumbilical ecchymosis. Studies useful in diagnosing and monitoring pancreatic injuries include CT scan, FAST, and laboratory studies. Current recommendations for treating pancreatic injuries involve monitoring and nonoperative management for most lower-grade injuries.[49]

Bowel Injuries

Bowel injuries may occur either immediately or over time, with resulting contusions, edema, rupture, or infarction. Continued abdominal assessment is valuable in early recognition of delayed or occult complications of abdominal trauma. It is important for the nurse to frequently reevaluate all patients with abdominal trauma when nonoperative management is chosen and to alert the team promptly when signs of deterioration begin to occur.[86]

Shock

Shock states can occur after the initial stabilization phase of trauma resuscitation from a variety of pathologies. Examples include new or worsening bleeding (hypovolemic), development of a tension pneumothorax (obstructive), worsening sequala following blunt cardiac injury (cardiogenic), and anaphylaxis after receiving an antibiotic (distributive). Other considerations in the post-resuscitation phase include anticipating the development of hypovolemic shock secondary to other processes. Examples of this include shifting of fluid into tissues from the vascular space, as with burns, sepsis, and occult or sudden hemorrhage. Specific assessments and goal-directed interventions in the post-resuscitation period are unique to each type of shock. See Chapter 6 for in-depth information regarding the pathology, signs and symptoms, and goal-directed interventions for hypovolemic, obstructive, distributive, and cardiogenic shock.

Special Consideration: Septic Shock

Assessment and intervention considerations for septic shock include the following[8]:

- Septic shock due to infection immediately after a traumatic injury is uncommon; its onset is usually delayed.
- Septic patients can be clinically difficult to distinguish from those in hypovolemic shock because both groups have tachycardia, peripheral vasoconstriction, decreased urinary output, and decreased blood pressure with a narrowed pulse pressure.
- An elevated temperature is often associated with septic patients; however, trauma patients may be febrile because of the inflammatory response to injury.
- Prophylactic antibiotic therapy may be indicated with open or contaminated injuries.

See the "Systemic Inflammatory Response Syndrome" and "Sepsis" sections in this chapter for additional information.

Disseminated Intravascular Coagulopathy

DIC begins when the body's clotting system is overwhelmed, such as in case of multiple traumas. In the patient with multiple injuries, platelets, plasma, and other vital components of the clotting cascade are lost to hemorrhage and dilution, and clotting factors become depleted through diffuse microvascular clot formation as a result of the inflammatory response to injury. Hypothermia may directly interfere by slowing the activity of coagulation and fibrinogen synthesis. Acidosis as a result of tissue hypoperfusion and hypoxia accelerates fibrinolysis, contributing to the development of DIC.[97]

Box 21-1 describes the laboratory findings in DIC. Treatment is aimed at rectifying the cause, though DIC is best treated by prevention. Administration of platelets and fresh frozen plasma can help control bleeding in the trauma patient and may limit the severity for the trauma patient with DIC.[1,96,97] Although DIC will not be present immediately after the traumatic injury, the treatments and interventions completed during the initial assessment can have a dramatic effect on its development.

Abdominal Compartment Syndrome

Abdominal compartment syndrome is a potentially lethal complication in trauma that was first identified approximately 25 years ago. In patients with this condition, massive interstitial edema within the abdomen from aggressive volume resuscitation or hematoma formation

---

BOX 21-1 Laboratory Trends in Disseminated Intravascular Coagulation

The trends include the following:

- Decreased platelet count
- Low platelet count
- Decreased fibrinogen
- Elevated fibrin degradation product
- Elevated D-dimer
- Prolonged prothrombin time
- Prolonged partial thromboplastin time

Data from Adelborg, K., Larsen, J. B., & Hvas, A.-M. (2021). Disseminated intravascular coagulation: Epidemiology, biomarkers, and management. *British Journal of Haematology, 192*(5), 803–818. https://doi.org/10.1111/bjh.17172

causes an abnormal increase in intra-abdominal pressures, causing intra-abdominal hypertension (IAH). IAH causes decreased blood flow to the kidneys and abdominal viscera, impaired ventilation, and reduced cardiac output. When combined, these effects contribute to progressive ischemia and multiple-organ dysfunction, which have a high mortality.[89]

Abdominal pressure is 2–7 mm Hg (.27–.93 kPa) in healthy patients and varies inversely with intrathoracic pressure in normal breathing. IAH is diagnosed with pressure greater than 12 mm Hg (1.60 kPa), and pressure greater than 20 mm Hg (2.67 kPa) in the context of new organ dysfunction is considered to be abdominal compartment syndrome. The risk for IAH is greater in patients who are morbidly obese, have chronic ascites, or are pregnant. Efforts to reduce the volume of crystalloid given during resuscitation have reduced the incidence of abdominal compartment syndrome.[89]

IAH can affect nearly all major body systems.

Abdominal Effects

Abdominal effects of IAH include the following[89]:

- Intra-abdominal bleeding from the spleen, liver, or mesentery is the most common cause of primary IAH. The distended abdomen acts like a pressure dressing, compressing the organs within its compartment. Secondary IAH can occur with massive blood loss from extra-abdominal sites, followed by resuscitation with large-volume crystalloid solution, leading to fluid shifts and peritoneal edema.
- As blood volume increases, so does intra-abdominal pressure (IAP), compressing abdominal structures and organs. This compression results in diminished perfusion and ischemia, acidosis, leaking capillaries, intestinal swelling, and splanchnic translocation.
- Decreased blood flow leads to poor healing.
- Hepatic hypoperfusion impairs liver function, glucose metabolism, and lactate clearance.

Cardiovascular Effects

Cardiovascular effects of IAH include the following[89]:

- The cardiovascular system is affected as increased IAP pushes up on the diaphragm, and increased intrathoracic pressures compress the heart and major vessels.
  - Measurement of central venous pressure may be falsely elevated because of increased intrathoracic pressure.
- The patient may appear well hydrated or even fluid overloaded in the presence of volume depletion.
- The increased intrathoracic pressure can cause a decrease in venous return, resulting in a decreased preload and loss of cardiac output.
- Rising intrathoracic pressure increases pulmonary vascular resistance and right ventricular afterload, which in turn increases the workload of the right ventricle and decreases left ventricular preload. Greater myocardial oxygen demand results in increased work of the heart.
- The femoral veins are compressed, causing venous stasis and increasing the risk of DVT.

Respiratory Effects

Respiratory effects of IAH include the following[89]:

- Increased thoracic pressure affects the pulmonary system.
- One of the first signs of abdominal compartment syndrome is pulmonary dysfunction.
  - Decreased lung expansion, limited respiratory excursion, and decreased tidal volume are all a result of increased intrathoracic pressure.
  - The result is hypoxemia and hypercarbia with respiratory acidosis.
- Atelectasis, ALI, or ARDS may develop.

Neurologic Effects

Neurologic effects of IAH occur when increased intrathoracic pressure causes pressure on the jugular veins; this decreases the drainage of cerebrospinal fluid and blood from the head, increasing ICP.[89]

Assessment Findings

Assessment findings for IAH and abdominal compartment syndrome include the following[89]:

- IAP measurement
  - One indirect method of monitoring IAP is measurement of urinary bladder pressure. A partially filled bladder accurately reflects IAP. Methods used to monitor urinary bladder pressure include the following[89]:
    - A transducer technique includes attaching a pressurized transducer and tubing to the urine specimen port of a urinary catheter.
  - A bladder scanner is a noninvasive alternative to confirm adequate urine volume prior to pressure measurement.
    - This limits the risk of contamination with backflow into the bladder.
    - Position the patient supine, with zero level established at the symphysis pubis.

- In addition to bladder pressure, abdominal girth may be beneficial as a trending device, although increased girth is not necessarily present with IAH.
- Low urinary output and hypotensive shock unresponsive to fluid resuscitation
- Tense, rigid, abdomen (distention may or may not be present)
- Increased peak airway pressures without thoracic injury
- Increased intracranial pressure without head injury
- Increased IAP (treatment is recommended when IAP exceeds 30 mm Hg (4 kPa) and the patient is symptomatic)

Rhabdomyolysis

Rhabdomyolysis is most commonly seen in patients with crush injuries or burns. Damage to tissues results in cellular destruction, which in turn releases myoglobin into the circulation. Myoglobin, an intracellular protein, obstructs renal perfusion and glomerular filtration. Sloughing of the renal tubular epithelium, myoglobin cast formation, and myoglobin in the urine produce the distinctive dark red- or brown-colored urine. Acute kidney injury results from obstruction and decreases in renal blood flow and glomerular filtration; the risk of acute kidney injury is as high as 42–74% as creatinine kinase levels increase.[70]

Hyperkalemia is a life-threatening complication of rhabdomyolysis.[57] It occurs when cell destruction releases intracellular potassium into the extracellular space, causing serum potassium levels to rise dramatically; this can result in ECG changes and cardiac irritability necessitating continuous cardiac monitoring.

Treatment for possible rhabdomyolysis begins with IV hydration. Fluid volume increases renal perfusion, prevents cast formation, and prevents additional ischemic kidney damage.[57] Fluid resuscitation aids in correction of acidosis resulting from hypoperfusion[57,90]:

- Begin aggressive fluid management to produce urine output of 100–300 mL/hr in adults. In pediatric patients, begin with an initial 20 mL/kg bolus and then twice the maintenance rate of IV fluids. Careful assessment of urine output should be calculated in both children and adults.
- Alkalization of the urine (urine pH > 8.0) with or without diuresis, through the administration of bicarbonate and osmotic diuretics, has been used, although evidence of its benefits has not been clearly established.
- Patients who develop renal failure may require hemodialysis, peritoneal dialysis, or renal replacement therapy. See Chapter 10, "Spinal and Musculoskeletal Trauma," for more information.
- Severe hyperkalemia is typically treated with calcium, insulin, and glucose.[57]
  - Substances that shift potassium from extracellular to intracellular spaces are only temporarily effective.[23]
  - Calcium does not affect potassium levels but protects against the cardiotoxic effects of hyperkalemia.
  - Other interventions may be necessary for definitive treatment[57]:
    - Diuresis
    - Intestinal potassium binders, such as sodium polystyrene sulfonate
    - Dialysis

Systemic Inflammatory Response Syndrome

Systemic inflammatory response syndrome (SIRS) is a generalized response to injury or illness that occurs because of an infection, trauma, or ischemia. If two or more of the following assessment findings are present, the patient meets the criteria for SIRS:

- Fever greater than 38°C (100.4°F) or less than 36°C (96.8°F)
- Heart rate greater than 90 beats/minute
- Respiratory rate greater than 20 breaths/minute or $PaCO_2$ less than 32 mm Hg (4.27 kPa)
- White blood cells greater than 12,000 cells/mcL or less than 4,000 cells/mcL or if there are greater than 10% band forms

The difference between SIRS and sepsis is that sepsis has an identified source of infection, and SIRS does not.[23]

Sepsis

In addition to the normal inflammatory process caused by trauma, patients can be at risk for developing an infection or sepsis. Sepsis is the presence of a systemic response, rather than a localized reaction or isolated infection.[23] Patients with a variety of conditions may be at risk for developing infection and sepsis, including the following groups[23]:

- Patients with penetrating injuries, open wounds, or contaminated wounds
- Those with blunt abdominal trauma or contamination of the peritoneal cavity by intestinal contents (bowel perforation or splanchnic translocation)
- Those experiencing surface or burn trauma with loss of the skin's protective barrier

Sepsis can produce widespread vascular damage:

- Endotoxin release leads to capillary leakage, shifting of fluid into the interstitial space, and edema.
- Increased viscosity of blood leads to clotting in the microcirculation and the development of coagulopathy.
- Tissue hypoxia can affect every organ and, if untreated or extreme, may cause multiple-organ dysfunction to develop.

Early recognition enables goal-directed therapy, including timely initiation of antibiotic therapy and improved patient outcomes.

Increased Intracranial Pressure

Cervical collars and flat, supine positioning may increase ICP in the patient with head injuries.[20,26] Methods for decreasing ICP include the following:

- Remove the cervical collar once the cervical spine is cleared.
- If unable to clear the cervical spine, consider alternative stabilization techniques that promote better venous return.
- Elevate the head of the bed unless contraindicated. Recent studies[26] indicate that in the intensive care setting, an individualized approach should be employed when determining degree of elevation because it may not be indicated in all patients.
- Maintain the patient's head in a neutral, midline position.
- Treat the patient for pain or anxiety.
- Promote diuresis, after any shock state has been controlled.
- Maintain normocarbia.
- Maintain normothermia.
- Reduce external stimuli by dimming lights, limiting noise, and clustering interventions.

Mental Health and Substance Use Disorders

Recognition of the psychological effects of trauma is an important aspect of the trauma care continuum. It is estimated that up to 21% of people experiencing a traumatic injury will develop posttraumatic stress disorder (PTSD) in the first year.[37] In addition to PTSD, there are other psychological sequelae of trauma, including depression and suicidal ideation.[25] According to Bulger et al., "Mental health, substance use, and other related problems such as firearm violence are common among injury survivors."[25(p283)] Trauma centers are expected to employ consistent use of evidence-based screening tools for mental health problems and substance use.[11] Trauma centers are further required to identify at-risk patients and provide interventions and appropriate referrals to a mental health provider.[11,25,37]

Alcohol Screening

Alcohol use/misuse is a common issue in trauma patients and can be present both before and after the traumatic event. According to the American College of Surgeons, "All trauma centers must screen all admitted trauma patients greater than 12 years old for alcohol misuse with a validated tool or routine blood alcohol content testing. Programs must achieve a screening rate of at least 80 percent."[11(p110)] Those who screen positive receive an appropriate intervention before being discharged.[11]

Between 31% and 47% of trauma patients report having ingested some form of intoxicant prior to injury.[92] Studies have shown that 1 in 4 to 5 patients admitted to the hospital have some degree of alcohol abuse or dependence.[2] The first clinical assessment findings of alcohol withdrawal include[2]:

- Autonomic hyperactivity
- Hand tremors
- Nausea or vomiting
- Psychomotor agitation
- Anxiety or restlessness

Additional assessment findings may include the following:

- Insomnia
- Transient hallucinations
- Generalized tonic-clonic seizure

Alcohol withdrawal syndrome is a life-threatening complication of patients withdrawing from alcohol.[100] The Clinical Institute Withdrawal Assessment for Alcohol-Revised (CIWA-Ar) tool is widely used to assess patients for severity of symptoms associated with alcohol withdrawal syndrome. However, this tool has limitations, particularly in the intensive care setting.[88] The nurse should be alert to the possibility of the trauma patient developing alcohol withdrawal and be ready to intervene appropriately to reduce the risk for the patient.

Treatment of alcohol withdrawal is individualized. Interventions include fluid and electrolyte replacement, supplemental thiamine, glucose, and multiple vitamins. Benzodiazepines to prevent delirium tremens may be prescribed to blunt the effects of withdrawal on the central nervous system.

Delirium

"Delirium is a neuropsychiatric syndrome that is common in critically ill adults and pediatric patients during an intensive care unit (ICU) stay."[60p1027] Consequences of delirium include longer ICU stays and increased mortality.[60] Routine delirium screening using a validated tool may reduce in-hospital mortality and patients' anxiety about their hospital stay.[60]

Musculoskeletal Trauma

Despite careful assessment, specific fractures may remain undiagnosed during the initial assessment, including those shown in **Table 21-3**.[7]

Consequences related to fractures can occur immediately, early, or late. Bones are highly vascular and prone to bleeding. In addition, sharp bone ends can damage surrounding muscle or blood vessels. A broken rib may result in a pneumothorax or lacerated liver. Early consequences related to fractures include the following:

- Infection
- Pneumonia
- DVT/pulmonary embolism
- Compartment syndrome (see Chapter 10)
- Fat embolism
- Pressure ulcers

Missed and Delayed Injuries

Although emergency and trauma physicians and nurses are trained to perform systematic and thorough assessments of trauma patients, the nature and variety of injury severity may not always allow for fully assessing patients and identifying all injuries at the time of admission. Understanding the mechanism of injury is useful for the trauma nurse, because different mechanisms of injury produce differing injury patterns with predictable associated underlying injuries and injury progression (see Chapter 3, "Biomechanics and Mechanisms of Injury," for more information). With such a patient, the trauma nurse will need to care for multiple injuries to multiple body systems, recognize the natural evolution of identified injuries and sequelae of resuscitative interventions, and be alert for commonly missed injuries.

An orderly, systematic approach to assessment and intervention for the priorities of airway, breathing, circulation, disability, and exposure/environmental control (ABCDE) helps to direct the resuscitative efforts for the trauma patient in the ED. In addition to an organized approach to assessment, some large medical centers have

TABLE 21-3 Undiagnosed Fractures

Injury	Missed/Associated Injury
› Clavicular fracture › Scapular fracture › Fracture and/or dislocation of shoulder	› Major thoracic injury, especially pulmonary contusion and rib fractures › Scapulothoracic dissociation
Fracture/dislocation of elbow	› Brachial artery injury › Median, ulnar, and radial nerve injury
Femur fracture	› Femoral neck fracture › Ligamentous knee injury › Posterior hip dislocation
Posterior knee dislocation	› Femoral fracture › Posterior hip dislocation
› Knee dislocation › Displaced tibial plateau	Popliteal artery and nerve injuries
Calcaneal fracture	› Spine injury or fracture › Fracture-dislocation of talus and calcaneus › Tibial plateau fracture
Open fracture	70% incidence of associated nonskeletal injury

Reproduced from American College of Surgeons. (2018). Musculoskeletal. In *Advanced trauma life support: Student course manual* (10th ed., pp. 148–167).

been using whole-body CT imaging to detect missed and delayed injuries in more severely injured patients. Missed injuries in these patients can include bowel perforation, splenic or liver contusion fractures, and brain injury. The implementation of this practice resulted in high sensitivity for detecting missed injuries in severely injured patients with an Injury Severity Score greater than 15.[106]

Post-resuscitation care reflects the same organized and systematic approach as the initial resuscitation, with the mindset of attempting to identify injuries not found (missed) or not present (delayed) on the initial trauma assessment.[87] The trauma nurse begins by reevaluating the ABCDE parameters and noting any change from the initial assessment, as well as known injuries, interventions performed, and trends in vital signs. Trauma nurses will anticipate and be able to recognize injury evolution and its likely consequences, so they can be prepared with appropriate interventions regardless of where they work, whether in the ED, ICU, post-anesthesia care unit, telemetry/intermediate care unit, or surgical care floor. Frequent, ongoing monitoring can help the trauma nurse to recognize changes in patient status and to intervene quickly.

Missed Injuries

Evaluating a trauma patient with multiple injuries is a challenge even for the most experienced clinician. Multiple factors may contribute to missed injuries, including equivocal radiologic results, inadequate or incomplete studies, simultaneous presentation of multiple patients, complicated patient presentation, or clinically inexperienced staff.[89] The presence of comorbid conditions can also produce a challenging injury assessment. Diseases such as hypertension and diabetes create pathophysiologic factors that may not be evident early in the course of trauma. Diabetes may alter the sensation of an injury because of neuropathy.

Although different institutions have different definitions for a missed injury, generally a missed injury is considered one that was not found during the initial assessment phase and is discovered when it begins to cause clinical symptoms, such as pain when a nonambulatory patient begins to walk for the first time after the injury.[78] It may become clinically significant when the injury contributes to morbidity or mortality or results in a delay in treatment. Patients with missed injuries experience higher Injury Severity Scores and longer hospital and ICU stays.[87]

It was found that as many as 11% of injuries are not discovered until outpatient follow-up after discharge.[87] The use of a tertiary survey has been shown to reduce missed injuries by 35%.[78] This survey consists of a complete examination performed following the primary and secondary surveys and within 24 hours after trauma to identify any injuries missed during the initial assessment. The tertiary survey includes a review of initial radiology studies, any additional indicated studies, standardized reevaluation of laboratory studies, and clinical assessment for the effective detection of hidden injuries.

Delayed Injuries

There is a distinct difference between missed injuries and delayed effects of injury. Missed injuries are present upon arrival at the ED but are not identified then. Delayed effects of injury may not be present upon arrival but develop over time as a result of the initial injury and should be considered part of the natural progression of the injury. It is absolutely critical to note new findings and identify deterioration in previous findings.

Data and quality metrics are a way of life for the modern healthcare practitioner. The Trauma Quality Improvement Program reviews the care delivered by trauma centers and has been implemented to "elevate the quality of care for trauma patients" in more than 800 trauma centers across the United States.[4] Care initiated by nurses in the ED—such as timely IV antibiotic administration for open fractures—will positively affect the patient and can demonstrate compliance with benchmarked standards, leading to better outcomes for trauma patients.

Emerging Trends

Health care is ever changing as both science and technology evolve at increasingly faster rates. Trauma nurses should be aware of emerging trends related to the care of the injured patient.

Extracorporeal Membrane Oxygenation

The use of veno-venous extracorporeal membrane oxygenation (ECMO) is an increasingly a viable option for patients with TBI and patients with respiratory failure who have failed routine ventilatory management. The use of veno-venous ECMO is a difficult decision requiring risk–benefit calculation. Complications of veno-venous ECMO include bleeding, infection, neurologic injury, and PTSD.[75]

An important advance in trauma care is the move toward caring more holistically for the patient and family. Just as the Screening, Brief Intervention, and Referral to Treatment tool is being used to evaluate patient alcohol use, so is the American College of Surgeons moving toward more comprehensive screening and intervention for PTSD in trauma patients. It is also of the utmost importance to recognize injury as a possible adverse childhood experience for children that can have lifelong consequences[30] and to employ trauma-informed care. Additionally, trauma survivor networks are working with trauma patients, families, and communities to help patients thrive after traumatic injury. Watch for these trends to expand as their benefits to trauma patients become more widely recognized.

Use of Whole Blood

In recent studies, the use of whole blood has been associated with the reduction in 24-hour mortality, major complications, and in hospital mortality. Using whole blood is correlated with outcome improvement in severely injured trauma patients in civilian and military populations. Further studies are needed to evaluate the use of whole blood during massive transfusion of trauma patients.[45]

Use of Thromoelastography

Thromboelastography (TEG) resuscitation protocols can assist in correcting coagulation abnormalities in severely injured trauma patients. The use of TEG has been shown to increase in-hospital and 28-day survival of trauma patients. Point-of-care testing expansion of TEG has resulted in faster decision making and could assist in optimizing care of severely injured patients.[79]

Summary

Trauma care does not end with the initial assessment Ongoing monitoring and observation are vital aspects of the care of the trauma patient after resuscitation and stabilization. Many complications develop in the post-resuscitative period, and the prepared nurse will anticipate them, intervening proactively. Even if the initial assessment is inconclusive, knowledge of mechanism of injury, coupled with predicted injury patterns, can aid the clinical team in their ongoing assessment as they look for subtle, associated changes that present in these patients. Assessment and reassessment are important for identified injuries and for potential or worsening injuries. The conditions described in this chapter and their consequences may or may not manifest while the trauma patient remains in the ED, in the ICU, or on the surgical care floor. Knowledge of injury patterns, tertiary assessment techniques, and the potential outcomes can be valuable in the critical thinking and decision making of the trauma nurse. Review of admission orders and knowledge of care pathways will promote early treatment and limit the risk of negative consequences, making the transition to definitive care smooth and efficient while enabling an individualized plan of care.

References

1. Adelborg, K., Larsen, J. B., & Hvas, A.-M. (2021). Disseminated intravascular coagulation: Epidemiology, biomarkers, and management. *British Journal of Haematology*, 192(5), 803–818. https://doi.org/10.1111/bjh.17172
2. Ahmed, N., & Kuo, Y. (2022). Risk of alcohol withdrawal syndrome in hospitalized trauma patients: A national data analysis. *Injury*, 53(1), 44–48. https://doi.org/10.1016/j.injury.2021.08.017
3. Al-Jeabory, M., Szarpak, L., Attila, K., Simpson, M., Smereka, A., Gasecka, A., Wieczorek, W., Pruc, M., Koselak, M., Gawel, W., Checinski, I., Jaguszewski, M. J., & Filipiak, K. J. (2021). Efficacy and safety of tranexamic acid in emergency trauma: A systematic review and meta-analysis. *Journal of Clinical Medicine*, 10(5), Article 1030. https://doi.org/10.3390/jcm10051030
4. American College of Surgeons. (n.d.). *Trauma Quality Improvement Program*. https://www.facs.org//quality-programs/trauma/tqp/center-programs/tqip
5. American College of Surgeons. (2018). Appendix B. In *Advanced trauma life support: Student course manual* (10th ed., p. 268).
6. American College of Surgeons. (2018). Head trauma. In *Advanced trauma life support: Student course manual* (10th ed., pp. 102–126).
7. American College of Surgeons. (2018). Musculoskeletal. In *Advanced trauma life support: Student course manual* (10th ed., pp. 148–167).
8. American College of Surgeons. (2018). Shock. In *Advanced trauma life support: Student course manual* (10th ed., pp. 42–61).
9. American College of Surgeons. (2018). Thoracic trauma. In *Advanced trauma life support: Student course manual* (10th ed., pp. 62–81).
10. American College of Surgeons. (2018). Transfer to definitive care. In *Advanced trauma life support: Student course manual* (10th ed., pp. 240–252).
11. American College of Surgeons. (2022). *Resources for optimal care of the injured patient: 2022 standards*. https://www.facs.org/quality-programs/trauma/quality/verification-review-and-consultation-program/standards/
12. Aminiahidashti, H., Shafiee, S., Zamani Kiasari, A., & Sazgar, M. (2018). Applications of end-tidal carbon dioxide ($ETCO_2$) monitoring in emergency department: A narrative review. *Emergency*, 6(1), e5. https://www.ncbi.nlm.nih.gov/pmc/articles/PMC5827051/
13. Anyanwu, C., & Reynal, S. (2018). Delayed splenic rupture resulting in massive intraperitoneal hemorrhage post ambulatory-related injury. *Cureus* 10(2), Article e2160. https://doi.org/10.7759/cureus.2160

14. Arumugam, S. K., Mudali, I., Strandvik, G., El-Menyar, A., Al-Hassani, A., & Al-Thani, H. (2018). Risk factors for ventilator-associated pneumonia in trauma patients: A descriptive analysis. *World Journal of Emergency Medicine, 9*(3), 203–210. https://doi.org/10.5847/wjem.j.1920-8642.2018.03.007
15. Bahloul, M., Dlela, M., Bouchaala, K., Kallel, H., Ben Hamida, C., Chelly, H., & Bouaziz, M. (2020). Post-traumatic pulmonary embolism: Incidence, physiopathology, risk factors of early occurrence, and impact outcome. A narrative review. *American Journal of Cardiovascular Disease, 10*(4), 432–443. https://www.ncbi.nlm.nih.gov/pmc/articles/PMC7675152/
16. Baiu, I., & Spain, D. (2019). Rib fractures. *JAMA, 321*(18), 1836. https://doi.org/10.1001/jama.2019.2313
17. Balas, M. C., Weinhouse, G. L., Denehy, L., Chanques, G., Rochwerg, B., Misak, C. J., Skrobik, Y., Devlin, J. W., & Fraser, G. L. (2018). Interpreting and implementing the 2018 Pain, Agitation/Sedation, Delirium, Immobility, and Sleep Disruption Clinical Practice Guideline. *Critical Care Medicine, 46*(9), 1464–1470. https://doi.org/10.1097/CCM.0000000000003307
18. Balvers, K., Van der Horts, M., Grauman, M., Boer, C., Binnerkade, J. M., Goslings, J. C., & Juffermans, J. P. (2016). Hypothermia as a predictor for mortality in trauma patients at admittance to the intensive care unit. *Journal of Emergencies, Trauma and Shock, 9*(3), 97–102. https://doi.org/10.4103%2F0974-2700.185276
19. Bauman, M., & Russo-McCourt, T. (2016). Caring for patients with spinal cord injuries. *American Nurse Today, 11*(5), 18–22. https://www.americannursetoday.com/caring-patients-spinal-cord-injuries/
20. Bazaie, N., Alghamdi, I., Alqurashi, N., & Ahmed, Z. (2021). The impact of a cervical collar on intracranial pressure in traumatic brain injury patients: A systematic review and meta-analysis. *Trauma Care, 2*(1), 1–10. https://doi.org/10.3390/traumacare2010001
21. Benson, A. B., & Moss, M. (2009). Trauma and acute respiratory distress syndrome: Weighing the risks and benefits of blood transfusions. *Anesthesiology, 110*(2), 216–217. https://doi.org/10.1097%2FALN.0b013e3181948ac0
22. Bläsius, F. M., Laubach, M., Andruszkow, H., Lübke, C., Lichte, P., Lefering, R., Hildebrand, F., & Horst, K. (2021). Impact of anticoagulation and antiplatelet drugs on surgery rates and mortality in trauma patients. *Scientific Reports, 11*(1), Article 15172. https://doi.org/10.1038/s41598-021-94675-7
23. Boka, K. (2020). Systemic inflammatory response syndrome (SIRS). *Medscape*. Retrieved May 7, 2022, from https://emedicine.medscape.com/article/168943-overview
24. Brain Trauma Foundation. (2016). *Guidelines for the management of severe traumatic brain injury* (4th ed.). https://braintrauma.org/uploads/03/12/Guidelines_for_Management_of_Severe_TBI_4th_Edition.pdf
25. Bulger, E. M., Johnson, P., Parker, L., Moloney, K. E., Roberts, M. K., Vaziri, N., Seo, S., Nehra, D., Thomas, P., & Zatzick, D. (2022). Nationwide survey of trauma center screening and intervention practices for posttraumatic stress disorder, firearm violence, mental health, and substance abuse disorders. *Journal of the American College of Surgeons, 234*(3), 274–287.
26. Burnol, L., Payen, J. F., Francony, G., Skaare, K., Manet, R., Morel, J., Bosson, J. L., & Gergele, L. (2021). Impact of head-of-bed posture on brain oxygenation in patients with acute brain injury: A prospective cohort study. *Neurocritical Care, 35*(3), 662–668. https://doi.org/10.1007/s12028-021-01240-1
27. Caprini, J. A. (2005). Thrombosis risk assessment as a guide to quality patient care. *Disease-a-Month, 51*(2–3), 70–78. https://doi.org/10.1016/j.disamonth.2005.02.003
28. Carnevale, J. A., Segar, D. J., Powers, A. Y., Shah, M., Doverstein, C., Drapcho, B., Morrison, J. F., Williams, J. R., Collins, S., Monteiro, K., & Assad, W. F. (2018). Blossoming contusions: Identifying factors contributing to the expansion of traumatic intracerebral hemorrhage. *Journal of Neurosurgery, 129*(5), 1305–1316. https://doi.org/10.3171/2017.7.JNS17988
29. Carpenter, C. R., Abrams, S., Courtney, D. M., Dorner, S. C., Dyne, P., Elia, T., Jourdan, D. N., Kaji, A. H., Martin, I., Mills, A. M., Nagasawa, K., Pillow, M., Reznek, M., Starnes, A., Temin, E., Wolfe, R., & Chekijian, S. (2022). Advanced practice providers in academic emergency medicine: A national survey of chairs and program directors. *Academic Emergency Medicine, 29*(2), 184–192. https://doi.org/10.1111/acem.14424
30. Centers for Disease Control and Prevention. (2021). *Adverse childhood experiences prevention strategy*. National Center for Injury Prevention and Control. https://www.cdc.gov/injury/pdfs/priority/ACEs-Strategic-Plan_Final_508.pdf
31. Cheng, T., Peng, Q., Jin, Y. Q., Yu, H. J., Zhong, P. S., Gu, W. M., Wang, X. S., Lu, Y. M., & Luo, L. (2022). Access block and prolonged length of stay in the emergency department are associated with a higher patient mortality rate. *World Journal of Emergency Medicine, 13*(1), 59–64. https://doi.org/10.5847/wjem.j.1920-8642.2022.006
32. Cremonini, C., Lewis, M. R., Jakob, D., Benjamin, E. R., Chiarugi, M., & Demetriades, D. (2022). Diagnosing penetrating diaphragmatic injuries: CT scan is valuable but not reliable. *Injury, 53*(1), 116–121. https://doi.org/10.1016/j.injury.2021.09.014
33. Dale, C. R., Kannas, D. A., Fan, V. S., Daniel, S. L., Deem, S., Yanez, N. D., III, Hough, C. L., Dellit, T. H., & Treggian, M. M. (2014). Improved analgesia, sedation, and delirium protocol associated with decreased duration of delirium and mechanical ventilation. *Annals of the American Thoracic Society, 11*(3), 367–374. https://doi.org/10.1513/AnnalsATS.201306-210OC
34. Dechert, R. E., Haas, C. F., & Ostwani, W. (2012). Current knowledge of acute lung injury and acute respiratory distress syndrome. *Critical Care Nursing Clinics of North America, 24*(3), 377–401. https://doi.org/10.1016/j.ccell.2012.06.006
35. DeMaio, A., & Semaan, R. (2021). Management of pneumothorax. *Clinics in Chest Medicine, 42*(4), 729–738. http://doi.org/10.1016/j.ccm.2021.08.008
36. de Moya, M., Nirula, R., & Biffl, W. (2017). Rib fixation: Who, what, when? *Trauma Surgery and Acute Care Open, 2*(1), 1–4. https://doi.org/10.1136/tsaco-2016-000059

37. deRoon-Cassini, T. A., Hunt, J. C., Geier, T. J., Warren, A. M., Ruggiero, K. J., Scott, K., George, J., Halling, M., Jurkovich, G., Fakhry, S. M., Zatzick, D., & Brasel, K. J. (2019). Screening and treating hospitalized trauma survivors for PTSD and depression. *Journal of Trauma Acute Care Surgery, 87*(2), 440–450. https://doi.org/10.1097/TA.0000000000002370
38. Eghbalzadeh, K., Sabashnikov, A., Zeriouh, M., Choi, Y. H., Bunck, A. C., Mader, N., & Wahlers, T. (2018). Blunt chest trauma: A clinical chameleon. *Heart, 104*(9), 719–724. https://doi.org/10.1136/heartjnl-2017-312111
39. Eipe, N., & Doherty, D. R. (2010). A review of pediatric capnography. *Journal of Clinical Monitoring and Computing, 24*(4), 261–268. https://doi.org/10.1007/s10877-010-9243-3
40. Frimpppong, K., Stollings, J. L., Carolo, M. E., & Ely, E. W. (2015). ICU delirium viewed through the lens of the PAD guidelines and the ABCDEF implementation bundle. In M. Balas, T. Clemmer, & K. Hargett (Eds.), *ICU liberation* (pp. 79–88). Society of Critical Care Medicine.
41. Geeraets, T., Velly, L., Abdennour, L., Asehnoune, K., Audibert, G., Bouzat, P., Bruder, N., Carrillon, R., Cottenceau, V., Cotton, F., Courtil-Teyssedre, S., Dahyot-Fizelier, C., Dailler, F., David, J. S., Engrand, N., Fletcher, D., Francony, G., Gergelé, L., Ichai, C., Javouhey, É., . . . Association des anesthésistes-réanimateurs pédiatriques d'expression française. (2017). Management of severe traumatic brain injury (first 24 hours). *Anesthesia, Critical Care and Pain Medicine, 37*(2), 171–186. https://doi.org/10.1016/j.accpm.2017.12.001
42. Gelbard, R. B., Karamanos, E., Farhoomand, A., Keeling, W. B., McDaniel, M. C., Wyrzykowski, A. D., Shafii, S. M., & Rajani, R. R. (2016). Immediate post-traumatic pulmonary embolism is not associated with right ventricular dysfunction. *American Journal of Surgery, 212*(4), 769–774. https://doi.org/10.1016/j.amjsurg.2015.08.027
43. Gowda, R., Jaffa, M., & Badjatia, N. (2018). Thermoregulation in brain injury. *Handbook of Clinical Neurology, 157*, 789–797. https://doi.org/10.1016/B978-0-444-64074-1.00049-5.
44. Grant, P. J., Greene, M. T., Chopra, V., Bernstein, S. J., Hofer, T. P., & Flanders, S. A. (2016). Assessing the Caprini score for risk assessment of venous thromboembolism in hospitalized medical patients. *American Journal of Medicine, 129*(5), 528–535. https://doi.org/10.1016/j.amjmed.2015.10.027
45. Hanna, K., Bible, L., Chehab, M., Asmar, S., Douglas, M., Ditillo, M., Castanon, L., Tang, A., & Joseph, B. (2020). Nationwide analysis of whole blood hemostatic resuscitation in civilian trauma. *Journal of Trauma and Acute Care Surgery, 89*(2), 329–335. https://doi.org/10.1097/ta.0000000000002753
46. Hazeltine, M. D., Guber, R. D., Buettner, H., & Dorfman, J. D. (2021). Venous thromboembolism risk stratification in trauma using the Caprini risk assessment model. *Thrombosis Research, 208*, 52–57. https://doi.org/10.1016/j.thromres.2021.10.016
47. Health Research and Educational Trust. (2018). *Preventing ventilator-associated events change package: 2018 update.* https://patientcarelink.org/wp-content/uploads/2018/09/preventing-ventilator-associated-events-change-package.pdf
48. Hinson, H., Rowell, S., Morris, C., Lin, A. L., & Schreiber, M. A. (2018). Early fever after trauma: Does it matter? *Journal of Trauma and Acute Care Surgery, 84*(1), 19–24. https://doi.org/10.1097/TA.0000000000001627
49. Ho, V. P., Patel, N. J., Bokhari, F., Madbak, F. G., Hambley, J. E., Yon, J. R., Robinson, B. R., Nagy, K., Armen, S. B., Kingsley, S., Gupta, S., Starr, F. L., Moore, H. R., III, Oliphant, U. J., Haut, E. R., & Como, J. J. (2017). Management of adult pancreatic injuries: A practice management guideline from the Eastern Association for the Surgery of Trauma. *Journal of Trauma and Acute Care Surgery, 82*(1), 185–199. https://doi.org/10.1097/ta.0000000000001300
50. Hoit, B. D. (2022). Constrictive pericarditis. *UpToDate*. Retrieved July 7, 2022, from https://www.uptodate.com/contents/constrictive-pericarditis
51. Hymel, G., Leskovan, J. J., Thomas, Z., Greenbaum, J., & Ledrick, D. (2020). Emergency department boarding of non-trauma patients adversely affects trauma patient length of stay. *Cureus, 12*(9), Article e10354. https://doi.org/10.7759/cureus.10354
52. Jensen, C. D., Stark, J. T., Jacobson, L. L., Powers, J. M., Joseph, M. F., Kinsella-Shaw, J. M., & Denegar, C. R. (2017). Improved outcomes associated with the liberal use of thoracic epidural analgesia in patients with rib fractures. *Pain Medicine, 18*(9), 1787–1794. https://doi.org/10.1093/pm/pnw199
53. Juffermans, N. P., Wirtz, M. R., Balvers, K., Baksaas-Aasen, K., van Dieren, S., Gaarder, C., Naess, P. A., Stanworth, S., Johansson, P. I., Stensballe, J., Maegele, M., Goslings, J. C., & Brohi, K., for the TACTIC partners. (2019). Towards patient-specific management of trauma hemorrhage: The effect of resuscitation therapy on parameters of thromboelastometry. *Journal of Thrombosis and Haemostasis, 17*(3), 441–448. https://doi.org/10.1111/jth.14378
54. Kagoura, M., Monden, K., Sadamori, H., Hioko, M., Ohno, S., & Takakura, N. (2022). Outcomes and management of delayed complication after severe blunt liver injury. *BMC Surgery, 22*, Article 241. https://doi.org/10.1186/s12893-022-01691-z
55. Kainoh, T., Iriyama, H., Komori, A., Saitoh, D., Naito, T., & Abe, T. (2021). Risk factors of fat embolism syndrome after trauma: A nested case-control study with the use of a nationwide trauma registry in Japan. *Chest, 159*(3), 1064–1071. https://doi.org/10.1016/j.chest.2020.09.268
56. Kirk, A., Elliott, J., Varma, D., & Kimmel, L. A. (2020). Fat embolism syndrome: Experience from an Australian trauma centre. *International Journal of Orthopaedic and Trauma Nursing, 36*, Article 100746. https://doi.org/10.1016/j.ijotn.2019.100746
57. Kodadek, L., Carmichael Ii, S. P., Seshadri, A., Pathak, A., Hoth, J., Appelbaum, R., Michetti, C. P., & Gonzalez, R. P. (2022). Rhabdomyolysis: An American Association for the Surgery of Trauma Critical Care Committee clinical consensus document. *Trauma Surgery & Acute Care Open, 7*(1), Article e000836. https://doi.org/10.1136/tsaco-2021-000836
58. Kodali, B. S. (2013). Capnography outside the operating rooms. *Anesthesiology, 118*(1), 192–201. https://doi.org/10.1097/ALN.0b013e318278c8b6

59. Kollef, M. (2021). Clinical presentation & diagnostic evaluation of ventilator-associated pneumonia. *UpToDate.* Retrieved July 1, 2022, from https://www.uptodate.com/contents/clinical-presentation-and-diagnostic-evaluation-of-ventilator-associated-pneumonia
60. Krewulak, K. D., Hiploylee, C., Ely, E. W., Stelfox, H. T., Inouye, S. K., & Fiest, K. M. (2021). Adaptation and validation of a chart-based delirium detection tool for the ICU (CHART-DEL-ICU). *Journal of the American Geriatrics Society, 69*(4), 1027–1034. https://doi.org/10.1111/jgs.16987
61. Leenellett, E., & Rieves, A. (2021). Occult abdominal trauma. *Emergency Medicine Clinics of North America, 39*(4), 795–806. https://doi.org/10.1016/j.emc.2021.07.009
62. Liu, J., Masiello, I., Ponzer, S., & Farrokhnia, N. (2018). Can interprofessional teamwork reduce patient throughput times? A longitudinal single-centre study of three different triage processes at a Swedish emergency department. *BMJ Open, 8*(4), Article e019744. https://doi.org/10.1136/bmjopen-2017-019744
63. Mallek, J. T., Inaba, K., Branco, B. C., Ives, C., Lam, L., Talving, P., & Demetriades, D. (2012). The incidence of neurogenic shock after spinal cord injury in patients admitted to a high-volume Level I trauma center. *American Surgeon, 78*(5), 623–626. https://doi.org/10.1177%2F000313481207800551
64. Marini, C. P., Petrone, P., Soto-Sánchez, A., García-Santos, E., Stoller, C., & Verde, J. (2021). Predictors of mortality in patients with rib fractures. *European Journal of Trauma and Emergency Surgery, 47*(5), 1527–1534. https://doi.org/10.1007/s00068-019-01183-5
65. McKenna, P., Heslin, S. M., Viccellio, P., Mallon, W. K., Hernandez, C., & Morley, E. J. (2019). Emergency department and hospital crowding: Causes, consequences, and cures. *Clinical and Experimental Emergency Medicine, 6*(3), 189–195. https://doi.org/10.15441/ceem.18.022
66. McNeill, M. M., & Hardy Tabet, C. (2022). The effectiveness of capnography versus pulse oximetry in detecting respiratory adverse events in the postanesthesia care unit (PACU): A narrative review and synthesis. *Journal of Perianesthesia, 37*(2), 264–269.E1. https://doi.org/10.1016/j.jopan.2021.03.013
67. Mitchell, C. (2016). Tissue oxygen monitoring as a guide for trauma resuscitation. *Critical Care Nurse, 36*(3), 12–70. https://doi.org/10.4037/ccn2016206
68. Mohr, N. M., Wessman, B. T., Bassin, B., Elie-Turenne, M. C., Ellender, T., Emlet, L. L., Ginsberg, Z., Gunnerson, K., Jones, K. M., Kram, B., Marcolini, E., & Rudy, S. (2020). Boarding of critically ill patients in the emergency department. *Journal of the American College of Emergency Physicians Open, 1*(4), 423–431. https://doi.org/10.1002/emp2.12107
69. Muthukumar, V., Karki, D., & Jatin, B. (2019). Concept of lethal triad in critical care of severe burn injury. *Indian Journal of Critical Care Medicine, 23*(5), 206–209. https://doi.org/10.5005/jp-journals-10071-23161
70. Nielsen, F. E., Cordtz, J. J., Rasmussen, T. B., & Christiansen, C. F. (2020). The association between rhabdomyolysis, acute kidney injury, renal replacement therapy, and mortality. *Clinical Epidemiology, 12*, 989–995. https://doi.org/10.2147/CLEP.S254516
71. Nieman, G. F., Gatto, L. A., Andrews, P., Satalin, J., Camporota, L., Daxon, B., Blair, S. J., Al-Khalisy, H., Madden, M., Kollisch-Singule, M., Aiash, H., & Habashi, N. M. (2020). Prevention and treatment of acute lung injury with time-controlled adaptive ventilation: Physiologically informed modification of airway pressure release ventilation. *Annals of Intensive Care, 10*(1), Article 3. https://doi.org/10.1186/s13613-019-0619-3
72. Nunn, M., Fischer, P., Sing, R., Templin, M., Avery, M., & Britton, A. (2017). Improvement of treatment outcomes after implementation of a massive transfusion protocol: A Level I trauma center experience. *American Surgeon, 83*(4), 394–398. https://doi.org/10.1177%2F000313481708300429
73. Ortega, R., Connor, C., Kim, S., Djang, R., & Patel, K. (2012). Monitoring ventilation with capnography. *New England Journal of Medicine, 367*(19), e27–e34. https://doi.org/10.1056/NEJMvcm1105237
74. Papazian, L. (2020). Ventilator-associated pneumonia in adults: A narrative review. *Intensive Care Medicine, 46*, 888–906. https://doi.org/10.1007/s00134-020-05980-0
75. Parker, B. M., Menaker, J., & Stein, D. M. (2022). ECMO safety in the setting of traumatic brain injury. In K. Wilson & S. O. Rogers (Eds.), *Difficult decisions in trauma surgery: An evidence-based approach*. Springer. https://doi.org/10.1007/978-3-030-81667-4_16
76. Paydar, S., Sabetien, G., Khalill, H., Fallahi, J., Tahami, M., Ziaian, B., Abbasi, H. R., Bolandparvaz, S., Ghaffarpasand, F., & Ghahramani, Z. (2016). Management of deep vein thrombosis (DVT) prophylaxis in trauma patients. *Bulletin of Emergency and Trauma, 4*(1), 1–7. https://beat.sums.ac.ir/article_44304_980a406b8c48fe278cf201b07865f3de.pdf
77. Platen, P. V., Pomprapa, A., Lachmann, B., & Leonhardt, S. (2020). The dawn of physiological closed-loop ventilation—A review. *Critical Care, 24*(1), Article 121. https://doi.org/10.1186/s13054-020-2810-1
78. Podolnick, J. D., Donovan, D. S., & Alanda, A. W., Jr. (2017). Incidence of delayed diagnosis of orthopedic injury in pediatric trauma patients. *Journal of Orthopedic Trauma, 31*(9), e281–e287. https://doi.org/10.1097/BOT.0000000000000878
79. Pressly, M., Parker, R. S., Neal, M. D., Sperry, J. L., & Clermont, G. (2020). Accelerating availability of clinically-relevant parameter estimates from thromboelastogram point of care device. *Journal of Trauma & Acute Care Surgery, 88*(5), 654–660. doi:10.1097/TA.0000000000002608
80. Rasouli, H. R., Esfahani, A. A., Nobakht, M., Eskandari, M., Mahmoodi, S., Goodarzi, H., & Abbasi Farajzadeh, M. (2019). Outcomes of crowding in emergency departments; A systematic review. *Archives of Academic Emergency Medicine, 7*(1), e52. https://doi.org/10.22037/aaem.v7i1.332
81. Rendeki, S., & Molnár, T. F. (2019). Pulmonary contusion. *Journal of Thoracic Disease, 11*(Suppl. 2), S141–S151. https://doi.org/10.21037/jtd.2018.11.53
82. Rothberg, D. L., & Makarewich, C. A. (2019). Fat embolism and fat embolism syndrome. *The Journal of the American Academy of Orthopaedic Surgeons, 27*(8), e346–e355. https://doi.org/10.5435/JAAOS-D-17-00571

83. Semple, J. W., Rebetz, J., & Kapur, R. (2019). Transfusion-associated circulatory overload and transfusion-related acute lung injury. *Blood, 133*(17), 1840–1853. https://doi.org/10.1182/blood-2018-10-860809

84. Shah, H., Ali, A., Patel, A. A., Abbagoni, V., Goswami, R., Kumar, A., Velasquez Botero, F., Otite, E., Tomar, H., Desai, M., Maiyani, P., Devani, H., Siddiqui, F., & Muddassir, S. (2022). Trends and factors associated with ventilator-associated pneumonia: A national perspective. *Cureus, 14*(3), Article e23634. https://doi.org/10.7759/cureus.23634

85. Silva, M., Moreira, N., Baiao, J., & Costa Almeida, C. (2021). Delayed splenic rupture and conservative management: Case series. *International Surgery Journal, 8*(11), 3407–3411. https://www.ijsurgery.com/index.php/isj/article/view/8065/5021

86. Smyth, L., Bendinelli, C., Lee, N., Reeds, M. G., Loh, E. J., Amico, F., Balogh, Z. J., Di Saverio, S., Weber, D., Ten Broek, R. P., Abu-Zidan, F. M., Campanelli, G., Beka, S. G., Chiarugi, M., Shelat, V. G., Tan, E., Moore, E., Bonavina, L., Latifi, R., Hecker, A., . . . Catena, F. (2022). WSES guidelines on blunt and penetrating bowel injury: Diagnosis, investigations, and treatment. *World Journal of Emergency Surgery, 17*(1), Article 13. https://doi.org/10.1186/s13017-022-00418-y

87. Stawicki, S. P., & Lindsey, D. E. (2017). Missed traumatic injuries: A synopsis. *International Journal of Academic Medicine, 3*(3), 13–23. https://doi.org/10.4103/ijam.ijam_5_17

88. Steel. T. L., Giovanni, S. P., Katsandres, S. C., Cohen, S. M., Stephenson, K. B., Murray, B., Sobeck, H., Hough, C. L., Bradley, K. A., & Williams, E. C. (2021). Should the CIWA-Ar be the standard monitoring strategy for alcohol withdrawal syndrome in the intensive care unit? *Addiction Science & Clinical Practice, 16*, Article 21. https://doi.org/10.1186/s13722-021-00226-w

89. Sugrue, M. (2017). Abdominal compartment syndrome and the open abdomen: Any unresolved issues? *Current Opinion in Critical Care, 23*(1), 73–78. https://doi.org/10.1097/MCC.0000000000000371

90. Szugye, H. S. (2020). Pediatric rhabdomyolysis. *Pediatrics in Review, 41*(6), 265–275. https://doi.org/10.1542/pir.2018-0300

91. Timon, C., Keady, C., & Murphy, C. G. (2021). Fat embolism syndrome—A qualitative review of its incidence, presentation, pathogenesis and management. *Malaysian Orthopaedic Journal, 15*(1), 1–11. https://doi.org/10.5704/MOJ.2103.001

92. Titus, D., Kowal-Vern, A., Porter, J., Matthews, M., Spadafore, P., & Vail, S. (2021). Trauma activation and substance use in an urban trauma center. *Surgical Science, 12*, 53–66. https://doi.org/10.4236/ss.2021.123008

93. van Veelen, M. J., & Brodmann Maeder, M. (2021). Hypothermia in trauma. *International Journal of Environmental Research and Public Health, 18*(16), Article 8719. https://doi.org/10.3390/ijerph18168719

94. Viccellio, P., Hochman, K. A., Semczuk, P., & Santora, C. (2018). Right focus, right solution: How reducing variability in admission and discharge improves hospital capacity and flow. In E. Litvak (Ed.), *Optimizing patient flow: Advanced strategies for managing variability to enhance access, quality, and safety* (pp. 97–112). The Joint Commission.

95. Vlaar, A. P. J., Toy, P., Fung, M., Looney, M. R., Juffermans, N. P., Bux, J., Bolton-Maggs, P., Peters, A. L., Silliman, C. C., Kor, D. J., & Kleinman, S. (2019). A consensus redefinition of transfusion-related acute lung injury. *Transfusion, 59*(7), 2465–2476. https://doi.org/10.1111/trf.15311

96. Wada, H., Matsumato, T., & Yamashita, Y. (2014). Diagnosis and treatment of disseminated intravascular coagulation (DIC) according to four DIC guidelines. *Journal of Intensive Care, 2*, Article 15. https://doi.org/10.1186/2052-0492-2-15

97. Wada, T., Shiraishi, A., Gando, S., Yamakawa, K., Fujishima, S., Saitoh, D., Kushimoto, S., Ogura, H., Abe, T., Mayumi, T., Sasaki, J., Kotani, J., Takeyama, N., Tsuruta, R., Takuma, K., Yamashita, N., Shiraishi, S. I., Ikeda, H., Shiino, Y., Tarui, T., . . . Otomo, Y. (2021). Disseminated intravascular coagulation immediately after trauma predicts a poor prognosis in severely injured patients. *Scientific Reports, 11*(1), Article 11031. https://doi.org/10.1038/s41598-021-90492-0

98. Waseem, M., & Bjerke. (2022). Splenic injury. *StatPearls*. StatPearls Publishing. https://www.ncbi.nlm.nih.gov/books/NBK441993/

99. Winkelmann, M., Soechtig, W., Macke, C., Schroeter, C., Clausen, J. D., Zeckey, C., Krettek, C., & Mommsen, P. (2018). Accidental hypothermia as an independent risk factor with poor neurological outcome in older multiply injured patients with severe traumatic brain injury: A matched pair analysis. *European Journal of Trauma and Emergency Surgery, 45*, 255–261. https://doi.org/10.1007/s00068-017-0897-0

100. Wolf, C., Curry, A., Nacht, J., & Simpson, S. A. (2020). Management of alcohol withdrawal in the emergency department: Current perspectives. *Open Access Emergency Medicine, 12*, 53–65. https://doi.org/10.2147/OAEM.S235288

101. Woodworth, L., & Holmes, J. F. (2019). Just a minute: The effect of emergency department wait time on the cost of care. *Economic Inquiry, 58*(2), 698–716. https://doi.org/10.1111/ecin.12849

102. Wu, X., Tao, Y., Marsons, L., Dee, P., Yu, D., Guan, Y., & Zhou, X. (2021). The effectiveness of early prophylactic hypothermia in adult patients with traumatic brain injury: A systematic review and meta-analysis. *Australian Critical Care, 34*(1), 83–91. https://doi.org/10.1016/j.aucc.2020.05.005

103. Wyrick, D., & Maxson, T. (2020). Thoracic trauma. In G. W. Holcomb, III, J. P. Murphy, & S. D. St. Peter (Eds.), *Holcomb and Ashcraft's pediatric surgery* (7th ed., pp. 224–235). Elsevier.

104. Xu, H. G., Kynoch, K., Tuckett, A., & Eley, R. (2020). Effectiveness of interventions to reduce emergency department staff occupational stress and/or burnout: A systematic review. *JBI Evidence Synthesis, 18*(6), 1156–1188. https://doi.org/10.11124/jbisrir-d-19-00252

105. Yarmohammadian, M. H., Rezaei, F., Haghshenas, A., & Tavakoli, N. (2017). Overcrowding in emergency departments: A review of strategies to decrease future challenges. *Journal of Research in Medical Sciences, 22*, Article 23. https://doi.org/10.4103/1735-1995.200277

106. Yoong, S., Kothari, R., & Brooks, A. (2019). Assessment of sensitivity of whole body CT for major trauma. *European*

Journal of Trauma and Emergency Surgery, 45(3), 489–492. https://doi.org/10.1007/s00068-018-0926-7

107. Zawadska, M., Szmuda, M., & Mazurkiewicz-Beldzinska, M. (2017). Thermoregulation disorders of central origin: How to diagnose and treat. *Anesthesiology Intensive Therapy, 49*(3), 227–234. https://doi.org/10.5603/AIT.2017.0042

108. Zhou, M., Xiao, M., Hou, R., Wang, D., Yang, M., Chen, M., & Chen, L. (2021). Bundles of care for prevention of ventilator-associated pneumonia caused by carbapenem-resistant Klebsiella pneumoniae in the ICU. *American Journal of Translational Research, 13*(4), 3561–3572. https://www.ncbi.nlm.nih.gov/pmc/articles/PMC8129229/

APPENDIX A

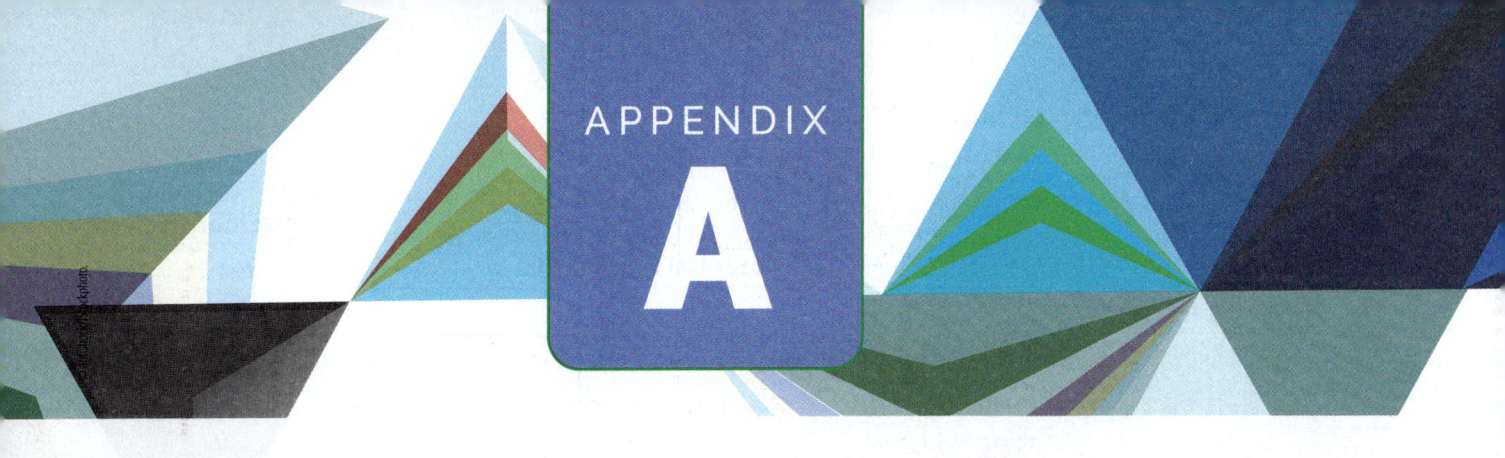

Trauma Nursing Process

Skill Steps	Potential Interventions	Demonstrated? Yes	No
Preparation and Triage			
1. Activate the team and assign roles.			
"Is there any specific equipment that you would prepare?"			
2. Prepare the trauma room.	May include, but not limited to, the following: › Bariatric equipment › Difficult airway or IV equipment › Fluid warmer › Pediatric equipment		
3. Don personal protective equipment (PPE).	Consider potential safety threats to the team or need for decontamination.		
"The patient has just arrived."			
General Impression			
4. Assess for obvious uncontrolled external hemorrhage or unresponsiveness/apnea and the need to re-prioritize to C-ABC.	When alterations are identified, intervene as appropriate and reassess. May include, but not limited to, the following: › Assess for a pulse. › Control external hemorrhage. › Initiate chest compressions. › Initiate IV resuscitation for significant blood loss with signs of very poor perfusion.		

(continues)

Appendix A Trauma Nursing Process

	Skill Steps	Potential Interventions	Demonstrated? Yes	No

Primary Survey

Airway and Alertness with Simultaneous Cervical Spinal Stabilization

Skill Steps	Potential Interventions	Demonstrated?
5. Assess level of consciousness using AVPU.	NOTE: If unresponsiveness was identified in Step 4, credit is also given here.	**
6. Open the airway.	May include, but not limited to, the following: › If cervical spinal injury is suspected, state the need for a second person to provide manual cervical spinal stabilization AND demonstrate manual opening of the airway using the jaw-thrust maneuver. › When the patient is alert and can cooperate, it is acceptable to ask the patient to open their mouth to assess the airway.	
7. Assess the patency and protection of the airway (identifies at least FOUR): › Bony deformity › Burns › Edema › Fluids (blood, vomit, or secretions) › Foreign objects › Inhalation injury (burns, singed nasal or facial hair, soot) › Loose or missing teeth › Sounds (snoring, gurgling, or stridor) › Tongue obstruction › Vocalization	When alterations are identified, intervene as appropriate and reassess. May include, but not limited to, the following: › Anticipate the need for intubation. › Insert an oral or nasopharyngeal airway. › Remove any loose teeth or foreign objects. › Suction the airway.	**

Breathing and Ventilation

Skill Steps	Potential Interventions	Demonstrated?
8. Assess breathing effectiveness (identifies at least FOUR): › Breath sounds › Depth, pattern, and general rate of respirations › Increased work of breathing › Open wounds or deformities › Skin color › Spontaneous breathing › Subcutaneous emphysema › Symmetrical chest rise and fall › Tracheal deviation or jugular venous distention	When alterations are identified, intervene as appropriate and reassess. May include, but not limited to, the following: › Anticipate need for a chest tube. › Anticipate need for drug-assisted intubation. › Anticipate need for decompression of pneumothorax. › Anticipate need for oxygen. › Provide bag-mask ventilations.	**

		Demonstrated?	
Skill Steps	**Potential Interventions**	Yes	No
9. If intubated, assess endotracheal tube placement (must identify ALL THREE): 　i. Attach a CO$_2$ detector device. After 5 to 6 breaths, assess for evidence of exhaled CO$_2$. 　ii. Simultaneously observe for rise and fall of the chest with assisted ventilations. 　iii. Auscultate over the epigastrium for gurgling AND lungs for bilateral breath sounds.	*NOTE:* If the learner chooses a capnography sensor instead of the one-time-use detection device, credit is given in Step 22.	**	
10. If intubated, assess ETT position by noting the number at the teeth or gums AND secure the ETT.			
11. If intubated, begin mechanical ventilation or continue assisted ventilation.			
Circulation and Control of Hemorrhage			
12. Assess circulation (must identify BOTH): 　› Inspect AND palpate the skin for color, temperature, and moisture. 　› Palpate a pulse.	When alterations are identified, intervene as appropriate and reassess. May include, but not limited to, the following: 　› Anticipate goal-directed therapy for shock. 　› Apply a cardiac monitor—credit given in Step 20. 　› Apply a pelvic binder. 　› Apply a traction splint. 　› Assess patency of prehospital IV line. 　› Compare central and peripheral pulses. 　› Consider sources of internal hemorrhage. 　› Control external hemorrhage. 　› Draw labs—credit given in Step 19. 　› Facilitate FAST and/or radiographs to identify source of internal hemorrhage. 　› Initiate chest compressions and advanced life support. 　› Obtain IV or IO access (two sites). 　› Palpate central pulse if peripheral pulse is absent. 　› Tilt pregnant patient or manually displace the uterus.	**	

(continues)

Appendix A Trauma Nursing Process

Skill Steps	Potential Interventions	Demonstrated? Yes	No
Disability (Neurologic Status)			
13. Assess neurologic status using the GCS: › Best eye opening › Best verbal response › Best motor response	When alterations are identified, intervene as appropriate and reassess. May include, but not limited to, the following: › Anticipate the need for a head CT. › Anticipate the need for drug-assisted intubation. › Assess bedside glucose (* with altered mental status). *NOTE:* The GCS is documented as nontestable if there is a factor, such as sedation or paralytics, interfering with communication.	**	
14. Assess pupils			
Exposure and Environmental Control			
15. Remove all clothing AND inspect for obvious injuries.	When newly identified life-threatening alterations are identified, intervene as appropriate and reassess. If a transport device is in place, it may be removed as soon as possible. If there are no contraindications, the patient may be turned to quickly assess the posterior. This is deferred until after the head-to-toe assessment and imaging if needed to evaluate spinal and pelvic stability.	**	
16. Provide warmth (identifies at least ONE): › Blankets › Increase room temperature › Warmed fluids › Warming lights			

NOTE: During testing, if the learner did not intervene to correct life-threatening findings in the primary survey and/or did not complete all double-starred criteria, the instructor will review the primary survey and notify the course director.

	Full Set of Vital Signs and Family Presence		
17. Obtain a full set of vital signs.	BP: / mm Hg MAP: mm Hg HR: beats/minute RR: breaths/minute T: °F (°C) SpO₂: %		
18. Facilitate family presence.			

Skill Steps	Potential Interventions	Demonstrated? Yes	No
Get Adjuncts and Give Comfort (LMNOP)			
19. **L**: Consider the need for laboratory analysis.	May include, but not limited to, the following: › Blood gases › Blood cross/type and screen › Coagulation studies › Complete blood count › Lactate › Metabolic panel › Pregnancy › Toxicology screen		
20. **M**: Attach the patient to a cardiac monitor.	Set monitor to record frequent blood pressures. Consider need for 12-lead ECG—credit given in Step 44.		
21. **N**: Consider the need for insertion of a nasogastric or orogastric tube.			
22. **O**: Assess oxygenation and continuous end-tidal capnography (if available).	May include, but not limited to, the following: › Increase or decrease the rate of assisted ventilation. › Wean oxygen (consider parameters other than oximetry due to hypothermia, vasoconstriction, and skin color's impact on pulse oximetry measurements). *NOTE:* Capnography is highly recommended for all patients and is vital for sedated or ventilated patients.		
23. **P**: Assess pain using an appropriate pain scale.		*	
24. Give appropriate nonpharmacologic comfort measures (identifies at least ONE): › Distraction › Family presence › Places padding over bony prominences › Repositioning › Splinting › Verbal reassurance › Other as appropriate	*NOTE:* Applying ice to swollen areas may be appropriate, but consider hypothermia risk for major trauma and pediatric patients.		

(continues)

Skill Steps	Potential Interventions	Demonstrated? Yes	No
25. Consider obtaining an order for analgesic medication.			

Consideration of Need for Definitive Care

"At this time, is there a need to consider transfer to a trauma center, surgery, or critical care?"

Secondary Survey

History and Head-to-Toe Assessment

26. Obtain pertinent history (identifies at least ONE): › Medical records/documents › Prehospital report › SAMPLE			

NOTE: The learner describes and demonstrates the head-to-toe assessment by describing appropriate inspection techniques and demonstrating appropriate auscultation and palpation techniques.

Skill Steps	Potential Interventions	Yes	No
27. Inspect AND palpate head for injuries.			
28. Inspect AND palpate face for injuries.			
29. Inspect AND palpate neck for injuries.	Demonstrate removal AND reapplication of cervical collar for assessment (if indicated).		
30. Inspect AND palpate chest for injuries.			
31. Auscultate breath sounds.			
32. Auscultate heart sounds.			
33. Inspect the abdomen for injuries.			
34. Auscultate bowel sounds.			
35. Palpate all four quadrants of the abdomen for injuries.			
36. Inspect and palpate the flanks for injuries.			
37. Inspect the pelvis for injuries.			
38. Apply gentle pressure over iliac crests downward and medially.			
39. Apply gentle pressure on the symphysis pubis (if iliac crests are stable).			
40. Inspect the perineum for injuries.			

Skill Steps	Potential Interventions	Demonstrated? Yes	No
41. Consider how to measure urinary output.	› Assess for contraindications for an indwelling urinary catheter. › Use an external catheter. › Weigh diapers (pediatrics and adults).	*	
42. Inspect and palpate all four extremities for neurovascular status and injuries.			

Inspect Posterior Surfaces

NOTE: If the patient has a suspected spinal or pelvic injury, imaging is obtained PRIOR to turning the patient. The log roll maneuver may cause secondary injuries, including spinal injury or hemorrhage.

Instructor prompt: *"Imaging has been performed, it is safe to turn the patient,"* or *"It is not safe to turn the patient."*

Skill Steps	Potential Interventions	Demonstrated? Yes	No
43. Inspect and palpate posterior surfaces.	Not required if suspected spinal or pelvic injury	*	

NOTE: Summarize injuries identified throughout the scenario and listed below. If the learner has not already identified them all, the instructor will ask for any additional noted at this time.

"What interventions or diagnostics can you anticipate for this patient?"

Skill Steps	Potential Interventions	Demonstrated? Yes	No
44. Identify at least THREE interventions or diagnostics.	May include, but not limited to, the following: › Antibiotics › Consults › Head CT for any alterations in mental status › Imaging (other radiographs, CT, US, interventional radiology as indicated) › Law enforcement › Mandatory reporting › Psychosocial support › Social services › Splinting › Tetanus immunization › Wound care		

Just Keep Reevaluating

"What findings will you continue to reevaluate while the patient is in your care?"

Skill Steps	Potential Interventions	Demonstrated? Yes	No
45. Reevaluate vital signs.			
46. Reevaluate all identified injuries and effectiveness of interventions.			

(continues)

Skill Steps	Potential Interventions	Demonstrated? Yes	No
47. Reevaluate the primary survey.			
48. Reevaluate pain.			
Definitive Care or Transport			
	"What is the definitive care for this patient?"		
49. Consider the need for transfer to a trauma center or admission.			

"Is there anything you would like to add at this time?"

Double-starred (**) criteria to be done in order—assessments and interventions must be completed prior to moving to the next step:

- **Alertness and airway
- **Breathing
- **Circulation
- **Disability
- **Exposure

Single-starred (*) criteria to be done—sequence is not critical:

- *Reassessment of primary survey interventions
- *Blood glucose if any alterations noted in Disability
- *Pain assessment using an appropriate scale
- *Inspect posterior surfaces (unless contraindicated by suspected spine or pelvis injury)

IV = intravenous; PPE = personal protective equipment; AVPU = Alert Verbal Pain Unresponsive (mnemonic); ETT = endotracheal tube; FAST = focused assessment with sonography for trauma; IO = intraosseous; GCS = Glasgow Coma Scale; CT = computed tomography; BP = blood pressure; MAP = mean arterial pressure; HR = heart rate; RR = respiratory rate; ECG = electrocardiogram; US = ultrasound.

Skills Performance Results

Evaluation Form

Evaluator _____

Learner _____

Demonstrated points   Number   Percentage

   Total possible   =   _____ / 100%

   Learner demonstrated   =   _____ _____

Demonstrated all ** steps in order   ❏ Yes   ❏ No

Demonstrated all * items   ❏ Yes   ❏ No

❏ Station successfully completed
- At least X of X points (points vary per scenario—passing score is 70%)
- All ** critical steps demonstrated in order

❏ Incomplete. Needs minimal instruction before reevaluation

❏ Incomplete. Needs considerable instruction before reevaluation

Potential instructor (must achieve 90%)   ❏ Yes   ❏ No

Note: Double-starred (**) criteria are completed in order before moving to the next step. The single-starred criteria (*) are essential skill steps and are expected to be performed during the skill station demonstration, but their sequence is not critical.

Index

Note: Page numbers followed by b, f, and t denote boxes, figures, and tables, respectively.

A

AAJT. See Abdominal Aortic Junctional Tourniquet (AAJT)
abandonment, 355
abdominal/pelvic trauma
  abdomen/pelvic vasculature, 166, 167t
  Abdominal Aortic Junctional Tourniquet (AAJT), 182
  anatomy and physiology of, 163–165
  bladder, 166, 176–177
  diagnostics and interventions for abdominal
    and angiography, 180–181
    computed tomography, 180
    diagnostic peritoneal lavage/diagnostic peritoneal aspiration, 181–182
    FAST examination, 180, 180f
    imaging studies, 179
    laboratory studies, 179
    radiologic evaluation, 182
  epidemiology, 168
  gallbladder, 165
  general interventions for patients with, 172
  large bowel, 165–166, 175–176
  liver, 165, 172–173, 174t
  male and female genitalia, 176
  mechanism of injury (MOI) for, 168–169t
    blunt trauma, 169–170
    penetrating trauma, 170
  nonoperative management of penetrating abdominal wounds, 181
  nursing care of the patient with
    laboratory monitoring, 171–172
    primary survey, 171
  pancreatic injuries, 175
  pathophysiological bases for assessment
    hemorrhage, 170
    pain, 170–171
  pelvic fractures, 177–178, 178–179f, 178t
  pelvic organs, 166
  pelvic ring injuries, 177, 177t
  pelvic structures, 166
  rectal injuries, 176
  reevaluation and post-resuscitation care, 182
  renal injuries, 179, 179t
  reproductive organs, 166, 176
  resuscitative endovascular balloon occlusion of the aorta, 181
  retroperitoneal organs
    kidneys, 166–167
    pancreas, 167
  secondary survey, 171–172
  small bowel, 165, 175–176
  spleen, 165, 173–175, 174t
  stomach injuries, 165
  ureters, 166
  urethra, 166, 176–177
  usual concurrent injuries, 170–171
Abdominal Aortic Junctional Tourniquet (AAJT), 182
abdominal cavity, 163–165
abdominal compartment syndrome, 445–447
  abdominal effects, 446
  assessment findings, 446–447
  cardiovascular effects, 446
  neurologic effects, 446
  respiratory effects, 446
abdominal effects, 446
abdominal injuries, 172–173t, 335, 359
abdominal trauma, 285, 444–445
  bowel injuries, 445
  hepatic injury, 444
  pancreatic injury, 444–445
  splenic injury, 444
ABGs. See arterial blood gases (ABGs)
abruptio placentae, 335–336
abusive behavior, patterns of, 350, 350f
acceleration, 26
ACEs. See adverse childhood experiences (ACEs)
acidosis, 94, 436
  metabolic acidosis, 436
  monitoring, 436
  respiratory acidosis, 436
acquired immunodeficiency syndrome (AIDS), 252
active shooter, 401–402
acute respiratory distress syndrome (ARDS), 442–443
acute stress disorder, 375–376
acute stress reaction, 374
acute subdural hematoma, 128
additional reevaluation measures, 343
adipose tissue, 193

adrenal gland response, 93
adult fluid replacement, 239–240
advance directives, 381–382
　　patient's right to choose, 381–382
　　right to be fully informed, 382
adverse childhood experiences (ACEs), 372
Affordable Care Act, 252
age-related anatomic/physiologic changes, 320–321
　　modifiable factors, 320–321
　　nonmodifiable factors, 320
agitated patients/families, caring for, 380–381
　　de-escalation, 380
　　mitigating violence, 380–381
　　preventing escalation, 380
AIDS. See acquired immunodeficiency syndrome (AIDS)
airway/ventilation, 63–77, 434–435. See also oxygenation and ventilation
　　airway obstruction, 66
　　anatomy and physiology of, 63–66
　　assessment findings, pathophysiology, 66–68
　　capnography devices, 80, 80f
　　capnography waveforms and their meanings, 81–82
　　　　breathing variation, 81
　　　　equipment malfunction, 83
　　　　intubation waveforms, 82
　　　　normal capnography waveform, 81
　　　　perfusion waveforms, 82
　　capnometry devices, 80, 80f
　　carbon dioxide monitoring, 76
　　　　qualitative devices, 76
　　　　quantitative monitors, 76
　　colorimetric devices, 80, 80f
　　definitive care or transport, 77
　　diagnostics and interventions for problems in, 77
　　diffusion, 66
　　lower airway, 64–65
　　mouth, structures in, 63, 64f
　　oxygenation and ventilation, 75–76
　　oxyhemoglobin dissociation curve, 75–76, 76f
　　patency, 237
　　perfusion, 66
　　physiology, 65–66
　　problems, nursing care of trauma patient, 68–76. See also breathing/ventilation
　　　　alertness and airway, 68–70
　　　　AVPU mnemonic, 68, 69t
　　　　cervical spinal motion restriction, 68
　　　　preparation, 68
　　　　primary survey, 68
　　　　safe practice, safe care, 68
　　　　triage, 68
　　pulse oximetry, 75
　　reevaluation and post-resuscitation care, 77
　　tube displacement/obstruction, 434–435
　　upper airway, 63–64
　　ventilation, 65–66

A–J mnemonic, 40, 267
alcohol screening, 448
alertness
　　and airway, 43–44, 68–70, 101
　　assessment of, 43–44
AMA. See American Medical Association (AMA)
American Burn Association's Burn Injury Referral Criteria, 241
American College of Surgeons
　　guidelines for screening patients with suspected spine injury, 214b
American Heart Association Guidelines for Emergency Cardiovascular Care, 436
American Medical Association (AMA), 251
American Psychiatric Association (APA), 251
amputation/penetrating injury, 217–218
ancillary team members, 17
ANS. See autonomic nervous system (ANS)
anterior cord syndrome, 201
aortic disruption, 158
aortic isthmus, 143
APA. See American Psychiatric Association (APA)
apoptosis, 94
applanation tonometry, 126
aqueous humor, 113
ARDS. See acute respiratory distress syndrome (ARDS)
arm/hand functions, 144, 145f
armed conflict and trauma, 8–9
　　wounded and sick in, intervention, 8, 9t
arterial blood gases (ABGs), 48, 75
articular cartilage, 194
ascending aorta, 143
asphyxia, 237
assault, 32
assertive statement, 20
assessment findings, 446–447
　　pathophysiology as a basis for, 66–68
assessment tools, 385
　　maslach burnout inventory, 385
　　The Professional Quality of Life, 385
assess proprioception, 215
associated injuries, 146t
at-risk individuals, tools for identification of, 355
Australia, trauma systems in, 6
autonomic nervous system (ANS), 191
autonomy, 382
autoregulation, 116
autotransfusion, 99, 156
AVPU mnemonic, 43–44, 68, 69t, 275
avulsion, 230

B

bariatric, defined, 297
basilar skull fracture, 124, 124f, 131, 131f
BBB. See blood–brain barrier (BBB)
BCI. See blunt cardiac injury (BCI)

Beck's triad, 157–158
β2-transferrin, 52
biologic agents, 404
biomechanics, 25–26
    energy forces and their effect, 25–26
    energy forms, 25, 25t
    kinetic energy (KE), 25–26
bite injuries, 358
bladder, 166
blast injuries, 213
blast trauma, 27, 34–37
    pressure effects on structure, 34, 34f
blood–brain barrier (BBB), 114
blood pressure, 167
blood pressure measurements, 102
blood supply, 195
    for head, 114, 115f
blunt cardiac injury (BCI), 157, 440
blunt esophageal injury, 151
blunt trauma, 27–28, 372
BMI. *See* body mass index (BMI)
body mass index (BMI), 297–298, 307
    levels, 300
bone
    classification of, 194
    structure of, 194, 194f
    and supporting structures, 192–193
    tissues, types of, 193
bony deformities, 51
bony pelvis functions, 166
bowel injuries, 445
bowel sounds, 171
Bowman space, 167
brachial plexus, 190
brain, 111–112, 111f
    lobes of, 111–112, 111f
    vascular supply to, 144f
brainstem, 112, 112f
breathing/ventilation, 45–46, 70–75, 101, 435
    assessment, 45
    breathing intervention (intubation) reassessment, 74–75
    breathing interventions, 70
    cricothyroidotomy, 73
    definitive airway, 46, 72–73
    difficult airways, 46, 73–74
    drug-assisted intubation (DAI), 74
    endotracheal tube (ETT), 73
    extraglottic airway (EGA) devices, 72
    intervention, 45
    nasopharyngeal airway (NPA), 71
    oropharyngeal airway (OPA), 71–72
    retroglottic airway (RGA), 72, 72f
    supraglottic airway (SGA), 72
    breathing intervention (intubation) reassessment, 74–75
Brown-Sequard syndrome, 202–203, 202t
bruises/ecchymosis, 358

bullet-related considerations, 33
burn injuries, 6
burn mass-casualty incident, 401
burnout, 383–384, 384t
burns, 358
    classification, 235
burn trauma, 285–286
    chemical burns, 246–247
    computerized protocol-driven resuscitation, 248
    electrical burns, 245–246
    epidemiology, 235
    escharotomy, 248
    mechanism of injury and biomechanics, 235
        chemical burns, 236
        electrical burns, 236
        radiation burns, 236
        thermal burns, 235–236
        usual concurrent injuries, 236
    nursing care of patient with
        primary survey and resuscitation adjuncts, 239–241
        reevaluation for transfer, 241–242
        secondary survey, 242–245, 243t, 244t
    pain management, 248
    pathophysiology as basis for assessment
        airway patency, 237
        capillary leak syndrome, 238
        hypothermia, 238–239
        hypoxia, asphyxia, and carbon monoxide poisoning, 237
        loss of skin integrity, 238, 238f
        mechanical obstruction, 238
        pulmonary injury, 237–238
    reevaluation of patient with, 247
    wound care, 247–248
burn wound, skin and depth of, 227, 228f

C

calcium chloride replacement, 99
Canadian C-Spine Rule, 219
cancellous tissue, 193
capillary dynamics, 229, 229t
capillary leak syndrome, 238
capillary membrane, 238
capnography, 438–439, 438t
capnography devices, 80, 80f
capnometry devices, 80, 80f
Caprini score, VTE, 441, 441t
carbon dioxide monitoring, 76
carbon monoxide poisoning, 237
cardiac output (CO), 142–143
    factors influencing, 142t
cardiac tamponade, 157–158, 158f, 440
cardiogenic shock (pump problem), 97
cardiovascular changes, 333
cardiovascular effects, 446
care filter, 415t

care of amputated part, 217
care of the trauma team, approach to, 385
    assessment tools, 385
cartilage, 193
cartilaginous joints, 194
catecholamines, 93
cavitation, 33-34
    caused by bullet, 33, 33f
    temporary cavity, 33
    traumatic cavitation of liver, 34, 34f
CBF. See cerebral blood flow (CBF)
CBRNE. See chemical, biological, radiological, nuclear/explosives (CBRNE) countermeasures
cellular response to shock, 90, 91f
central cord syndrome, 201-202
cerebral autoregulation, 116
cerebral blood flow (CBF), 114-115, 118
cerebral contusion, 126-127
cerebral perfusion pressure (CPP), 115-116, 116t
cerebral response to shock, 94
cerebrospinal fluid (CSF), 111
cervical plexus, 190
cervical spine injury (CSI), 284-285
cervical spinal motion restriction, 43, 68
cervical spinal stabilization/spinal motion restriction, 148, 300, 303
cervical spine, 219
    Canadian C-Spine Rule, 219
    clearance, 213
    NEXUS criteria for, 225
cervical vertebrae, 191
chemical agents, 402-404
chemical, biological, radiological, nuclear/explosives (CBRNE) countermeasures, 402-405
    biologic agents, 404
    chemical agents, 402-404
    decontamination, 402, 403f, 403t
    explosives, 404-405
    personal protective equipment, 402
    radiologic/nuclear events, 404, 404f
chemical burns, 236, 246-247
chest, 53, 213
    drainage systems, 159-160, 159t
    tube drainage, 160
child maltreatment, 350-351
children in, disaster, 398
chronic subdural hematoma, 128-129
circulation and control of hemorrhage, 46-47, 101-102
circulation care, 435
circumferential burns, 243-244
cisgender, 255
clear messaging, 20
The Clinical Institute Withdrawal Assessment for Alcohol-Revised (CIWA-Ar) tool, 448
closed-loop communication, 20
closed-loop mechanical ventilation, 438

CO. See cardiac output (CO)
coagulation, zone of, 238
coagulopathy, 95, 437-438
collagen, 228
colon, 165-166
colorimetric devices, 80, 80f
communication, 17-20
    assertive statement, 20
    brief, 19
    clear messaging, 20
    closed-loop communication, 20
    debrief, 19
    huddle, 19
    interpreter services, 379
    knowledge sharing, 19
    mutual respect, 20
    shared mental model, 18
    techniques during trauma resuscitation, 19-20
    trauma bay, effective communication in, 19-20
comorbidities, 195
compact bone, 193
compartment pressure measurement tool, 209, 210f
compartment syndrome, 207-208, 209f, 218
compassion fatigue, 382, 383t
compensated shock, 92, 102
computed tomography (CT) scan, 307, 342
computerized protocol-driven resuscitation, 248
concurrent injuries, 197
concussion, 129
conjunctiva, 112-113
contusion, 230
cord concussion, 198
cord contusion, 198
cord transection, 198
core team members, 17
cornea, 113
corneal injury, 132, 133t
cortical sensation, 189
corticospinal tracts, 188, 188f
coup/contrecoup injury, 126, 127f
COVID-19 pandemic, 382, 393, 394
CPP. See cerebral perfusion pressure (CPP)
cranial nerves, 112, 113f
craniofacial fractures, 130-132, 131f
cricothyroidotomy, 73
crisis, 374-375, 375t
crisis standards of care, 396
critical incidents, 384, 385t
crush injuries, 207, 213, 218
crush syndrome, 207
CSF. See cerebrospinal fluid (CSF)
CSI. See cervical spinal injury (CSI)
CT. See computed tomography (CT) scan
Cullen's sign, 171
cultural humility, 260-261
cyanosis, 275

D

DAI. *See* diffuse axonal injury (DAI)
DAI. *See* drug-assisted intubation (DAI)
damage control resuscitation (DCR), 47, 98
damage control surgeries for shock, 100
data/quality metrics, 450
DCR. *See* damage control resuscitation (DCR)
deadnaming, 259
deceleration, 26
decompensated/hypotensive shock, 90, 92
decontamination, 402, 403f, 403t
deep sensation, 189
deep vein thrombosis (DVT), 440–441
de-escalation, 380
defibrillation, 305
definitive airway, 46, 72–73
    types of, 73
definitive care/transport, 325–326, 343
    head trauma, 137
    musculoskeletal trauma, 218
    pediatric trauma, 287
    pelvic fractures, 177–178
    rib fractures, 325–326, 326f
    stay/adverse events, length of, 325
    surface trauma, 235
    thoracic and neck trauma, 160
delirium, 448–449
dense connective tissue, 193
depressed skull fracture, 130–131
depression, 351
dermatomes, 189–190, 190f
dermis, 228
developing resilience, 386, 386b
DFSA. *See* drug-facilitated sexual assault (DFSA)
diabetes, 300
diagnostic peritoneal lavage (DPL), 283, 342
diagnostic procedures, 341–342, 341t
diaphragmatic injury, 440
diaphysis, 194
diencephalon, 112, 112f
difficult airways, 46, 73–74
diffuse axonal injury (DAI), 130
diffuse injuries
    concussion, 129
    diffuse axonal injury (DAI), 130
    postconcussive syndrome, 129–130
diffusion, 66, 146
direct injury, 198
disability/neurologic status, 47–48, 102, 435
disaster
    definition of, 393
    disaster life cycle, 394f
    FDNY-START Triage, 413
    JumpSTART, 410
    management, 286
    mitigation, 394

    preparedness, 394–395
        hospital disaster preparedness plans, 394–395
        incident command system, 395
    recovery, 398–399
        family reunification, 398–399
        mass-fatality incidents, 398
        psychological triage, 399
    response, 395–398, 396b
        children in, 398
        crisis standards of care, 396
        disaster triage, 396–397, 397t
        evacuation, 397
        patient surge, 395–396
        shelter-in-place, 397–398
    SALT Triage, 411
    SEIRV Triage, 412
    Simple Triage and Rapid Treatment (START) triage, 409
    triage comparison, 414–416
    types of, 399–405
        emerging trends, 405
        human-made disasters, 401–405, 403f, 403t
        natural disasters, 399–401
disaster life cycle, 394f
disaster mortuary operational response team (DMORT), 398
disaster triage, 396–397, 397t
dislocations, 203, 204t
disorders, mental health and substance use, 448–449
    alcohol screening, 448
    delirium, 448–449
disseminated intravascular coagulopathy, 445, 445t
distributive shock (pipe problem), 97
    anaphylactic shock, 97
    neurogenic shock, 97
    septic shock, 97
DMORT. *See* disaster mortuary operational response team (DMORT)
DOPE mnemonic, 77
double-starred criteria, 42–48
DPL. *See* diagnostic peritoneal lavage (DPL)
driving under the influence (DUI), 4
drowning, 6
drug-assisted intubation (DAI), 74
    medications, 85t
        etomidate, 86t
        fentanyl, 86t
        ketamine, 86t
        midazolam, 86t
        propofol, 86t
        rocuronium, 86t
        succinylcholine, 86t
        vecuronium, 87t
drug-facilitated sexual assault (DFSA), 352
DUI. *See* driving under the influence (DUI)
DVT. *See* deep vein thrombosis (DVT)

E

ears, 52
earthquake, 400
eclampsia, 334
ECMO. *See* extracorporeal membrane oxygenation (ECMO)
ED. *See* emergency department (ED) boarding
edema formation, 238
EDs. *See* emergency departments (EDs)
EF. *See* Enhanced Fujita (EF) Scale
EGA. *See* extraglottic airway (EGA) devices
ejection, 29
elder abuse, 354–355
   abandonment, 355
   emotional abuse, 354
   financial abuse, 355
   neglect, 354–355
      emotional neglect, 355
      physical neglect, 355
elder maltreatment, 326–327
electrical burns, 236, 245–246
electronic indentation tonometry, 126, 126f
emergency department (ED) boarding, 382, 434
emergency management, 394
Emergency Nurses Association (ENA), 271
emergency resuscitation, 305
emerging trends, 327–328, 405, 450–451
   extracorporeal membrane oxygenation, 450–451
   resources, 387
   thromboelastography, 451
   use of whole blood, 451
emotional abuse, 354
emotional neglect, 355
ENA. *See* Emergency Nurses Association (ENA)
endotracheal tubes (ETTs), 73, 275, 434
energy forms, 25
   acceleration, 26
   bending, 27, 27t
   bone, 26
   combined loading, 27, 27t
   compression, 27, 27t
   deceleration, 26
   energy forces, 27, 27t
   external energy, 26
   muscle density, 27
   organ structures, 27
   shearing, 27, 27t
   strain, 26
   stress, 26
   tension, 27, 27t
   torsion, 27, 27t
   types of, 26–27
energy transfer, physics of, 23–25
England, trauma systems in, 7
Enhanced Fujita (EF) Scale, 401
EOMs. *See* extraocular eye movements (EOMs)
epidermis, 227–228
epidural hematoma, 127
epinephrine, 93
epiphyseal plate, 194
epiphysis, 194
epithelial tissue, 193
escharotomy, 248
ethical considerations, 381–382
   advance directives, 381–382
   organ and tissue donation, 382
ETTs. *See* endotracheal tubes (ETTs)
evacuation, 397
expanding, 33
explosion-related injuries, 36, 36t
explosions effects on human body, 34, 35t
   auditory, 36, 36t
   digestive, 36, 36t
   eye, orbit, face, 36, 36t
   primary, 34, 35t
   quaternary, 34, 35t
   quinary, 34, 35t
   respiratory, 36, 36t
   secondary, 34, 35t
   tertiary, 34, 35t
explosives, 404–405
exposure/environmental control, 48, 102, 435
exposure *vs.* contamination, 402
external energy, 26
extracorporeal membrane oxygenation (ECMO), 450–451
extraglottic airway (EGA) devices, 72
extraocular eye movements (EOMs), 51, 52f, 125, 125f
extremities, 215
eyes, 51–52, 112–114, 114f
   anatomy of, 114f
   fundus of, 114f
eye injuries
   corneal injury, 132, 133t
   globe rupture, 132, 134t
   ocular burns, 132–133, 134t
   orbital fracture, 132, 133t
   retrobulbar hematoma, 132, 133t

F

face, anatomy of, 112, 113f
facility preparation, 273
fall injuries, 6
falls, 31–32, 213, 314–316
   risk, 195
family-centered care, 379, 380t
family information centers (FICs), 399
family presence, 48, 379–380
   full set of vital signs and, 48–49, 102
family reunification, 398–399
FAST. *See* Focused Assessment with Sonography for Trauma (FAST)
fat embolism, 205–206, 442

fat embolism syndrome, 442
FDNY-START triage, 413, 415t
fear/anxiety, 377
feet burns, 244
femur fractures, 204–206
fibrous joints, 194
FICs. See Family information centers (FICs)
field triage of injured patients, national guideline for, 40, 41f, 42, 2021
financial abuse, 355
FLACC (face, legs, activity, cry, consolability) scale, 281, 281t
flail chest, 152–153, 153f, 439
flat bones, 194
floods, 401
fluid dynamics, 229, 229t
fluid resuscitation, 98–99
FMJ. See full metal jacket (FMJ)
focal brain injuries
  cerebral contusion, 126–127
  epidural hematoma, 127
  herniation syndrome, 129, 129f
  intracerebral hematoma, 127
  subdural hematoma, 127–129
Focused Assessment with Sonography for Trauma (FAST), 46, 103, 283, 307, 342, 440
  in thoracic trauma, 149f
forensic evidence collection, 367–368
FOUR score, 120, 122–123, 122f
  vs. Glasgow Coma Scale, 121t
fractures, 130–132, 131f, 204t
  atlas/axis, 203
  basilar skull, 124, 124f, 131, 131f
  classification of, 205t
  craniofacial, 130–132, 131f
  depressed skull, 130–131
  femur, 204–206
  Le Fort, 124, 124f
  linear skull, 130
  mandibular, 132
  maxillary, 131–132, 131f
  open, 206
  orbital, 132, 133t
  patella, 197
  pelvic. See pelvic fractures
  rib, 152
  skull, 130–131
  sternal, 152
  thoracic skeletal, 146t
  thoracic vertebral, 205t
  types of, 206f
  vertebral body, 203–204
frangible bullets, 33
freeze-dried plasma, 105
frostbite, 233
  interventions, 233b
full metal jacket (FMJ), 33

G

gallbladder, 165
gastrointestinal changes, 334
GCS. See Glasgow Coma Scale (GCS)
general impression, 42
geriatric trauma patient, nursing care of, 321–324
  preparation and triage, 321
  primary survey, 321–323
  reevaluation, 324
  resuscitation adjuncts, 321–324
Germany, trauma systems in, 7
Ghana, trauma systems in, 7–8
Glasgow Coma Scale (GCS), 120, 122t
  vs. FOUR score, 121t
global burden of road traffic deaths, 5, 5f
global trauma, 1–9
  armed conflict and trauma, 8–9
  burn injuries, 6
  drowning, 6
  epidemiology of, 1–2
  fall injuries, 6
  global impact, 2–9
  globe rupture, 132, 134t
  glomerular filtrate rate (GFR), 167
  injury risk factors, 2–3
  intentional injuries, 1–2
  leading causes of death
    1981–2020, 2, 3f
    from preventable injuries, 2, 3f
  special considerations, 5
  unintentional injuries, 1–2
  violence against
    children, 6
    older people, 6, 7t
    against women, 6
  younger individuals, death causes, 2, 2f
goal-directed therapy, 97
Grey Turner's sign, 171
grief, bereavement/mourning, 377–380, 378t
  additional psychosocial care considerations, 379
  communication/interpreter services, 379
  cultural considerations of grief, 378
  family-centered care, 379, 380t
  family presence during resuscitation/invasive procedures, 379–380
  grief assessment, 378
  grief interventions, 378–379
ground substance, 228
GSWs. See gunshot wounds (GSWs)
gunshot wounds (GSWs), 168, 195

H

halo sign, 52, 124–125
hands burns, 244

hazard vulnerability analysis (HVA), 394
head, 213
head injuries, 358head-on impacts
　continuous ICP monitoring, 136
　coup/contrecoup injury, 126, 127f
　craniofacial fractures, 130–132, 131f
　definitive care/transport, 137
　diagnostics and interventions for
　　laboratory studies, 136
　　radiographic studies, 136
　diffuse injuries
　　concussion, 129
　　diffuse axonal injury (DAI), 130
　　postconcussive syndrome, 129–130
　eye injuries
　　corneal injury, 132, 133t
　　globe rupture, 132, 134t
　　ocular burns, 132–133, 134t
　　orbital fracture, 132, 133t
　　retrobulbar hematoma, 132, 133t
　focal brain injuries
　　cerebral contusion, 126–127
　　epidural hematoma, 127
　　herniation syndrome, 129, 129f
　　intracerebral hematoma, 127
　　subdural hematoma, 127–129
　head trauma
　　anatomy and physiology, 109, 110f
　　blood–brain barrier (BBB), 114
　　blood supply for head, 114, 115f
　　brain, 111–112, 112f
　　cerebral blood flow, 114–115
　　cerebral perfusion pressure (CPP), 115–116, 116t
　　cranial nerves, 112, 113f
　　eyes, 112–114, 114f
　　face, 112, 113f
　　intracranial pressure, 115, 116f
　　meninges, 111
　　scalp, 109
　　skull, 109–111, 110f
　　tentorium, 111
　interventions for patient with, 133–135
　mandibular fractures, 132
　maxillary fractures, 131–132, 131f
　middle meningeal artery embolization, 137
　nursing care of the patient with
　　intraocular pressure (IOP), 126, 126f
　　ophthalmoscope examination, 126
　　preparation and triage, 119
　　primary survey and resuscitation adjuncts, 119–123
　　pupil examination, 125–126
　　reevaluation for transfer, 123
　　secondary survey and diagnostics and therapeutics for, 123–126
　　visual acuity, 125, 125f
　penetrating injuries, 130

point of care ocular ultrasonography, 137
reevaluation and post-resuscitation care, 136
head-on/topside impacts of crash, 30
head-to-toe assessment, 51–54
　abdomen/flanks, 53
　bony deformities, 51
　chest, 53
　ears, 52
　extraocular eye movements, 51, 52f
　extremities, 54
　eyes, 51–52
　general appearance, 51
　head and face, 51
　neck and cervical spine, 53
　nose, 53
　pelvis/perineum, 53–54
　soft-tissue injuries, 51
healthcare providers, management of stress in, 387
Heart Association's Advanced Cardiac Life Support Guidelines, 305
heart, great vessels, 142–143, 142t
heart rate, 102
hematologic changes, 334
hematoma, 230
　formation, 207
hemorrhage, 170, 304
　in abdomen and pelvic trauma, 167t
　circulation and control of, 120
　pelvic fracture and, 167
hemostatic resuscitation, 98
hemothorax, 156, 440
hepatic injury, 444
herniation syndrome, 129, 129f
HICS. See Hospital Incident Command System (HICS)
high-impact trauma, 197
high-performance trauma teams, 17, 17f
high side crash, 30
HIV. See human immunodeficiency virus (HIV)
HIV/AIDS, 252, 253t
H–J steps in the secondary survey, 50
hollow-point bullets, 33
homelessness, 254–255
hospital disaster preparedness plans, 394–395
hospital evacuations, 397
Hospital Incident Command System (HICS), 395
human immunodeficiency virus (HIV), 252
human-made disasters, 401–405, 403f, 403t
　active shooter, 401–402
　chemical, biological, radiological, nuclear/explosives countermeasures, 402–405
　　biologic agents, 404
　　chemical agents, 402–404
　　decontamination, 402, 403f, 403t
　　explosives, 404–405
　　personal protective equipment, 402
　　radiologic/nuclear events, 404, 404f

human trafficking, 254, 353, 354f, 369–370
hurricane, 400
HVA. *See* hazard vulnerability analysis (HVA)
hydrogen cyanide, 237
hydrostatic pressure, 229
hypercapnia, 118
hypercarbia, 118
hyperemia, 238
hyperkalemia, 210, 447
hyperoxia, 66, 67t
hyperthermia, 323
hyperventilation, 118
hypodermis, 228
hypotension, 118, 199, 277b
　　Pediatric Advanced Life Support (PALS) guidelines for, 277b
hypotensive resuscitation, 98
hypothermia, 94, 219, 238–239, 279, 436, 437f
hypovolemic shock, 95–97, 277
hypoxemia, 66, 67t
hypoxia, 118, 237
　　signs and symptoms of, 118

I

IAH. *See* intra-abdominal hypertension (IAH)
ICS. *See* incident command system (ICS)
immersion burns, 235
immune response, 200
incident command system (ICS), 395
incomplete spinal cord lesion, 201–203, 201f, 202t
incomplete spinal cord syndromes, 201f
increased intracranial pressure, 448
ineffective circulation, 147
ineffective ventilation, 146–147
initial assessment, 39–57, 355–362, 356b. *See also* primary survey; secondary survey
　　of airway, inspect, auscultate, and palpate, 44
　　A-J Mnemonic, 40
　　of alertness, 43–44
　　AVPU mnemonic, 43–44
　　breathing and ventilation, 45–46
　　care of patients with physical abuse, special considerations for, 357–359
　　computer-aided decision-making, 56
　　danger and lethality assessment, 361
　　definitive care or transport, 56
　　double-starred criteria, 42
　　emerging trends, 56
　　general impression, 42
　　interventions, 44
　　mandated reporting, 361
　　National Protocol for Sexual Assault Medical Forensic Examinations, 359–361
　　pharmacologic treatment to pro-survival phenotype, 56–57
　　post-resuscitation care, 56
　　preparation, 40
　　red criteria, 40, 41f, 42
　　reevaluation, 50
　　rehabilitation, 361–362, 362f
　　right resources, 41
　　right time, 40
　　right trauma facility, 40
　　safe care, 40
　　safe practice, 40, 355–356, 356b
　　triage, 42
　　uncontrolled hemorrhage, 42
　　yellow criteria, 40, 41f, 42
The Injured Trauma Survivor Screen, 376
Injured Trauma Survivor Screen (ITSS), 376, 377t
injuries
　　biomechanics and mechanisms of, 145
　　in burns, 238, 238f
　　cerebral blood flow, 118
　　hypercarbia, 118
　　hypotension, 118
　　hypoxia, 118
　　intracranial pressure, 118–119, 119t
　　mechanism of, 117
　　penetrating trauma, 130
　　risk factors, 117
　　types of, 117–118
　　usual concurrent injuries, 117
injuries, biomechanics and mechanisms of, 23–37. *See also* biomechanics; kinematics of injury; motor vehicle collisions (MVCs)
　　blast trauma, 27, 34–37
　　blunt trauma, 27–28
　　bullet-related considerations, 33
　　cavitation, 33–34
　　emerging trends, 37
　　falls, 31–32
　　mechanism of, 28–31
　　motor vehicle collisions (MVCs), 28
　　penetrating trauma, 27, 32
　　thermal trauma, 27, 34
　　types of, 27–37
injury/biomechanics, mechanisms of, 332–333
injury prevention, 4
　　three Es of injury control, 4
　　　　education, 4
　　　　enforcement and legislation, 4
　　　　engineering, 4
　　World Health Organization, 4
injury risk factors, 2–3
Injury Severity Scores, 439, 450
intentional injuries, 1–2
interfacility transports, 428–429
internal defibrillation, 149
The International Disaster Database, 393
The International Federation of Red Cross and Red Crescent Societies, 393

internet resources, 288t
interpersonal violence
  abusive behavior, patterns of, 350, 350f
  at-risk individuals, tools for identification of, 355
  epidemiology, 348, 348f
  forensic evidence collection, 367–368
  initial assessment, 355–362, 356b
    care of patients with physical abuse, special considerations for, 357–359
    danger and lethality assessment, 361
    mandated reporting, 361
    National Protocol for Sexual Assault Medical Forensic Examinations, 359–361
    rehabilitation, 361–362, 362f
    safe practice, 355–356, 356b
  intimate partner violence (IPV)/human trafficking, 369–370
  prevention, 362
  risk factors, 348–350, 349t
  types of, 350
    child maltreatment, 350–351
    drug-facilitated sexual assault, 352
    elder abuse, 354–355
    human trafficking, 353, 354f
    interpersonal violence during pregnancy, 352, 353f
    intimate partner violence, 351
    Lesbian, Gay, Bisexual, Transgender, Asexual, and Questioning Populations, 353
    physical assault/abuse, 351–352
    sexual assault, 352
interpersonal violence during pregnancy, 352, 353f
interventions, 341, 373–374, 374b
intervertebral discs, 192
intimate partner violence (IPV), 351, 369–370
intra-abdominal hemorrhage, 274
intra-abdominal hypertension (IAH), 446
intracerebral hematoma, 127
intracranial hemorrhage, 274
intracranial pressure, 115, 116f, 118–119, 119t
intrafacility transport, 428
intraocular pressure (IOP), 126, 126f
ionizing radiation, 404
IOP. See intraocular pressure (IOP)
irregular bones, 194
irreversible shock, 90, 92–93
ITSS. See Injured Trauma Survivor Screen (ITSS)

J

jaw-thrust maneuver, 69, 69f
joint dislocations, 210–211
JumpSTART, 146t, 410

K

KE. See kinetic energy (KE)
Kehr's sign, 171
kidneys, 166–167

kinematics of injury, 23–25
  Newton's First Law of Motion, 24
  Newton's Second Law of Motion, 24
  Newton's Third Law of Motion, 24
  physics of energy transfer, 23–25
  terminology, 23, 24t
kinetic energy (KE), 25–26

L

laboratory studies, 342–343
LACE (soft-tissue injuries), 51
laceration, 230
large bowel injuries, 165–166, 175–176
lateral (T-bone) impact injury patterns, 29
lateral or angular impacts of crash, 30
lateral transfer devices, 307
Law of Conservation of Energy, 24
Le Fort classification system, 131, 131f
Le Fort fractures, 124, 124f
LEMON mnemonic, 74, 74t
Lesbian, Gay, Bisexual, Transgender, Asexual, and Questioning Populations (LGBTQ+), 353
  additional care considerations, 260–261
  definition, 255t
  diversity, 261
  epidemiology, 252
  equity, 261
  gender expression, 255
  gender identity, 255
  healthcare disparities and access to healthcare, 252
  history of, 251–252
  HIV/AIDS, 252, 253t
  homelessness, 254–255
  human trafficking, 254
  inclusion, 261
  internet resources, 262t
  mental health, 254
  nursing care, 256
    family presence, 260
    pronouns, importance of, 260, 260t
    transgender health, 257–258, 257t, 258–259t
  reevaluation and ongoing care, 261–262
  reproductive care, 253
  risk-taking behaviors, 254
  sexual and reproductive health, 252
LET. See low-energy trauma (LET)
ligaments, 192, 194
limb salvage, 207
linear skull fracture, 130
lipophilic medications, 300
liver, 165
  injuries, 172–173, 174t
LMNOP mnemonic, 49–50
long bones, 194
  structural components of, 194, 194f
low-energy trauma (LET), 314

lower airway, 64–65
low side crash, 30
lumbar plexus, 191

M

magnetic resonance imaging, 307
male/female genitalia, 176
maltreatment, 285
mandibular fractures, 132
mangled extremity, 207, 208t
Mangled Extremity Severity Score (MESS), 207, 208t
MAP. See mean arterial pressure (MAP)
maslach burnout inventory, 385
mass-casualty event (MCE), 394
mass-fatality incidents, 398
massive transfusion, 99
maternal cardiopulmonary arrest, 336–337
maternal stabilization, 341
maxillary fractures, 131–132, 131f
MCE. See mass-casualty event (MCE)
MCI. See multiple casualty incident (MCI)
MDCT. See multidetector computed tomography (MDCT)
mean arterial pressure (MAP), 116
mechanical obstruction, 238
mechanical ventilators, 438
mechanisms of injury (MOIs), 332
    for abdominal and pelvic trauma, 168–169t
        blunt trauma, 169–170
        penetrating trauma, 170
    and associated patterns of injury in pediatric patients, 268t
    burn trauma, 235
        chemical burns, 236
        electrical burns, 236
        radiation burns, 236
        thermal burns, 235–236
        usual concurrent injuries, 236
medications, 218
medulla, 112
medullary cavity, 194
melanocytes, 227–228
meninges, 111
MESS. See Mangled Extremity Severity Score (MESS)
metabolic acidosis, 436
midbrain, 112
middle meningeal artery embolization, 137
midline retroperitoneum, 167t
missed abdominal injuries, 444
missed/delayed injuries, 449–450
missile injuries, 232
mitigating violence, 380–381
mitigation, disaster, 394
modifiable factors, 320–321
Modified Lund and Browder Chart, 243, 244t
MOIs. See mechanisms of injury (MOIs)

monitoring, 436
monitoring adjuncts, 438–439
    capnography, 438–439, 438t
    mechanical ventilators, 438
Monro–Kellie doctrine, 115, 116f
moral injury, 382
mortality, 144
motorized recreational vehicles (MRVs), 29–30
    head-on or topside impacts, 30
    high side crash, 30
    lateral or angular impacts, 30, 30f
    low side crash, 30
motor spinal nerve tracts, 188, 188f
motor vehicle collisions (MVCs), 4, 28, 117, 144, 316–317, 316f, 317t, 318–320t
    up/over pathway, 29
    down and under pathway injuries, 29
    ejection, 29
    first impact of, 28, 28f
    injury mechanism, 28–31
    lateral (T-bone) impact injury patterns, 29
    motor vehicle (auto), 29
    potential injury patterns in, 28–31
    rollover collisions, 29
    rotational impacts, 29
    second impact of, 28, 28f
    third impact of, 28, 29f
    vehicle-versus-pedestrian injuries, 30–31
mouth, structures in, 63, 64f
MRVs. See motorized recreational vehicles (MRVs)
mucosa, 165
multidetector computed tomography (MDCT), 43
multiple casualty incident (MCI), 394
muscularis, 165
musculoskeletal changes, 334
musculoskeletal injuries
    classification of, 197t
musculoskeletal trauma, 285, 449, 449t
    amputations, 207
    blood and nerve supply, 195
    bones and supporting structures, 192–193
    classification of bones, 194
    compartment syndrome, 207–208, 209f
    concurrent injuries, 197
    crush injury, 207
    definitive care/transport, 219
    diagnostics and interventions for, 218
    epidemiology, 195
    fall risk, 195
    fat embolism syndrome, 205–206
    femur fractures, 204–206
    hyperkalemia, 210
    joint dislocations, 210–211
    joints, tendons, and ligaments, 194, 195f
    mangled extremity, 207, 208t
    mechanisms of injury

478 Index

musculoskeletal trauma (*Continued*)
    concurrent injuries, 197
    fall risk, 195
    types of, 196–197, 197*t*
    nursing care of patient with
        interventions, 215–218, 216–217*f*
        primary survey, 211–212
        secondary survey, 212–215
    open fractures, 206
    pathophysiology as basis for assessment
        alterations in neurovascular exam, 200
        hypotension, 199
    reevaluation, 219
    rhabdomyolysis, 210
    structure of bone, 194, 194*f*
    types of, 196–197, 197*t*
    types of injuries, 196–197, 197*t*
mushrooming, 33
MVCs. *See* motor vehicle collisions (MVCs)

N

nasal trumpet, 71
nasopharyngeal airway (NPA), 71
National Center on Elder Abuse, 354
National Clearinghouse on Abuse in Later Life (NCALL), 328
National Disaster Medical System, 398
National Highway Traffic Safety Administration (NHTSA), 37
natural disasters, 399–401, 400*f*, 400*t*
    burn mass-casualty incident, 401
    earthquake, 400
    flood, 401
    hurricane, 400
    tornado, 400–401
NCALL. *See* National Clearinghouse on Abuse in Later Life (NCALL)
neck, 213
    anatomy of, 143–144, 144*f*
    and cervical spine, 53
    injuries, 144, 146
    trauma, 151
needle decompression, insertion sites for, 156, 156*f*
neglect, 354–355
    emotional, 355
    physical, 355
Nepal, trauma systems in, 8
nerve plexuses, 190–191
nerve supply, 195
nervous system response, 199–200
nervous tissue, 194
Netherlands, trauma systems in, 8
neurogenic shock, 199, 199*t*
neurologic changes, 334
neurologic effects, 446
neurologic status, 435

NEXUS criteria, for cervical spine clearance, 225
NHTSA. *See* National Highway Traffic Safety Administration (NHTSA)
nonfatal strangulation, 351
nonmodifiable factors, 320
nonverbal communication, 261
norepinephrine, 93
normal vital signs ranges, 271, 272*t*
nose, 53
NPA. *See* nasopharyngeal airway (NPA)
nurse, psychosocial care of, 382–385
    burnout, 383–384, 384*t*
    compassion fatigue, 382, 383*t*
    critical incidents, 384, 385*t*
    moral injury, 382
    secondary traumatic stress, 383, 383*t*
    social media, 384
    vicarious trauma, 384
    workplace violence, 384
nursing care, 337–343
    interventions, 341
    primary survey, 338–340, 339*t*
    reevaluation, 341–343
    secondary survey, 340–341, 341*f*
    triage and prioritization, 337–338
Nursing Code of Ethics, 381

O

obese trauma patient
    definitive care or transport, 308
    emerging trends, 308
    epidemiology, 298, 298*f*
    mechanisms of injury and biomechanics, 298–299
    nursing care, 300
        computed tomography, 307
        FAST exam, 307
        magnetic resonance imaging, 307
        preparation, 300
        primary survey and resuscitative measures, 300–305
        radiographs, 307
        reevaluation measures, 306–307
        secondary survey, 306
        ultrasound, 307
    pathophysiologic differences, 299–300, 299*f*, 301–302*t*
    patient dignity, 307–308
    post-resuscitation care, 308
    reevaluation, 308
    staff and patient safety, 307
obesity, defined, 297
obesity hypoventilation syndrome (OHS), 300
obstructive shock (mechanical problem), 97
ocular burns, 132–133, 134*t*
OHS. *See* obesity hypoventilation syndrome (OHS)
older trauma patient

age-related anatomic/physiologic changes, 320–321
  modifiable factors, 320–321
  nonmodifiable factors, 320
 definitive care/transport, 325–326
  rib fractures, 325–326, 326f
  stay/adverse events, length of, 325
 elder maltreatment, 326–327
 emerging trends, 327–328
 epidemiology, 313–314, 314f
 geriatric trauma patient, nursing care of, 321–324
  preparation and triage, 321
  primary survey, 321–323
  reevaluation, 324
  resuscitation adjuncts, 321–324
 mechanisms of injury in, 314–320, 315t
  falls, 314–316
  motor vehicle collisions, 316–317, 316f, 317t, 318–320t
  pedestrian-related collisions, 317, 320
 post-resuscitation care, 325
 reevaluation, 324–325
 secondary survey, 324–325
 violence against, 6, 7t
OPA. *See* oropharyngeal airway (OPA)
open fractures, 206, 217
open pneumothorax, 154, 154f
open wounds, 206
operational considerations, 433–434
 ED boarding, 434
 throughput, 434
ophthalmoscope examination, 126
OPOs. *See* organ procurement organizations (OPOs)
orbital fracture, 132, 133t
organ procurement organizations (OPOs), 382
organ/tissue donation, 382
orogastric tube, 280
oropharyngeal airway (OPA), 71–72
oxygenation and ventilation, 66–68, 75–76, 103, 280
 inadequate, 66–68
 terminology, 66, 67t
oxygen delivery, 435
oxyhemoglobin dissociation curve, 75–76, 76f

P

pain, 170–171, 200, 209
 management, 248
  nonpharmacologic approaches for, 281, 281t
 scale, 281t
pallor, 209
pancreas, 167
 exocrine cells, 167
pancreatic injury, 175, 444–445
pancreatic islets, 167
pancreato-biliary system, 165
paralysis, 209
paresthesia, 209

PAT. *See* Pediatric Assessment Triangle (PAT)
patella fractures, 197
patient dignity, 307–308
patient's right to choose, 381–382
patient surge, 395–396
pattern burns, 235
PE. *See* pulmonary embolism (PE)
PECARN algorithm, 284f, 287
pedestrian-related collisions, 317, 320
pedestrian struck by vehicle, 213
Pediatric Assessment Triangle (PAT), 273
pediatric fluid replacement guidelines, 241
Pediatric Glasgow Coma Scale, 271, 272–273t
pediatric resuscitative endovascular balloon occlusion of the aorta, 287
pediatric trauma
 abdominal trauma, 285
 anatomic and physiologic differences from adults, 270
 burn trauma, 285–286
 childhood growth and development, 269–270, 292–294
 definitive care/transport, 287
 diagnostics and interventions, 283
 disaster management, 286
 emerging trends, 287
 epidemiology, 267–268
 guidelines for care in emergency department, 295–296
 maltreatment, 285
 mechanisms of injury and biomechanics, 268, 268t
 motor vehicle design to reduce, 287
 musculoskeletal trauma, 285
 nursing care of, 270–286
 reevaluation and post-resuscitation care, 286–287
 resuscitative endovascular balloon occlusion of the aorta, 287
 secondary survey, 281–283
  head-to-toe, 282–283
  history, 282
 traumatic brain injury, 287
Pediatric Trauma Score, 281
pediatric triage tape, 416t
PEEP. *See* positive end-expiratory pressure (PEEP)
pelvic binders, 178, 178–179f
pelvic cavity, 163–165
pelvic fractures, 177–178, 178–179f, 178t, 335
 assessment findings, 177
 classification of, 178t
 definitive care/transport, 177–178
 and hemorrhage, 167
pelvic organs, 166
pelvic retroperitoneum, 167t
pelvic ring injuries, 177, 177t
pelvic stability, 172
pelvic structures, 166
pelvic vasculature, 166
pelvis/perineum, 53–54, 213

penetrating trauma, 27, 32
  expanding, 33
  frangible bullets, 33
  full metal jacket (FMJ), 33
  hollow-point bullets, 33
  mushrooming, 33
  point of impact, 32
  proximity, 32
  soft-nose bullets, 33
  velocity and speed of impact, 32
PEP. *See* post-exposure prophylaxis (PEP)
performance improvement and trauma care, 20–21
  continuous process of, 20, 20*f*
perfusion, 66, 146
pericardiocentesis, 158, 158*f*
perineal burns, 244
periosteum, 194
PERRL. *See* pupils for equality, roundness, and reactivity to light (PERRL)
personal protective equipment (PPE), 402
physical assault/abuse, 351–352
physical neglect, 355
pneumonia/aspiration, 443–444
pneumothorax, 440
poikilothermia, 209
point of care ocular ultrasonography, 137
point of impact, 32
Poison Control Center and Safety Data Sheets, 402
pons, 112
portable radiograph, 50, 103
portal hepatic/retrohepatic inferior vena cava, 167*t*
positive end-expiratory pressure (PEEP), 443
postconcussive syndrome, 129–130
posterior cord syndrome, 201
posterior hip, 210*f*
post-exposure prophylaxis (PEP), 253*t*
post-resuscitation care, 56, 325, 343
  emerging trends, 450–451
    extracorporeal membrane oxygenation, 450–451
    thromboelastography, 451
    use of whole blood, 451
  missed/delayed injuries, 449–450
  monitoring adjuncts, 438–439
    capnography, 438–439, 438*t*
    mechanical ventilators, 438
  operational considerations, 433–434
    ED boarding, 434
    throughput, 434
  primary assessment, 434–435
    airway, 434–435
    breathing/ventilation, 435
    circulation, 435
    disability, 435
    exposure/environmental control, 435
  selected injuries/illnesses, 439–449
    abdominal compartment syndrome, 445–447
    abdominal trauma, 444–445
    acute lung injury/acute respiratory distress syndrome, 442–443
    blunt cardiac injury, 440
    cardiac tamponade, 440
    deep vein thrombosis, 440–441
    diaphragmatic injury, 440
    disorders, mental health and substance use, 448–449
    disseminated intravascular coagulopathy, 445, 445*t*
    fat embolism, 442
    flail chest, 439
    hemothorax, 440
    increased intracranial pressure, 448
    musculoskeletal trauma, 449, 449*t*
    pneumonia/aspiration, 443–444
    pneumothorax, 440
    pulmonary contusion, 439–440
    pulmonary embolism, 442
    rhabdomyolysis, 447
    rib fractures, 439
    sepsis, 447–448
    shock, 445
    systemic inflammatory response syndrome, 447
    venous thromboembolism, 441, 441*t*
  trauma triad of death, 435–438
    acidosis, 436
    coagulopathy, 437–438
    hypothermia, 436, 437*f*
post-RSI hypotension and hypoxemia, 87
posttraumatic stress disorder (PTSD), 351, 352
posttraumatic stress disorder, 376
The Power and Control Wheel, 350, 351*f*
PPE. *See* personal protective equipment (PPE)
pre-exposure prophylaxis (PrEP), 253*t*
pregnant trauma patient
  anatomic/physiologic changes, 333–334
    cardiovascular changes, 333
    gastrointestinal changes, 334
    hematologic changes, 334
    musculoskeletal changes, 334
    neurologic changes, 334
    renal/genitourinary changes, 334
    reproductive changes, 334
    respiratory changes, 333–334
  definitive care/transport, 343
  epidemiology, 332
  injury/biomechanics, mechanisms of, 332–333
  nursing care, 337–343
    interventions, 341
    primary survey, 338–340, 339*t*
    reevaluation, 341–343
    secondary survey, 340–341, 341*f*
    triage and prioritization, 337–338
  reevaluation/post-resuscitation care, 343
  selected injuries/emergencies, 335–337
    abdominal/pelvic injuries, 335

abruptio placentae, 335–336
  maternal cardiopulmonary arrest, 336–337
  preterm labor, 335
  uterine rupture, 336
PrEP. See pre-exposure prophylaxis (PrEP)
preparation and triage, 321
preparedness, disaster, 394–395
  hospital disaster preparedness plans, 394–395
  incident command system, 395
pressure, 209
preterm labor, 335
preventing escalation, 380
prevention, 362
Primary Response Incident Scene Management (PRISM) Processes, 403t
primary survey, 43–50, 321–323, 338–340, 339t
  alertness and airway, 43–44
  assessment of alertness, 43–44
  breathing and ventilation, 45–46
  cervical spinal motion restriction, 43
  circulation and control of hemorrhage, 46–47
  damage control resuscitation (DCR), 47
  definitive airway, 46
  difficult airways, 46
  disability (neurologic status), 47–48
  exposure and environmental control, 48
  full set of vital signs and family presence, 48–49
  get adjuncts and give comfort, 49–50
  LMNOP mnemonic, 49–50
PRISM Processes. See Primary Response Incident Scene Management (PRISM) Processes
The Professional Quality of Life (ProQOL), 385promoting self-awareness, 387
pronouns, importance of, 260, 260t
ProQOL. See The Professional Quality of Life (ProQOL)
psychological triage, 399
psychosocial aspects, of trauma care
  agitated patients/families, caring for, 380–381
    de-escalation, 380
    mitigating violence, 380–381
    preventing escalation, 380
  care of the trauma team, approach to, 385
    assessment tools, 385
  emerging trends/resources, 387
  ethical considerations, 381–382
    advance directives, 381–382
    organ and tissue donation, 382
  nurse, psychosocial care of, 382–385
    burnout, 383–384, 384t
    compassion fatigue, 382, 383t
    critical incidents, 384, 385t
    moral injury, 382
    secondary traumatic stress, 383, 383t
    social media, 384
    vicarious trauma, 384
    workplace violence, 384

responses to trauma, 371–372
selected psychosocial trauma reactions, 374–380
  acute stress reaction, 374
  crisis, 374–375, 375t
  fear/anxiety, 377
  grief, bereavement/mourning, 377–380, 378t
  traumatic stress disorders, 375–376, 377t
trauma patient, psychosocial nursing care of, 372–374
  adverse childhood experiences, 372
  interventions, 373–374, 374b
  secondary survey, 372–373
trauma team, support/strategies for, 386–387
  developing resilience, 386, 386b
  healthcare providers, management of stress in, 387
  promoting self-awareness, 387
The PsySTART mental health triage, 399
PTSD. See posttraumatic stress disorder (PTSD)
pulmonary contusion, 156–157, 439–440
pulmonary embolism (PE), 442
pulmonary injury, 237–238
pulmonary response to shock, 94
pulse oximetry, 75, 103
pulses, 209
puncture wound, 232
pupils for equality, roundness, and reactivity to light (PERRL), 48
push-pull technique, for intravenous fluid administration, 278b, 278f

R

radiation, 287
  burns, 236
radiographic studies, 218
radiologic/nuclear events, 404, 404f
ramped position, 303, 303f
rapid sequence intubation (RSI), 74, 84
RAS. See reticular activating system (RAS)
REBOA. See resuscitative endovascular balloon occlusion of the aorta (REBOA)
recovery, disaster, 398–399
  family reunification, 398–399
  mass-fatality incidents, 398
  psychological triage, 399
rectal injuries, 176
reevaluation, 50, 324–325, 341–343
  additional reevaluation measures, 343
  CT scan, 342
  diagnostic peritoneal lavage, 342
  diagnostic procedures, 341–342, 341t
  FAST exam, 342
  laboratory studies, 342–343
  patient transfer, 50
  portable radiograph, 50
  REBOA, 342
  ultrasound, 342
reflexes, 217

renal injuries, 179, 179t, 334
    scale, 179t
reproductive care, LGBTQ+, 253
reproductive changes, 334
reproductive organs, 166, 176
residual limb, 217
respirations, 102
respiratory acidosis, 436
respiratory changes, 333–334
respiratory effects, 446
respiratory system, 141–142, 142f, 200
response, disaster, 395–398, 396b
    children in, 398
    crisis standards of care, 396
    disaster triage, 396–397, 397t
    evacuation, 397
    patient surge, 395–396
    shelter-in-place, 397–398
resuscitation adjuncts, 321–324
resuscitation-associated coagulopathy, 94
resuscitative endovascular balloon occlusion of the aorta (REBOA), 98, 100, 149–150, 181, 342
resuscitative thoracotomy, 149
reticular activating system (RAS), 112
retina, 113
retrobulbar hematoma, 132, 133t
retroglottic airway (RGA), 72, 72f
retroperitoneal organs
    kidneys, 166–167
    pancreas, 167
return of spontaneous circulation (ROSC), 149
RGA. See retroglottic airway (RGA)
rhabdomyolysis, 210, 361, 447
rib fractures, 152, 325–326, 326f, 439
right to be fully informed, 382
Ringer's lactated solution, 240
risk-taking behaviors, 254
road traffic deaths, global burden of, 5, 5f
rollover collisions, 29
ROSC. See return of spontaneous circulation (ROSC)
rotational elastometry, 438
rotational impacts, 29
RSI. See rapid sequence intubation (RSI)
rule of nines in adult, 243, 245f
ruptured diaphragm, 158–159, 159f

S

sacral sparing, 200, 203, 217
safe care, 40
safe practice, 40
SAMPLE mnemonic, 50, 282
SBP. See systolic blood pressure (SBP)
scald burns, 236
scalp, 109
SCI. See spinal cord injury (SCI)
sclera, 112–113

screening tools, 376, 377t
secondary survey, 324–325, 340–341, 341f, 372–373, 50–56. See also head-to-toe assessment
    additional diagnostic tests or interventions, 55–56
    history, 50
    H–J steps in secondary survey, 50
    inspect posterior surfaces, 54–55
    just keep reevaluating, 55
    SAMPLE mnemonic, 50
secondary traumatic stress (STS), 383, 383t
SEIRV triage, 412, 415t
sensory function, 189
    cortical sensation, 189
    reflex arc, 189
        structures of, 189
sensory spinal nerve tracts, 188, 188f
sepsis, 447–448
septic shock, 445
serosa, 165
serum lactate, 75
sesamoid bones, 194
severe traumatic brain injury, 120, 120t
sexual and reproductive health, LGBTQ+, 252
sexual assault, 352
SGA. See supraglottic airway (SGA)
shared mental model, 18, 18f
shelter-in-place, 397–398
shock, 89–105, 447. See also hypovolemic shock
    adrenal gland response, 93
    aerobic cellular metabolism, 89, 90f
    anaerobic cellular metabolism, 89, 90f
    autotransfusion, 99
    bleeding control education and training for community, 105
    body's compensatory response to, 93–94
        baroreceptor activation, 93
        chemoreceptor activation, 93
    calcium chloride replacement, 9
    cardiogenic shock (pump problem), 97
    cellular response to, 90, 91f
    cerebral response, 9
    classification of, 95–98
    damage control surgeries, 100
    definitive care and transport, 104
    distributive shock (pipe problem), 97
        anaphylactic shock, 97
        neurogenic shock, 97
        septic shock, 97
    emerging trends, 104–105
    etiology, classification of, 95, 96t
        cardiogenic, 95, 96t
        distribution, 95, 96t
        hypovolemic, 95, 96t
        obstructive, 95, 96t
    fluid resuscitation, 98–99
    freeze-dried plasma, 105

management strategies, 98–100
  damage control resuscitation, 98
  hemostatic resuscitation, 98
  hypotensive resuscitation, 98
  tourniquets, 98
massive transfusion, 99
nursing care of the patient in, 101–104
  alertness and airway, 101
  blood pressure measurements, 102
  breathing and ventilation, 101
  circulation and control of hemorrhage, 101–102
  disability (neurologic status), 102
  exposure and environmental control, 102
  full set of vital signs and facilitate family presence, 102
  get adjuncts and give comfort, 102–103
  heart rate, 102
  interventions, 101–102
  laboratory studies, 102–103
  monitor, 103
  oxygenation, 103
  preparation and triage, 101
  primary survey and resuscitation adjuncts, 101–103
  respirations, 102
  safe practice, safe care, 101
obstructive shock (mechanical problem), 97
pathophysiology of, 89–90
pulmonary response, 94
reevaluation and post-resuscitation care, 104
renal response, 94
resuscitative endovascular balloon occlusion of the aorta, 100
secondary survey, 103
  computed tomography, 104
  diagnostic peritoneal aspiration and lavage, 103
  diagnostic studies, 103–104
stages of, 90–93, 92f
  compensated, 90, 92
  decompensated/hypotensive, 90, 92
  irreversible, 90, 92–93
systemic inflammatory response syndrome, 94
tranexamic acid (TXA), 100
trauma diamond of death, 105
trauma triad of death, 94–95
viscoelastic testing, 104–105
whole blood, 105
short bones, 194
simple pneumothorax, 153–154
Simple Triage and Rapid Treatment (START) triage, 409, 414t
single-starred criterion, 49
SIRS. See systemic inflammatory response syndrome (SIRS)
skeletal injuries, 358–359
skeletal muscle, 194
skin integrity, loss of, 238, 238f
skull, 109–111, 110f
  fractures, 130–131

sleep apnea, 298, 299, 304, 306
small bowel injuries, 165, 175–176
SMR. See spinal motion restriction (SMR)
social media, 384
soft-nose bullets, 33
soft-tissue injuries, 51
Sort–Assess–Lifesaving Interventions–Treatment and/or Transport (SALT) triage, 411, 416t
spinal cord
  autonomic nervous system (ANS), 191
  cross-section of, 188f
  motor function, 188–189, 188f, 189t
  nerve plexuses, 190–191
  sensory function, 189
  spinal nerves, 189–190, 190f, 191t
spinal cord injury (SCI), 43
  level of, 201
  severity of neurologic deficit, 201–203, 201f, 202t
  vertebral column injuries, 203, 204t
    atlas and axis fractures, 203
    subluxation or dislocation, 203
    vertebral body fractures, 203–204
    vertebral fracture stability, 203, 204t
spinal motion restriction (SMR), 68, 219
spinal nerves, 189–190, 190f, 191t
  segments, 189, 191t
spinal shock, 199t, 200
spinal structures, effects of force on, 197, 198f
spinal trauma
  definitive care/transport, 219
  emerging trends
    hypothermia, 219
    spinal motion restriction, 219
    stem cell research, 219
  epidemiology, 195
  mechanisms of injury and biomechanics, 195, 196t
  nursing care of patient with
    preparation and triage, 211
    primary survey and resuscitation adjuncts, 211–212
    safe care, 211
    safe practice, 211
    secondary survey, 212–215, 215t
  pathophysiology as basis for assessment, 197, 198f
    immune (inflammatory) response, 200
    nervous system response, 199–200
    pain, 200
    primary injury, 198
    respiratory system, 200
    secondary injury, 198–200, 198f
    vascular system response, 199, 199t
  reevaluation and post-resuscitation care, 219
  spinal cord injuries
    level of injury, 201
    severity of neurologic deficit, 201–203, 201f, 202t
  types of injuries, 196–197
    usual concurrent injuries, 197

spine, 193f
spleen injuries, 165, 173–175, 174t, 444
  grading, 174t
splinting, 215, 216f
stab wounds, 170
START triage. See Simple Triage and Rapid Treatment (START) triage
stasis, zone of, 238
stay/adverse events, length of, 325
stem cell research, 219
sternal fractures, 152
stomach, 165
  injuries, 176
"Stop the Bleed" campaign, 219, 220f
strain, 26
strangulation, 358
stress, 26
STS. See secondary traumatic stress (STS)
subdural hematoma, 127–129
  acute, 128
  chronic, 128–129
subluxation, 203
submucosa, 165
supraglottic airway (SGA), 72
surface trauma
  abrasion, 230
  anatomy and physiology of, 228f
    capillary and fluid dynamics, 229, 229t
    dermis, 228
    epidermis, 227–228
    hypodermis, 228
    wound healing, 228–229
  avulsion, 230
  contusion and hematoma, 230
  definition of, 230
  definitive care/transport, 235
  diagnostics and interventions for
    laboratory studies, 234
    radiographic studies, 233
    wound care, 234
  frostbite, 233
  laceration, 230
  mechanisms of injury (MOI), 230
  missile injuries, 232
  nursing care of patient with
    interventions, 233
    primary survey, 230
    secondary survey, 230–231
  pathophysiology as basis for assessment, 230
  puncture wound, 232
  reevaluation and post-resuscitation care, 235
sympathetic and parasympathetic stimulation, effects of, 191, 192t
synovial joints, 194
systemic inflammatory response syndrome (SIRS), 94, 447

systemic vasoconstriction, 277
systolic blood pressure (SBP), 277b

T

tachycardia, 277
targeted temperature management, 436
TasP. See treatment as prevention (TasP)
TBI. See traumatic brain injury (TBI)
TCRN. See Trauma Certified Registered Nurse (TCRN)
team leader, 16–17
TeamSTEPPS (Team Strategies and Tools to Enhance Performance and Patient Safety), 18
  core competencies, 18, 18t
TEG. See thromboelastography (TEG)
TEM. See thromboelastometry (TEM)
temperature monitoring, hypothermia, 436
tenderness, flanks for, 171–172
tendons, 194
tension pneumothorax, 155, 155f
tentorium, 111
thermal burns, 235–236
thermal trauma, 27, 34
thoracic and neck trauma
  aortic disruption, 158
  biomechanics and mechanisms of injury, 145
  blunt cardiac injury (BCI), 157
  blunt esophageal injury, 151
  cardiac tamponade, 157–158, 158f
  definitive care/transport, 160
  emerging trends, 160
  epidemiology, 144
  flail chest, 152–153, 153f
  heart and thoracic great vessels, 142–143, 142t
  hemothorax, 156
  nursing care of the patient with
    cervical spinal stabilization/spinal motion restriction, 148
    primary survey, 147–150
    secondary survey, 150
  open pneumothorax, 154, 154f
  pathophysiology as basis for assessment findings
    ineffective circulation, 147
    ineffective ventilation, 146–147
  pulmonary contusion, 156–157
  reevaluation
    chest drainage systems, 159–160, 159t
    imaging studies, 159
    and post-resuscitation care, 160
  respiratory system, 141–142, 142f
  rib and sternal fractures, 152
  ruptured diaphragm, 158–159, 159f
  simple pneumothorax, 153–154
  tension pneumothorax, 155, 155f
  tracheobronchial injury, 150–151
  usual concurrent injuries, 145–146, 146t
thoracic cavity, 141

thoracic skeletal fractures, 146t
thoracic surface landmarks, 142, 142f
thoracic vasculature, 143, 143f
thoracic vertebrae, 191
thoracic vertebral fractures, 205t
three-sided dressing, 154, 154f
thromboelastography, 438
thromboelastography (TEG), 451
thromboelastometry (TEM), 104
thromboembolism prevention, 306–307
throughput, 434
tibiofibular joint, 195f
TIC. See trauma-informed care (TIC)
TICLS mnemonic, 274, 274b
TNP. See trauma nursing process (TNP)
tornado, 400–401
tourniquets, 98, 217
tracheobronchial injury, 150–151
tranexamic acid (TXA), 100
trans broken arm syndrome, 261
transgender, 255
transgender health, 257–258, 257t, 258–259t
transition of care, for trauma patient
   decision to transport, 427, 428t
   emergency department boarding, 431
   Emergency Medical Treatment and Active Labor Act (EMTALA), 426–427
   emerging trends, 431
   modes of transport, 428, 429t
   require transport, 427
   risks of transport, 430–431
      equipment for, 430–431
      nursing considerations, 430
   transport considerations, 427
   transport team composition, 428–430
      interfacility, 428–430
      intrafacility, 428
trauma around the world, 1–9. See also global trauma
trauma bay, effective communication in, 19–20
Trauma Certified Registered Nurse (TCRN), 14
trauma diamond of death, 105
trauma-informed care (TIC), 372–373
trauma nursing, 13–14
   education position statement, 14
trauma nursing process (TNP), 39
trauma patient, psychosocial nursing care of, 372–374
   adverse childhood experiences, 372
   interventions, 373–374, 374b
   secondary survey, 372–373
trauma, preparing for, 13–21
The Trauma Quality Improvement Program, 450
trauma resuscitation, communication techniques during, 19–20
trauma room, preparation in, 42
trauma system/programs, 14–17
   across the globe, 6–8

   Australia, 6
   England, 7
   Germany, 7
   Ghana, 7–8
   Nepal, 8
   Netherlands, 8
   snapshots, 6–8
   trauma triad of death, 94–95
ancillary team members, 17
communication, 17–20
core team members, 17
elements of, 14, 14f
high-performance trauma teams, 17, 17f
nurse roles and responsibilities, 15–16
nursing, 13–14
shared mental model, 18
team leader, 16–17
team structure and roles, 16–17
trauma center level expectations, 15
trauma nursing education position statement, 14
trauma team activities, 15
trauma team, support/strategies for, 386–387
   developing resilience, 386, 386b
   healthcare providers, management of stress in, 387
   promoting self-awareness, 387
traumatic brain injury (TBI), 117, 287
traumatic stress disorders, 375–376, 375–377, 377t
   acute stress disorder, 375–376
   posttraumatic stress disorder, 376
   screening tools, 376, 377t
trauma triad of death, 435–438
   acidosis, 436
   coagulopathy, 437–438
   hypothermia, 436, 437f
treatment as prevention (TasP), 253t
triage, 42, 68
triage and prioritization, 337–338
triage comparison, 414–416
tube displacement/obstruction, 434–435
tumbling, 33
TXA. See tranexamic acid (TXA)

U

ultrasound, 307, 342
uncontrolled hemorrhage, 42
unintentional injuries, 1–2
The United Nations Office for Disaster Risk Reduction, 397
upper airway, 63–64, 64f
upper lateral retroperitoneum, 167t
ureters, 166
urethra, 166
The U.S. Department of Homeland Security, 402
U.S. National Center for Missing and Exploited Children, 353

usual concurrent injuries, 117, 145–146, 146t, 170, 236
uterine rupture, 336

V
VAP. *See* ventilator-associated pneumonia (VAP)
vascular supply, 192
vehicle-versus-pedestrian injuries, 30–31
venous thromboembolism (VTE), 441, 441t
ventilation, 65–66, 146
ventilator-associated pneumonia (VAP), 443
vertebrae, 193f
vertebral column injuries, 191, 193f, 203, 204t
    atlas and axis fractures, 203
    cervical vertebrae, 191
    ligaments and intervertebral discs, 192
    lumbar, sacral, and coccygeal vertebrae, 191
    subluxation or dislocation, 203
    thoracic vertebrae, 191
    vascular supply, 192
    vertebral body fractures, 203–204
    vertebral fracture stability, 203, 204t
vicarious trauma, 384
violence
    against children, 6
    against older people, 6
    against women, 6
VIPP mnemonic, 55
viscoelastic testing, 104–105
visual acuity exam, 125, 125f
vitreous humor, 113
VTE. *See* venous thromboembolism (VTE)

W
Waddell triad, 31, 31f
whole blood, 105
whole blood, use of, 451
Wildfires, 401
women, violence against, 6
workplace violence, 384
World Health Organization, 4
wounds
    care, 247–248
    differentiating depth of, 243t
    healing, 234
        phase process, 228–229
    irrigation, 234